Community Health Nursing

A Canadian Perspective Second Edition

Edited by Lynnette Leeseberg Stamler and Lucia Yiu

PEARSON

Prentice
Hall

Toronto

This book is written in memory of my parents who were both educators; to Allan for everlasting support; and to the students, colleagues and clients who inspire me to love both nursing and teaching.

—*L. L. Stamler*

To my parents; my three daughters, Tamara, Camillia, and Tiffany; my lifelong mentor, Dr. Donna Foley; my students; and always our clients.

—*Lucia Yiu*

Library and Archives Canada Cataloguing in Publication

Community health nursing: a Canadian perspective/edited by Lynnette Leeseberg Stamler, Lucia Yiu—2nd ed.

Includes index.
ISBN 978-0-13-234066-3

1. Community health nursing—Canada—Textbooks. I. Stamler, Lynnette Leeseberg, 1952– II. Yiu, Lucia, 1951–

RT98.C644 2008   610.73'430971   C2007-905252-5

ISBN-13: 978-0-13-234066-3
ISBN-10: 0-13-234066-6

Vice President, Editorial Director: Gary Bennett
Acquisitions Editor: Michelle Sartor
Marketing Manager: Colleen Gauthier
Developmental Editor: John Polanszky
Production Editor: Imee Salumbides
Copy Editor: Kelli Howey
Proofreader: Audrey Dorsch
Production Coordinator: Patricia Ciardullo
Composition: Joan M. Wilson
Photo and Permissions Research: Lisa Brant
Art Director: Julia Hall
Cover and Interior Design: Geoff Agnew
Cover Image: Getty Images/Gay Bumgarner

Care has been taken to confirm the accuracy of information presented in this book. The authors, editors, and the publisher, however, cannot accept any responsibility for errors or omissions or for the consequences from application of the information in this book and make no warranty, expressed or implied, with respect to its contents.

For permission to reproduce copyrighted material, the publisher gratefully acknowledges the copyright holders listed beneath photos, figures, and tables throughout, which are considered an extension of this copyright page.

Statistics Canada information is used with the permission of Statistics Canada. Users are forbidden to copy the data and redisseminate them, in an original or modified form, for commercial purposes, without permission from Statistics Canada. Information on the availability of the wide range of data from Statistics Canada can be obtained from Statistics Canada's Regional Offices, its World Wide Web site at http://www.statcan.ca, and its toll-free access number 1-800-263-1136.

6   11 10

Printed and bound in the United States of America.

Brief Contents

Contents

List of Canadian Research Boxes

Preface

We would like to begin by thanking both students and faculty who welcomed our first edition and provided excellent and insightful feedback for the new edition. We are delighted that this book has been useful not only at multiple levels within a basic or post-RN curriculum, but also in preparation for the Canadian Nurses Association certification examination in community health. Also, to know that the first edition was informative, easy to read, and had challenged their thinking made developing this new edition even more meaningful.

In the preface to the first edition we posed the question, "why should we choose to write a community health nursing book from a Canadian perspective?" The response to the first edition has solidified our perceptions. We believe that there are historical, political, legislative, cultural, and social influences that are unique to Canadians. They have shaped the evolution of Canadians as a society, our definitions of health, and our expectations relative to health care delivery. Community health nurses are both a product of those influences and an influence themselves. It is not surprising that community health nursing has evolved differently in Canada than in other countries. We believe that new practitioners in community health nursing must understand these influences to continue to practice in and shape community health nursing.

As before, *Community Health Nursing: A Canadian Perspective*, Second Edition, has been written with the undergraduate student in mind. Each topic is written with the understanding that this will be the student's first foray into the community nursing spectrum. We have chosen to incorporate individual, family, and community as client perspectives throughout the text.

OUR APPROACH

Over time there has been much discourse on community health nursing versus public health nursing versus community-based nursing. A variety of authors have offered different definitions that attempt to discriminate amongst these terms. They base their conclusions on factors such as who is the client, what is the setting, what is the educational preparation of the nurse, and who is the employer. Historically, "community health nursing" was used to describe all nursing outside the hospital setting. In this book, community health nursing is defined as a specialty in nursing that encompasses a number of sub-specialties, such as public health nursing and home health nursing. The client may be an individual, group, community, or population, but care is rendered with an eye to the health of the population. The setting may be a home, institution, community, or an agency serving the population. The

common academic preparation is the basic education leading to the designation Registered Nurse; however, it is clear that additional educational preparation is frequently required. The employer may be an individual, family, community, government, or non-governmental agency. Whether the chapter authors are addressing a specific health issue or a specific population or aggregate, all are speaking about a segment within the larger whole of community health nursing.

It is our belief that community health nursing functions within a multiplicity of theories and understandings. Some theories are common to all facets of the nursing profession, such as ethical treatment of clients, family assessment, or the meaning of health. In some cases, nursing drove the development of the theory; in others, we have used the work of theorists in other disciplines. This text reflects that multiplicity, and the authors have described how the theories relate to community health nursing.

We continue to hear that faculty and students are looking for an overview text. While space does not permit an exhaustive perusal of each of the topics, important as they are, we have made every effort to provide as broad and comprehensive an overview of this field as possible. Each chapter has been updated to provide the basics of the content area and point the student to additional sources of information through the chapter features.

NEW TO THE SECOND EDITION

The new edition brings many changes. As is appropriate to the pace of change in community health and community health nursing, you will notice that the chapters have been extensively updated, with new content, statistics, and Canadian research. In response to readers, we have added five new chapters to this edition. They are (in order of appearance): Chapter 15: Information Technology; Chapter 16: School Health; Chapter 19: Clients in Rural Areas; Chapter 23: Gay, Lesbian, Bisexual and Transgender Clients; and Chapter 24: Disaster Nursing and Emergency Preparedness.

Several other chapters have changed in terms of direction. These include Chapter 3: Roles and Functions of Community Health Nurses in Practice Settings, which incorporates material from the old Chapter 26. The chapter on hospice and respite care from the first edition has been expanded to include additional related topics and now appears as Chapter 17: Long Term Care. Chapter 18: Clients in the Community Mental Health System now also includes topics previously covered in the old chapter on suicide. The topic of hunger has been added to the discourse on poverty and homelessness in Chapter 27: Poverty, Hunger, and Homelessness.

Research and cases throughout the text have been thoroughly updated in an effort to keep the book as current as possible. Many chapters have also benefited from the contribution of new authors who were able to offer a fresh perspective and new insights.

We have also continued to build on the features of the second edition, with the addition of discussion notes in the Instructor Manual for all the questions in the Canadian Research Boxes.

ABOUT THE CONTRIBUTORS

The contributors are as many and varied as the topics. This second edition brings new and repeat authors to the book. As before, some hold academic positions, some are in management or policy positions, while others are frontline practitioners. All came with a desire to contribute to a Canadian community health nursing text. Each brought expertise and knowledge to a particular chapter and topic. Each has presented the various historical, geographical, and theoretical perspectives that assist in explaining and describing community nursing practice. We believe that all have made a meaningful contribution to introducing nursing students to this specialty. You will find a list of the contributors, their affiliations, and the chapters they authored following the preface. To provide context on the varied experience and expertise of our contributors, we have also provided a short biographical sketch for each contributor immediately following the chapter(s) they wrote.

CHAPTER ORGANIZATION

The chapters in *Community Health Nursing: A Canadian Perspective* are organized into four parts:

- Part I: Perspectives on Community Health Nursing in Canada
- Part II: Foundations and Tools for Community Health Nursing Practice
- Part III: Community Clients with Special Needs
- Part IV: Common Community Health Issues

Part I: Perspectives on Community Health Nursing in Canada introduces students to the general topic area. **Chapter 1: The Origins of Community Health Nursing** presents an historical perspective on Canadian community health nursing so that students may be enlightened by lessons from the past. **Chapter 2: Financing, Policy, and Politics of Health Care Delivery** presents the administration of community health from legislative, cultural, and political perspectives. **Chapter 3: Nursing Roles, Functions, and Practice Settings** presents a discussion of the variety of settings, roles, and functions germane to community health nursing, incorporating the roles previously outlined in Chapter 26 from the first edition. The authors in **Chapter 4: Advocacy, Ethical, and Legal Considerations** have used the Standards of Practice for Community Health Nursing (found in Appendix A) to frame a discussion on legal and ethical issues for CHNs. These chapters form the underpinning for the subsequent sections.

Part II: Foundations and Tools for Community Health Nursing builds the base upon which the sub-specialties rest. It begins in **Chapter 5: Concepts of Health** with a discourse on health from a variety of perspectives. Health promotion is examined from a variety of theoretical frameworks in **Chapter 6: Population Health Promotion Models and Strategies**, demonstrating how the philosophy and framework can influence the decisions about interventions. **Chapter 7: Primary Health Care** provides an examination of primary health care as it was in the past and is in the present with a section on international and global health. **Chapter 8: Epidemiology** describes the science of epidemiology and how it can inform community health nurses' practice. This is followed by a discussion of communicable diseases and their assessment and control in **Chapter 9: Communicable Diseases**. In **Chapter 10: Family Care** the authors explore individual and family care within the context of community, whereas in **Chapter 11: Community Care** the community is defined as the client and introduces a new community health promotion model. Occupational health and related issues such as workplace safety are explored in **Chapter 12: Occupational Health**. **Chapter 13: Community Health Planning, Monitoring, and Evaluation** examines specifics around planning, monitoring, and evaluating community health programs. Guided information on finding, using, and participating in community health nursing research is the focus of **Chapter 14: Research**. Part II concludes with **Chapter 15: Information and Communication Technology** and a new discussion on information technology and how it contributes to community nursing practice. We believe the topics in Parts I and II are essential for an understanding of community health nursing.

Parts III and IV, composed of focus chapters, provide the details that make the picture of community health nursing more complete. In each focus chapter, a specific health issue or population is presented. In **Part III**, the focus is on **Community Clients with Special Needs**. The chapters in this part are: **Chapter 16: School Health, Chapter 17: Long-Term Care, Chapter 18: Clients in the Community Mental Health System, Chapter 19: Clients in Rural Areas, Chapter 20: Multicultural Clients, Chapter 21: Aboriginal Clients, Chapter 22: Clients in the Correctional Setting, Chapter 23: Gay, Lesbian, Bisexual, and Transgender Clients,** and **Chapter 24: Disaster Nursing and Emergency Preparedness**. In each case the focus is on the population, with a discussion on health issues frequently seen in each population.

In contrast, **Part IV** focuses on **Common Community Health Issues** that may apply to a variety of populations. Here we have chosen to focus on five specific issues: Adolescent Sexual Health and Pregnancy in **Chapter 25,** Family Violence in **Chapter 26**), Poverty, Hunger, and Homelessness in **Chapter 27,** Substance Abuse in **Chapter 28,** and Sexually Transmitted Infections and Blood Borne Pathogens in **Chapter 29**). In these chapters, the authors have explored the issue first and then identified the populations most affected.

The text concludes with a brief look at where the field of community health nursing is headed and the coming opportunities and challenges in **Chapter 30: Future Directions**.

As you read through the book, you will notice that some concepts and items are mentioned in several of the chapters. This is because they are often seminal documents or definitions that may be viewed through the lenses of the various topics and authors. For instance, many of the chapters will talk about the Lalonde Report, the Epp Report, or the *Declaration of Alma Ata*. You will note that each author views the reports differently, depending on the chapter topic. For example, proponents of health promotion may view some of the reports from one perspective, while the author of the chapter on primary health care may discuss a slightly different perceived influence of the same report. Similarly, cross-cultural nursing is mentioned in the family chapter and the multicultural chapter, but may also be mentioned in the Aboriginal Canadians chapter and the family violence chapter. We anticipate that students and teachers will not see this as redundancy, but rather as an example of multiple perspectives and how and why a multiplicity of theory and practice exists in community health nursing.

A Note on Appendices

We are pleased to offer two appendices to the second edition. As in the first edition, we include an excerpt from the Canadian Community Health Nursing Standards of Practices. Released in May 2003, this document explicitly reflects the current practice standards for Canadian community health nurses. In our appendix, we have included the Canadian Community Health Nursing Practice Model, along with a complete outline and description of the standards. In several chapters, contributors have made reference to the standards to enhance the discussion.

Secondly, we also have included the core competencies for public health. These have been developed with broad national consultation over the last few years. Core Competencies for Public Health in Canada are the essential knowledge, skills and attitudes necessary for the practice of public health. The practice of public health is both an art and a science. A set of core competencies helps to explain the nature of public health and the kinds of common knowledge, skills and attitudes that public health professionals use in their work. The core competencies are based on the core functions of public health: population health assessment, health surveillance, disease and injury prevention, health promotion and health protection and are organized under seven categories: public health sciences; assessment and analysis; policy and program planning, implementation and evaluation; partnerships, collaboration and advocacy; diversity and inclusiveness; communication; leadership. The competencies have been included in partnership with the Public Health Agency of Canada.

Chapter Features

A special effort has been made with this book to incorporate features that will facilitate learning and enhance an understanding of community health nursing in Canada.

- **Chapter Objectives** outline the salient points of the chapter and clarify the skills and knowledge to be learned in that chapter.
- **Canadian Research Boxes** present specific studies from the literature or the authors' knowledge to illustrate or augment the material covered in the chapter. Either the researchers themselves are nurses, or we have chosen health research that community health nurses can use in their practice. Each Research Box is followed by a few Discussion Questions to assist students in using the results.

Canadian Research Box 11.1

Yiu Matuk, L., & Ruggirello, T. (2007). Culture connection project: Promoting multiculturalism in elementary schools. *CJPH, 98*(1), 26–29.

This school-based community project aimed to promote multiculturalism among grade-school students through drama education in Windsor-Essex County, Ontario. Participants included a total of 665 Grade 3 to 6 students from 6 targeted schools, with 158 lead-class students representing each school. Using a non-experimental design approach, cultural themes from group discussions with

---

- **Case Studies** illustrate a practice application of the information presented in the chapter, followed by Discussion Questions. In Chapter 14: Research, the case studies and the research boxes have been combined to illustrate a practice question, followed by a literature search and application of research found.

Case Study: Testing Website Accessibility

Identify your favourite health information website or your current clinical placement agency website. Once you have located the website, highlight and copy the URL (Universal Resource Locator—a unique identifier that provides an address for an internet site). Then proceed to an accessibility checker website. Three popular web accessibility checker sites are http://webxact.watchfire.com, www.cynthiasays.com, and http://checker.atrc.utoronto.ca (a Canadian site recently developed at the University of Toronto). Paste in the URL at the checker site. It will analyze your site and

---

- **Key Terms** are boldfaced where they are introduced in the body of the text. For convenience, all of the key terms are listed at the end of each chapter in the order in which they appear.
- **Study Questions** test students' knowledge of the facts and concepts in the chapter. Answers to the study questions are included at the end of the book.

STUDY QUESTIONS

1. Name four community settings where CHNs work, and describe their role and functions.
2. What are the characteristics of a healthy community?
3. What nursing process skills will you use to promote the health of the community?
4. What assessment components are used when assessing community health?
5. Define population health, community engagement, com-

- **Individual** and **Group Critical Thinking Exercises** challenge students to reflect on the content of the chapter and apply it in different situations.

INDIVIDUAL CRITICAL THINKING EXERCISES

1. Why is it important for the nurse to provide care to the community?
2. How does the community health nursing process differ from the individual nursing process?
3. How would you work with your community to identify their health needs and share their community experiences?
4. In developing a health profile for a community, what assessment questions would you ask for each category of the community components? Where and how would you collect the needed data?
5. Why is it important to use participatory tools for community planning?

GROUP CRITICAL THINKING EXERCISES

1. Based on the community needs matrix tool (Table 11.3), what

- **References** cited in the chapter are presented in APA format. A complete list of the research box citations has been highlighted at the end of the book.
- **Additional Resources** direct students to further information on the chapter topic. These include references to books, journal articles, and websites. Students will also find references to specific government and non-governmental agencies relevant to the chapter topics.

Teaching Support

The following supplements are designed to aid instructors in presenting classes, fostering classroom discussion, and encouraging learning.

- **Instructor's Resource Manual** This comprehensive resource has been extensively revised for the new edition. Each chapter begins with an overview, a list of learning objectives from the text and an outline. This is followed by detailed discussion points for the Individual and Group Critical Thinking Exercises found at the end of each chapter, as well as the discussion questions found in the Case Studies and Canadian Research Boxes throughout the text. New features to the second edition Instructor's Resource Manual are lecture suggestions, classroom activities, and out-of-class assignments tied to each of the four parts in the text. The Instructor's Resource Manual with Solutions is available for download from Pearson Education Canada's online catalogue at **http://vig.pearsoned.ca** and on the Instructor's Resource CD-ROM that accompanies this textbook.

- **TestGen Testbank** This computerized testbank contains over 1000 questions made up of a mix of true/false, multiple choice, short answer, essay and CRNE-type questions. Questions can be searched and identified by question type, chapter heading, and level of difficulty. Each question has been checked for accuracy and is available in the latest version of TestGen software. This software package allows instructors to custom design, save, and generate classroom tests. The test program permits instructors to edit, add, or delete questions from the test bank; edit existing graphics and create new ones; analyze test results; and organize a database of tests and student results. This software allows for greater flexibility and ease of use. It provides many options for organizing and displaying tests, along with search and sort features. This TestGen testbank is available for download from Pearson Education Canada's online catalogue at **http://vig. pearsoned.ca** and on the Instructor's Resource CD-ROM that accompanies this textbook.

- Both the Instructor's Manual and the TestGen are provided in electronic format on the **Instructor's Resources CD-ROM (ISBN-10: 0135152534).**

ACKNOWLEDGEMENTS

In the creation of a book such as this, there are so many people to thank. First, we need to thank students and colleagues for encouraging us to start the project and then move on to a second edition. As the second edition began to take shape, we were thankful for the many authors who once again agreed to contribute to the book or suggested others who had the expertise we required. Many of our authors took time from other projects to add their knowledge to the book, making this book a priority. We would also like to extend a special thank you to the authors who contributed to the first edition, but were unable to participate this time including:

E. Merilyn Allison
Lynn J. Anderson
Dauna Crooks
Margaret England
Bonnie Kearns
Sue LeBeau
Ann Malinowski
Patricia Malloy
Joanne K. Olson

At Pearson Education Canada, Mr. Maurice Esses, Ms. Lori Will, Mr. John Polanszky, and Ms. Michelle Sartor guided us through the whole process. Ms. Kelli Howey, provided expertise, ideas, and support, which were invaluable in moving through production. The reviewers, who were nameless to us at the time, contributed significant time and effort in assisting us to make this text strong and representative of Canadian community health nursing. Their names are listed below. Each of us had particular friends and family members who were supportive as we moved through the process of completing a major text. We are grateful to all of you. Finally, as teachers, we thank our students, who were guiding forces in considering the project at all.

Many nurses across the country have contributed countless hours to portray community health nursing with passion and pride. We are very excited with this new edition. We hope teachers and learners will also be excited as they continue to learn, explore, and discuss community health nursing as a distinct specialty in Canadian nursing.

Lynnette Leeseberg Stamler and Lucia Yiu

REVIEWERS

Megan Aston, Dalhousie University

Pamela J. Dietrich, University of Western Ontario

Lina Dumais, Bow Valley College

Lenore Duquette, Humber College Institute of Technology and Advanced Learning

Helen Harrison, Fanshawe College

Corinne Hart, Ryerson University

Geraldine Macdonald, University of Toronto

Jo-Ann MacDonald, University of Prince Edward Island

Christina Murray, Mount Royal College

Alison Nelson, University of Calgary

Cathy O'Brien Larivee, University of New Brunswick

Joanne Ricci, University of British Columbia

Maureen Sullivan-Bentz, University of Ottawa

Holly Wallace, University of Western Ontario

Contributors

Rhonda J. King Blood, RN, BScN, MA
Health Promotions Specialist, Urban Aboriginal Mental
Health Program, Chinook Health, Lethbridge, Alberta
Chapter 21—Aboriginal Clients

Kathleen Carlin, RN, MSc, PhD
Assistant Professor, Philosophy Department,
Ryerson University
Chapter 4—Advocacy, Ethical, and Legal Considerations

Sharon L. Chadwick, RN, BScN, MSc,
COHN(C), COHN-S
Senior Manager, WHS Program Planning, Research and
Audit, Workplace Innovation and Continuous Improvement
Branch, Government of Alberta
Chapter 12—Occupational Health

Donna Ciliska, RN, PhD
Professor, School of Nursing, McMaster University;
Nursing Consultant, Hamilton Public Health and
Community Services
Chapter 14—Research

Sue Coffey, RN, PhD
Associate Professor, School of Nursing, York University
Chapter 2—Financing, Policy, and Politics of
Health Care Delivery

Benita Cohen, RN, PhD
Assistant Professor, Faculty of Nursing, University of Manitoba
Chapter 6—Population Health Promotion Models and
Strategies

Cathy Crowe, RN, BAAN, MEd
Co-founder, Toronto Disaster Relief Committee
Chapter 27—Poverty, Hunger, and Homelessness

Bernice Doyle, RN, COHN(C)
Manager, Workplace Health and Safety Policy and Standards
Branch, Government of Alberta
Chapter 12—Occupational Health

Kathryn Edmunds, RN, BN, MSN, PhD (C)
Doctoral Student, School of Nursing, University
of Western Ontario
Chapter 10—Family Care
Chapter 20—Multicultural Clients

Nancy Edwards, RN
Full Professor, School of Nursing and Department of
Epidemiology and Community Medicine, University
of Ottawa
Chapter 13—Community Health Planning, Monitoring,
and Evaluation

Josephine Etowa, RN
Associate Professor, School of Nursing, Dalhousie University
Chapter 13—Community Health Planning, Monitoring,
and Evaluation

Adeline R. Falk-Rafael, RN, PhD
Professor, School of Nursing, York University
Chapter 2—Financing, Policy, and Politics of Health Care
Delivery

Linda Ferguson, RN, PhD
Full Professor, College of Nursing, University of
Saskatchewan
Chapter 15—Information and Communication Technology

Irene Buckland Foster, RN, BScN, MScN
Manager, Child Health Team, Family Health Services,
Middlesex-London Health Unit, London, Ontario
Chapter 16—School Health

Elizabeth Battle Haugh, RN, BA, MScN
Director of Health Promotion, Windsor-Essex County
Health Unit; Adjunct Professor, Faculty of Nursing,
University of Windsor
Chapter 3—Nursing Roles, Functions, and Practice Settings

Janet B. Hettler, RN, DipN, BScN, MN
Manager, Crisis Nursery, Calgary Children's Cottage Society
Chapter 29—Sexually Transmitted Infections and Blood
Borne Pathogens

Joan Wharf Higgins, PhD
Associate Professor, School of Physical Education, University
of Victoria
Chapter 5—Concepts of Health

Lori Jacobson, BA
Nursing Program, University of Ottawa
Chapter 7—Primary Health Care

Anne Katz, RN, PHD
Adjunct Professor, University of Manitoba
Chapter 23—Gay, Lesbian, Bisexual, and Transgender
Clients

Margaret Ann Kennedy, RN
Assistant Professor, School of Nursing, St. Francis Xavier
University
Chapter 13—Community Health Planning, Monitoring,
and Evaluation

Elizabeth Kinnaird-Iler, RN, BScN, MSc
Manager, Healthy Babies Healthy Children Program,
Windsor-Essex County Health Unit
Chapter 20—Multicultural Clients

Judith C. Kulig, RN, DNSc
Professor, Nursing Program, School of Health Sciences,
University of Lethbridge
Chapter 19—Clients in Rural Areas

Yvette Laforêt-Fliesser, RN, BScN, MScN
Associate Professor, University of Western Ontario; Manager,
Young Adult Program, Middlesex-London Health Unit,
London, Ontario
Chapter 16—School Health

Wendi Lokanc-Diluzio, BN, MN
Sexual Health Specialist, Calgary Health Region
Chapter 29—Sexually Transmitted Infections and Blood
Borne Pathogens

Carol MacDougall, RN, BSc, MA
Public Health Manager, School and Sexual Health, Perth
District Health Unit, Stratford, Ontario
Chapter 16—School Health

Martha L.P. MacLeod, RN, PHD
Associate Professor, Nursing and Community Health
Sciences Programs, University of Northern British Columbia
Chapter 19—Clients in Rural Areas

Margaret M. Malone, RN, PHD
Associate Professor, School of Nursing, Ryerson University
Chapter 26—Violence in Families

Cynthia Mannion, MSc, PHD
Assistant Professor, Faculty of Nursing, University of Calgary
Chapter 25—Adolescent Sexual Health and Pregnancy

Sheila Marchant-Short, RN, BScN, MScN
Manager, Communicable Disease Control Program, North
Bay, Ontario
Chapter 9—Communicable Diseases

Lori Schindel Martin, BA, BScN, MScCHN, PHD
Associate Professor, School of Nursing, Faculty of
Community Health Services, Ryerson University
Chapter 17—Long-Term Care

Marion McKay, RN, PHD
Faculty of Nursing, University of Manitoba
Chapter 1—The Origins of Community Health Nursing
in Canada

Barbara L. Mildon, RN, MN, CHE
Chief Nurse Executive and VP Professional Practice and
Integration, Fraser Health Authority, Surrey, British
Columbia
Chapter 3—Nursing Roles, Functions, and Practice Settings

Elaine Mordoch, RN, PHD
Instructor, Faculty of Nursing, University of Manitoba
Chapter 18—Clients in the Community Mental Health
System

Alison Nelson, RN, BScN, MN
Co-chair, Alberta Society for the Promotion of Sexual
Health; Decision Support and Evaluation Manager,
Screening Programs, Population Health and Information,
Alberta Cancer Board
Chapter 29—Sexually Transmitted Infections and Blood
Borne Pathogens

Linda J. Patrick, RN, BScN, MA, MSc, PHD
Undergraduate Coordinator, Faculty of Nursing, University
of Windsor
Chapter 10—Family Care

Elizabeth Peter, RN, BScN, BA, MScN, PHD
Associate Professor and Associate Dean, Academic Programs,
Faculty of Nursing, University of Toronto
Chapter 4—Advocacy, Ethical, and Legal Considerations

Cindy Peternelj-Taylor, RN, MSc
Professor, College of Nursing, University of Saskatchewan
Chapter 22—Clients in the Correctional Setting

Roger Pitblado, PHD
Senior Research Fellow, Centre for Rural and Northern
Health Research, Laurentian University
Chapter 19—Clients in Rural Areas

Rose Alene Roberts, RN, BScN, MSc, PHD
Assistant Professor, College of Nursing, University of
Saskatchewan
Chapter 21—Aboriginal Clients

Joanne Shaw, RN, BN
Chapter 22—Clients in the Correctional Setting

Mary Anne Simpson, RN, BScN, MSc
Manager of Vaccine Preventable Diseases, Communicable
Diseases and Sexual Health Services, Middlesex-London
Health Unit, London, Ontario
Chapter 24—Disaster Nursing and Emergency Preparedness

Dawn Smith, RN, BScN, MN, PhD
Assistant Professor, School of Nursing, University of Ottawa
Chapter 7—Primary Health Care

Lynnette Leeseberg Stamler, RN, BSN, MEd, PhD
Professor and Graduate Chair, College of Nursing,
University of Saskatchewan
Chapter 8—Epidemiology
Chapter 30—Future Directions

Norma J. Stewart, RN, PhD
Professor and Associate Dean, College of Nursing, University
of Saskatchewan
Chapter 19—Clients in Rural Areas

Louise R. Sweatman, RN, BScN, LLB, MSc
COO, Assessment Strategies Inc., Canada's Testing
Company
Chapter 4—Advocacy, Ethical, and Legal Considerations

Helen Thomas, RN, MSc
Associate Professor, School of Nursing, McMaster
University; Clinical Consultant, Hamilton Public Health
and Social Services, Public Health Research Education and
Development (PHRED) Program
Chapter 14—Research

Ruta Valaitis, RN, PhD
Associate Professor, School of Nursing, McMaster
University

Chapter 15—Information and Communication
Technology

Janet L. Wayne, RN, BScN, MN
Quality Improvement Consultant, Calgary Health Region
Chapter 29—Sexually Transmitted Infections and Blood
Borne Pathogens

Leeann Whitney, RN, BScN, MAEd
Director of Infectious Diseases, North Bay Parry Sound
District Health Unit
Chapter 9—Communicable Diseases

Hélène Philbin Wilkinson, RN, BScN, MN
Program Manager, Forensic Mental Health Program,
Northeast Mental Health Centre, North Bay, Ontario
Chapter 28—Substance Abuse

Phil Woods, RPN, PhD
Associate Professor, College of Nursing, University of
Saskatchewan
Chapter 22—Clients in the Correctional Setting

Lucia Yiu, RN, BScN, BA, BSc, MScN
Associate Professor, Faculty of Nursing, University of Windsor;
Educational and Training Consultant
Chapter 7—Primary Health Care
Chapter 9—Communicable Diseases
Chapter 11—Community Care
Chapter 24—Disaster Nursing and Emergency Preparedness
Chapter 30 –Future Directions

Lynne Young, RN, PhD
Associate Professor, School of Nursing, University of
Victoria
Chapter 5—Concepts of Health

The Origins of Community Health
Nursing in Canada

Marion McKay

OBJECTIVES

After studying this chapter, you should be able to:

1. Identify the social conditions and beliefs that were the impetus for the development of community health nursing in Canada.

2. Discuss the theoretical and practical distinctions between the practices of visiting nurses and public health nurses.

3. Describe how the emergence of the welfare state shaped the evolution of public health and visiting nursing programs.

4. Discuss the role that women played in the development of public health and visiting nursing programs.

5. Compare and contrast the work of community health nurses in urban, rural, and remote areas of Canada.

INTRODUCTION

The purpose of this chapter is to explore the history of community health nursing programs delivered by professionally educated nurses. From their origins in the late nineteenth century, community health nursing programs have been profoundly influenced by a variety of social, political, and economic forces. The **public health movement**, well established in Canada by the beginning of the twentieth century, put the health of Canadians on the public agenda. **Maternal feminists**, who believed that the unique nurturing capacity of women made them particularly suited to the development of programs to assist women and children (Ladd-Taylor, 1994), also played a major role in the creation of the Canadian welfare state. Their searching critiques of the prevailing social order sparked many of the social reform programs established in early-twentieth-century Canada, including the child welfare movement, services for child-bearing women, and the establishment of mothers' allowances and other programs to assist families in need (Christie & Gauvreau, 1996). In addition, social beliefs about gender and appropriate roles for women shaped the social system in which community health nurses (CHNs) lived and practised. Finally, the tensions between professional medicine and nursing created both

opportunities for and barriers to the development of nursing practice in the community.

It is impossible in the space of a single chapter to describe and analyze the development of community health nursing in each Canadian province and territory. Instead, this chapter will trace trends in the development of community health nursing by using specific examples drawn from published sources and from research in progress. It will trace the evolution of community health nursing from its dual origins in philanthropic health care organizations and publicly funded municipal health departments, examining the role that the evolving concepts of charity and citizenship played in shaping current models of community health nursing. It will also examine the challenges that confronted nurses as they carved out a role in the community. In the final analysis, community health nursing was always both a response to and a product of its particular time and place.

THE ORIGINS OF COMMUNITY HEALTH NURSING IN CANADA

Community health nursing evolved in two streams. The earliest form was **district nursing** or **visiting nursing**, which evolved in late-nineteenth-century Britain, the United States, and Canada. Charitable agencies, often organized and operated by maternal feminists, employed visiting nurses (VNs) to provide care to poor and destitute families. Working-class and lower-middle-class families also were recipients of visiting nursing services. These families could not afford to hire full-time private duty nurses, and their homes were not large enough to provide accommodation for a nurse during the term of her employment. In Canada, visiting nursing services were organized at both the national and the local level. The best known of these, the Victorian Order of Nurses for Canada (VON), was founded in 1897 "to supply nurses, thoroughly trained in Hospital and District Nursing, and subject to one Central Authority, for the nursing of the sick who are otherwise unable to obtain trained nursing in their own homes, both in town and country districts" (Lady Aberdeen, cited in Gibbon, 1947, p. 8).

The public health nurse (PHN) was a civil servant employed by the local, provincial, or federal government. **Public health nursing** emerged in Canada in the early twentieth century when civic departments of health established health education and preventive programs to combat communicable disease, infant mortality, and morbidity in school-age children. Nurses were perceived as the ideal professionals to deliver these programs because of their medical knowledge and their ability to interact with women and children in private homes and in the public school setting (Sears, 1995).

Although these definitions are theoretically distinct, in practice there was considerable blurring of the boundaries between the practices of VNs and PHNs. For example, in some Canadian cities the VON provided programs on behalf of the local health department. In other communities, the VON provided public health programs to supplement those provided by the local government. PHNs in rural and remote areas of the country, however, often provided bedside nursing care and obstetrical care because no VNs were available to undertake this work.

In her analysis of twentieth-century Canadian nursing, McPherson (1996) divides the profession into three sectors: hospital nurses, private duty nurses, and public health (including visiting) nurses. During the late nineteenth and early twentieth centuries, when community health nursing emerged as a distinct specialty, the majority of all nurses were self-employed as private duty nurses. Public health and visiting nurses were counted among the profession's elite. Employment in this specialty practice required additional clinical skills such as midwifery training and, particularly after World War I, post-diploma training at a university (Baldwin, 1997; Green, 1974; McPherson, 1996; Miller, 2000; Penney, 1996). Myra (Grimsley) Bennett, who worked for 50 years as a nurse along Newfoundland's northwestern coast, took two courses in midwifery prior to leaving England (Green, 1974).

As an occupational group, nurses came from a variety of social backgrounds, including middle-class, working-class, and agricultural families. The majority were female, white, and Canadian or British born. Nursing, one of the few respectable careers available to women, offered young women seeking autonomy from their family the prospect for both financial independence and social status (McPherson, 1996). Many women married and left the profession soon after completing their hospital training programs. Others, usually those who remained single or those whose marriages had ended, forged life-long careers in nursing.

Public health and visiting nurses were different from nurses employed in other sectors of the health care system in several ways. They tended to remain in their community practices longer than those employed in hospitals and private duty nursing. They also enjoyed greater financial stability and higher salaries (McPherson, 1996). Published biographical material also indicates that these nurses actively sought opportunities that combined challenging work with travel and adventure. "I had always wanted to travel," wrote Margaret Giovannini, another Newfoundland outpost nurse, "...and when the opportunity arose to work as well as travel I liked it" (Giovannini, 1988, p. 1). Other pioneer CHNs wrote of their eagerness to find a place where they could fulfill their desire to use their hard-won knowledge and skills in a meaningful way (Colley, 1970; Miller, 2000). "When I first arrived at my

little northern hospital in Granite Springs," wrote Mary E. Hope, "I felt that my search for the end of the rainbow was over.... With my shining new public health nursing diploma under my arm, I was a consecrated scientist about to enlighten this benighted wilderness village.... This was my kingdom" (Hope, 1955, pp. 5–6). Still others sought a practice free (or at least more distant) from the hierarchy and constraints of supervisors and large institutions (Green, 1974). Bessie J. Banfill, who worked in rural Saskatchewan, found that her work among that province's settlers, many of whom were immigrants from Eastern Europe, fulfilled a deep personal need. "[I]mpulsive by nature, and restless and dissatisfied with hospital routine and nursing patients surrounded by luxury, I longed for more challenging adventure and freedom" (Banfill, 1967, p. 9). Many genuinely enjoyed interaction with people and embraced opportunities to learn about other cultures (Baldwin, 1997). Banfill (1967) wrote that her "Scottish blood boiled" in response to comments that foreigners were not welcome in Canada. Their sense of adventure, independence, courage, and humanitarianism led pioneering Canadian CHNs to offer their services in Canada's poorest urban districts and most isolated rural communities. These qualities also placed them at the forefront of efforts to place health care within reach of all Canadians.

HEALTH, THE INDIVIDUAL, AND THE STATE

The idea that health care was a right of citizenship, rather than a privilege based upon social rank and income, developed slowly during Canada's first century. The British North America Act (1867) made only limited provisions for the establishment and maintenance of a health care system. The Act specified that the federal government was responsible for quarantine and for the establishment of Marine Hospitals. All other responsibilities for the organization of health care, including public health services, devolved to the provinces. These responsibilities were not specified within the Act, nor did the provinces, in the early years after Confederation, make much effort to undertake them. Such organized health care as did exist was provided at the local (municipal) level through public welfare or, more frequently, charitable organizations. Many provinces passed enabling legislation in the late nineteenth century, which allowed for the establishment of local and provincial departments of health. However, even at the local level, there was considerable reluctance to provide public health services on an ongoing basis. Most early health departments were organized in response to specific local emergencies. When the emergency was over, they were dissolved (Bilson, 1980; Bliss, 1991). Similarly, medical officers of health (MOHs) were appointed on a part-time basis until the 1880s. Toronto, for example, appointed its first full-time MOH in 1883 (MacDougall, 1990). Nurses were an even later addition to the staff of local health departments.

These arrangements were consistent with the social attitudes of the time. The state neither undertook nor was expected to undertake any responsibility for the health care of individuals and families. Those who could afford to pay for their own health care did so. Those who did not have the financial means to make these arrangements either went without care or, if sufficiently desperate or destitute, turned to local governments or charitable organizations for assistance. The poverty, poor health, and social unrest created by industrial capitalism, immigration, and urbanization demonstrated the inadequacy of nineteenth-century assumptions about individual and collective responsibility for the provision of health care. They also shaped the organization and financing of the public health system and the nature of community health nursing.

The Emergence of the Public Health Nurse

The Rise of Urban Health Departments The establishment of urban health departments was fraught with controversy. In an era when individuals were expected to provide for their own health care and governments were not permitted to intrude into the personal lives of individual citizens, health departments threatened to blur the boundaries between the private and public domains. Further, they did so at considerable expense to the public purse. A.J. Douglas, Winnipeg's first full-time MOH, summed up the challenges of his office as follows:

> [W]hen I first took office, the health officer, in my community at least, was looked upon by most people as a rather unnecessary appendage to the municipal pay-roll—not only unnecessary, but very often pernicious, for sometimes he had the temerity to interfere with citizens, particularly the so-called best citizens' inalienable right to do as they please.... It was considered that his proper sphere was to supervise the collection of city wastes, to keep the streets clean, to juggle with statistics (always with a view to emphasizing the salubrity of his own locality), and to occasionally show some activity during outbreaks of the more serious communicable diseases.... He was always to use discretion as to whose toes he trod upon; he was not to point out glaring sanitary defects in his community as this spoiled business and kept visitors away. (Douglas, 1912, p. 85)

At the end of the nineteenth century, Canada's major urban centres faced a health crisis that matched in substance, if not quite in magnitude, that of cities in the United States and Great Britain. Major Canadian cities such as Montreal, Toronto, and Winnipeg possessed inadequate or non-existent sanitary infrastructures at the time of their most rapid expansion (Artibise, 1975; Bliss, 1991). The problems were most acute in areas populated by new immigrants and the working poor. The unsanitary living conditions, overcrowding, and inadequate nutrition created by urban poverty were a recipe for disaster. Infant and maternal mortality rates in all European and North American cities climbed steadily at the end of the nineteenth century and remained a significant public health issue in the early part of the twentieth century (Meckel, 1990). Winnipeg consistently reported one of the highest infant mortality rates in Canada during the first two decades of the twentieth century. (See Figure 1.1.) Periodic

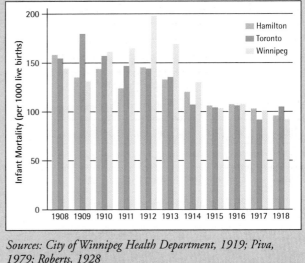

FIGURE 1.1 Infant Mortality Rates (per 1000 Live Births) in Selected Canadian Cities, 1908–1918

Sources: City of Winnipeg Health Department, 1919; Piva, 1979; Roberts, 1928

Note: Infant mortality statistics were not regularly reported for many other Canadian cities until the early 1920s.

outbreaks of communicable diseases such as smallpox, cholera, typhoid, and influenza killed thousands of Canadians. Tuberculosis (TB) emerged as the leading cause of death for urban dwellers who had survived early infancy (Humphreys, 1999).

The first cohort of Canadian public health officials focused their efforts on creating adequate systems of waste disposal and a safe water supply. In addition, drawing on the new science of bacteriology, efforts were directed toward establishing a safe food supply. Particular attention was focused on the health hazards created by unpasteurized milk. Many Canadian cities enacted by-laws that required the inspection of meat, milk, and bread sold within the city limits and hired inspectors to enforce these regulations.

In the early twentieth century, public health officials identified health education as another strategy to combat unnecessary disease and death. It was at this point that nurses were first employed as civil servants in local health departments. Although the exact chronology varies from one city to another, the first PHNs were responsible for TB control, child hygiene programs, or school inspection programs. (See Table 1.1.) Two important trends can be identified from these pioneering initiatives. First, the employment of nurses by civic authorities was often undertaken with considerable reluctance and only after voluntary programs had foundered in the face of overwhelming need and inadequate financial resources. Second, early PHNs were appointed to single specific programs rather than to a generalist practice.

From Voluntary to Civic Public Health Programs In 1907 in Toronto, the first civic nurse was employed to provide health education and nursing care in the home to TB patients. However, this nurse and her predecessors had previously been employed by the Toronto General Hospital through a special fund donated by a concerned Toronto citizen. When this

TABLE 1.1
Evolution of Community Health Nursing Programs in Canada

1891–1900: Laying the Groundwork for Community Health Nursing

1897	Victorian Order of Nurses for Canada founded	Ottawa
1897	District nurse employed by general hospital outpatient department	Winnipeg
1898	First VON local branch established	Ottawa

1901–1910: Emergence of Specialized Community Health Nursing Programs

1901–10	Milk depots and child hygiene programs established by voluntary agencies	Toronto, Montreal, Winnipeg
1901	National anti-tuberculosis society founded	Ottawa
1904	Margaret Scott Nursing Mission founded	Winnipeg
1905	TB nurse employed by general hospital outpatient department	Toronto
1906	TB nurse employed by City Health Department	Ottawa
1907	Medical inspection of school children inaugurated by school board	Montreal
1909	Nurses employed by school board for school inspection program	Winnipeg
1909	Lethbridge Nursing Mission founded	Lethbridge, AB
1910	Civic funding provided to support child hygiene program and milk depot	Winnipeg

1911–1930: Elaboration and Consolidation of Community Health Nursing Programs

1914	Child Hygiene program transferred to City Health Department	Toronto, Winnipeg
1914	School Board nurses transferred to City Health Department	Toronto
1914	Public Health Nursing reorganized as a generalist program	Toronto
1916	First provincial public health nurses employed	Manitoba
1918–20	VD control programs established under federal-provincial program	Canada
1919	Provincial District Nursing Service established	Alberta
1919	Red Cross funding supports establishment of public health nursing programs at five Canadian universities	Canada
1920	Provincial school health program established with Red Cross funding	Prince Edward Island
1920	County nursing program established with Red Cross funding	Nova Scotia
1920	Provincial public health nurses employed to work in Northern Ontario	Ontario
1920	First full-time provincial health unit in Canada established	Saanich, BC
1921	Provincial child hygiene program established with Red Cross funding	New Brunswick

1931–1980: Community Health Nursing in the Evolving Welfare State

1941–42	Buck Commission recommends major reorganization of public health and visiting nursing programs	Manitoba
1943	Margaret Scott Nursing Mission closes	Winnipeg
1943	VON transfers prenatal, postnatal, and child health programs to provincial health department	Manitoba
1968–70	VON establishes home care demonstration projects	Ontario
1973	*Pickering Report* recommends VON be mandated to deliver home care programs in Canada	Canada
1974	VON included in first publicly funded provincial home care program	Manitoba

Note: Events identified are those found in current literature and may not, in all instances, be the first such program established in Canada.

arrangement ended, Toronto's city council agreed to include the salary of the TB nurse in the health department's budget. Her work went on virtually unchanged, except that she was now required to report to the MOH twice a week (Royce, 1983). That same year in Montreal, the Tuberculosis League hired a nurse from the VON to provide instruction to those suffering from TB (Gibbon, 1947). In Winnipeg, TB nursing was established in 1909 by the Anti-Tuberculosis Society, a voluntary association of physicians and interested citizens (City of Winnipeg Health Department, 1910). The health visiting and health education provided by the Society's TB nurse was carefully coordinated with the city's sanitation and health inspection programs. The Winnipeg Health Department took over the TB nursing program in 1914. A major reason for the change from voluntary to civic funding was to enable the TB nurses to "have the power to make people carry out our regulations where at present persuasion and argument are about the only weapons she can personally use" (City of Winnipeg Health Department, 1915, p. 7).

In other cities, the first PHNs participated in initiatives to preserve and promote the health of school-age children. As working-class children were removed from economic production and placed in the public school system, the significant health problems from which they suffered became fully visible (Peikoff & Brickey, 1991). In the opinion of public officials and social reformers, this situation was intolerable. Ill health detracted from the child's educational attainment, and, worse still, the sickly child of the present was destined to become the poverty-stricken and dependent citizen of the future. Programs for the medical inspection of school children were established in major cities across Canada. School-based inspections were often augmented by home visits to educate the parents and to ensure that all recommendations were followed (Sutherland, 1981). In many cities, such as Montreal, Toronto, Winnipeg, and Vancouver, school health programs were initially established by the board of education. They were subsequently taken over by the health department as part of the process of consolidating all public health programs under one jurisdiction (City of Winnipeg Health Department, 1910; MacDougall, 1990).

Finally, many early PHNs were employed in programs to reduce infant mortality. Despite all efforts to improve urban sanitation and to regulate food and milk supplies, infant mortality rates in Canadian cities did not begin to decline significantly until well into the second decade of the twentieth century. What made this state of affairs a national crisis rather than a family tragedy was a shift in beliefs about the role that children played in industrial society and in the process of nation building. Every child, even the Canadian-born child of an Eastern European immigrant, became a precious element in the patriotic process of nation building (Peikoff & Brickey, 1991). An equally powerful concern, which particularly preoccupied Canadian-born, Anglo-Celtic members of the elite and middle classes, was the fear that they would soon be overwhelmed as a social and political force by the waves of immigrants arriving from Southern and Eastern Europe (McLaren & McLaren, 1997). As the failure of sanitarian and bacteriological strategies

to reduce infant mortality became evident, MOHs across North America and Western Europe re-examined their assumptions about its etiology and the role that public health might legitimately play in its reduction. Their experiences with poor and immigrant populations convinced them that other factors, particularly those embedded in family and cultural practices, also influenced infant mortality (Meigs, 1916).

Canadian efforts to reduce infant mortality were initiated by elite and middle-class women. Their desire to alleviate the suffering of women and children was inspired by both the **social gospel movement** and maternal feminism. The social gospel movement, which placed priority on the quality of human life on earth, united clergy, politicians, and ordinary citizens in efforts to reform Canadian society (Merkley, 1987). The movement found important allies among maternal feminists, who were also advocating sweeping social reform, particularly to protect the interests of women, children, and families (Christie & Gauvreau, 1996).

Public health officials and maternal feminists also turned their attention to the care that infants received from their mothers (Meigs, 1916). They concluded that many parents, particularly the mothers, were "ignorant" and barely capable of providing a safe and healthy environment for the nation's future citizens. Because removing children from their parents was no longer a viable option, educating mothers about infant feeding and hygiene became the intervention of choice (Peikoff & Brickey, 1991). Infant/child welfare/hygiene programs were carried out at milk depots, well baby clinics, and in private homes (Locke, 1918; MacNutt, 1913). VNs staffed the clinics and visited the homes of newborn infants in the early postpartum period. They assessed the health of both the infant and mother, the family's childcare practices, and hygienic conditions in the home. A major focus was to promote the breastfeeding of newborn infants.

In Toronto, a variety of women's groups, settlement houses, and church missions established milk depots and well baby clinics for the city's poorest citizens (MacDougall, 1990; Royce, 1983). Twenty "gouttes de lait" (clinics where mothers unable to breastfeed learned how to properly use cow's milk) were established in Montreal by the Fédération nationale Saint-Jean-Baptiste between 1910 and 1912 (Baillargeon, 2002). In 1915, the VON undertook responsibility for child welfare work in Edmonton, and in 1922 a similar program was established in Ottawa (Gibbon, 1947). In Winnipeg, a child hygiene program was founded in 1910 by the Margaret Scott Nursing Mission (MSNM) with funding from the city's health department.

Although voluntary programs confirmed the overwhelming need for both milk depots and child hygiene programs, they could not be sustained. In Winnipeg, for example, the Margaret Scott Nursing Mission encountered such severe financial problems that the health department took over the program in 1914. A similar pattern of municipal takeover of voluntary programs occurred in other Canadian cities, with PHNs taking the place of VNs in the delivery of child hygiene and milk depot services.

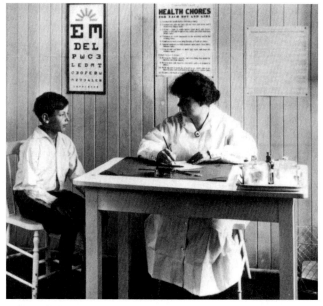

Photo 1.1

In Winnipeg, the first public health nurses were hired by the school board to carry out medical inspections of school-age children. This 1923 photograph shows a provincial public health nurse conducting a health inspection of a school boy in Brooklands, a working-class suburb of Winnipeg.

Credit: Provincial Archives of Manitoba: Public Health Collection 63 (N13039)

From Specialist to Generalist Practice In the second decade of the twentieth century, urban PHNs began to deliver general rather than specialized services in the community. This change was pioneered in Toronto, where the community health system had gradually evolved into a confusing mix of programs under the auspices of a variety of private and civic organizations. School health nurses were employed by the board of education. VNs were employed by philanthropic organizations to staff milk depots and child hygiene programs. PHNs employed by the health department were assigned to several programs, including TB control, measles control, and child welfare. In 1914, Toronto's Child Hygiene and the Communicable Disease programs were amalgamated at the service delivery level and each PHN provided direct care in the home for both programs. The rationale for this reorganization was that the family, rather than the individual, was the basic unit of intervention in public health nursing. "We decided to specialize in homes rather than diseases," stated Eunice Dyke, superintendent of Toronto's PHNs, "and to safeguard the interests of the medical specialist by office organization rather than multiplication of health visitors" (cited in Royce, 1983, p. 49). In 1917, the board of education nurses were transferred to the City of Toronto Health Department, and their responsibilities were integrated into the role of the generalist PHN (Royce, 1983). Visiting nursing services continued to be provided by the VON and the St. Elizabeth Visiting Nursing Association. These were coordinated with the preventive and health education programs provided by the PHNs (MacDougall, 1990).

Canadian Research Box 1.1

Gleason, M. (2002). Race, class, and health: School medical inspection and "healthy" children in British Columbia, 1890–1930. *Canadian Bulletin of Medical History/Bulletin Canadien d'histoire de la médecine, 19*(1), 95–112.

This historical analysis examines the efforts of social reformers and public health professionals to impose urban, Anglo-Celtic, middle-class values about health on school-age children and their parents. Interventions in the school setting included daily personal hygiene inspection of the children by teachers, a regular program of medical inspections, health education, communicable disease control, and home visits by school/public health nurses to ensure that families both understood and complied with health professionals' recommendations to improve identified medical and health problems. Rural families and those of Aboriginal, Asian, Eastern European, and East Indian origin were the primary targets of these programs because their health practices and beliefs were more likely to deviate from the standards set by the white urban middle class. The author concludes (1) that the standards for school health programs and medical inspection of school children could not be attained in rural and working-class school districts, (2) that these programs stigmatized children whose families were unwilling or unable to conform to white middle-class models of health, (3) that reform programs that targeted non-Anglo-Celtic families were powerful instruments to strengthen and legitimize the existing social and political system, and (4) that public health professionals contributed to this process, both deliberately and inadvertently, through their paternalistic and sometimes judgmental interactions with both children and parents.

Discussion Questions:

1. How do these findings compare with other descriptions you have read about the impact of public health programs on school-age children and their families?

2. If you were asked to plan a school health program, how would you use the findings of this study?

The Establishment of Rural Public Health Nursing Public health services in rural and small-town Canada were relatively unorganized until after World War I. A severe shortage of nurses occurred during and after the war (Riddell, 1991), and the majority of available nurses were unprepared for work in public health nursing. Post-diploma programs to prepare nurses for public health work were unavailable in Canada. The VON had established training centres in several Canadian cities, including Ottawa, Toronto, and Winnipeg, to prepare registered nurses interested in joining the Order (Gibbon, 1947). However, the impact of the training centres was constrained by the Order's limited financial resources.

Fiscal constraints were another factor that delayed the development of rural public health services. Urban centres with a reasonably large tax base found it difficult enough to fund health departments. The challenge of raising sufficient

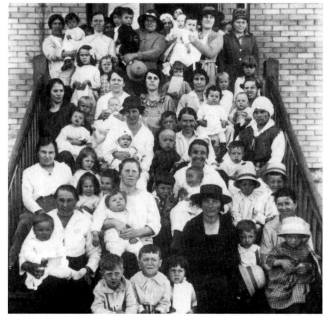

Photo 1.2

Child hygiene programs offered public health officials an opportunity to both monitor the health of young children and encourage their mothers to adopt Canadian child-rearing practices. This group, which includes 34 infants and children, gathered on the steps of All People's Mission, Winnipeg, in 1921 after having attended a child health clinic staffed by Dr. Ellen Douglas and several nurses.

Credit: Provincial Archives of Manitoba: L.B. Foote Collections 1452 (N2377)

Canadian Research Box 1.2

McPherson, K. (2003). Nursing and colonization: The work of Indian Health Service nurses in Manitoba, 1945–1970. In G. Feldberg, M. Ladd-Taylor, A. Li, & K. McPherson (Eds.). *Women, health, and nation: Canada and the United States since 1945* (pp. 222–246). Montreal & Kingston: McGill–Queen's University Press.

This article analyzes the work of Indian Health Service (IHS) nurses working in Zone 6 of the IHS after 1945. It first reviews historical approaches to the "complex relationship of gender, professionalism, and colonization" (p. 223) and then discusses how these categories of analysis have been used to examine the experiences of nurses working with government-sponsored Aboriginal health programs in the United States and Canada. Drawing on this body of literature, McPherson argues that nurses working in Aboriginal communities have had an ambiguous impact on the health and cultural practices of the populations that they served. For example, because of their gender, nurses could forge closer relationships with Aboriginal women than could male physicians and Indian agents, and were thus more able to offer "medical" care and health teaching. As members of a profession often subordinated to medicine, nurses working in isolated Aboriginal communities often

enjoyed considerable autonomy and had many opportunities to practise in expanded roles. Their role within the larger colonial project is more problematic. Given that medicine was a primary tool by which European settlers sought to undermine Aboriginal peoples' cultural beliefs and practices, IHS nurses were full participants in the process of imposing Western cultural practices upon Canada's indigenous populations. However, depending on their own attitudes and beliefs, nurses could also choose to support or at least tolerate the use of traditional healing practices in the communities in which they worked.

McPherson and others caution against an inappropriately benign interpretation of the impact of Westernized health care services in Aboriginal communities. All nurses, they argue, wielded professional, cultural, and racial power over Aboriginal people. Their interventions drew on middle-class standards of hygiene and childcare, which often had little relevance to populations experiencing poverty, cultural disruption, the depletion of traditional sources of food, and environmental pollution. As well, Canadian IHS nurses worked within a bureaucracy that both defended and perpetuated a system of health care based on charity, not citizenship.

Using Zone 6 as a case study, McPherson draws additional examples and provides further analysis of how gender, professional status, and colonialism both helped and hindered the work of IHS nurses working in Manitoba and Northwestern Ontario. Further analysis, she argues, is needed to understand the extent to which individual nurses may have "managed to work around racism and colonialism" (p. 240) to forge gender-based bonds with Aboriginal women. In the final analysis, sweeping generalizations about the impact of IHS nurses contribute little to the debate. "Understanding women's relationships with the state and with medicine demands that we ask, which women in what historical circumstances and in what relations of power?" (p. 241).

Discussion Questions:

1. To what extent do you think that today's health education and health promotion programs contain cultural, racial, and gender biases that limit their effectiveness and create barriers between community health nurses and the populations that they serve?

2. What forums would you use to lobby for reform of current community-based health care programs?

funds in small towns and unorganized rural districts was nearly insurmountable. As well, power over the allocation of scarce financial resources rested with far fewer individuals in non-urban settings. Both Stuart (1987) and Riddell (1991) contain first-person accounts by early rural PHNs about the impact that "penny pinching" local officials had on the development of local public health programs.

Popular conceptions about the relative healthiness of urban and rural settings also delayed the development of rural

Photo 1.3

Immunization of school-age children was an important part of a rural PHN's work. Small schools and long distances made this a challenging task. In 1932, public health nurse Ina Grenville and an unidentified physician were photographed immunizing a group of school children at Algoma School in Northern Ontario.

Credit: Archives of Ontario. Reference code: RG 10-30-2 (I0005225) Immunizing Children, Algoma, Ontario, 1932

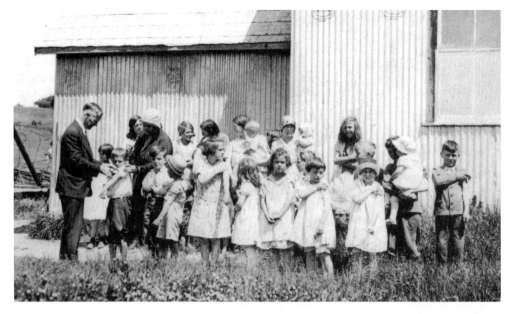

public health programs. Prior to the war, cities had been perceived as more unhealthy environments (Stuart, 1987). The visibility of urban squalor and the relative invisibility of its rural equivalent lulled many social reformers into believing that the pastoral nature of rural life was a healthy antidote to the evils of the city.

After World War I, the development of public health nursing was facilitated by a change in the mandate of the International Red Cross. To support more general efforts at rebuilding social structures in the post-war era, the International Red Cross prioritized the development of public health nursing (Hutchinson, 1996). The Canadian Red Cross possessed a substantial fund that had originally been earmarked to support the war effort (VON Minutes, Feb 1920). In the immediate post-war period, it used these funds to establish cottage hospitals and public health nursing services in rural and isolated communities (Miller, 2000; Riddell, 1991; Stuart, 1987), to support visiting nursing services in urban centres (MSNM Minutes, Feb 1920; VON Minutes, Feb 1920), and to provide funding for post-diploma programs in public health nursing at several Canadian universities (Riddell, 1991; Stuart, 1987). In British Columbia, for example, successive classes of nurses graduating from the University of British Columbia's post-diploma and baccalaureate nursing programs accelerated the pace at which rural public health programs could be established (Green, 1984; Riddell, 1991; Zilm & Warbinek, 1995).

The poor health of many military personnel recruited from rural Canada and the horrific loss of life during World War I also redirected political and public attention to the establishment of rural public health programs (Stuart, 1987). The agrarian protest movement in Ontario and the Prairie Provinces also accelerated the development of rural public health services in the post-war era. In Ontario, for example, the election of an agrarian/labour coalition government in 1919 was rapidly followed by the implementation of rural public health programs (Stuart, 1987).

At the local level, rural women's groups such as the Women's Institute and the United Farm Women made community development and the development of health care services a priority. These women lobbied local officials, served tea at child welfare clinics, sewed layettes for destitute families, provided transportation, made referrals, raised funds, and in untold other ways tried to enable the PHNs to fulfill their professional obligations to the fullest extent possible (Miller, 2000; Riddell, 1991; Stuart, 1987).

Unlike their counterparts in urban settings, the first rural PHNs were generalists. Blurring the boundaries between visiting nursing and public health nursing, these nurses delivered programs in health education, school health, maternal/child health, communicable disease control, social welfare, dental health, and medical/surgical nursing (Riddell, 1991; Stuart, 1987). In addition, they delivered babies and provided emergency medical, dental, and even veterinary assistance on the frequent occasions when these professionals were not available (Giovannini, 1988; Miller, 2000; Riddell, 1991; Stuart, 1987).

To accomplish this work, rural PHNs faced formidable challenges created by distance and climate. Although their urban counterparts, particularly in the early years, often walked many miles to visit homes at considerable distances from streetcar routes, urban nursing districts were measured in mere city blocks. Rural districts were enormous. As Olive Matthews reported in *The Canadian Nurse* in 1920: "I have a car for my school inspection, given voluntarily by Argyle and Clear Lake districts. It is the only way of covering 925 miles twice a year and paying home visits" (Matthews, 1920, p. 16). The first-hand accounts of early rural PHNs contain vivid descriptions of the various modes of transportation used in the course of their work and the dangerous road and weather conditions in which they travelled (Colley, 1970; Giovannini, 1988; Miller, 2000; Nevitt, 1978).

In the interwar years, the development of public health services was uneven and often unsuccessful. The time available to follow up on individuals and families needing health education or preventive services was limited, and the nurses' ability to provide long-term follow-up in complex situations was significantly constrained. The need for primary care in rural and isolated areas also limited the successful establishment of public health nursing programs. Many communities wanted VNs who provided bedside nursing care, rather than PHNs who focused on health education and prevention of illness (Matthews, 1920; Stuart, 1987).

On the other hand, local physicians sometimes did not support public health programs because they feared that the PHNs would provide primary care and thus compete with them for both patients and income. It took considerable effort on the part of the nurses to assuage these concerns. Stuart (1987), in her analysis of rural public health nursing in northern Ontario, found that PHNs often avoided giving advice to families about the prevention of communicable diseases even when they knew more about immunization programs than did the local physicians. One of the strategies employed to mute the protests of local physicians was to refer all individuals found to have "abnormal" conditions to the attending physician for further follow-up, even in cases where the nurses could have provided this care themselves (Riddell, 1991).

However, tensions surrounding which level of government should finance the public health system likely had the most negative impact on the development of PHN services in rural areas in the interwar years. For example, the nurses sent out to establish a public health system in northern Ontario were not permanently stationed in a community. Instead, they were expected to provide a short-term "demonstration" of the benefits of public health programs, then move on to another location. Should the local authorities agree that these services were necessary, the financing to continue them was to be allocated at the local level. Local authorities were often very happy to accept the services of PHNs financed by the provincial government but reluctant to employ them out of local funds (Stuart, 1987).

Visiting Nursing in Canada

As is evident from the preceding discussion, previously private health concerns, such as TB and infant hygiene, were redefined as public health concerns in the early part of the twentieth century. In some communities, public health programs replaced services pioneered by visiting nursing organizations. In others, visiting nursing organizations either entered into contractual arrangements with local health departments to provide these services or continued to provide them on their own initiative in the absence of government action. In addition to their occasional involvement in public health programs, visiting nursing organizations also continued to fulfill their original mandate to provide bedside nursing care in the home. This section will examine the experiences and challenges of Canadian visiting nursing organizations between 1897 and 1945.

Established in 1897, the VON is Canada's only national community health nursing organization. Its capacity to respond to local needs and opportunities stemmed from its organizational structure. Local branches were established in communities that had enough volunteers to sustain the organization. They reported to the central board, located in Ottawa, which set out guiding principles for the operation of local branches. It also encouraged local branches to seize opportunities to extend their work and to demonstrate the VON's capacity to deliver the whole range of community health nursing services. Visiting nursing services were the backbone of the local branches. In most communities, bedside nursing care was provided to a full range of destitute, working-class, and middle-class families who could not afford to hire private-duty nurses. Families paid what they could for these services. The difference between the actual cost of the service and what was paid in fees was underwritten by charitable donations, fundraising, and, in some cases, grants from city or provincial governments. In this way, the local branches fulfilled a dual mandate: charitable work among the poor and the provision of affordable nursing care to the working and middle classes. The history of the VON has been documented in two monographs, one written on the occasion of its 50th anniversary (Gibbon, 1947) and one to celebrate its 100th year of service in Canada (Penney, 1996). The experience of the Winnipeg Branch of the VON will be used as a case study to illustrate how the unique characteristics of specific communities shaped the services offered by the local branches.

In Winnipeg, charitable visiting nursing was pioneered by the Margaret Scott Nursing Mission, founded in 1904 to support the charitable work that Margaret Scott had been carrying out in the immigrant districts of Winnipeg since the 1890s (MSNM Minutes, May 1904). Scott was not a nurse, but in the course of her visits she encountered many people requiring medical and nursing assistance. The Mission performed an important role in preventing the admission of indigent patients to the charity wards of the Winnipeg General Hospital, thus reducing the cost of their care for local taxpayers. In keeping with the goals of the social gospel movement and maternal feminism, the majority of the Mission's patients in the early years were children and pregnant women. After hospital-based obstetrical care became the norm even for poor women, the majority of individuals receiving services from the MSNM were elderly or chronically ill.

The incursion of the Winnipeg branch of the VON into visiting nursing in 1905 forced the two organizations to coordinate their work so that they would not duplicate services. Ultimately, they agreed that the VON would provide services to those who "...did not wish to be classed as charity patients & who were willing to pay moderately for the services of a nurse," while the MSNM would continue to focus its attention on Winnipeg's poor and destitute populations (MSNM Minutes, May 1910). For the first few years, the Winnipeg Branch struggled to establish a non-charitable visiting nursing program in the city and the growth of the organization was relatively slow.

However, new life was injected into the Winnipeg Branch after WWI. In 1919, a new superintendent of nurses brought fresh ideas gleaned from her extensive experience in other communities. In 1920, the local Red Cross Society

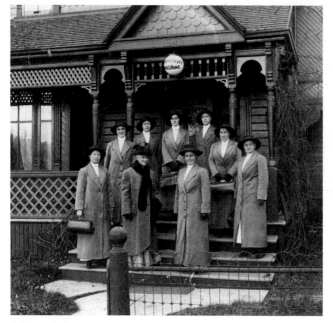

Photo 1.4

The Margaret Scott Nursing Mission provided charitable visiting nursing services to Winnipeg's poor and immigrant citizens from 1904–1943. It was located at 99 George St. on the south edge of Winnipeg's famous North End. This photograph, circa 1914, was taken just prior to the takeover of their child hygiene program by the City Health Department. Margaret Scott is front row centre.

Credit: Allan D. McKay (private collection)

provided the funds to put some of these ideas into action. Between 1919 and 1925, the Winnipeg Branch expanded its visiting nursing services into several suburbs adjacent to Winnipeg. It also established child welfare clinics, mothercraft classes, special clinics for immigrant women, and prenatal visiting in urban and suburban Winnipeg. It pioneered the use of mothers' helpers to assist mothers whose primary need was respite rather than nursing care. In addition, the Winnipeg Branch entered into agreements with two major Winnipeg employers to provide industrial (occupational health) nursing services to their employees and opened a dental clinic to provide dental care to working-class and indigent families. In 1923, they inaugurated an hourly nursing service for middle-class families who could afford to pay nurses on an hourly basis but not full-time (VON Minutes, May 1923). The enlarged scope of their programs was coordinated with other agencies such as the city and provincial PHNs, the outpatient departments of the Winnipeg General and Children's Hospitals, and the MSNM.

One very important function distinguished VNs employed by charitable organizations from publicly employed PHNs. This was the VNs' responsibility to ensure that the nursing care they provided did not **pauperize** their clients by diminishing their personal initiative and rendering them permanently dependent on the state. Because the provision of charitable health and welfare services was a responsibility of

local governments and the wealthy elite (Taylor, 1987), the possibility that charitable assistance might be given indiscriminately was a significant concern for its providers. Charity relieved the suffering of the poor, but it might also pauperize them. Because PHNs were paid out of public funds, they were, at least in theory, required to assist all who requested their services. Visiting nursing services, however, were at least partially funded by charitable donations. Part of their responsibility, therefore, was **investigation work**, which involved the financial assessment of the family and the determination of what portion of the cost of the nursing visit the family could afford. Paying at least part of the cost mitigated the humiliation of accepting charity and enabled families to avoid being classified as paupers. Thus, the VON's major role in their Winnipeg dental clinic was to visit the homes of the clinic patients and determine their ability to pay. In the same vein, the nurses of the Lethbridge Nursing Mission (LNM) could provide charitable assistance to destitute families in addition to providing bedside nursing care, because they had the necessary mandate and experience (Richardson, 1997). Even the MSNM encouraged its clients to pay anything, even a penny, for the services of its nurses.

By the beginning of World War II, the essential elements of community health nursing services had been put in place across the country. Provincial health departments had been organized and local health departments operated in the majority of Canadian cities. The scope of work in health education and prevention of illness had enlarged to include such programs as mental health, venereal disease control, preschool health, and prenatal education. The VON continued to flourish by using its success in the provision of bedside nursing care in the home as a springboard to also provide public health programs in communities where local attitudes and gaps in services made this possible. The only irony was that, although it had been envisioned by its founders as a nursing service for those living in rural and isolated "country districts," the VON had attained its greatest success and stability in Canada's urban centres.

COMMUNITY HEALTH NURSING IN THE WELFARE STATE

The Political and Economic Context

Even prior to World War II, the provision of health care services had undergone significant change in Canada. The federal, provincial, and local governments now funded, albeit at times reluctantly, many services that had previously been the responsibility of the individual, the family, or a charitable organization. The provision of publicly funded health and social welfare programs by federal and provincial governments is known as the **welfare state**. The transition from laissez-faire government to the welfare state gained momentum during the 1930s. The Great Depression dramatically demonstrated the limited capacity of local and provincial governments to provide health and

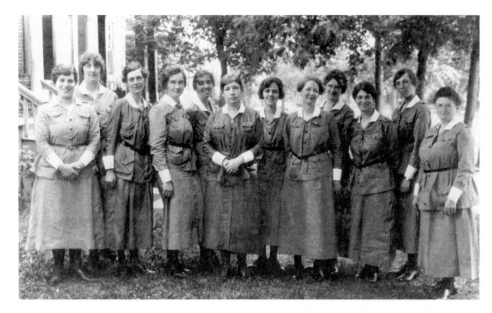

Photo 1.5

Annah L. Prichard, District Superintendent, with the nursing staff of the Winnipeg Branch VON. Prichard served in this capacity between 1919 and 1925, during an era of rapid expansion of the Winnipeg Branch.

Credit: Victorian Order of Nurses, Manitoba Branch Photographic Collection

social welfare services during times of greatest need. However, the federal government's ability to intervene was limited under the provisions of the BNA Act. In 1937, the Royal Commission on Dominion-Provincial Relations was appointed to determine how federal and provincial powers might be modified to improve the social welfare of all Canadians. It tabled its report in 1940, recommending that the federal government assume responsibility for unemployment insurance and old age pensions and that the provincial governments retain responsibility for public health programs and hospital care (Owram, 1986). However, concerns about how the government could protect citizens from the economic consequences of prolonged illnesses persisted. Several private and provincial medical and hospital insurance programs evolved after World War II, but these did not provide all Canadians with equitable access to health care. In 1948, the federal government established health grants for a variety of health programs offered at the provincial level (Shillington, 1972). Universal insured medical and hospital services were established with the passage of the Hospital Insurance and Diagnostic Services Act in 1957 and the Medical Care Insurance Act in 1968.

However, community and public health agencies across Canada never benefited from federal legislation and funding in the same way as did the acute and long-term health care sector. Despite the recommendations of the 1943 Report of the Advisory Committee on Health Insurance (the Heagerty Report), the funding of the Canadian public health system remained the responsibility of local and provincial governments (Government of Canada, 1943). In many instances, provincial legislation concerning the establishment of local health units was enabling rather than mandatory. Funding to support these health units was usually obtained though cost-sharing arrangements between the local and provincial governments, with the latter providing anywhere from one-third to two-thirds of the necessary funding. In some instances, charitable organizations such as the Canadian Red Cross and the Rockefeller Foundation provided funding to establish local or provincial public health programs and/or health units (Archives of Manitoba, The Garson Papers, 1942; Baldwin, 1997; Canadian Public Health Association [CPHA], 1940; Miller, 2000). Thus, public health services were available only in communities that possessed both the interest to request them and the financial resources to fund them (CPHA, 1940; Government of Canada, 1943). Federal financial contributions to the public health system were confined to specific programs, often for specific periods of time. For example, the venereal disease campaign received federal funding between 1919 and 1932. More recently, the National Immunization Strategy, a five-year federal transfer program, was established in 2003. Despite the limited federal support for the community health sector, federal/provincial cost-sharing arrangements for the acute and long-term health care sector had a significant impact on the programs offered by both public health nursing and visiting nursing programs.

New Roles for Visiting Nurses: The Emergence of Home Care Programs

Publicly funded health care programs changed the organization and work of visiting nursing associations in several ways. First, philanthropic support of local VNAs such as the MSNM and the LNM waned. Most closed in the decade immediately following World War II, unable to sustain either their funding or the quality of their nursing programs (MSNM, 1943; Richardson, 1997).

Although the VON continued to grow during the postwar years, it was also forced to respond to the changing face of health care in Canada. Expanded local and provincial departments of health took over public health programs that previously had been provided by the VON (Penney, 1996). Hospital admission became the norm for most Canadians requiring obstetrical, medical, or surgical care. This development shifted the VON visiting nursing caseloads to the care of convalescent and chronically ill individuals. Further, the erosion of charitable donations, which had at least partially offset the cost of caring for the poor in the past, meant that VNs were more likely to be providing care to those who could afford to pay for these services either directly or through third-party insurance arrangements.

In the early 1970s, rising hospital costs created both an opportunity and a crisis for the VON. Patients were discharged from hospital earlier and required longer and more complex follow-up care in the community. However, these individuals were often unable to obtain bedside nursing care in their homes during their convalescence. No publicly insured programs for home care services existed until 1974, when the first such program was established in Manitoba (Shapiro, 1997). The VON realized that participation in publicly insured home care programs was an opportunity to both consolidate and strengthen their organization. It commissioned a national report, which recommended that Canada's oldest and most experienced visiting nursing organization be given the mandate to deliver publicly insured home care programs (Pickering, 1976). However, individual provincial governments made a variety of decisions about the organization and funding of home care programs, and these did not always include the VON (Penney, 1996). Today, as it did in the past, the VON continues to function by offering a mix of services shaped by local circumstances, with a particular focus on creating programs to respond to unmet needs among specific segments of the population (Penney, 1996).

New Mandates for Public Health Nurses

Increased government responsibility for the health care of Canadians also had a significant impact on public health nursing. Between 1940 and 1970, health departments focused on the elaboration of existing programs. However, this process also included a general shift of emphasis from traditional programs such as child health, immunization, and communicable disease control to programs focusing on the reduction of morbidity and mortality from chronic illnesses and injuries. Early postpartum discharge programs, a modification of the traditional postpartum home visit, placed significant demands on the time and resources of PHNs. In some instances, staffing patterns in health units and community health centres were modified to provide seven-day-a-week early postpartum services to mothers and neonates.

The reduction in government spending during the 1980s and 1990s affected PHNs both directly and indirectly. Static or reduced nursing staffs decreased levels of service for many programs. Infrastructures for communicable disease control were particularly hard hit. The loss of capacity to monitor, identify, and follow up on communicable diseases has been identified as one of the major reasons for the resurgence of TB and the recent emergence of new diseases, such as AIDS and SARS (Garrett, 1994, 2000).

Challenges Old and New

Community-based nurses have always been conscious of the impact that political, economic, and other macro systems have on individual, family, aggregate, and population health. Knowledge development in health promotion, healthy public policy, and the determinants of health enabled nurses to shape their practices in ways that sought to engage both health care professionals and community members in finding new and innovative ways to achieve health for all. More about these ideas and their application to the practices of community-based nurses will be found in subsequent chapters of this book.

In a similar vein, working with individuals, families, and groups from diverse cultures, traditions, and languages has always been an integral part of the practices of both VNs and PHNs. Health-seeking behaviours are enmeshed in both cultural and scientific knowledge. Thus, avoiding the imposition of health care practices that simply reflect the beliefs and values of the dominant culture requires sensitivity, adaptability, and openness on the part of nurses who practise in their clients' homes and neighbourhoods. History provides us with many examples of well-meaning individuals and groups who failed to recognize and/or respond to the health care needs of specific populations in a culturally appropriate manner. Rather than creating a false sense of complacency about the progress of nursing knowledge and practices, these examples should remind today's nurses that embracing and nurturing the cultural diversity of contemporary Canadian society is both a privilege and an ongoing challenge.

Summary

At the end of the twentieth century, many aspects of community health nursing had come full circle. Publicly funded home care programs have created a tremendous growth in the number of nurses working in community settings. However, the role of home care nurses, who provide bedside nursing care and health education to the sick and convalescent, is similar to that fulfilled by the VNs of the late nineteenth and early twentieth centuries. The number of PHNs, on the other hand, has remained relatively stable. Their mandate has continued to emphasize health promotion, communicable disease control, healthy child development, prevention of chronic illness, and the identification of other factors that create morbidity and mortality in the population. What has changed is their visibility. Although PHNs have worked in the community for nearly a century, their small numbers and the presence of many other community-based service providers have rendered them less visible and more likely to be overlooked by both the funders and the users of the health care system. The challenge for the community health nurses of the future is to regain the visibility of their predecessors and to continue to demonstrate the capacity of nurses to provide leadership in the community-based health care systems of tomorrow.

KEY TERMS

public health movement
maternal feminist
district nursing
visiting nursing
public health nursing
social gospel movement
pauperize
investigation work
welfare state

STUDY QUESTIONS

1. Describe the two forms of community health nursing that evolved in Canada in the early twentieth century.

2. What social movements supported the emergence of community health nursing?

3. Which segments of the population were the focus of early community nursing programs?

4. Briefly describe the three earliest public health programs in which nurses were involved and the reasons for their implementation.

5. How did the British North America Act (1867) and nineteenth-century beliefs about the role of government influence the development of community-based health care services?

6. Describe the emergence of the Canadian welfare state.

7. Describe the role that non-governmental organizations, such as the VON, the Red Cross, and local philanthropic agencies, played in the development of community-based nursing programs.

INDIVIDUAL CRITICAL THINKING EXERCISES

The sources listed at the end of each question are cited in full in either the References or the Additional Resources section of this chapter. Each source will provide additional insights into the controversies and debates surrounding the history of public health and visiting nursing.

1. Meryn Stuart (1989), in her analysis of the development of rural public health nursing in northern Ontario, states that "The Board's focus on health education, however delivered by the nurses, would not erase the effects of poverty.... Health education was a facile solution to the serious problem of the lack of permanent human and material resources" (p. 111). Analyze the apparent lack of congruency between the needs of the populations that public health programs served and the typical services that these programs offered. (Sources: Piva, 1979; Stuart, 1989)

2. Physicians and nurses assumed different roles in early community health organizations. What role did gender play in the assignment of these roles? (Sources: McPherson, 1996, Chapter 1; Stuart, 1992)

3. Community health nursing has frequently been described as more autonomous than nursing practice in institutional settings. However, Eunice Dyke, Toronto's first supervisor of public health nursing, once stated that "...public health nursing has in the medical profession its greatest friend and not infrequently its greatest stumbling block." How autonomous was the practice of early community health nurses? (Sources: Comacchio, 1993, Chapter 7; Stuart, 1992)

4. What role did middle-class ideas about class, ethnicity, and gender play in the development of public health programs to protect the health of infants and children? (Sources: Comacchio, 1993, Chapter 3; Gleason, 2002)

5. Reflect on the constraints/limits on the scope of practice of PHNs in the 1920s and '30s. Do you see any parallels in the practice of PHNs today? Are there recurring patterns, and, if so, what are they? (Sources: Stuart, 1989, 1992)

6. The major target groups of early public health and visiting nursing organizations were the poor, the working class, and recently arrived immigrants. However, there is little published analysis of how these groups responded to the interventions of middle-class social reformers and public health officials. What do you think some of their responses might have been?

GROUP CRITICAL THINKING EXERCISES

1. Social historians such as Alan Hunt (1999) argue that charity, philanthropy, and welfare programs are essentially efforts by the elite and middle classes to impose their behaviour, values, and culture upon others. Hunt describes these programs of moral or social regulation as being inspired by "...the passionate conviction that there is something inherently wrong or immoral about the conduct of others" (p. ix). Locate an issue of an early public health or nursing journal such as *The Public Health Journal* (now the *Canadian Journal of Public Health*) or *The Canadian Nurse* (particularly the section on public health). Conduct a brief content analysis of the issue, paying close attention to how the recipients of public health interventions are described. What conclusions can be drawn about the attitudes of health care professionals? What anxieties seem to underlie the interventions they describe and recommend to other health care practitioners?

2. Nurses were the intermediaries between the clients they served and the social and political elite who employed them to work in the community. However, their perspective on the objectives and effectiveness of community-based health care programs is often absent from published histories of public health. To fill this gap in the historical record, do one of the following: (1) locate a biographical account written by an early visiting or public health nurse, (2) locate an oral history of an early visiting or public health nurse in an archive, or (3) interview a retired visiting or public health nurse. How does their account resemble and differ from the history of community-based

nursing presented in this chapter? How would you account for any differences you identify?

3. Based on what you have learned about the history of community health nursing in Canada, what do you believe are the greatest challenges facing nurses in this practice setting today and in the future?

PRIMARY SOURCES

Archives of Manitoba, The Garson Papers, P2357, Folder 11, Dr. Carl Buck. Notes on Meeting of Council dated January 21, 1942.

Margaret Scott Nursing Mission, Board of Management. (n.d.). *Minutes 1904–1943.* (Archives of Manitoba. MG10 B9 Box IV).

Victorian Order of Nurses for Canada, Winnipeg Branch. (n.d.). *Minutes of Board Meetings 1901–1927.*

REFERENCES

Artibise, A. F. (1975). *Winnipeg: A social history of urban growth, 1874–1914.* Montreal: McGill–Queen's University Press.

Baillargeon, D. (2002). Entre la "Revanche" et la "Veillée" des berceaux: Les médecins québécois francophones, la mortalité infantile et la question nationale, 1910–40. *Canadian Bulletin of Medical History/Bulletin Canadien d'histoire de la médecine, 19*(1), 113–137.

Baldwin, D. O. (1997). *She answered every call: The life of public health nurse Mona Gordon Wilson (1894–1981).* Charlottetown: Indigo Press.

Banfill, B. J. (1967). *Pioneer nurse.* Toronto: Ryerson Press.

Bilson, G. (1980). *A darkened house: Cholera in nineteenth-century Canada.* Toronto: University of Toronto Press.

Bliss, M. (1991). *Plague: A story of smallpox in Montreal.* Toronto: HarperCollins.

Canadian Public Health Association. (1940). *The development of public health in Canada.* Toronto: University of Toronto Press.

Christie, N., & Gauvreau, M. (1996). *A full-orbed Christianity: The Protestant churches and social welfare in Canada.* Toronto: University of Toronto Press.

City of Winnipeg Health Department. (1910). *Annual report for the year ending December 1909.* Winnipeg: City of Winnipeg.

City of Winnipeg Health Department. (1915). *Annual report for the year ending December 1914.* Winnipeg: City of Winnipeg.

City of Winnipeg Health Department. (1919). *Annual report for the year ending December 1918.* Winnipeg: City of Winnipeg.

Colley, K. B. (1970). *While rivers flow: Stories of early Alberta.* Saskatoon: Prairie Books.

Douglas, A. J. (1912). Chairman's address, Section of Municipal Health Officers, American Public Health Association. *American Journal of Public Health, 2*(2), 85–86.

Garrett, L. (1994). *The coming plague: Newly emerging diseases in a world out of balance.* New York: Penguin Books.

Garrett, L. (2000). *Betrayal of trust: The collapse of global public health.* New York: Hyperion Press.

Gibbon, J. M. (1947). *The Victorian Order of Nurses for Canada: 50th anniversary, 1897–1947.* Montreal: Southam Press.

Giovannini, M. (1988). *Outport nurse.* St. John's: Memorial University, Faculty of Medicine.

Government of Canada. (1943). Report of the advisory committee on health insurance [the Heagerty Report]. Ottawa: Minister of Pensions and National Health.

Green, H. G. (1974). *Don't have your baby in the dory!: A biography of Myra Bennett.* Montreal: Harvest House.

Green, M. (1984). *Through the years with public health nursing: A history of public health nursing in the provincial government jurisdiction British Columbia.* Ottawa: Canadian Public Health Association.

Hope, M. E. (1955). *Lamp on the snow.* London, UK: Angus & Robertson.

Humphreys, M. (1999). Tuberculosis: The "consumption" and civilization. In K. F. Kiple (Ed.), *Plague, pox & pestilence: Disease in history* (pp. 136–141). London, UK: Phoenix Illustrated.

Hutchinson, J. F. (1996). *Champions of charity: War and the rise of the Red Cross.* Boulder, CO: Westview Press.

Ladd-Taylor, M. (1994). *Mother-work, women, child welfare and the state, 1890–1930.* Urbana, IL: University of Illinois Press.

Locke, H. L. F. (1918). The problem of our infant population with special reference to the opportunity of the welfare nurse. *American Journal of Nursing, 18*(7), 523–526.

MacDougall, H. (1990). *Activists & advocates: Toronto's Health Department, 1883–1983.* Toronto: Dundurn Press.

MacNutt, J. S. (1913). The Board of Health nurse: What she can do for the public welfare in a small city. *American Journal of Public Health, 3*(4), 1913.

Matthews, O. (1920). Child welfare. *The Canadian Nurse, 16*(1), 15–16.

McLaren, A., & McLaren, A. T. (1997). *The bedroom and the state: The changing practices and politics of contraception and abortion in Canada, 1880–1997* (2nd ed.). Oxford, UK: Oxford University Press.

McPherson, K. (1996). *Bedside matters: The transformation of Canadian nursing, 1900–1990.* Toronto: Oxford University Press.

Meckel, R.A. (1990). *Save the babies: American public health reform and the prevention of infant mortality 1850-1929.* Baltimore: Johns Hopkins University Press.

Meigs, G. L. (1916, August). Other factors in infant mortality than the milk supply and their control. *American Journal of Public Health, 6,* 847–853.

Merkley, P. (1987). The vision of the good society in the social gospel: What, where and when is the kingdom of God? *Historical Papers: Canadian Historical Association,* pp. 138–145.

Miller, G. L. (2000). *Mustard plasters and handcars: Through the eyes of a Red Cross outpost nurse.* Toronto: Natural Heritage/Natural History.

Nevitt, J. (1978). *White caps and black bands: Nursing in Newfoundland to 1934.* St. John's, NL: Jefferson Press.

Owram, D. (1986). *The government generation: Canadian intellectuals and the state, 1900–1945.* Toronto: University of Toronto Press.

Peikoff, T., & Brickey, S. (1991). Creating precious children and glorified mothers: A theoretical assessment of the transformation of childhood. In R. Smandych, G. Dodds, & A. Esau (Eds.), *Dimensions of childhood: Essays on the history of children and youth in Canada* (pp. 29–61). Winnipeg: Legal Research Institute of the University of Manitoba.

Penney, S. (1996). *A century of caring: The history of the Victorian Order of Nurses for Canada.* Ottawa: Victorian Order of Nurses for Canada.

Pickering, E. A. (1976). *A case for the VON in home care.* Ottawa: Victorian Order of Nurses for Canada.

Piva, M. J. (1979). *The condition of the working class in Toronto, 1900–1921.* Ottawa: University of Ottawa Press.

Richardson, S. (1997). Women's enterprise: Establishing the Lethbridge Nursing Mission, 1909–1919. *Nursing History Review, 5,* 105–30.

Roberts, J. (1928). Twenty-three years of public health. *The Public Health Journal, 19,* 554.

Riddell, S. E. (1991). *Curing society's ills: Public health nurses and public health nursing in rural British Columbia, 1916–1946.* Unpublished master's thesis, Simon Fraser University, Vancouver.

Royce, M. (1983). *Eunice Dyke: Health care pioneer: From pioneer public health nurse to advocate for the aged.* Toronto: Dundurn Press.

Sears, A. (1995). Before the welfare state: Public health and social policy. *Canadian Review of Sociology and Anthropology/Revue canadienne de sociologie et d'anthropologie, 32*(2), 169–188.

Shapiro, E. (1997). *The cost of privatization: A case study of home care in Manitoba.* Ottawa: Canadian Centre for Policy Alternatives.

Shillington, C. H. (1972). *The road to medicare in Canada.* Toronto: Del Graphics.

Stuart, M. E. (1987). *"Let not the people perish for lack of knowledge": Public health nursing and the Ontario rural child welfare project, 1916–1930.* Unpublished doctoral dissertation, University of Pennsylvania, Philadelphia, PA.

Sutherland, N. (1981). "To create a strong and healthy race": School children in the public health movement, 1880–1914. In S. E. D. Shortt (Ed.), *Medicine in Canadian society: Historical perspectives* (pp. 361–393). Montreal: McGill–Queen's University Press.

Taylor, M. G. (1987). *Health insurance and Canadian public policy.* Montreal: McGill–Queen's University Press.

Zilm, G., & Warbinek, E. (1995). Early tuberculosis nursing in British Columbia. *The Canadian Journal of Nursing Research, 27*(3), 65–81.

ADDITIONAL RESOURCES

Websites

American Association for the History of Nursing
www.aahn.org

AMS Nursing History Research Unit
www.health.uottawa.ca/nursinghistory/

B.C. History of Nursing Group
www.bcnursinghistory.ca/bchn.html

Canadian Association for the History of Nursing
www.cahn-achn.ca

College & Association of Registered Nurses of Alberta
www.nurses.ab.ca/museum/intro.html

Margaret M. Allemang Centre for the History of Nursing
www.allemang.on.ca

Nurses Association of New Brunswick
www.nanb.nb.ca

United Kingdom Centre for the History of Nursing
www.ukchnm.org

Monographs and Articles

Buhler-Wilkerson, K. (1989). *False dawn: The rise and decline of public health nursing, 1900–1930.* New York: Garland.

Buhler-Wilkerson, K. (2001). *No place like home: A history of nursing and home care in the United States.* Baltimore, MD: Johns Hopkins University Press.

Comacchio, C. (1993). *Nations are built of babies: Saving Ontario's mothers and children 1900–194*0. Montreal: McGill–Queen's University Press.

Copp, T. (1981). Public health in Montreal, 1870–1930. In S. E. D. Shortt (Ed.), *Medicine in Canadian society: Historical perspectives.* Montreal: McGill–Queen's University Press.

Gleason, M. (2002). Race, class and health: School medical inspection and "healthy" children in British Columbia, 1890–1930. *Canadian Bulletin of Medical History/Bulletin Canadien d'histoire de la médecine, 19*(1), 95–112.

Hunt, A. (1999). *Governing morals: A social history of moral regulation.* Cambridge, UK: Cambridge University Press.

Stuart, M. (1989). Ideology and experience: Public health nursing and the Ontario Rural Child Welfare Project, 1920–25. *Canadian Bulletin of Medical History/Bulletin Canadien d'histoire de la médecine, 6,* 111–131.

Stuart, M. (1992). "Half a loaf is better than no bread": Public health nurses and physicians in Ontario, 1920–1925. *Nursing Research, 41*(1), 21–27.

FURTHER READING

A comprehensive synthesis of the history of community health nursing in Canada has never been written. This chapter does not fill that gap. It focuses almost exclusively on the work of "trained nurses" and their work in formal community health programs, both of which originated in the late nineteenth century. While facilitating a thematic approach to the subject, this approach also has limitations. It omits the significant contributions of lay and religious women who visited and cared for the sick in their homes from the time that the first European settlers arrived in Canada. The contributions of national and regional community nursing organizations such as the VON, the Saint Elizabeth Visiting Nurses' Association of Ontario, and the Lethbridge Nursing Mission receive limited attention. The chapter also does not discuss in any detail the experiences and practices of outpost nurses working with, for example, the Canadian Red Cross, the Grenfell Mission (Labrador), le service medical aux colons (Quebec), and Alberta's District Nursing Service. Although the influence of maternal feminist lay women is discussed in some detail in this chapter, the role of other non-governmental groups instrumental in the establishment of community and public health nursing is not discussed in any detail. For example, both the Red Cross and the Rockefeller Foundation funded demonstration projects in public health nursing in several Canadian provinces. These programs were eventually integrated into provincial public health systems.

This chapter is also limited by the existing historiography. Most of the existing monographs and articles focus on the development of public health and community health nursing programs prior to 1970. This is not entirely unexpected. For many historians, contemporary developments in community health nursing are not yet history and these changes await historical analysis. Finally, the historiography of community health nursing in Canada is unevenly developed. Some provinces and regions have been blessed with historians who have written extensively on the subject. Others have not. The following bibliography provides further resources for those interested in learning more about the history of community health nursing in Canada, particularly those aspects of the subject that are not adequately discussed in the chapter itself.

Canada

Allemang, M. (2000). Development of community health nursing in Canada. In M. Stewart (Ed.), *Community health nursing in Canada* (2nd ed.) (pp. 329). Toronto: W. B. Saunders.

Arnup, M. K. (1991). *Education for motherhood: Women and the family in twentieth century English Canada.* Unpublished doctoral dissertation, University of Toronto.

Bates, C., Dodd, D., & Rousseau, N. (2005). *On all frontiers: Four centuries of Canadian nursing.* Ottawa: University of Ottawa Press.

Buckley, S., & McGinnis, J. D. (1982). Venereal disease and public health reform in Canada. *Canadian Historical Review, 63*(3), 337–354.

Dodd, D. (1991) Advice to parents: The Blue Books, Helen MacMurchy, MD, and the Federal Department of Health, 1920–34. *Canadian Bulletin of Medical History, 8*(2), 203–230.

Duncan, S. M., Leipert, B. D., & Mill, J. E. (1999). Nurses as health evangelists?: The evolution of public health nursing in Canada, 1918–1939. *Advances in Nursing Science, 22*(1), 40–51.

Emory, F. H. M. (1953). *Public health nursing in Canada.* Toronto: Macmillan.

Harrison, H. E. (2001). *"In the picture of health": Portraits of health, disease and citizenship in Canada's public health advice literature, 1920–1960.* Unpublished doctoral dissertation, Queen's University, Kingston, ON.

Lewis, J. (1986). The prevention of diphtheria in Canada and Britain 1914–1945. *Journal of Social History, 20*(1), 163–176.

McCuaig, K. (1999). *The weariness, the fever, and the fret: The campaign against tuberculosis in Canada, 1900–1950.* Montreal: McGill–Queen's University Press.

Nesmith, T. (1985). The early years of public health: The Department of Agriculture, 1867–1918. *Archivist, 12*(5), 13.

Newfoundland and Labrador

House, E. (1990). *The way out: The story of NONIA, 1920–1990.* St. John's: Creative Publishers.

Neary, P. (1998). Venereal disease and public health administration in Newfoundland in the 1930s and 1940s. *Canadian Bulletin of Medical History, 15*(1), 129–151.

Neary, P. (1998). "And gave just as much as they got": A 1941 American perspective on public health in Newfoundland. *Newfoundland Studies, 14*(1), 50–70.

Nova Scotia

Farley, J. (2002). The Halifax diphtheria epidemic (1940 to 1944): A disaster waiting to happen or a blessing in disguise? *Journal of the Royal Nova Scotia Historical Society, 5,* 44–63.

Gregor, F. (2005) "Home nursing has continued to present problems": The St. John Ambulance Home Nursing Program in Nova Scotia. In J. Fingard & J. Guildford (Eds.), *Mothers of the municipality: Women, work, and social policy in post 1945 Halifax* (pp. 226–252). Toronto: Toronto University Press.

Gregor, F. (2004). Mapping the demise of the St John Ambulance Home Nursing Program in Nova Scotia, 1950–1975. *Canadian Bulletin of Medical History, 21*(2), 351–75.

Penney, S. (1990). *Inventing the cure: Tuberculosis in twentieth century Nova Scotia.* Unpublished doctoral dissertation, Dalhousie University, Halifax.

Twohig, P. (2001). Public health in industrial Cape Breton, 1900–1930s. *Journal of the Royal Nova Scotia Historical Society, 4,* 108–131.

Twohig, P. (2005). The Rockefellers, the Cape Breton Island Health Unit and public health in Nova Scotia. *Journal of the Royal Nova Scotia Historical Society, 5,* 122–133.

Prince Edward Island

Beck, B., & Townshend, A. (1993). The Island's Florence Nightingale. *Island Magazine, 34,* 16.

Baldwin, D. (1995). Interconnecting the personal and public: The support networks of Public Health Nurse Mona Wilson. *Canadian Journal of Nursing Research 27*(3), 19–37.

Baldwin, D. (1990). The volunteers in action: The establishment of government health care on Prince Edward Island, 1900–1931. *Acadiensis, 19*(2), 121–147.

Baldwin, D. (1993). Amy MacMahon and the struggle for public health. *Island Magazine, 34,* 20–27.

Lanigan, H., & Beck, B. (2005). The great white plague: Tuberculosis on Prince Edward Island. *Island Magazine, 57,* 22–29.

Palmer, D. (2005). Public health nursing on Prince Edward Island in the 1930s. *Island Magazine 57,* 30–33.

Quebec

Baillargeon, D. (2002). Care of mothers and infants in Montreal between the wars: The visiting children's nurses of the Metropolitan Life, milk deposits and maternal assistance. In M. D. Behiels (Ed.). *Quebec since 1800: Selected readings* (pp. 93–209). Toronto: Irwin Publishing.

Baillargeon, D. (1998). Gouttes de lait et soif de pouvoir. Les dessous de la lutte contre la mortalité infantile à Montréal, 1910–1953. *Canadian Bulletin of Medical History, 15*(1), 27–57.

Baillargeon, D. (1993). Les infirmières de la Métropolitaine au service des Montréalaises. In Les bâtisseuses de la cité, Actes du colloque "Les bâtisseuses de la cité," Section d'études féministes, congrès de l'Acfas, Montréal, ACFAS, Les cahiers scientifiques no. 79, 1993, pp. 107–120.

Baillargeon, D. (1996). Fréquenter les gouttes de lait: L'expérience des mères Montréalaises, 1910–65. *Revue d'Histoire de l'Amérique Française, 50*(1), 29–68.

Braithwaite, C., Keating, P., & Viger, S. (1996). The problem of diphtheria in the Province of Quebec: 1894–1909. *Histoire Sociale, 29*(57), 71–95.

Cohen, Y., & Gélinas, M. (1989). Les infiermières hygiénistes de la Ville de Montréal: Du service privé au service civique. *Histoire Sociale, 22*(44), 219–246.

Cohen, Y. (2004). Rapports de genre, de classe et d'ethnicité: l'Histoire des infirmières au Québec. *Canadian Bulletin of Medical History, 21*(2), 387–409.

Copp, T. (1981). Public health in Montreal, 1870–1930. In S. E. D. Shortt (Ed.), *Medicine in Canadian society: Historical perspectives.* Montreal: McGill–Queen's University Press.

Daigle, J., & Rousseau, N. (1998). Le service médical aux colons: Gestation et implantation d'un service infirmier au Québec (1932–1943). *Revue d'Histoire de l'Amérique Française, 52*(1), 47–72.

Desrosiers, G., Gaumer, B., & Keel, O. (1998). La santé publique au Québec: Histoire des unités sanitaires de comté: 1926–1975. Montreal: University of Montreal Press.

Gaumer, B., Desrosiers, G., & Keel, O. (2002). *Histoire du Service de Santé de la Ville de Montréal, 1865–1975.* SainteFoy, QC: University of Laval Press.

Gagnon, F. (1994). État, médecine et santé communautaire au Québec (1970–1988): La construction d'un discours. Unpublished doctoral dissertation, University of Laval, Quebec City.

Goulet, D., Lemire, G., & Gauvreau, D. (1996). Des bureaux d'hygiène municipaux aux unités sanitaires le conseil d'hygiène de la province de Québec et la structuration d'un système de santé publique, 1886–1926. *Revue d'Histoire de l'Amérique Française, 49*(4), 491–520.

Guérard, F. (1996). L'hygiène publique au Québec de 1887 à 1939: Centralisation, normalisation et médicalisation. *Recherches Sociographiques, 37*(2), 203–227.

Guillaume, P. (1990). Épiscopat Québecois et santé publique dans la deuxième moitié du XIXe siècle. *Revue d'Histoire Moderne et Contemporaine, 37*(Apr–June), 324–336.

Merrick, E., Daigle, J., Rousseau, N., & Saillant, F. (1993). Des traces sur la neige: La contribution des infirmières au développment des régions isolées du Québec au XXe siècle. *Recherches féministes, 6*(1), 93–103.

Rousseau, N., & Daigle, J. (2000). Medical service to settlers: The gestation and establishment of a nursing service in Quebec, 1932–1943. *Nursing History Review, 8,* 95–116.

Ontario

Bator, P. (1979). *"Saving lives on the wholesale plan": Public health reform in the City of Toronto, 1900–1930.* Unpublished doctoral dissertation, University of Toronto, Toronto.

Comacchio, C. (1993). *Nations are built of babies: Saving Ontario's mothers and children 1900–1940.* Montreal: McGill–Queen's University Press.

Comacchio, C. (1988). "The mothers of the land must suffer": Child and maternal welfare in rural and outpost Ontario, 1918–1940. *Ontario History, 80*(3), 183–205.

Dodd, D. (2001). Helen MacMurchy, MD: Gender and professional conflict in the medical inspection of Toronto schools, 1910–1911. *Ontario History, 93*(2), 127–149.

Dehli, K. (1990). Health scouts for the state? School and public health nurses in early twentieth-century Toronto. *Historical Studies in Education, 2*(2), 247–264.

Gagan, R. (1989). Mortality patterns and public health in Hamilton, Canada, 1900–14. *Urban History Review, 17*(3), 161–175.

Rafael, A. R. F. (1999). The politics of health promotion: Influences on public health in Ontario, Canada from Nightingale to the nineties. *Advances in Nursing Science, 22*(1), 23–39.

Risk, M. (1973). *The origins and development of public health nursing in Toronto, 1890–1973.* M.A. Thesis, University of Toronto, Toronto.

Stuart, M. (1992). "Half a loaf is better than no bread": Public health nurses and physicians in Ontario, 1920–1925. *Nursing Research, 41*(1), 21–27.

Stuart, M. (1989). Ideology and experience: Public health nursing and the Ontario Rural Child Welfare Project, 1920–25. *Canadian Bulletin of Medical History, 6*(2), 111–131.

Stuart, Meryn. (1994). Shifting professional boundaries: Gender conflict in public health 1920–1925. In D. Dodd & D. Gorham (Eds.), *Caring and curing: Historical perspectives on women and healing in Canada* (pp. 49–70). Ottawa: University of Ottawa Press.

The Prairies

Bramadat, I., & Saydak, M. (1993). Nursing on the Canadian Prairies, 1900–1930: Effects of Immigration. *Nursing History Review, 1,* 105–117.

Kozak, N. (2005). Advice ideals and rural prairie realities: National prairie scientific motherhood advice, 1920–1929.

In Unsettled pasts: Reconceiving the West through women's history. Calgary: University of Calgary Press.

Manitoba

Jones, E. (2003). *"Searching for the springs of health": Women and working families in Winnipeg's 1918–1919 influenza epidemic.* Unpublished doctoral dissertation, University of Manitoba, Winnipeg.

McKay, M. (2005). *Saints and sanitarians: The role of women's voluntary agencies in the development of Winnipeg's public health system, 1882–1945.* Unpublished doctoral dissertation, University of Manitoba, Winnipeg.

McKay, M. (2006). "The tubercular cow must go": Business, politics, and Winnipeg's milk supply, 1894–1922. *Canadian Bulletin of Medical History, 23*(2), 355–380.

McPherson, K. (2003). Nursing and colonization: The work of Indian Health Service Nurses in Manitoba, 1945–1970. In G. Fedlberg, M. Ladd-Taylor, A. Li, & K. McPherson (Eds.), *Women, health, and nation: Canada and the United States Since 1945* (pp. 223–246). Montreal: McGill–Queen's University Press.

Saskatchewan

Drees, L. M., & McBain, L. (2001). Nursing and Native Peoples in Northern Saskatchewan: 1930s–1950s. *Canadian Bulletin of Medical History, 18*(1), 43–65.

Lux, M. (1997). "The Bitter Flats": The 1918 influenza epidemic in Saskatchewan. *Saskatchewan History, 49*(1), 313.

Alberta

Gahagan, A. C. (1979). *Yes father: Pioneer nursing in Alberta.* Manchester, NH: Hammer Publications, 1979.

Stewart, I. (1979). *These were our yesterdays: A history of district nursing in Alberta.* Altona: D. W. Friesen and Sons.

Richardson, S. (1998). Frontier health care: Alberta's District Nursing Service. *Alberta History, 46*(1), 2–9.

Richardson, S. (2002). Alberta's provincial travelling clinic. *Canadian Bulletin of Medical History, 19*(1), 245–263.

Richardson, S. (1998). Political women, professional nurses, and the creation of Alberta's District Nursing Service, 1919–1925. *Nursing History Review, 6,* 25–50.

British Columbia

Davies, M. (2005). Night soil, cesspools, and smelly hogs on the streets: Sanitation, race, and governance in early British Columbia. *Histoire Sociale, 38*(75), 135.

Gleason, M. (2002). Race, class, and health: School medical inspection and "healthy" children in British Columbia, 1890 to 1930. *Canadian Bulletin of Medical History, 19*(1), 95–112.

Hayes, M., & Foster, L. (2002). Too small to see, too big to ignore: Child health and wellbeing in British Columbia. *Canadian Western Geographical Series,* no. 35. Victoria: Western Geographical Press.

Northwest Territories/Yukon

Crnkovich, M. (Ed.). (1990). *Gossip: A spoken history of women in the North.* Ottawa: Canadian Arctic Resources Committee.

Goodwill, J. (1988). Indian and Inuit Nurses of Canada. *Saskatchewan Indian Federated College Journal 4*(1), 93–104.

Goodwill, J. (1984). Nursing Canada's Indigenous People. *Canadian Nurse 80*(1), 6.

Scott, J. K., with Kieser, J. E. (Ed.). (2002). *Northern nurses: True nursing adventures from Canada's North.* Oakville, ON: Kokum Publications.

Zelmanovits, J. (2003). "Midwife preferred": Maternity care in outpost nursing stations in Northern Canada, 1945–1988. In G. Fedlberg, M. Ladd-Taylor, A. Li, & K. McPherson (Eds.), *Women, health, and nation: Canada and the United States Since 1945* (pp. 161–188). Montreal: McGill–Queen's University Press.

VOLUNTARY ORGANIZATIONS

Canadian Red Cross

Elliott, J. (2004). *"Keep the flag flying": Medical outposts and the Red Cross in Northern Ontario, 1922–1984.* Unpublished doctoral dissertation, Queen's University, Kingston.

Elliott, J. (2004). Blurring the boundaries of space: Shaping nursing lives at the Red Cross outposts in Ontario, 1922–1945. *Canadian Bulletin of Medical History 21*(2), 303–325.

Massie, M. (2004). Ruth Dulmage Shewchuk: A Saskatchewan Red Cross outpost nurse. *Saskatchewan History, 56*(2), 35–44.

Perry, A. A. (1930). Guarding settlers on outposts of North: How railway Red Cross hospitals and hospital car on Canadian National System watch over welfare of pioneer families. *Canadian National Railways Magazine, 16,* 89, 33.

Sheehan, N. (1987). The Red Cross and relief in Alberta, 1920s–1930s. *Prairie Forum, 12*(2), 277–293.

Grenfell Mission

Bulgin, I. (2001). *Mapping the self in the utmost purple rim: Published Labrador memoirs of four Grenfell nurses.* Unpublished doctoral dissertation, Memorial University, St. John's.

Coombs, H. (2004). "I guess I should have been a suffragette!!!!": A profile of Lesley Diack, nurse with the Grenfell Mission, 1950–1988. *Newfoundland Quarterly, 97*(2), 28–32.

Diack, Lesley. (1963). *Labrador nurse.* London: Victor Gollancz Ltd.

Merrick, Elliott. (1942). *Northern nurse.* New York: Charles Scribner's Sons.

Perry, J. (1997). *Nursing for the Grenfell Mission: Maternal and moral reform in Northern Newfoundland and Labrador, 1894–1938.* Unpublished M.A. thesis, Memorial University, St. John's.

Victorian Order of Nurses for Canada

Bienvenue, L. (1998). Le Victorian Order of Nursing dans la croisade hygiéniste Montréalaise, 1897–1925. *Bulletin d'Histoire Politique, 6*(2), 64–73.

Boutilier, B. (1994). *Gender, organized women, and the politics of institution building: Founding the Victorian Order of Nurses for Canada, 1893–1900.* Unpublished doctoral dissertation, Carlton University, Ottawa.

MacDonald, C. (1997). From founding to frontier: The VON in the Klondike. *Beaver, 77*(5), 13–18.

Religious Groups

Duchaussois, P. (1919). *The Grey Nuns in the far North (1867–1919).* Toronto: McClelland & Stewart.

Mitchell, E. (c.1987). *The Grey Nuns of Montréal at the Red River, 1844–1984.* Sine Locum: Sine Nomen.

Paul, P. (1994). The contribution of the Grey Nuns to the development of nursing in Canada: Historiographical issues. *Canadian Bulletin of Medical History, 11*(1), 207–217.

About the Author

Marion McKay, RN, PhD, holds a bachelor's and master's degree in nursing and an MA and PhD in history. She is currently involved in two Social Sciences and Humanities Research Council (SSHRC) research projects, one exploring contemporary PHNs' experiences in working with families living in poverty, and the other exploring how nurses and their work contributed to changing notions of health, citizenship, and national belonging in Canada. Prior to joining the Faculty of Nursing at the University of Manitoba, she worked for several years as a public health nurse.

The author acknowledges with deep gratitude the assistance and advice of several valued colleagues and friends, including Meryn Stuart, Nicole Rousseau, Janet Beaton, Benita Cohen, and Sandra Gessler. Special thanks to Ulysses Lahaie, who translated several articles written in French and got hooked on nursing history in the process. Thank you also to the anonymous reviewers whose comments did much to improve previous drafts of this chapter. A SSHRC Doctoral Fellowship supported the research necessary for the preparation of this manuscript and is acknowledged with thanks.

Financing, Policy, and Politics of Health Care Delivery

CHAPTER

2

Adeline Falk-Rafael and Sue Coffey

OBJECTIVES

After studying this chapter, you should be able to:

1. Summarize milestones in the development of the Canadian health care system.
2. Identify federal, provincial, municipal, and regional responsibilities for the delivery of health care in Canada.
3. Examine delivery models and funding mechanisms for health care in Canada, specifically those that apply to community health care.
4. Critique current health care reform initiatives and their implications for community health nursing practice.

INTRODUCTION

> To many Canadians, the Canada Health Act provides for a health care system that helps to define this country. The Act symbolizes the values that represent Canada; it articulates a social contract that defines health care as a basic right and it describes the features of the health care system. (Auditor General of Canada, 2002, chap. 29, p. 13)

The Canadian health care system, **Medicare,** is a feature of Canadian culture that expresses its unique value system. Evolving from the traditions of the religious orders that first provided health care in Canada, Medicare reflects values of social justice, equity, and community. The fundamental principle that all members of our society, including the most vulnerable, are entitled to receive the health care they need contrasts sharply with the American system, which is grounded in the value of individuality and the belief that health care is a commodity to be sold to those who can afford it.

Yet there are increasing pressures to "Americanize" the Canadian health care system. Almost every day, reports in the media suggest that health care in Canada is in a crisis state, that spending is spinning out of control, and that drastic changes are needed to ensure its sustainability. A recent Supreme Court of Canada ruling (the Chaoulli decision) restricting Quebec's ability to ban private insurance for publicly insured services may, some fear, eventually affect other jurisdictions. Waiting times, at the heart of the Supreme Court decision, are of increasing concern to Canadians (Pollara Research, 2005; Rachlis, 2004). It is important for community health nurses (CHNs) to understand how our health care system evolved; how the funding, allocation, and delivery of community health services differ from medical and hospital care; and what factors are driving health care reform in this country.

BIRTH OF CANADIAN MEDICARE

Although the 1867 Constitution Act (also known as the British North America Act) did not explicitly assign responsibility for health policy to either the federal or provincial governments, historically both levels of government have been involved in ensuring the availability of health services and funding those services. Deber (2000) notes that because the Constitution assigned responsibility for hospitals exclusively to provinces, health care in Canada has been erroneously interpreted to fall under provincial jurisdiction. With only a few exceptions, such as the direct health services provided by the federal government to Aboriginal populations, veterans, and military personnel, provincial governments have assumed responsibility for the delivery of health care. However, funding for health care is another matter. The Canadian Constitution contains an equalization clause requiring provinces to provide "reasonably comparable levels of public service for reasonably comparable levels of taxation" (Sullivan & Baranek, 2002, p. 21). Because provincial and territorial wealth varies considerably, the federal government's involvement has been necessary to equalize services across provinces. Since 1957, the federal government has done that by contributing money (in effect, transferring money from wealthier to poorer provinces) and by stipulating specific conditions the provinces must meet in order to receive that money. Before further discussing the Canadian health care system, a review of key points in the evolution of the system is warranted.

In 1919, access to medical care was of sufficient concern that Mackenzie King, then leader of the Liberal party, convinced his party to include national health insurance as part of its platform (Rachlis & Kushner, 1994). Rachlis and Kushner note that, partly because of provincial objections to federal involvement in health care, attempts to implement national insurance for both hospital and physicians' services were initially unsuccessful. North America's first universal health insurance program was actually implemented at a provincial level. In Saskatchewan in 1947, Tommy Douglas and the Co-operative Commonwealth Federation (CCF) party introduced legislation to institute Medicare. For his role in bringing about this historic change, Tommy Douglas is still sometimes referred to as the father of Medicare. It was not until 1957 that similar legislation, the Hospital Insurance and Diagnostic Services Act (HIDS), was passed by the federal government (Rachlis & Kushner, 1994).

The HIDS provided financial incentives for the provinces to establish hospital insurance plans. It ensured that if provincial plans included five key principles, the federal government would pay half the costs. Those principles, still the legal cornerstones of Medicare, are **comprehensiveness**, **accessibility**, **universality of coverage**, **public administration**, and **portability of benefits**. The incentive provided powerful motivation for the provinces' participation and resulted in both the rapid expansion of cost-shared institutional care and the neglect of programs that focused on home care support and health promotion.

In 1962, Saskatchewan once again led the country with legislation providing universal, publicly funded medical insurance. In 1966, the federal government followed suit with the passage of the National Medical Care Insurance Act (Medicare). This Act, enshrining the right of Canadians to physicians' services, stipulated that the same five principles were necessary to ensure the federal government's payment of 50% of provincial health care costs. The Act was implemented in 1968, and by 1971 all provinces were fully participating (Rachlis & Kuschner, 1994).

The blanket 50/50 cost-sharing quickly placed a great strain on the federal budget and made fiscal planning increasingly difficult (Rafael, 1997). As a result, in 1977, the federal government passed the Established Programs Financing Act (EPF), which changed the federal share of health costs from a 50/50 split to per capita block grants. These grants were tied to economic performance through being linked to the gross national product (GNP) and consisted of both cash and tax points, which allowed the provincial governments a greater share of collected taxes (Rachlis & Kushner, 1994). This new cost-sharing arrangement was adjusted several times over the next 20 years, with each adjustment decreasing the federal contribution (Bégin, 1987). Both the Liberal and Conservative parties slashed cash contributions, clearly benefiting federal coffers. However, the changes might also have represented deliberate attempts to decrease federal involvement in health care. Former Minister of Health and Welfare the Honourable Monique Bégin reflected on the difficulties that the EPF created:

> The EPF legislation had not repealed the two pillars of Medicare: HIDS and the Medical Care Act. So their conditions and regulations...still applied, with one major drawback: the feds could no longer refuse to reimburse their half of the costs when it was felt there was a problem, for we [now had a transfer process]...with no enforcement mechanism. (Bégin, 2002, p. 2)

The Canada Health Act

Soon after the passage of the EPF, Bégin was appointed federal Minister of Health and Welfare (Bégin, 2002). She quickly became aware that extra-billing by physicians and user fees by provincial institutions were rising dramatically. Her analysis revealed a number of factors: (a) the popularity of neo-conservative economics, which generally promoted a reduced role for governments and a larger role for the private sector, (b) partisan politics with a liberal government at the federal level and conservative governments in 8 of 10 provinces, and (c) wage and price controls, which had included physicians' incomes. Bégin believed the extra-billing and user-fee trends posed a serious threat to Medicare and so on December 12, 1983, introduced to Parliament Bill C-3, the Canada Health Act.

Passage of the **Canada Health Act (CHA)** in April 1984 was a proud moment in Canadian nursing history. Bégin faced tough opposition to the Act from lobby groups, opposition parties, and even from members of the Liberal cabinet (Bégin, 2002). Intense lobbying and support by the Canadian Nurses Association (CNA) was instrumental in the bill's passage. In the words of Bégin: "Nursing became a big player during the Canada Health Act. They made the difference; it's as simple as that" (Rafael, 1997). Not only were nurses instrumental in passing the CHA into law, but they were also successful in amending it. As it was introduced into Parliament in 1983, Bill C-3 identified only physicians as providers of insurable services. The CNA amendment changed the language to include other health care workers as potential providers of insurable services (Mussallem, 1992). To date, no provincial legislation has been enacted to allow nurses to bill provincial health insurance plans directly.

The purpose of the CHA was to ban extra-billing and user fees by providing the federal government with the legal authority to penalize provinces that permitted such practices (Canada, House of Commons, 1984). Under the CHA, federal funding for essential medical services would continue as long as the provinces' health insurance plans met the criteria of being *publicly administered* (administered by a public authority accountable to the provincial government), comprehensive (must cover necessary in-hospital, medical, and surgical-dental services), universal (100% of residents must be covered), portable (available after a maximum of three months of residency and no extra charge for care out of province), and accessible (no user fees, and health care providers must be reimbursed adequately). These five principles of Medicare will be discussed more fully later in the chapter. The CHA represented a significant accomplishment in ensuring that Canadians' access to health care continued regardless of ability to pay or province of residence. It also perpetuated, however, the dominance of a biomedical approach to health care by identifying only essential medical and hospital services as those qualifying for federal cost-sharing.

The EPF continued to be the mechanism for transferring money from federal to provincial governments for health care until 1996. At that time, the EPF and the existing payment plan for welfare, the Canada Assistance Plan (CAP), were replaced by the Canada Health and Social Transfer (CHST) block fund, which included federal transfer payments for health, postsecondary education, and welfare (Sullivan &

Baranek, 2002). Allocations to provinces continued in the same proportion as the previous combined EPF and CAP entitlements (Canada, Department of Finance, 2002). However, the EPF funding formula had been severely cut by Prime Minister Mulroney's Conservative government between 1986 and 1991, reducing its growth to 3% less than the GNP growth (Rachlis & Kushner, 1994). As a result, the actual amount of the federal transfer in combined tax points and cash declined steadily until it reached a new low of $25.8 billion in 1997–1998—less than 50% of the CHST.

Changes since that time have improved the situation considerably. First, revisions to CHST funding for the years 1998–2003 included an increase to the CHST, a revision of the funding formula to account for provincial population growth rates, and adjustments to narrow funding disparities (Canada, Department of Finance, 2002). Second, in response to recommendations of the Commission on the Future of Health Care (Romanow, 2002a), the 2003 First Ministers' Accord separated out the health expenditures from the CHST in a new fund called the Canada Health Transfer (CHT) and identified an additional Health Reform Fund to address home care, primary care, and catastrophic drugs (Health Council of Canada, 2005a). Third, in their 2004 10-Year Plan to Strengthen Health Care, the first ministers allocated funding for additional specific priorities, such as wait times and selected home care services (Health Council of Canada, 2005a). As a result, the federal contribution to health care has risen significantly since its low point in 1998 (Marchildon, 2006).

Assessment of the Canada Health Act In assessing the degree to which the CHA was successful in ensuring that all Canadians have access to the health care they need, we need to look first at the express purpose of the Act. Second, it is important to examine the extent to which other aspects of health care have been implemented. Finally, the performance of the Canadian health care system should be compared with health care in other countries.

Express Purpose of the CHA Has the Canada Health Act accomplished what it set out to do, that is, "establish criteria and conditions in respect of insured health services and extended health care services provided under provincial law that must be met before a full cash contribution may be made" (Canada, House of Commons, 1984, Introduction)? Within the first three years of the CHA's passage (1984–1987), penalties amounting to $245 million had been levied against 7 of 10 provinces (Auditor General of Canada, 2002). When each of the penalized provinces abolished extra-billing and user fees, all penalties were reimbursed, as provided for in the Act. Thus, with respect to these issues, the CHA fulfilled its purpose. However, the issue of provincial/territorial non-compliance with the five criteria of the Act remains to be adequately addressed. The 1999 Auditor General's report chastised the federal government for not even collecting sufficient information to ensure compliance, noting that, "parliament cannot readily determine the extent to

which each province and territory has satisfied the criteria and conditions of the Canada Health Act" (Auditor General of Canada, 2002, p. 17). This criticism points out a shortcoming of the Canada Health Act that has been echoed in federal and provincial reports on health care since then—it lacks specific mechanisms to ensure accountability and transparency (Fooks & Lewis, 2002).

The intent of the CHA was to relate federal cash contributions not only to insured health services but also to extended health care services. The CHA defines the latter as "nursing home intermediate service, adult residential care service, home care services, and ambulatory health care services" (Canada, House of Commons, 1984, Section 2). However, funding for extended health care was not linked to compliance with the five principles of Medicare. As a result, provinces can decide what they want to spend. Sullivan and Baranek (2002) report a "threefold variation in public spending support across the provinces in extended health services like home care and pharmaceuticals" (p. 23). Thus, one would have to conclude that the CHA has not been effective with respect to the growing fields of home care and pharmaceuticals. Recognition of these limitations was evident in the final report of the Commission on the Future of Health Care and in the priorities set by the 2003 and 2004 first ministers' agreements on health reform.

A Broader Focus on Health In addition to its stated purpose, the Act also implicitly and explicitly suggests a broader purpose. For example, Section 3 of the Act strongly endorses health promotion, stating that the "primary objective of Canadian health care policy" is twofold: to facilitate reasonable access to health services and "to protect, promote and restore the physical and mental well-being of residents of Canada" (Canada, House of Commons, 1984, Section 3). Despite this, the Act limited its focus to medically necessary hospital and physicians' services (and dental services in hospitals). Protective, promotive, and preventive services were not required to meet the five criteria of Medicare and were not subject to the conditions of the Act. Thus these services, which were provided largely by provincial public health systems and which added a critical balance to the treatment-focused insured services addressed by the CHA, were left unprotected by federal legislation. As a result, the extent to which these services are offered may vary considerably from one province/territory to another, in violation of the very intent of the Act.

International Comparisons The two aspects of the Canadian health care system that can be compared with other countries are the level of health Canadians enjoy and the relative cost of their health care system. The Organisation for Economic Co-operation and Development (OECD) provides data that are helpful in making such international comparisons. Table 2.1 reports selected health outcomes by country for specific years. Canada's life expectancies for both women and men rank among the highest in the world. Although Canadian infant mortality rates have dropped significantly since 1990, the

TABLE 2.1
Comparisons of Health Outcomes by Country

	Infant Mortality Rate/1000		Life Expectancy at Birth—Females		Life Expectancy at Birth—Males	
	1990	2003	1990	2000	1990	2000
Australia	8.2	4.8	80.1	82	73.9	76.6
Canada	6.8	5.3	80.8	81.9	74.4	76.7
Germany	7.0	4.2	78.4	81	72	75
Japan	4.6	3.0	81.9	84.6	75.9	77.7
New Zealand	8.4	6.2*	78.3	81.1	72.4	76.3
Sweden	6.0	3.1	80.4	82	74.8	77.4
United Kingdom	7.9	5.3	78.5	80.2	72.9	75.4
United States	9.2	6.9	78.8	79.5	71.8	74.1

Source: OECD Health Data, 2006 (Organisation for Economic Co-operation & Development, 2006)

* 2002 figure—2003 not available

TABLE 2.2
Comparisons of Health Expenditures Data by Country

	Total Expenditures Per capita in US$ PPP***		Total Health Expenditures % of GDP		Public Expenditure % Total Health Expenditure	
	1970	2003	1970	2003	1970	2003
Australia	188	2876	4.5	9.2	57.2	67.5
Canada	299	2998	7.0	9.9	69.9	70.1
Germany	269**	3005	6.2**	10.9	72.8**	78.2
Japan	149	2249	4.5	8.0*	69.8	81.5*
New Zealand	211	1902	5.1	8.0	80.3	78.3
Sweden	312	2745	6.8	9.3	86.0	85.4
United Kingdom	163	2347	4.5	7.9	87.0	85.4
United States	352	5711	7.0	15.2	36.5	44.6

Source: OECD Health Data, 2006 (Organisation for Economic Co-operation & Development, 2006)

* Estimate
** Data refer to West Germany
*** PPP is adjustment for purchasing power parity

2003 rate of 5.3 deaths per 1000 live births is still higher than in a number of other developed countries.

When comparing health outcomes to expenditures, one message is very clear: increased spending on health care does not result in better health. In 2003, the United States spent more per capita on health care than any of the other 29 countries compared by the OECD. Health expenditures in the U.S. also represented the highest percentage of GDP. Yet American health outcomes rank among the lowest compared with other countries. Japan, on the other hand, spent less than half as much per capita on health as the U.S. yet ranks first on all three measures of health. Canada's per capita spending in 2003

was about 52% that of the U.S., and health care spending amounted to 9.9% of the GDP, compared with 15.2% in the U.S. However, on all three health outcomes, Canada fared substantially better than the United States. Perhaps this is related to the fact that the American health care industry relies to a larger extent on private funding than any of the other 29 countries compared. (See Table 2.2, last column.)

These and more comprehensive data analyses suggest that Canada's universal health coverage is less costly and more effective than the privatized health system of our U.S. neighbour (Alberta Association of Registered Nurses, Canadian Nurses Association, Ontario Nurses Association, Registered

Nurses Association of Ontario, & United Nurses of Alberta, 2000; Deber, 2000; Rachlis, Evans, Lewis, & Barer, 2001; Sullivan & Baranek, 2002). Recent research also provides some support for this conclusion. (See Canadian Research Box 2.1.) There is still room for improvement, however, as noted by the Commissioner on the Future of Health Care:

> First and foremost, I am convinced that the Medicare house needs remodelling but not demolishing. Medicare was, and continues to be, the right choice. But the mix of publicly available health services currently covered under Medicare needs to be adapted to today's medical realities and delivery systems. When we first started debating Medicare 40 years ago, "medically necessary" health care could be summed up in two words: hospitals and doctors. Today, hospital and physician services account for less than half of the total cost of the system. More money is spent on drugs than on physicians. There are more specialists and more care is delivered in homes, in communities, and through a wide array of health care providers. In short, the practice of health care has evolved. And despite efforts to keep pace, Medicare has not. (Romanow, 2002b, p. 2)

To address the need for "remodelling" of the Medicare house that had become so widely apparent, Canada's first ministers reached key agreements for health care renewal in 2003 and 2004. The creation of the Health Council of Canada was the result of the 2003 agreement. (See Canadian Research Box 2.2.)

THE FEDERAL ROLE IN HEALTH PROMOTION

When the legislative pillars of Canadian Medicare were enacted in 1957, 1966, and 1984, the biomedical model dominated public and political thinking about health. The clinical definition of health was the absence of disease, and the term "health promotion" was often used interchangeably with "disease prevention." Labelling the illness-centred, treatment-focused physicians' and hospital services that were insured under the Acts as "health care" attests and contributes to this confusion. As challenges to the idea that health was related exclusively to a country's health care emerged, the federal government provided some leadership in the development of health promotion policies and resources.

The first federal acknowledgement of the limitations of the primacy of the funded medical/treatment system in Canada was *The Lalonde Report* of 1974 (Lalonde, 1974). It explicitly presented a vision for health promotion services as a critical component of this country's health care system. The Report was influenced significantly by McKeown's 1958 British research (McKeown, 1979). McKeown asserted that improvements in sanitation, nutrition, and the ability to space pregnancies were much stronger determinants of health than

health care alone. The influence of his thinking is evident in the health framework proposed in the Lalonde Report, which identified four **determinants of health**: environment, lifestyle, human biology, and the health care system.

Despite its identification of environment as a determinant of health, the Lalonde Report is often linked primarily to an emphasis on lifestyle. Some have suggested that the report was less a critique of the dominance of a biomedical approach to health than an attempt to undermine Medicare. However, the Lalonde Report was revolutionary in its time, leading a global reconceptualization of health promotion.

Four years later, Canada and other countries around the world met at the International Conference on Primary Health Care in Alma Ata, USSR. They urged governments to take action to "protect and promote the health" of the people of the world by issuing the *Declaration of Alma Ata* (World Health Organization, 1978), to which Canada was a signatory.

In the years following Alma Ata, federal leadership in health promotion policy continued. In 1986, the federal Minister of Health at the time, the Honourable Jake Epp, published the document *Achieving Health for All: A Framework for Health Promotion* (Epp, 1986). The Epp Framework expanded Lalonde's definition of health promotion; incorporated some of the tenets of primary health care; and emphasized the role of broad social, environmental, and political determinants of health. The document concluded with a denouncement of strategies that focus on individual responsibility for health, or "blaming the victim," while ignoring the social and economic conditions that contribute to disease and disability.

The Epp Framework formed the basis for the Ottawa Charter for Health Promotion that emerged from the First International Conference on Health Promotion, hosted by the federal government in November 1986 (World Health Organization, Canadian Public Health Association, & Health and Welfare, 1986). The Charter, authored jointly by Health Canada, the Canadian Public Health Association (CPHA), and the World Health Organization (WHO), identified prerequisites for health, strategies for promoting health, and outcomes of those strategies. The Charter acknowledged that caring for oneself and others is conducive to health and identified caring, holism, and ecology as essential concepts in health promotion.

The federal government has continued to support health promotion through the development of resources. Its Health Promotion and Programs Branch, which later evolved into the Population and Public Health Branch, produced a number of resources, such as the *Population Health Template* (Health Canada, 2001) and the *Population Health Promotion Model* (Hamilton & Bhatti, 1996). However, despite providing documents that emphasize the barriers to health created by broad social, economic, and political factors, the federal government has been less progressive in introducing the policy changes necessary to redress these factors.

Canadian Research Box 2.1

Devereaux, P. J., Choi, P. T. L., Laccjetto, C., Weaver, B., Schunemann, H. J., Haines, T., et al. (2002). A systematic review and meta-analysis of studies comparing mortality rates of private for-profit and private not-for-profit hospitals. *Canadian Medical Association Journal, 166*(11), 1399–1406.

Devereaux, P. J., Schunemann, H. J., Ravindran, N., Bhandari, M., Garg, A. X., Choi, P. T. L., et al. (2002). Comparison of mortality between private for-profit and private not-for-profit hemodialysis centers: A systematic review and meta-analysis. *JAMA: The Journal of the American Medical Association, 288*(19), 2449–2457.

Devereaux, P. J., Heels-Ansdell, D., Lacchetti, C., Haines, T., Burns, K., Cook, D. J., et al. (2004). Payments for care at private for-profit and private not-for-profit hospitals: A systematic review and meta-analysis. *Canadian Medical Association Journal,170*(12), 1817–1824.

Until recently, the debate about private for-profit versus private not-for-profit health care delivery has been largely theoretical speculation. Researchers led by Dr. P. J. Devereaux of McMaster University have published three studies comparing costs and/or mortality rates in private for-profit agencies with those in private not-for-profit agencies (Devereaux, Choi et al., 2002; Devereaux, Schunemann et al., 2002; Devereaux et al., 2004).

The first study examined the relative effect of private for-profit versus private not-for-profit delivery of hospital care on patient mortality (Devereaux, Choi et al., 2002). Strict screening processes reduced the 8665 citations to 805 publications, which were evaluated against eligibility criteria. Thirteen publications reporting 15 studies met the criteria. Those studies, all in the U.S., involved more than 26 000 hospitals and 38 million patients between 1982 and 1995. The pooled analysis showed that private for-profit hospitals were associated with relative increase in risk of death of 2%.

A second study made a similar comparison of mortality in private for-profit and private not-for-profit hemodialysis centers (Devereaux, Schunemann et al., 2002). Again, a broad literature search identifying more than 7000 citations was narrowed to 7 publications, representing more than 500 000 patient-years of data, that met the eligibility criteria. The meta-analysis demonstrated an 8% increased risk of death in for-profit dialysis centres. The researchers calculated, based on the 208 000 Americans receiving in-centre hemodialysis each year, that approximately 2500 deaths could be avoided each year if all received care in a private not-for-profit centre.

The third study examined the relative costs of receiving care at private for-profit and private not-for-profit hospitals (Devereaux et al., 2004). From the more than 7000 citations, 8 studies fulfilled the eligibility criteria, involving more than 350 000 patients. The researchers' meta-analysis demonstrated that care in private for-profit hospitals was 19% more costly than that received at private not-for-profit hospitals. Based on the findings, the researchers calculated that if Canada were to convert half of its hospitals to private for-profit agencies, costs for hospital care would increase by $3.6 billion annually.

The studies by Devereaux et al. strongly refute the argument that a "profit motive optimizes care and minimizes cost" (Woolhandler & Himmelstein, 2004). Woolhandler and Himmelstein, two Harvard researchers, shed some light on why care in investor-owned facilities is so much higher. Incentives to increase profits, they argue, actually drive up costs. Fraudulent practices, high administrative costs, and exorbitant CEO salaries and benefits all contribute to higher costs while diverting money away from care. Investor ownership, they conclude, embodies a new value system that "views patients as commodities [and] marks the triumph of greed" (p. 1815).

Discussion Questions:

1. What do you expect would be the effect of investor ownership on nursing care; that is, how could money being diverted from care affect the ability of nurses to provide high-quality care?

2. The studies Devereaux et al. used involved U.S. institutions. To what extent do you think the same results would be found in Canada, if we moved to a parallel system for acute care services?

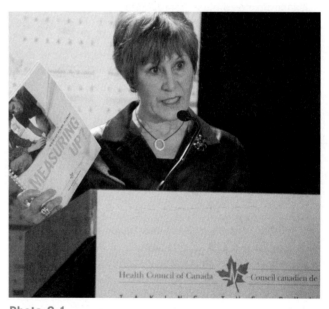

Photo 2.1

Canada's First Ministers established the Health Council of Canada in 2003 amid national recognition that health system renewal and significant investments were needed to improve the quality, accessibility and sustainability of our public health care system. Through insightful monitoring, public reporting, and facilitating informed discussion, the Council shines a light on what helps or hinders health care renewal. (See Canadian Research Box 2.2.) Pictured: Health Council Chair Jeanne Besner releases the Health Council's third annual report in February 2007.

Credit: Gary Beechey, BDS Studios

Canadian Research Box 2.2

Health Council of Canada. (2006a). *Health care renewal in Canada: Clearing the road to quality.* Retrieved October 22, 2006, from http://www.healthcouncilcanada.ca/en/index.php?option=com_content&task=view&id=70&Itemid=72.

Health Council of Canada. (2006b). *The Health Council at work: Shining a light on health care renewal.* Retrieved September 5, 2006, from http://healthcouncilcanada.ca/docs/rpts/2006/2006_Corporate_Annual_Report.pdf.

The creation of the Health Council of Canada sprang from recommendations of federal reports (Romanow, 2002b; Standing Senate Committee on Social Affairs, Science and Technology, 2002) on the status of the Canadian health care system. In response, the first ministers created the Health Council of Canada as part of the 2003 First Ministers' Accord on Health Care Renewal to monitor and report on renewal of the health care system and to ensure transparency and accountability (Health Council of Canada, 2006b). The next year, the 2004 First Ministers' Accord expanded those responsibilities to include reporting annually on health status and health outcomes.

The Health Council of Canada was created in December 2003 and consists of 26 councillors: 12 to represent their respective jurisdictional governments, and 14 non-government representatives. Those representatives bring a broad range of expertise in health care delivery, systems, and economics. Currently, the Chair of the Council is Dr. Jeanne Besner, a nurse from Alberta. The Council accomplishes its work through the work of the councillors and the support of a highly skilled secretariat.

The Health Council is funded by Health Canada and operates as a non-profit organization, reporting to the Canadian public (Health Council of Canada, 2006a). The Council has been involved in numerous consultations and has issued a number of publications, available on its website (www.healthcouncilcanada.ca). To date, two annual reports on progress made in the country toward the commitments to health care renewal made by the first ministers in 2003 and 2004 have been issued. The first (Health Council of Canada, 2005b), in January 2005, identified four areas for attention: health human resources; the health of First Nations, Métis, and Inuit peoples; primary health care reform; and the modernization of health records to electronic formats. In addition to the report on progress on key elements of the first ministers' agreements, the second report (Health Council of Canada, 2006a) acknowledges that despite large investments the four areas for attention identified in the 2005 report remain challenges. To address them, it identifies three pathways:

■ **Improve access to health care.** Five areas for action are identified in this pathway. They include efforts to improve primary health care through faster implementation of interdisciplinary teams and increased use of telehealth technologies; to address health human resource issues by ensuring adequate numbers of health care workers are adequately prepared and are able to work to the full potential of their respective scopes of practice; to expand the range of publicly funded home care services and broaden the compassionate care benefits program; to manage pharmaceuticals through standardizing public coverage for prescription medications and banning direct-to-consumer advertising of prescription drugs; and to improve wait list management.

■ **Improve the quality of care.** Specific areas for attention are strengthening patient safety; accelerating development and use of linked electronic records; increasing quality improvement training and high-quality reporting of patient outcomes; and increasing transparency of reporting on the health of Canadians and the performance of the health care system.

■ **Improve population health.** Three aspects of population health are identified: improving chronic disease prevention and management; providing funding to attain Canada's public health goals with appropriate measurement of progress; and reducing health inequalities.

The 2006 report emphasizes that access to health care is not enough—quality of services, sufficient attention to prevention, and reduction of health inequities must also be addressed. It concludes that the identified pathways require sustained, coordinated, and accountable effort.

Discussion Questions:

1. Discuss the five areas for action the Health Council identified to improve access to health care. What would be your highest priority and why?

2. Discuss which action areas in the Health Council's three pathways you think would most improve the health of communities. Provide rationale to support your decision.

CANADIAN HEALTH CARE: FUNDING, ALLOCATION, AND DELIVERY

Health care services in Canada, including community services, are provided through an array of programs with vastly different philosophies, funding mechanisms, and goals. Hospital and physicians' services are largely publicly financed. Public-sector revenue (taxes collected by federal, provincial, and municipal governments) accounts for approximately 70% of the money spent on health care, with out-of-pocket expenses or private health-insurance claims accounting for the remainder. (See Table 2.3.) The proportion of services paid for through public funding has shifted substantially since the inception of Medicare. In 1960, prior to Medicare, fewer than half of health services were publicly funded. Public funding for health services reached its peak in the mid-1970s and stayed stable at just over 75% for the next decade. Since the mid-1980s, the portion of publicly funded services has steadily declined.

TABLE 2.3
Percentage of Canadian Health Care Costs Publicly and Privately Funded Health Since Inception of Medicare

Year	% Publicly Funded	% Privately Funded
1960	42.6	57.4
1970	69.9	30.1
1980	75.6	24.4
1995	71.4	28.6
2000	70.3	29.7
2004*	69.8	30.2

Source: OECD Health Data, 2006 (Organisation for Economic Co-operation & Development, 2006)

*Estimate

The actual distribution of funds is also an important consideration. Table 2.4 reflects the emphasis on funding essential medical and hospital services stipulated in the CHA. Table 2.4 shows that although hospital and institutional funding have decreased somewhat, comparable increases in home care funding, for example, are not evident. Although they have quadrupled since 1992 (Sullivan & Baranek, 2002), home care expenditures remain somewhat invisible in the Canadian Institute for Health Information (CIHI) statistics. Public health expenditures, contrary to the emphasis on health promotion in federal policy statements, remain a minute portion of total health spending. Although selected home health services were agreed to in the 2004 first ministers' health accord, they are far from a national home care program (Rachlis, 2004).

In order to understand and evaluate the effectiveness of the various means of providing community health services, it is critical to use an appropriately broad framework. Deber (2000) proposes three key elements—financing, delivery, and allocation—for such a framework. For the purposes of this chapter, these three central components are defined in the following way:

1. *Financing* refers to the methods by which money is collected by governments, insurers, and providers (e.g., taxes, premiums) as well as to the decisions about the extent of coverage (e.g., what kinds of services are covered and who receives that coverage).

2. *Delivery* refers to the way in which health care services are organized and the mechanisms by which they are provided.

3. *Allocation* refers to the links created between financing and delivery. Decisions about how providers are reimbursed and the incentives inherent in the way providers are paid are considered when one examines allocation of services.

Application of this model to the case of acute care hospitals sheds light on these interrelated components. *Financing* is derived largely from public funds (Deber, 2000). Provincial/territorial governments then determine funding formulae to *allocate* this money to boards of directors of the hospitals. In those jurisdictions in which regionalization has occurred, monies flow to regional governments to be allocated to hospital boards.

Deber (2000) points out that hospital care is primarily privately *delivered* in Canada. Although Canadian hospitals are frequently referred to as "public hospitals," they are run by private boards and their employees are not government workers. To be consistent with the meaning of "public funding," the term public hospital should be reserved for those institutions that are administered and staffed by employees of various levels of government, such as many psychiatric hospitals. Such is the case in countries in which the health system is socialized, for example, the U.K. and Scandinavia, in which health care providers are government employees (Deber).

TABLE 2.4
Selected Health Expenditures by Use of Funds Over Time (current dollars; % total health expenditures)

	Hospitals	Other Institutions	Other*	Physicians	Other Professionals**	Drugs	Public Health	Admin.
1975	44.7 %	9.2%	1.9%	15.1%	9.0%	8.8%	3.3%	2.8%
1985	40.8	10.3	2.5	15.2	10.4	9.5	3.8	2.4
1995	34.4	9.7	4.5	14.4	11.5	13.6	4.5	3.3
2000	31.1	9.5	4.7	13.2	11.8	15.4	5.3	3.4
2004	30.3	9.4	4.2	13.1	11.2	16.6	5.5	4.0

Source: Based on data from the Canadian Institute for Health Information (2006). National health expenditure trends, 1975–2006. Retrieved May 15, 2007, from http://secure.cihi.ca/cihiweb/dispPage.jsp?cw_page=AR_31_E.

* Home care, medical transportation services, medical appliances and others
** Dental care, vision care, and others

Clarity about these three aspects of health care is important in understanding current health-care-reform initiatives. Some changes referred to as "privatization" are rather a shift from **not-for-profit** private delivery to **for-profit** private delivery (Deber). The distinction will become more fully apparent as Deber's framework is used to analyze public health, primary care, and home care services in Canada.

HEALTH CARE IN THE COMMUNITY

This section will examine the financing, allocation, and delivery of three community health services: primary care/primary health care, public health, and home care or home health nursing. A number of models used in different areas of the country will be highlighted.

Primary Care/Primary Health Care

The terms primary care and primary health care are often erroneously used interchangeably. The definition of primary health care in the *Declaration of Alma Ata* can be summarized as accessible, acceptable, affordable health care (World Health Organization, 1978). Other specific tenets of primary health care identified in the charter include its basis in research; its breadth, encompassing the full spectrum of services from promotive to rehabilitative; the identification of health education, proper nutrition, disease prevention and control, and maternal and child health care as minimum services; the recognition that intersectoral and interdisciplinary approaches are necessary for success; and an emphasis on community participation and empowerment.

Primary care, on the other hand, refers simply to the services that a person commonly accesses at the first point of contact with the health care system. In many "developed" countries, primary care services have been dominated by medicine and thus have focused mainly on acute care and treatment of disease. While the largest group of primary care providers in Canada continues to be physicians, other providers include nurse practitioners, dentists, chiropractors, pharmacists, dietitians, midwives, optometrists, and, to some extent, public health nurses. The medicalized focus of primary care is reflected in our current funding mechanisms that overtly favour physicians as privileged health care providers. Most Canadians access primary care in the community in physicians' offices, commonly through a family or general practitioner (GP), who is most often reimbursed on a fee-for-service basis (Marchildon, 2006; Rachlis, 2004). A small portion of the Canadian population receives primary care services through community health centres, walk-in clinics, or emergency rooms (Shah, 1998).

Legislation As noted previously, the effect of legislation has been to limit the influence of the federal government, define services in terms of physician and hospital care, and maintain physicians at the centre of the decision-making system (Hutchison, Abelson, & Lavis, 2001; Tuohey, 2002).

Financing Both the funding and focus of primary care services are directly related to the provisions of the CHA. Because essential medical services are the only primary care services identified as eligible for federal/provincial cost-sharing, physicians have enjoyed a monopoly in the provision of such services, severely disadvantaging other primary care providers and the public.

Physicians' fees account for 13.1% of total health care costs. (See Table 2.4.) The most expensive form of remuneration for physicians' services is fee-for-service (FFS), yet an average of 83% of physician remuneration in Canada is FFS (Marchildon, 2006). Increasing criticism for this traditional and costly model of primary care has led to significant innovations over the past quarter century, with alternative models of payment using some combination of salary, capitation, and FFS being used in varying degrees in each province. However, substantial differences exist among provinces: Alberta's FFS reimbursement of physicians is the highest in the country at 91%, while FFS reimbursement in Newfoundland and Labrador is only 63%, the lowest in Canada (Marchildon, 2006).

Delivery Like hospitals, primary care services in Canada are largely publicly funded and privately delivered. It is widely recognized that the most cost-effective and comprehensive models of primary care delivery involve the provision of services by salaried, multidisciplinary teams (Rachlis, 2004). Although admitting to widespread resistance to such models by physicians, Rachlis describes exemplars of multidisciplinary team practices in a number of provinces. Among these are the networks of Centres Locaux de Services Communautaires (CLSCs) in Quebec and Community Health Centres in Ontario.

The emphasis on primary health care in many of the reports on the health system in recent years, combined with an influx of federal money dedicated to primary health care reform, has begun to create shifts with the potential to change primary care delivery significantly (Marchildon, 2006). Among those shifts are the move toward replacing FFS remuneration of physicians with alternative payment structures and the expansion of telehealth services, particularly in rural and remote areas of the country. Another development is the enactment of legislation in many provinces to enable nurse practitioners to deliver primary care services. However, it should be noted that to date no province has established associated funding mechanisms for their reimbursement. This has resulted in the slow growth and severe underutilization of nurse practitioners. The Canadian Nurse Practitioner Initiative (CNPI), funded by Health Canada through the Primary Health Care Transition Fund, has developed recommendations with the goal of sustained integration of nurse practitioners in the Canadian health care system (CNPI, 2006).

Allocation Allocation of funds and resources (the decisions that tie funding to delivery) is based on many factors, which may include availability of resources (e.g., ratio of health care professionals to the population), characteristics of the community that affect the need for service (e.g., age distribution), personal factors that affect the need for service (e.g., education, income), and characteristics of the health care system (e.g., points of entry, accessibility of resources, cost, and barriers to care) (Shah, 1998). At the present time, allocation decisions are generally provincial responsibilities and are carried out by regional authorities (Marchildon, 2006), who forward them to providers. Among the exceptions to the devolution of funding from the province to regional health authorities are remuneration of physicians and payment for prescription drugs; all provinces maintain control over allocation of those costs (Marchildon, 2006). Examples of types of regional authorities include health regions (BC, NS, PEI, NB), regional health authorities (MB, AB, NL) and local health integration networks (ON), regional health and social service authorities (NWT), and agences de santé et des services sociaux (PQ).

As noted, physicians' fees account for 13.1% of total health costs, and the overwhelming majority of physicians earn almost all of their income this way. Hutchison et al. (2001) noted that "for the 89% of Canadian family physicians/GPs who receive some FFS income, FFS payments account for an average of 88% of their total income" (p. 117). Increasing criticism for this traditional and costly model of primary care has led to significant innovations over the past quarter century.

Public Health

Whereas hospital and physicians' services have been governed by federal legislation for at least the last half of the twentieth century, public health was decentralized at the outset so that sole responsibility for public health rested with the provinces (Ostry, 1995). Yet the same principles of comprehensiveness, universality, portability, public administration, and accessibility characterized Canadian public health services until the late twentieth century. Public health augmented Medicare by ensuring that health promotion and protection services were among the affordable, acceptable, essential health services that were "universally accessible to individuals and families in the community" (World Health Organization, 1978). Together, Canada's public health services and national health care system provided health services that were consistent with the tenets of primary health care.

Over the past decade, however, the public health infrastructure in Canada has been severely eroded. In 1996, the Canadian Public Health Association (CPHA) warned of the erosion by noting that in some jurisdictions "Public Health units and specific categories of workers (e.g., Public Health nurses) are disappearing" (CPHA, 1996, pp. 1–12). Further warnings were issued by Justice Horace Kreever's report in 1997 and the auditor general's report in 1999 (Canadian Medical Association [CMA], 2002). However, all admonitions seemed to fall on deaf ears, and the deepening crisis recently prompted editors of the *Canadian Medical Association Journal* to devote an entire issue to exposing a Canadian public health system "on the ropes" (CMA, 2002). Sullivan (2002) reported the key findings of a report of the Federal, Provincial, and Territorial Advisory Committee on Population Health that identified severe problems in public health in Canada, such as disparities among provinces and regions, severely inadequate and decreasing funding, critical human resource problems, and the development of public health policies without consideration of relevant data. There was a consensus that the water contamination in Walkerton, Ontario, in 2000 was a wake-up call for Canadian public health, occurring because "institutions vital to the infrastructure of public health were neglected" (Schabas, 2002, p. 1282).

Less than a year after that warning, a new public health crisis in the form of the SARS outbreak in Toronto again pointed to the inadequacy of Canada's public health infrastructure to protect the public's health. In May 2003 the federal government commissioned The National Advisory Committee on SARS and Public Health to assess "current public health efforts and lessons learned for ongoing and future infectious disease control" (National Advisory Committee on SARS and Public Health, 2003). The investigation and resultant report (often referred to as the Naylor Report) resulted in significant actions focused on strengthening the emergency preparedness of Canada through its public health infrastructure. A key recommendation was the creation of the Public Health Agency of Canada (PHAC). PHAC's two main pillars in Winnipeg and Ottawa are connected to a network of specialized centres across the country; the agency has responsibility for infectious diseases, emergency preparedness, and chronic diseases. At the same time, the government established six collaborating centres across the country, each with a specific focus ranging from determinants of health in Atlantic Canada to environmental health in British Columbia (Health Canada, 2004).

Legislation The PHAC was created by an Order in Council in September 2004 (Health Canada, 2006b). Bill C-5, the Public Health Agency of Canada Act, underwent third reading in the House of Commons in June 2006 and is currently before the Senate. The bill provides the legislative authority for the PHAC and transfers the supervision of the Population and Public Health Branch of Health Canada to the PHAC (Library of Parliament, 2006). Although the PHAC has the mandate to coordinate six functions of public health (population health assessment, health promotion, health protection, disease and injury control and prevention, surveillance, and emergency preparedness and response) (Marchildon, 2006), public health is primarily a jurisdictional responsibility outlined by legislation at the provincial/territorial level. Each province/territory has one primary piece of legislation that governs public health functions (CPHA, 1997). However, often other provincial/territorial acts may include aspects of public health function (e.g., environmental or occupational health).

In addition to Bill C-5, the federal Quarantine Act was revised in 2005, also in response to outbreaks of SARS, West Nile virus, and avian influenza (Public Health Agency of Canada, 2004). This update expands the federal government's power to screen, examine, and detain people, goods, and carriers that are arriving in or departing from Canada and that pose a health risk to Canadians or people elsewhere in the world.

Financing In the past few years, federal funding for public health has increased somewhat. In addition to transferring $400 million from Health Canada to the PHAC, the federal government committed $650 million over three years to national public health functions (Canadian Coalition for Public Health in the 21st Century, 2005). However, funding to support and enhance the large majority of public health work, which is carried out at the jurisdictional level, is funded as part of the overall provincial and/or municipal health budgets. None of the existing or new transfer payments committed to in the 2004 first ministers' 10-year plan are designated specifically for public health (Canadian Coalition for Public Health in the 21st Century, 2005). Table 2.4 shows that the percentage of health expenditures for public health has increased somewhat over the past 30 years, but it remains a very small amount of total health care expenditures. A survey conducted by the Canadian Public Health Association in 1997 identified significant differences in funding among provinces and territories (CPHA, 2000). That is unlikely to have changed; despite the progress that has been made, Canada still does not have a national public health program, and provinces are free to make changes in funding and allocation mechanisms that can deepen disparities among and within provinces.

Delivery Not surprisingly, therefore, the delivery of public health services also varies considerably across the country (CPHA, 1997). Public health in Canada is delivered largely by municipal, regional, or provincial employees, including a wide variety of public health professionals, such as public health nurses, public health inspectors, nutritionists, dentists and dental hygienists, and health promoters. However, in the decline of the public health infrastructure that occurred in the 1990s, some services were contracted out to private companies (e.g., water testing), while the elimination of others created a market for private delivery of services that once were publicly available (e.g., school nursing services).

In the post-SARS era and the context of public health renewal, attention was focused on the need to build the capacity of the public health workforce (National Advisory Committee on SARS and Public Health, 2003). The development of core competencies, common to all public health professionals, was undertaken for that purpose and led by the PHAC (PHAC, 2006). Some disciplines have also undertaken to develop competencies specific to their discipline in order to augment the common core competencies. For example, the Community Health Nurses Association of Canada (CHNAC) had developed national standards of practice (CHNAC, 2003) before the SARS outbreak and the Naylor Report's recommendation to do so (National Advisory Committee on SARS and Public Health, 2003). The standards formed the basis for designating community health nursing (including both public health and home health nursing) as a practice specialty by the Canadian Nurses Association. The standards also provided a framework from which core community nursing competencies were identified and that formed the basis for a certification exam, written for the first time in 2006.

Allocation Allocation of funds for public health services depends in large part on provincial governance and delivery structures. Funds may be generated by provincial taxes and distributed to regions and municipalities through funding formulas. In such shared funding arrangements, there may be dual approval mechanisms at the provincial and regional/municipal level for allocation of funds. On the other hand,

regional governments may have the complete authority to allocate funding. In those cases, public heath services often compete for funds with other health services such as acute care.

Home Care/Home Health Nursing

Home care generally refers to a range of services provided by health professionals (e.g., nurses, physiotherapists), homemaking or personal support services, and/or social services (Sullivan & Baranek, 2002). Home care services generally fall into three categories: supportive home care, focused on supporting clients with chronic illnesses to remain at home; long-term home care, which provides an alternative for residential or long-term care institutionalization; and post-acute hospitalization (Le Goff, 2002). Some provinces also provide palliative care services or services to specialized populations, such as pediatric home care (Health Canada, 2006a).

The use of home care services has been growing exponentially in Canada since 1980, increasing at an average annual rate of 11.3% (Le Goff, 2002). The Goff Report prepared for the Government of Canada, however, notes that estimates of home care expenditures may not be completely accurate since they are compiled by various agencies by using different methods and, as shown in Table 2.4, are combined with other services in the breakdown of "other" health expenditures (Health Canada, 2006a). The increase in expenditures is not surprising given the increased emphasis on early discharge and decrease in hospital expenditures that occurred over the same time period. Other societal factors may also have contributed to the increased demand for home care services.

Legislation Despite the focus in federal reports on improving and standardizing home care services, and despite the priority given to home care in the 2004 first ministers' 10-year plan for health care renewal (Health Council of Canada, 2005a), Canada still does not have a national home care plan, and so differences in funding, access, and delivery of home care services exist across jurisdictions (Rachlis, 2004). Currently, nine provinces have legislation that addresses the financing and provision of home care services at provincial and regional levels, although other provinces and territories have Orders in Council or guidelines that govern the delivery of home care services (Canadian Home Care Association, 2006). To complicate matters further, professional services may be governed by different legislation or regulations than are homemaker services (Health Canada, 2006a).

Financing Financing of home care is the responsibility of provincial/territorial governments, with few exceptions. (Home care for veterans and First Nations peoples is funded and delivered by the federal government.) However, significant differences exist among provinces and territories with respect to the percentage of total health budget designated for home care—from less than 2% in Yukon to more than 5% in Manitoba, Ontario, New Brunswick, Nova Scotia, and Newfoundland and Labrador (Health Canada, 2006a). Other differences among provinces and territories are eligibility for services criteria, extent of services provided, and use of co-payments (Le Goff, 2002). Because of these differences, the proportion of privately funded home care varies considerably from an average of 22% of total health expenditures across provinces and territories (Le Goff, 2002). This is of particular concern because home care services have replaced at least some health services that were previously provided in hospitals and 100% publicly funded. Shifting funding for such services from public to personal responsibility reduces access for those who are unable to pay for private insurance or out-of-pocket expenses and thus creates a two-tier system for home care within provinces and territories. Differences in the proportion of privately funded home care services across provinces and territories create further inequities among provinces and territories.

Delivery Most provinces and territories have delegated responsibility for service delivery decisions to regional or local health authorities, while still maintaining control over policy guidelines, standards for regional service delivery, reporting requirements, and monitoring outcomes. Services are delivered using four basic frameworks (Health Canada, 2006a). The models, summarized in Table 2.5, all utilize a single-point-of-entry system. Jurisdictions differ in the degree to which contracting out services to private agencies (both not-for-profit and for-profit) occurs. In recent years there has been an increase in the prevalence of private for-profit home care services (Marchildon, 2006).

Allocation Home care funding is devolved in most provinces and territories to regional health authorities. In 2005, Ontario introduced regionalization through its 14 Local Health Integration Networks (LHINs), while Prince Edward Island eliminated its regional authorities (Marchildon, 2006). A recent trend for using a population needs–based funding model is an attempt to make the allocation of home care funds more equitable.

Within their total budget, each region/province and territories must decide how much is allocated to home care versus acute care and other health services, how much is set aside for support services, and which programs receive support. Funding for home care is then provided to single-point-of-

entry home care organizations that streamline referrals and deliver home care services. Case managers are then required to make further funding decisions at the individual level.

HEALTH CARE REFORM IN CANADA

Marchildon (2006) identifies two phases of Canadian health reforms. The first phase, 1988–1996, was characterized by cost-cutting. Hospital beds were closed, services were rationalized through regionalization, many nurses lost their positions, and provincial governments and educational institutions actively strove to decrease the number of nurses, contributing to the current shortage. In contrast, physicians experienced zero growth, due as much to an additional year of practitioner training as to a freeze on their fee schedules (Marchildon, 2006).

The second phase of health reform in Canada extends from 1997 to the present time (Marchildon, 2006). It has been marked by a concern for fiscal sustainability of the health care system and characterized by numerous provincial (e.g., Fyke, Mazankowski) and national (e.g., Romanow, Kirby, Naylor) reports directed toward sustaining and improving Canadian health care. Specific concerns have centred on wait times; specific services, such as home care, First Nations health care, and catastrophic drug insurance; and an adequate supply of health human resources.

Canada's health care system clearly has some problems. Such issues as the skewed distribution of funding toward acute care and curative services, the dominance of a biomedical approach in insured services, and increasing inequities in uninsured services warrant substantial changes to create the equitable, accessible, integrated health care system that was envisioned when Medicare was initially conceived.

Increasing concerns about waiting lists were crystallized in the 2005 Supreme Court of Canada decision on what has become known as the "Chaoulli" case. Chaoulli is a Quebec physician who complained that Quebec's ban on private insurance for publicly insured services resulted in unacceptable wait times and violated Quebec's Charter of Rights and Freedoms (McIntosh, 2006; Shaw, 2005). The decision, although

---

TABLE 2.5
Models of Home Care Delivery Across Provinces

Professional Services	Home Support Services	Provinces and Territories Using the Model in 1999*
Provided by public employees	Provided by public employees	Saskatchewan, Quebec, Prince Edward Island, Yukon, Northwest Territories
Provided by public employees	Contracted out	New Brunswick, Newfoundland and Labrador, British Columbia, Alberta
Some provided by public employees; some contracted out	Contracted out	Nova Scotia, Manitoba
Contracted out	Contracted out	Ontario

Source: Adapted from a report by Mireille Dumon-Lemasson, Carol Donovan, Maggie Wyle with the assistance of the Federal-Provincial-Territorial Advisory Committee on Health Services Working Group on Continuing Care, June 1999.

* The most recent data available, from Health Canada, 2006a

specific to Quebec, has raised concern that it is a "Trojan Horse" decision that will create an opportunity for multinational insurance companies and health care providers to gain entry to the Canadian health care "market" through the provisions of international trade agreements (Sinclair, 2005).

It is important to understand that not all pressure for health care reform is simply a desire for a better system. The Canadian health care system's values of social justice, equity, and community are incompatible with others such as individualism and market economics. Privatization of Canadian health care offers a substantial opportunity to for-profit providers. In one analysis, if the private portion of health care rose only 20%, an additional $16 billion per year would be available to health care businesses (Registered Nurses' Association of Ontario, 1999). Such a potentially lucrative market is attractive to the large for-profit health care corporations that monopolize the American health care industry. As globalization trends continue, threats that international trade agreements may be able to compromise Canadian sovereignty in determining the structure and scope of its own health care system need to be taken seriously (Barlow, 2002).

The value conflict between those who favour a sustainable, universally accessible health care system and those who favour privatization and a market-driven health care system are summed up in the words of an American cardiologist. Speaking of the decline of American health care, he describes a situation familiar to current Canadian health care debates:

> Like most social transformations, there were ample warnings of an impending crisis. It was not precipitated by an invasion of barbarians scaling down the ramparts of an ethical profession. Rather, it began when doctors were seduced by financial incentives, with unquestioning third-party payers providing an open till.... For-profit health care is an oxymoron. The moment care is rendered for-profit, it is emptied of genuine caring. This moral contradiction is beyond repair. It entails abandoning values acquired over centuries of professionalizing health care into a humanitarian service. (Lown, 1999)

Common Arguments against Continuance of a Publicly Funded, Not-for-Profit Delivered Health System

A common argument for change in health care is the increased demand expected because of the greying of Canadians. This argument does not stand up in the face of empirical Canadian and international research, which demonstrates that aging, per se, has accounted for little increase in health care expenditures in the past (Barer, Evans, Hertzman, & Johri, 1998). Barer et al. suggest that the myth that an aging population will escalate spending makes intuitive sense, but changing medical practices with relation to elders has more bearing on health care costs than aging. They are supported by recent research conducted in Manitoba that suggests it is healthy seniors, rather than sick ones, who are responsible for significant increases in health care use (Canadian Health Services Research Foundation [CHSRF], 2001a).

Another frequently advanced argument is that user fees will make the health care system more efficient by eliminating abuse of the system. However, most health care spending is beyond patients' control and requires the order of a physician (CHSRF, 2001b). In analyzing the results of the Rand Health Insurance Study in the U.S., the CHSRF reported that medical services declined for everyone, but more so among poor people. They noted that "sick people were more likely to die when user charges were installed." The CHSRF pamphlet also reports Saskatchewan's experience with user fees between 1968 and 1975 in which similar barriers to care occurred, and the province's overall health care costs did not decrease! Barer et al. (1998) point out that unlike taxation, which draws contributions most heavily from people with the highest income, user fees take a larger share from those with the lowest incomes.

The third commonly advanced argument is for a parallel health system in which those who could afford to pay would have the "choice" to pay out-of-pocket and jump waiting lists. This argument was the essence of the Chaoulli decision. Such a parallel system, the argument goes, would relieve pressure on the public health care system. Like most arguments, this one has an intuitive appeal but others counter this argument by noting not only that the measurement of waiting lists has been inaccurate and their management poor (CHSRF, 2002b) but also that numerous exemplars of successful wait list management approaches exist in Canada (Rachlis, 2004). Moreover, after examining parallel systems already in place, CHSRF researchers concluded that rather than shortening waiting lists, a secondary system actually increases waiting times because practitioners working in the private system are no longer available in the public one. Thus, the increased "choice" a private system affords is a luxury available only for those with higher income levels.

Another myth to advance the argument for privatization is that it would lead to more efficiency. Again, experiences in the U.S. and in Alberta suggest otherwise. According to a CHSRF analysis, cataract surgeries in Calgary, which now are all purchased from private companies, are more expensive and create longer waiting lines that those in neighbouring cities (CHSRF, 2002a). As noted in Canadian Research Box 2.1, studies of not-for-profit and for-profit institutions in the U.S. suggest that the quality of care is better when the profit motive is not at cross-purposes with care.

The debate about privatization is not about private delivery, since most health care in Canada is already privately provided (Alberta Association of Registered Nurses et al., 2000; Deber, 2000). However, as Evans, Barer, Lewis, Rachlis, & Stoddart (2000) observe, the concern is about for-profit delivery. Most hospitals are run by private boards. Most physicians, dentists, and other health care entrepreneurs are, in fact, private businesses. And some long-standing home nursing associations, such as St. Elizabeth Health Care, are private, for-profit agencies. The concern is that in investor-owned health care insurance and delivery organizations responsibilities to shareholders for profit margins supersede those to patients, and that clinical decisions move away from the provider–patient partnership and rest instead with business administrators. It is in protecting profit margins that "cherry-picking" (that is, restricting eligibility for insurance to those

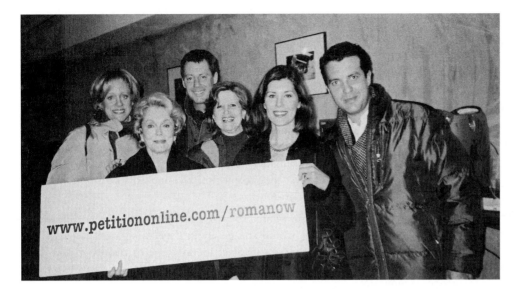

Photo 2.2

RNAO executive director Doris Grinspun (centre) joins Canadian celebrities in giving health care a helping hand. From left, Fiona Reid, Shirley Douglas, Dan Lett, Doris Grinspun, Sonja Smits, and Rick Mercer. The actors took to the virtual stage at a Toronto internet café, joining tens of thousands of other Canadians who have signed an online petition urging the federal and provincial governments to quickly implement the full Romanow Report.

Credit: Registered Nurses' Association of Ontario

who are at lowest risk) becomes problematic. Expensive redundancies enter the equation when services are increased to avoid waiting lines. And increased competition adds duplication and increased administrative expenses to overall costs.

One recent trend that occurred during these periods of reform in Canada and elsewhere was the use of public–private partnerships (3Ps) to construct and operate hospitals. In such a model, the government contracts a private agency to build and operate the hospital. McKee, Edwards, & Atun (2006) undertook a review of such partnerships for the World Health Organization and concluded that although 3P models are more likely to get hospitals built on time and within budget, they do so at the expense of quality and, in the long run, are more likely to cost taxpayers more.

Case Study: Establishing a Nursing Centre

Primary health care has been slow to be realized in Canada. The Comox Valley Nursing Centre is an example of an innovative approach to health care that has successfully met a community's needs.

In the early 1990s, the Registered Nurses' Association of British Columbia secured funding from the provincial government to establish the Comox Valley Nursing Centre as a 16-month primary health care project that would demonstrate the "breadth of nursing practice when constraints were removed" (Attridge , Budgen, Hilton, McDavid, Molzahn, & Purkis, 1997, p. 34).

The next step was to establish a steering committee, consisting of nurses and a community representative. Planning was centred on achieving the following goals (Attridge et al., 1997):

- increasing coordination and integration of health services,
- providing essential health care,
- increasing client self-reliance and participation in health care,
- addressing social determinants of health, and
- providing health care that gave good fiscal and clinical outcomes.

A few months later, a Community Advisory Committee (CAC) was established to represent more voices from the community, and the steering committee was replaced by a Nursing Practice Council (NPC). The Centre opened approximately eight months after receipt of the funding.

One full-time coordinator and four part-time nurses, along with 31 volunteers, provided a range of health promotion services to the community (Attridge et al., 1997). Over the 16-month demonstration project period, 437 individuals visited the centre with a wide range of health issues, including acute or chronic physical complaints; psychological, spiritual, or social concerns; and/or a need for health counselling, health assessment, or health networking. Support groups, advocacy groups, and therapeutic groups, such as a group of compulsive over-eaters, were formed (Attridge et al., 1997). In addition, the nursing staff were involved with more than 30 community outreach projects, such as foot-health groups for seniors, health promotion sessions at shopping malls, and asthma information sessions.

The impact of the nursing centre was evaluated by researchers at the University of Victoria. Written questionnaires indicated that the clients' average satisfaction rating was 33.9 in a possible range of 9–36. Interviews likewise revealed very positive client experiences. Clients valued being respected, not rushed, and obtaining better information than they had in previous encounters with the health system. Eighty-nine percent reported positive physical health changes that could be attributed to visiting the nursing centre; none reported any negative physical changes (Attridge et al., 1997). Cost-effectiveness was difficult to demonstrate because of the lack of comparable services.

Clarke and Mass (1998) analyzed the project's evaluation reports and examined how collaboration and empowerment manifested themselves in the nurses' practice. Various antecedents and outcomes of collaboration were identified. Empowering nursing practice ranged from personal empowerment, small-group development, community organization, and coalition advocacy to political action. The authors concluded that clients were empowered in large part because of the empowerment nurses felt in being able to practise the full scope of nursing. They reflect on a reality that many nurses experience:

> When professionals are not granted professional status, they have great difficulty in establishing an empowering contract with their clients because they lack enough voice in the situation to be able to do so. The Comox Valley Nursing Centre Demonstration Project provided the context for nurses to practice autonomously, to be independent, self-directing, and self-governing, and to be accountable for their own decisions and actions within a project that was responsible to expressed community needs. (Clarke & Mass, 1998, p. 222)

The Comox Valley Nursing Centre received funding to extend its services for an additional 16 months. It ended in December 1996 (Attridge et al., 1997). According to the evaluations, the Nursing Centre was highly successful and had the potential to make an important contribution in the provision of health care.

Discussion Questions

1. The Comox Valley Nursing Centre was established because the Registered Nurses' Association of British Columbia capitalized on an opportunity: the provincial government's reform initiatives. What opportunities exist at the present time to establish a nursing centre in your area?

2. If you wanted to establish a nursing centre in your area, how would you go about developing a proposal? Who would you involve? Identify one or two goals that the project might have.

3. Discuss Clarke and Mass's conclusion that an empowering nursing practice was possible because the nature and structure of the nursing centre empowered the nurses who practised there. To what extent do you agree that nurses' ability to facilitate the empowerment of clients is dependent on their own empowerment?

LOOKING TO THE FUTURE

The Canadian health care system has been described as a fusion of public, private, and mixed public–private health care (Marchildon, 2006). Assessment of the performance of the public part of the system against the stated goals of the Canada Health Act is quite favourable. Numerous reports on the state of the health care system have, however, identified serious concerns regarding the scope of the public aspect of health care (e.g., health promotion services at the population level, home care, and pharmacare) and the increasing barriers to access posed by long wait lists for primary care as well as some diagnostic and treatment services. Some of these issues are directly related to the sustainability of funding and health human resources. Commitments to addressing these issues are, at least to some extent, evident in the 2003 and 2004 federal–provincial agreements on health care renewal and can be seen in the priorities and work of the Health Council of Canada (Canadian Research Box 2.2). Hopefully the principles of public consultation, transparency, and accountability that underpin these efforts will ensure that the necessary changes are made to the scope and delivery of public health care in Canada to ensure its sustainability in the future.

One aspect of sustainability pertains to funding. The single-payer system that characterizes the public aspect of Canadian health care has been pivotal to its success in maintaining costs (Church & Barker, 1998). It, however, has been challenged by the Chaoulli decision, even though that decision for now pertains only to Quebec (Marchildon, 2006). Regionalization may also pose a challenge to cost containment ability (Church & Barker, 1998). Although the issues Church and Barker raised were early in the Canadian regionalization experience, many are still valid. One relates to the economy of scale that was hoped to be achieved through global regional budgeting but that requires more densely populated regions than are possible through current regional structures. Without achieving this economy of scale, they warn, regionalization may actually increase health care expenditures.

In assessing the mixed public–private facet of Canadian health care, Marchildon includes many of the aspects of health care discussed above as limitations of the scope of Medicare (Marchildon, 2006). Evaluating them, he observes, is difficult because they are part of dramatically different systems across jurisdictions that use neither standardized data collection nor program evaluation methods. With respect to funding for drug expenditures, Marchildon notes the escalation in drug expenditures (Table 2.4) that has contributed significantly to the increasing proportion of privately funded Canadian health care (Table 2.3). This trend certainly threatens some of the underpinning principles of Medicare.

Private health care in Canada, Marchildon (2006) observes, has not been systematically studied and is often invisible to the public because some private services are supported or subsidized by public funds. Important in examining private health care is the differentiation of for-profit and not-for-profit delivery, such as the work done by Devereaux and colleagues (refer to Canadian Research Box 2.1).

Marchildon (2006) concludes his analysis of the Canadian health care system by observing that during the 1980s Canadians were more satisfied with their health care system than any other OECD comparator country. To regain that satisfaction, he warns, "governments and health organizations must be prepared to initiate major reforms—some of which will threaten existing stakeholders as well as change the scope of practice boundaries for providers—and invest more public money" (p. 133). The satisfaction of patients who received services within the public health care system actually increased between 2001 and 2003 (Marchildon, 2006), despite concerns with its shortcomings.

Summary

To varying degrees, all levels of government are involved in Canadian health care. A universally accessible, publicly funded, not-for-profit-delivered health care system is steeped in Canadian values and embraced by the Canadian public. Efforts to enshrine those values in federal legislation began as early as 1919. The present legislation, the Canada Health Act, is limited in that its principles of comprehensiveness, accessibility, universality of coverage, public administration, and portability of benefits apply only to essential medical and hospital services. Nevertheless, the publicly funded and largely privately delivered health care system has served Canadians well with respect to both health outcomes and cost-effectiveness.

Pressures to reform Canadian Medicare have come not only because of its narrow focus but also from individuals and groups who favour augmenting the public system with services provided by the for-profit sector. Numerous reports at provincial and federal levels over the past 10 years have recommended reforms to the health care system. Health care renewal in a number of key areas, such as primary health care and home care, has been committed to and initial efforts to reform these aspects of health care have begun. Wait time reduction has become an increasing focus for reform, particularly after a 2005 Supreme Court decision ruled that wait times violated Quebec's Charter of Rights and Freedoms.

The federal government has played a global leadership role in developing health promotion strategies. However, a coordinated approach to implementing health promotion policy at the community and population levels has been hampered by the lack of a national public health plan and often a lack of political will. Attention to Canada's public health system post SARS has led to the establishment of the PHAC and efforts to build Canada's capacity in infectious disease management and emergency preparedness. Whether this more biomedical and epidemiological emphasis will shift attention and resources from public health nursing services that promote the health of individuals, families, and communities remains to be seen.

Medicare, as it was conceptualized more than 35 years ago and re-entrenched in the Canada Health Act of 1984, has by and large performed well. The arguments advanced for an increased role of the private, for-profit sector in health care do not hold up well under scrutiny and seem to be motivated less by evidence than by ideology and greed. It remains to be seen whether current efforts to renew Canada's public health care system will be sufficient both to meet the needs of twenty-first century Canadians and to withstand the pressures of forces anxious for a share of the profits a market-driven health system would create.

KEY TERMS

Medicare
comprehensiveness
accessibility
universality of coverage
public administration
portability of benefits
Canada Health Act (CHA)
determinants of health
not-for-profit
for-profit

STUDY QUESTIONS

1. Identify the origins of Medicare in Canada and summarize the essential provincial/territorial and federal laws that created the present Canadian health care system.

2. What role did organized nursing play in the passage of the Canada Health Act?

3. Discuss the federal and provincial/territorial responsibilities for health according to the Canadian Constitution Act.

4. Contrast the funding mechanisms for public health and home health nursing services.

5. Describe how the Canada Health Act was or was not successful in achieving the intended goals.

6. Discuss the purpose, membership, and activities of the Health Council of Canada.

INDIVIDUAL CRITICAL THINKING EXERCISES

1. How would your life be different if health care in this country were provided based on ability to pay, rather than need?

2. How can you as a nursing student protect the public and not-for-profit nature of the Canadian health care system?

3. How is access to health care in Canada now both different from and the same as it was for your parents? for your grandparents?

4. How do your own values fit with the societal values that are reflected in the five funding criteria described in the Canada Health Act (1984)?

5. This chapter has shown that health policy decisions may leave a legacy for generations. Describe briefly one policy revision you would make in the areas of primary care/primary health care, public health, and home care.

6. In an ideal world, create a health care system designed to provide the best care, to the most people, in the most cost-effective manner. Describe mechanisms for financing, allocation, and delivery. Compare and contrast this system with the current Canadian system.

GROUP CRITICAL THINKING EXERCISES

1. Who stands to gain from health care privatization? How? Who stands to lose?

2. Discuss the advantages and disadvantages of opening up the Canada Health Act to introduce changes to Medicare.

3. What would be the advantages and disadvantages of a national home care program?

4. The Government of Canada has introduced a child fitness tax credit that, beginning in 2007, allows a non-refundable tax credit of up to $500 per child under 16 (maximum $1500 per family) for parents to cover costs of enrolling their children in physical activities. What impact do you expect that to have on children's health?

REFERENCES

Alberta Association of Registered Nurses, Canadian Nurses Association, Ontario Nurses Association, Registered Nurses' Association of Ontario, & United Nurses of Alberta. (2000). *Towards a sustainable, universally accessible health-care system.* A discussion paper prepared for the National Nursing Forum.

Attridge, C., Budgen, C., Hilton, A., McDavid, J. C., Molzahn, A., & Purkis, M. E. (1997). The Comox Valley Nursing Centre. *Canadian Nurse,* February, 34–38.

Auditor General of Canada. (2002). *1999 Report of the Auditor General of Canada to the House of Commons* (chapter 29). Retrieved April 15, 2007, from http://www.oag-bvg.gc.ca/domino/reports.nsf/html/99menu_e.html.

Barer, M. L., Evans, R. G., Hertzman, C., & Johri, M. (1998). *Lies, damned lies, and health care zombies: Discredited ideas that will not die* (HPI Discussion Paper #10). Houston, TX: University of Texas, Health Policy Institute.

Barlow, M. (2002). *Profit is not the cure: A call to citizens' action to save Medicare.* Retrieved April 15, 2007, from http://www.canadians.org/healthcare/documents/profit_not_cure.pdf.

Bégin, M. (1987). *Medicare: Canada's right to health.* Montreal: Optimum.

Bégin, M. (2002). *Revisiting the Canada Health Act (1984): What are the impediments to change?* Address to the Institute for Research on Public Policy, 30th Anniversary Conference, Ottawa.

Canada, Department of Finance. (2002). *A brief history of the Canada Health and Social Transfer (CHST).* Retrieved April 15, 2007, from http://www.fin.gc.ca/FEDPROV/hise.html.

Canada, House of Commons. (1984). An Act Relating to Cash Contributions by Canada in Respect of Insured Health Services Provided Under Provincial Health Care Insurance Plans and Amounts Payable by Canada in Respect of Extended Health Care Services and to Amend and Repeal Certain Acts in Consequence Thereof. (The Canada Health Act). Ottawa: Government of Canada.

Canadian Coalition for Public Health in the 21st Century. (2005). *Beyond the Naylor gap: Public health and productivity.* Retrieved November 2, 2006, from http://www.cpha. ca/english/policy/briefs/prevente/CCPH21_brief_october_ 2005_.pdf.

Canadian Health Services Research Foundation. (2001a). *Myth: The aging population will overwhelm the healthcare system.* Ottawa: Author.

Canadian Health Services Research Foundation. (2001b). *Myth: User fees would stop waste and ensure better use of the healthcare system.* Ottawa: Author.

Canadian Health Services Research Foundation. (2002a). *Myth: For-profit ownership of facilities would lead to a more efficient healthcare system.* Ottawa: Author.

Canadian Health Services Research Foundation. (2002b). *Myth: A parallel private system would reduce waiting times in the public system.* Ottawa: Author.

Canadian Home Care Association. (2006). *Home care facts: Governance and legislation.* Retrieved November 3, 2006, from http://www.cdnhomecare.ca/content.php?doc=79.

Canadian Institute for Health Information. (2006). *National health expenditure trends, 1975–2006.* Retrieved May 15, 2007, from http://secure.cihi.ca/cihiweb/dispPage. jsp?cw_page=AR_31_E.

Canadian Medical Association. (2002). Public health on the ropes. (Editorial). *Canadian Medical Association Journal, 166*(10), 1245.

Canadian Nurse Practitioner Initiative (2006). *Nurse practitioners: The time is now. A solution to improving access and reducing wait time in Canada.* Retrieved October 27, 2006, from http://www.cnpi.ca/documents/pdf/ Nurse_Practitioners_The_Time_is_Now_e.pdf.

Canadian Public Health Association (1996). *Focus on health: Public health in health services restructuring.* Ottawa: Author.

Canadian Public Health Association. (1997). *Public health infrastructure in Canada: Summary document.* Ottawa: Author.

Canadian Public Health Association. (2000). *An ounce of prevention: Strengthening the balance in health care reform.* Ottawa: Author.

Church, J., & Barker, P. (1998). Regionalization of health services in Canada: A critical perspective. *International Journal of Health Services, 28*(3), 467–486.

Clarke, H. F., & Mass, H. (1998). Comox Valley Nursing Centre: From collaboration to empowerment. *Public Health Nursing, 15*(3), 216–224.

Community Health Nurses Association of Canada. (2003). *Canadian Community Health Nursing Standards of Practice.* Retrieved April 28, 2007, from http://www. communityhealthnursescanada.org/Standards.htm.

Deber, R. B. (2000). Getting what we pay for: Myths and realities about financing Canada's health care system. *Health Law in Canada, 21*(2), 9–56.

Epp, J. (1986). *Achieving health for all: A framework for health promotion.* Ottawa: Health and Welfare Canada.

Evans, R. G., Barer, M. L., Lewis, S., Rachlis, M., & Stoddart, G. (2000). *Private highway, one-way street: The deklein and fall of Canadian medicare?* Retrieved April 14, 2007, from http://www.chspr.ubc.ca/node/321.

Fooks, C., & Lewis, S. (2002). *Romanow and beyond: A primer on health reform issues in Canada.* Retrieved October 31, 2006, from http://www.cprn.com/en/doc.cfm?doc=130.

Hamilton, N., & Bhatti, T. (1996). *Population health promotion.* Ottawa: Health Canada, Health Promotion and Development Division.

Health Canada. (2001). *The population health template: Key elements and actions that define a population health approach.* Retrieved April 27, 2007, from http://www.phac-aspc.gc.ca/ph-sp/phdd/pdf/discussion_paper.pdf.

Health Canada. (2004). *News Release: Government of Canada announces details of new Public Health Agency of Canada and appoints acting chief public health officer.* Retrieved January 11, 2006, from http://www.phac-aspc.gc.ca/media/nr-rp/2004/2004_01_e.html.

Health Canada. (2006a). *Provincial and territorial home care programs: A synthesis for Canada.* Retrieved November 3, 2006, from http://www.hc-sc.gc.ca/hcs-sss/pubs/care-soins/1999-pt-synthes/synth_e.html.

Health Canada. (2006b). *Public Health Agency of Canada sustainable development strategy 2007–2010: Toward sustainable development in public health.* Retrieved September 5, 2006, from http://www.phac-aspc.gc.ca.

Health Council of Canada. (2005a). *Elements of the 2003 First Ministers' Accord on health care renewal and the 2004 10-Year Plan to Strengthen Health Care.* Retrieved September 5, 2006, from http://healthcouncilcanada.ca/docs/AccordComparisonEN.pdf

Health Council of Canada. (2005b). *Health care renewal in Canada: Accelerating change.* Retrieved November 6, 2006, from http://www.healthcouncilcanada.ca/en/index.php?option=com_content&task=view&id=32&Itemid=32.

Hutchison, B., Abelson, J., & Lavis, J. (2001). Primary care in Canada: So much innovation, so little change. *Health Affairs, 20*(3), 116–131.

Lalonde, M. (1974). *A new perspective on the health of Canadians: A working paper.* Ottawa: Health and Welfare Canada.

Le Goff, P. (2002). *Home care in Quebec and Ontario: Structures and expenditures.* Retrieved November 3, 2006, from http://dsp-psd.communication.gc.ca/Collection-R/LoPBdP/BP/prb0231-e.htm

Library of Parliament. (2006). *Legislative Summaries Bill C-5 Public Health Agency of Canada Act.* Retrieved November 1, 2006, from http://www.parl.gc.ca/common/bills_ls.asp?lang=E&ls=c5&source=library_prb&Parl=39&Ses=1.

Lown, B. (1999, August 1). For-profit care's morbid results. *Boston Sunday Globe,* pp. E1, E5.

Marchildon, G. (2006). *Health systems in transition: Canada.* Toronto: University of Toronto Press.

McIntosh, T. (2006). *Don't panic: The hitchiker's guide to Chaoulli, wait times, and the politics of private insurance.* Retrieved September 5, 2006, from http://www.cprn.org/en/doc.cfm?doc=1394.

McKee, M., Edwards, N., & Atun, R. (2006). *Public–private partnerships for hospitals.* Retrieved November 10, 2006, from http://www.who.int/bulletin/volumes/84/11/06-030015.pdf.

McKeown, T. (1979). *The role of medicine: Dream, mirage or nemesis?* Princeton, NJ: Princeton University Press.

Mussallem, H. K. (1992). Professional nurses' associations. In A. J. Baumgart & J. Larsen (Eds.), *Canadian nursing faces the future* (2nd ed., pp. 495–518). Toronto: Mosby.

National Advisory Committee on SARS and Public Health. (2003). *Learning from SARS: Renewal of public health in Canada.* Retrieved November 1, 2006, from http://www.phac-aspc.gc.ca/publicat/sars-sras/naylor/.

Organisation for Economic Co-operation & Development. (2006). *OECD health data 2006: Statistics and indicators for 30 countries.* Retrieved October 23, 2006, from http://www.oecd.org/document/30/0,2340,en_2649_37407_12968734_1_1_1_37407,00.html.

Ostry, A. (1995). The history of public health in Canada: Differences in the history of public health in nineteenth century Canada and Britain. *Canadian Journal of Public Health, 86*(1), 5–6.

Pollara Research. (2005). *Health care in Canada survey.* Retrieved October 30, 2006, from http://www.mediresource.com/e/pages/hcc_survey/pdf/2005_hcic.pps.

Public Health Agency of Canada. (2004). *Questions and answers: Updated Quarantine Act.* Retrieved November 2, 2006, from http://www.phac-aspc.gc.ca/media/nr-rp/2004/2004_54bk1_e.html.

Public Health Agency of Canada. (2006). *Core competencies for public health.* Retrieved November 2, 2006, from http://www.phac-aspc.gc.ca/php-psp/core_competencies_for_ph_e.html.

Rachlis, M., Evans, R. G., Lewis, P., & Barer, M. L. (2001). *Revitalizing medicare: Shared problems, public solutions.* Tommy Douglas Research Institute. Retrieved April 27, 2007, from http://www.chspr.ubc.ca/node/262.

Rachlis, M. (2004). *Prescription for Excellence.* Toronto: HarperCollins.

Rachlis, M., & Kushner, C. (1994). *Strong medicine: How to save Canada's health care system.* Toronto: Harper Perennial.

Rafael, A. R. F. (1997). *Every day has different music: An oral history of public health nursing in Southern Ontario, 1980–1996.* Unpublished doctoral dissertation, University of Colorado, Denver.

Registered Nurses' Association of Ontario. (1999). *The Canada Health Act: To preserve and protect.* Toronto: Author.

Romanow, R. (2002a). *Building on values: The future of health care in Canada.* Retrieved October 4, 2007, from http://www.hc-sc.gc.ca/english/pdf/romanow/pdfs/HCC_Final_Report.pdf.

Romanow, R. (2002b). *Shape the future of health care: Interim report.* Retrieved April 27, 2007, from http://dsp-psd.pwgsc.gc.ca/Collection/CP32-76-2002E.pdf.

Schabas, R. (2002). Public health: What is to be done? *Canadian Medical Association Journal, 166*(10), 1282–1283.

Shah, C. P. (1998). *Public health and preventive medicine in Canada* (4th ed.). Toronto: University of Toronto Press.

Shaw, J. (2005). Wrestling with wait times. *Registered Nurse Journal, 17,* 12–15.

Sinclair, S. (2005). *Supreme Court health ruling oblivious to trade treaty threats.* Retrieved May 9, 2006, from http://www.policyalternatives.ca/index.cfm?act=news&call=1138&do=article&pA=BB736455.

Standing Senate Committee on Social Affairs, Science and Technology. (2002). *The health of Canadians—The federal role final report.* Retrieved October 21, 2006, from http://

www.parl.gc.ca/37/2/parlbus/commbus/senate/com-e/
soci-e/rep-e/repoct02vol6-e.htm.

Sullivan, P. (2002). Canada's public health system beset by
problems: Report. *Canadian Medical Association Journal,
166*(10), 1319.

Sullivan, T., & Baranek, P. (2002). *First do no harm: Making
sense of Canadian health reform.* Toronto: Malcolm Lester
& Associates.

Tuohey, C. H. (2002). The costs of constraint and prospects
for health care reform in Canada. *Health Affairs, 21*(3),
32–46.

Woolhandler, S., & Himmelstein, D. (2004). The high costs
of for-profit care. *Canadian Medical Association
Journal,170*(12), 1814–1815.

World Health Organization. (1978). *Declaration of Alma Ata.*
Retrieved April 27, 2007, from http://www.euro.who.int/
AboutWHO/Policy/20010827_1.

World Health Organization, Canadian Public Health Association,
& Health and Welfare Canada. (1986). *Ottawa Charter for
health promotion.* Ottawa: Health and Welfare Canada.

ADDITIONAL RESOURCES

Readings

Canadian Health Services Research Foundation. (Various
years). *Mythbuster Series: A series of essays giving the research
evidence behind Canadian health care debates.* http://www.
chsrf.ca/mythbusters/index_e.php.

Deber, R. B., Millan, K., Shapiro, H., & McDougall, C. W.
(2006). A cautionary tale of downloading public health in
Ontario: What does it say about the need for national
standards for more than doctors and hospitals? *Healthcare
Policy, 2,* 60–75.

Falk-Rafael, A. R., Fox, J., & Bewick, D. (2005). Health care
reforms in Ontario, Canada: Moving toward or away from
primary health care? Report of a 1999 survey of public

health nurses. *Primary Health Care Research and
Development, 6*(2), 172–183.

Fooks, C., & Maslove, L. (2004). *Rhetoric, fallacy, or dream?
Examining the accountability of health care to Canadians.*
Retrieved September 5, 2006, from http://www.cprn.org/
en/doc.cfm?doc=549.

Health Canada. (2005). Canada's Health Care System.
Retrieved August 14, 2007, from http://www.hc-sc.gc.ca/
hcs-sss/alt_formats/hpb-dgps/pdf/pubs/2005-hcs-sss/2005-
hcs-sss_e.pdf. Look at the timeline of important health
legislation.

Rachlis, M. (2005). *Public solutions to health care wait lists.*
From Canadian Centre for Policy Alternatives Website:
http://www.policyalternatives.ca/documents/National_
Office_Pubs/2005/Health_Care_Waitlists.pdf.

About the Authors

Adeline R. Falk-Rafael, RN, PhD, is a Professor in the
School of Nursing at York University, Toronto, where she
currently teaches in the graduate and undergraduate programs. Her program of research has focused on power and
empowerment in public health nursing, and her findings
have been reported in such journals as *Advances in Nursing
Science, Public Health Nursing,* and the *Journal of
Professional Nursing.* She is a past president of the
Registered Nurses' Association of Ontario.

Sue Coffey, RN, PhD, is an Associate Professor in the
School of Nursing at York University, Toronto. In addition
to extensive experience working in acute care settings, Ms.
Coffey has a master's degree in community health nursing.
She has worked with aggregates experiencing acute and
chronic health conditions as well as with those focusing on
health promotion.

Appendix 2A

Funding for Health Services for First Nations and Inuit in Canada ROSE ALENE ROBERTS

The First Nations and Inuit Health Branch (FNIHB) is a branch
within Health Canada (HC) that is responsible for the delivery of
health services in Aboriginal communities. Services are federally
funded and regionally managed. FNIHB is divided into seven
regions (Atlantic, Quebec, Ontario, Manitoba, Saskatchewan,
Alberta, and British Columbia) that roughly correspond to the
provincial boundaries. Atlantic region includes all four Atlantic
provinces. Yukon, the Northwest Territories, and Nunavut are over-
seen by the Northern Secretariat.

FNIHB regions are separate, parallel structures to the HC
regional offices that exist in each region. Regional authority is decentralized and each region has its own unique organizational structure
and relationship to its First Nations (FN) constituents. Most of the
First Nations and Inuit (FN/I) communities in Atlantic, Quebec,
and British Columbia regions manage their own health care services

in whole or in part. In the remainder, the non-transferred community-based health services are managed by the regional office.

First Nations and Inuit people are Canadian citizens and, as
such, have access to provincially and territorially funded health services that fall under the Canada Health Act, 1984. Aboriginal people
are included in the per capita allocations of federal funding that are
transferred to the provinces for "medically necessary" health services.
First Nations communities (formerly termed "reserves") below the
60th parallel, however, are considered to be federal or crown land.
For this reason, the federal government has historically funded public health and primary health care services on reserves. "North of 60"
Aboriginal people compose most of the population of the Canadian
territories; reserves are largely absent; and health services for
Aboriginal people are completely integrated into the health and
social services systems.

Indian Health Policy, 1979

The Federal Indian Health policy is one of the cornerstones of current policy regarding First Nations people and the Canadian Government. The Indian Health Policy of 1979 stated that it was based on the special relationship of the Indian people to the federal government and to the Crown. This relationship is committed to addressing access issues and health disparities that exist for Aboriginal people.

Policy for federal programs for Indian people (of which the health policy is an aspect), flows from constitutional and statutory provisions, treaties, and customary practice. It also flows from the commitment of Aboriginal people to preserve and enhance their culture and traditions. It recognizes the intolerable conditions of poverty and community decline, which affect many Aboriginal communities, and seeks a framework in which communities can remedy these conditions. The federal government recognizes its legal and traditional responsibilities to Aboriginal populations and seeks to promote the ability of Aboriginal communities to pursue their aspirations within the framework of Canadian institutions (Health Canada-FNIHB, 2005a).

Many Aboriginal communities exhibit conditions that are comparable to the level of poverty and community decline present in many rural and remote parts of Canada. Combined with this economic disadvantage are cultural isolation and the effects of a colonial past. For this reason, addressing the determinants of health is a key feature of federal policy for FN communities. Thus, the Indian Health Policy of 1979 noted that improving the level of health in First Nations communities is founded on three pillars:

- community development (socioeconomic, cultural, and spiritual) to remove the conditions of poverty and powerlessness that prevent the members of the community from achieving a state of physical, mental, and social well-being;

- the traditional relationship of the First Nations people to the federal government, in which the federal government promotes the capacity of First Nations communities to manage their own local health services; and

- the Canadian health system consisting of specialized and interrelated services funded by federal, provincial, or municipal governments, First Nations bands, or the private sector.

The federal role lies in public health activities on reserves, health promotion, and the detection and mitigation of hazards to health in the environment. The most significant provincial and private roles are in the diagnosis and treatment of acute and chronic disease and in the rehabilitation of the sick (Health Canada-FNIHB, 2005a).

In 1989, the "Treasury Board approved authorities and resources to support the transfer of Indian health services from Medical Services, Health and Welfare Canada (now Health Canada) to First Nations and Inuit wishing to assume responsibility" (Health Canada-FNIHB, 2005b). This "transfer process" (also called the "transfer initiative"):

- permits health program control to be assumed at a pace determined by the community, that is, the community can assume control gradually over a number of years through a phased transfer;

- enables communities to design health programs to meet their needs;

- requires that certain mandatory public health and treatment programs be provided; and

- strengthens the accountability of Chiefs and Councils to community members.

Further, the transfer process:

- gives communities the financial flexibility to allocate funds according to community health priorities and to retain unspent balances,

- gives communities the responsibility for eliminating deficits and for annual financial audits and evaluations at specific intervals,

- permits multi-year (three- to five-year) agreements,

- does not prejudice treaty or Aboriginal rights,

- operates within current legislation, and

- is optional and open to all First Nations communities south of the 60th parallel (Health Canada-FNIHB, 2005b).

Financial Highlights

FNIHB is responsible for funding the delivery of community-based health services to 638 Aboriginal communities and about 765 000 persons, most south of the 60th parallel. FNIHB directly manages health services in about half those communities and administers integrated agreements and transfer agreements for the rest, who manage their own health services in whole or in part following the process outlined above.

The total budget for FNIHB in 2004–2005 was $1.7 billion and was projected to increase to $2.0 billion by 2007–2008. FNIHB also funds an extended health benefit program, the Non-Insured Health Benefits program (NIHB). The NIHB is a payer of last resort for health services that are not covered under the Canada Health Act for all status Indians in Canada, both on and off reserve. This includes, for example, drugs, dental care, eyeglasses, other assistive devices, short-term crisis intervention mental health services and medical transportation. Approximately 48%, or $837 million, was allocated to the NIHB program. Pharmaceuticals (45%), transportation (28%), and dental costs (18%) were the three major expenses in the 2004–2005 NIHB budget (Health Canada-FNIHB, 2005c).

Health services resources accounts for 51% of the budget ($896 million) and includes community nursing, alcohol/drug counselling, Brighter Futures, transfer initiatives, as well as other administrative expenses. The operation of FNIHB hospitals accounts for the remaining 1.4% ($24 million) (Health Canada-FNIHB, 2005c).

Recently, FNIHB implemented a home care program that receives about $90 million annually in federal funding. Home care services are community based and band managed. As First Nations and Inuit assume greater control of health services through such mechanisms as integrated agreements and transfer agreements, the involvement of FNIHB in direct service delivery has steadily declined.

Demographic Highlights: South of the 60th Parallel

There are 609 FN/I communities that receive services through the First Nations and Inuit Health Branch in the provincial regions as outlined above. Delivery of health services is administered in First Nations and Inuit communities in various ways. Those communities interested in having more control of their health services can decide from a menu of approaches: health services transfer, integrated community-based health services, and self-government, based on their eligibility, interests, needs, and capacity.

Since 1989, when the transfer process was initiated, 79% of eligible First Nations communities are now involved in the First Nations Control Process; 46% have signed Community-Based

Transfer Agreements; and 33% have signed Integrated Community-Based Health Services Contribution Agreements. Furthermore, 21% of all treatment services have been transferred, along with 19% of National Native Alcohol and Drug Abuse Program (NNADAP) Treatment Centres, and 40% of hospitals (two out of five hospitals, three hospitals have been closed) (Health Canada-FNIHB, 2006).

Community Types

In order to better allocate resources, communities have been classified according to their degree of access to provincial or territorial health services. For example, a remote-isolated community may require professional nursing services 24/7. However, funding for these services also depends on community size.

Type 1: Remote-Isolated: No scheduled flights, minimal telephone or radio services, and no road access.

Type 2: Isolated: Scheduled flights, good telephone services, and no year-round road access.

Type 3: Semi-Isolated: Road access greater than 90 km to physician services.

Type 4: Non-Isolated: Road access less than 90 km to physician services.

Remote, isolated communities of fewer than 200 people may have only a lay community health representative (CHR) on site, who consults with a community health nurse in a neighbouring community nursing station. Alternatively, a nurse may visit for one or more days a month. Larger centres may have a nursing station with two or more nurses. Nurses in these settings function in an expanded role and provide essential public health, primary care, and physician and pharmacist replacement services on a 24-hour-a-day, seven-day-per-week basis. FNIHB has more than 800 FTE-registered nurse employees working in 76 nursing stations and more than 195 health centres (Health Canada-FNIHB, 2007). Larger, less isolated communities have community health centres that provide more typical public health and primary care services during standard business hours. A physician may visit on a regular basis and/or clients are referred out for doctor visits. Rarely, a community health centre may provide expanded role nursing services after hours.

In both cases, FNIHB's Non-insured Health Benefits (NIHB) program provides funding for medical transportation for the community member to visit a doctor or a hospital when required.

Other Federally Funded Programs

Health Canada currently funds 52 NNADAP Treatment Centres with approximately 700 beds, and 10 National Youth Solvent Abuse Treatment Programs (NYSATP) with an additional 120 beds through FNIHB. NNADAP provides more than 550 programs including prevention, intervention and aftercare activities. More than 700 workers, the majority of whom are First Nations and Inuit, are employed by NNADAP (Health Canada-FNIHB, 2005c).

Health Canada also provides funding for early childhood development and targeted programs for fetal alcohol syndrome/fetal alcohol effects, Aboriginal Head Start, Brighter Futures, tobacco reduction, food safety, HIV/AIDS, diabetes, tuberculosis elimination, and the Canada Prenatal Nutrition Program. Many of these programs are allocated to the communities on a per capita basis, which can result in very small sums for tiny communities. FNIHB also provides funds for scholarships for FN/I who are pursuing careers in the health field. These funds are administered by the National Aboriginal Achievement Foundation (NAAF), a non-governmental organization.

Other government departments and branches provide funding to FN/I communities that contributes to addressing determinants of health. FNIHB and Indian and Northern Affairs Canada (INAC) jointly resource on-reserve water quality: FNIHB is accountable for monitoring and testing and INAC for infrastructure. There was $600 million for five years allocated in the 2003 budget for water management in First Nations communities (Indian and Northern Affairs Canada, 2005). INAC is responsible for housing and community-based education. The Solicitor General funds community policing or support from the Royal Canadian Mounted Police. Human Resources Development Canada has an Aboriginal division that works with FN/I communities on strategies to improve access to trades.

In these ways, the federal government attempts to address determinants of health while FNIHB ensures access to community-based health services and supports community development.

REFERENCES

Health Canada-First Nations and Inuit Health Branch. (2005a). *Indian health policy 1979.* Accessed April 23, 2007, from http://www.hc-sc.gc.ca/fnih-spni/services/indi_health-sante_poli_e.html.

Health Canada-First Nations and Inuit Health Branch. (2005b). *Ten years of health transfer First Nations and Inuit control.* Accessed April 23, 2007, from http://www.hc-sc.gc.ca/fnih-spni/pubs/agree-accord/10_years_ans_trans/2_intro_e.html #History_of_transfer.

Health Canada, First Nations and Inuit Health Branch. (2005c). *Non-Insured Health Benefits Program: 2004–2005 Annual Report.* Retrieved April 12, 2007, from http://www.hc-sc.gc.ca/fnih-spni/pubs/nihb-ssna/2005_rpt/index_e.html.

Health Canada, First Nations and Inuit Health Branch. (2006). *Transfer status as of December 2006.* Retrieved April 12, 2007, from http://www.hc-sc.gc.ca/fnih-spni/finance/agree-accord/trans_rpt_stats_e.html.

Health Canada, First Nations and Inuit Health Branch. (2007). *Nursing.* Retrieved April 20, 2007, from http://www.hc-sc.gc.ca/fnih-spni/services/nurs-infirm/index_e.html.

Indian and Northern Affairs. (2005). *First Nations water top priority for Government of Canada.* Retrieved April 20, 2007, from http://www.ainc-inac.gc.ca/nr/prs/m-a2003/2-02304_e.html.

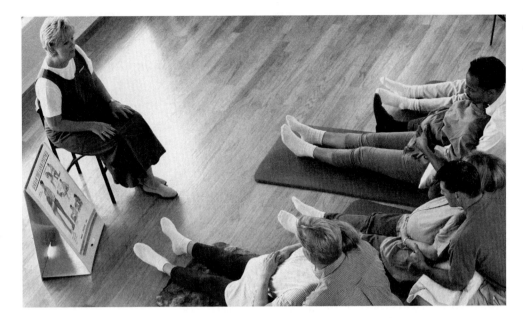

Photo 3.1

Parents' anxiety is reduced by preparing for parenthood before the birth of the baby.

Credit: © Purestock/MaXx Images

Some very large groups can be termed *populations* because they share a common characteristic such as a place of work or study. PHNs working within the school setting have an opportunity to provide comprehensive health promotion strategies to their school populations on several levels. (See Chapter 16.) Decisions about which health promotion issues to address are made with staff, parents, and students, and are based on epidemiological principles and health status data. PHNs may deliver teacher workshops and classroom presentations, or organize interactive health fairs where students visit booths and play games to raise awareness about lifestyle issues, sexual health, or injury prevention. To be most effective, health education needs to be incorporated into other aspects of the general curriculum and supported with healthy school policy. Knowledge acquisition about a particular health issue frequently does not translate into a behaviour change. For example, safer sex behaviours among youth are rarely the result of direct education; they require social support and skills such as comfort with condom use and an environment that facilitates access to condoms (Rew et al., 2002). Likewise, teaching children about the benefits of a healthy diet, physical activity, and a smoke-free lifestyle are not effective unless they are reinforced within the school environment through opportunities for physical activity throughout the day, healthy food choices in the cafeteria, and smoke-free school grounds. Teaching students about the importance of wearing bike helmets is meaningless if not supported by school policy and environment supports to ensure the availability of helmets. The PHN can be a key player in policy advocacy within the school setting by working with parent councils and school staff to develop healthy school policies and resulting healthy school environments.

The same process can be used within the workplace setting. Comprehensive workplace wellness programs (see Chapter 12) include a combination of education and policy support for a healthy work environment. Often, health screening is incorporated into a workplace model. A health fair that includes education about physical activity, nutrition, and tobacco cessation may also entail the opportunity for employees to have their blood pressure and blood cholesterol checked to rule out potential cardiovascular problems. Large community health fairs are another means of engaging the general population in health promoting behaviours. Although an education strategy, the target is very broad, and awareness of services is the general outcome.

Community as Client   A community is generally viewed as comprising many subgroups or sub-populations. It can be as big as an entire city or a municipal or provincial region serviced by a public health department or regional health authority. It can be very large in geographical size and small in population, such as in a rural outpost region in the far north of Canada. It can be as small as a school community. Working with an entire community provides an opportunity for very broad or macro health promotion strategies to complement the direct education done with smaller groups or populations. As previously discussed in dealing with groups, it is acknowledged that education sessions in isolation from other reinforcers are not effective in changing health behaviours. Broader or more macro strategies are required.

A comprehensive approach entails social marketing, in which mass media are used in conjunction with community events and promotional material to raise community awareness and motivate people to create a social change. **Social marketing** has been described as a process to influence the acceptability of a social idea or cause. (See Chapter 6.) These initiatives, as all macro strategies, are based on epidemiological evidence of a need for a behaviour change from health status data. Plans for a social marketing campaign are designed within a multidisciplinary team of strategic communication specialists for process and messaging design, and health professionals, including PHNs, for the content. The plans are detailed and are developed with built-in evaluation components. Formative evaluation or focus testing is used to assess the reliability of the message with a small group of individuals from the target population. Social marketing involves the classic "Four P" model (Weinrich, 2003). **Product** is the message or concept you are trying to sell. An example may be injury prevention in children. **Price** means what it will cost to adopt the injury-prevention behaviours. It could be time energy to constantly monitor a toddler or the financial cost of a safety gate. **Place** means channel of distribution of the product to the target population. It could be ways to reach out to the young parents at a community centre or an entire community. **Promotion** usually involves a multidimensional communication campaign targeting a segment of the community, although the community at large may benefit from the message with increased awareness. Under optimal resource allocations, this may involve paid electronic media messages supported by print media, posters, pamphlets, and community forums or workshops for professionals or the public. The ultimate goal is to achieve some positive behaviour change. But at the least, it does create awareness of an issue. One example of a PHN-led injury-prevention campaign targeted to caretakers of children 0 to 6 years old involved all the previously mentioned components. A campaign entitled "Hold, Follow, Watch" (see Figure 3.1) included a brand design and catchy tune to remind parents and caretakers that these three simple strategies were required to prevent falls in children, the primary cause of injuries within the 0 to 6 population. Content was reinforced in parenting classes and in workshops with professionals. "Turn off the Screen—Turn on the Family" was a similar project targeted at parents; the product was increase in physical activity among the school-aged population. Additional *Ps* included in other models are *policy* and *partnerships*, both of which are integral to any successful health promotion initiative (Windsor Essex County Health Unit, 2006).

Community mobilization is a term that describes a process of activating a community to achieve healthy public policy and/or enhancing the capacity of a community to sustain a positive change. PHNs are often involved in this through coalitions with community partners. They can provide the research and epidemiological data to support the cause from a health perspective. An example of mobilizing a community through a coalition is tobacco policy advocacy. Although the federal government enforces the issue of sales of tobacco products to minors and many provincial governments have province-wide smoking restrictions, in some provinces local governments are responsible for their own control of environment tobacco smoke in public places. PHNs join forces with other local health agencies, such as the Lung Association, Heart and Stroke Foundation, and Cancer Society to create awareness in the community. Local champions of the cause are recruited to generate media coverage; eventually, a groundswell of residents get involved and make their voices heard by local politicians and a smoking by-law is created that fits the health culture of that community. Similar initiatives have been orchestrated for walking trail and bike path advocacy in communities looking for more environmental support to promote physical activity.

Community development is a less concrete strategy that PHNs are often involved in to facilitate a community's efforts

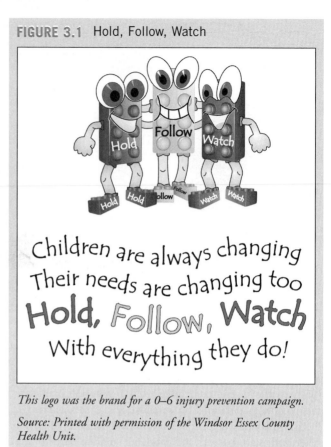

FIGURE 3.1 Hold, Follow, Watch

Children are always changing
Their needs are changing too
Hold, Follow, Watch
With everything they do!

This logo was the brand for a 0–6 injury prevention campaign.
Source: Printed with permission of the Windsor Essex County Health Unit.

to establish its goals and take steps to achieve positive change. The nurse could assume a strong facilitating role in this process, but the community members must own the change for sustainability purposes. (See Chapters 7 and 11.) Reducing youth crime and illegal drug use in an urban housing project is an example of a goal of a particular community development strategy. The PHN may help community members to lobby local politicians and find resources to build a youth activity centre and to recruit volunteers to act as mentors for local youth. But this type of project must be in the total control of the community members themselves, while the nurse acts as a consultant or facilitator. Although broad, the role of the PHN in this type of community involvement is often elusive. PHNs are often quite integrated in the community, or doing the macro health promotion strategies directed at the community as a whole, and therefore they and their work are not as visible and measurable as other community health nurses who provide direct care and hands-on interventions within the curative aspect of health promotion. PHNs working with community partners and coalitions need to be cognizant that they are using the nursing process in their work, and documentation of this may take untraditional forms. Minutes of meetings must be significantly detailed to reflect the PHN's actions. The PHN's daily planner, emails, and telephone logs are evidence of assessing, planning, and implementation as much as tools to organize time efficiently. Project plans must be clear in identifying the role of the PHN and expected outcomes.

All of the most common macro health promotion strategies described above can be effective in reinforcing the need for policy change to create supportive environments for healthy communities. From healthy food policies in schools, to family-friendly workplace policies, to no-smoking by-laws, healthy public policy is a sustainable means of reinforcing health behaviour. Nurses have an important role in advocating for public policy, but PHNs are especially effective because of their knowledge of specific communities. All of these macro strategies can work in synergy to ensure that prerequisites for healthy communities exist.

Evaluation to ensure continuous quality improvement in nursing practice is just as vital for these larger-scale projects as it is at the individual or small-group level. Although formal evaluation of outcomes is usually done by program evaluation specialists, the PHN must be aware of the outcomes of the nursing interventions. Evaluation of nursing interventions beyond the individual or family level in public health has often been problematic as behaviours focusing on prevention can be difficult to measure. Nonetheless, it is important for the PHN to follow the steps in the nursing process and incorporate effective evaluation strategies into the macro or population-based projects.

Home Health Nursing

Home health nursing is a specialized area of nursing practice in which the nurse provides care in the client's home, school, or workplace. Clients and their designated caregivers are the focus of home health nursing practice. The goal is to initiate, manage, and evaluate the resources needed to promote the client's optimal level of well being and functioning. Nursing activities necessary to achieve this goal may warrant preventive, maintenance, and restorative emphasis to prevent potential problems from developing.

Although the role of the **home health nurse** (HHN) is commonly categorized as generalist in nature, the trend to well-informed consumers who increasingly expect care from nurses specializing in the relevant clinical area has given rise to numerous specialty roles for HHNs. These include wound ostomy resource nurse, psychogeriatric nurse, continence adviser, diabetes nurse educator, palliative care nurse consultant, respiratory nurse specialist, and many others. These specialty home health care nurses ideally do not take over client care, but rather provide expert client assessment and care plan guidance that contributes to client care excellence while augmenting the generalist nurse's knowledge base and competencies. Thus, the specialty nursing roles promote client satisfaction while also positively influencing career satisfaction for both the specialty nurse (by offering career diversity) and the generalist nurse (by contributing to practice confidence and competence).

Individual as Client The separation of home health nursing from what is now recognized as public health nursing has occurred over the years as an outcome of health system development and funding structures. Accordingly, while the focus of home health nursing today is the client, their family, and/or their caregivers, care is provided within the context of the principles of primary health care, with an emphasis on health promotion and clinical care services. The majority of care is delivered in the practice settings of client's home, school, or community clinic.

The home health nurse's relationship with the client is based on the understanding that the nurse is a "guest in the house" and therefore adapts all care according to the client's environment and direction. Holistic health assessment skills are critical in order to determine not only the physical and psychosocial needs of the client but also, as importantly, the role played by the family/caregivers and home environment in supporting or challenging the client's achievement of health goals. A collaborative approach based on a nurse–client partnership model is a hallmark of the home health nurse's work with clients to identify the client's desired health goals, develop the care plan, and obtain consent for the care.

Clinical expertise in a wide range of tasks and interventions is another requisite for the home health nurse. With the high rates of day surgery and the short lengths of hospital stay that characterize today's health care system, home health nurses manage the full spectrum of acute treatment regimens such as intravenous drug therapies (including chemotherapy) via a host of venous access devices and infusion pumps, complex wounds, chest drainage systems, new tracheotomy care regimes, and post cerebral vascular and cardiac event monitoring and treatment programs. HHNs also possess considerable competency in the nursing care of chronic conditions, including peritoneal dialysis, respiratory disease (including ventilator-dependent clients), long-term mental health and psychogeriatric conditions, acquired brain injuries, and infants/children with complex and life-long care needs. These clinical aspects of home health care demand highly effective critical-thinking and problem-solving skills.

Family as Client Home health nursing views the family as inseparable from the client as the focus of care. Assessing the strengths and needs of the family is foundational to maximizing the self-care abilities of the client/family. Accordingly, an understanding of family theory is a prerequisite for home health nurses. Home health nurses mobilize and/or augment the ability of family members to assist the client in meeting the health goals. Where the health support needs of the client are short-term, home health nurses may teach family members about the particular health alteration and implications (e.g., care considerations for diabetes), specific skills (e.g., wound care), reportable signs and symptoms, and appropriate community supports. Situations where the HHN has a long-term relationship with the family, for example when providing care to a chronically ill child over months or years, require an in-depth understanding of alterations in the family dynamics arising from changes in family roles and functioning.

The HHN's role in palliative care in the home is particularly delicate. **Palliative care** focuses on symptom management for untreatable conditions, usually in the last six months of a person's life. Research into end-of-life or palliative care indicates that dying in a hospital is one indicator of poor quality end-of-life care (Barbara et al., 2006). If possible, a planned, supported, natural death in the comfort of home is usually viewed as a better option for the sake of the entire family. Once aggressive treatment has been stopped, the HHN helps the family get the supports in place to provide for an optimal end-of-life experience.

Hospice programs exist in most communities to provide palliative care in the home. HHNs may be employed by hospice agencies or liaise with them through their roles in home care agencies. The goal is to ensure a pain- and symptom-controlled environment for the patient and comfort for the family. Family members often feel helpless and fearful of the unknown. The HHN can provide answers to assist with family decision making and help prepare the family for the death of their loved one in a climate of respect, dignity, and comfort. These care situations may be stressful for both nurses and family, as though the nurses may be seen as supportive and helpful, they may also be viewed by the family as strangers in the family environment. In addition, the closeness and longevity of the relationship may lead to a blurring of the nurse–client boundaries requiring the nurse to be vigilant in avoiding boundary violations.

The complexity of HHNs' family-centred care is further illustrated by the need for the nurse to be knowledgeable and responsive to any indications of child, elder, or spousal abuse. Numerous success indicators provide evidence of the effectiveness of home health nurses in caring for clients and families in home and school environments. These indicators include observable improvements in caregivers' confidence and knowledge in providing care, reductions in the stress levels of clients and caregivers, remediation of abusive situations, and the appreciation of clients/caregivers as expressed by verbal and written thanks, often to employers, newspapers, or regulatory colleges.

Group as Client Although opportunities for HHNs to work with groups as the focus of care are limited, some such roles are now in existence. Examples include a home health nurse who was contracted to work in a school setting where the student body comprised children with complex and long-term health needs. The role of the nurse was to provide client-specific care interventions such as medication administration, tube feedings, etc., as well as to consider and provide for the overall health needs of all school children. This latter aspect of the role involved assessing the safety of the school environment, planning activities for the entire school population, and acting as an adviser to the teachers on the intersection of the child's health needs and classroom performance.

In another role involving care to a group, an HHN provides clinical care to individual residents of a religious residence, but also contributes to the overall health care and well-being of all residents as a member of the facility's planning committee. Table 3.2 presents some of the broader roles of CHNs where the general attributes may vary due to the diversity of their practices across Canada. Table 3.3 highlights more specific roles

of nurses working in the community, such as primary health care nurse practitioners, nurse entrepreneurs, faith community nurses, and forensic nurses. (See the case study below.)

TABLE 3.2
Roles of CHNs

CHN Roles	PHN	HHN
Caregiver/educator/consultant	✓	✓
Facilitator/communicator/collaborator	✓	✓
Researcher/evaluator	✓	✓
Resource manager/planner	✓	✓
Public policy formulator	✓	X
Social marketer	✓	X
Community developer	✓	X
Surveillance and epidemiology data manager	✓	X

Case Study

You are a nursing student in your final year of study to obtain your baccalaureate degree in nursing. After writing your registration examination, you will apply for nursing positions in your area. You have enjoyed the community clinical experiences in your nursing education and would like to pursue a career in that area. You are aware of the diversity in practice settings in the community, but the concept of working autonomously, which seems to be a consistent feature in most of them, really appeals to you. You want to make the position a good match for your personality as well as your clinical interests and skills.

Discussion Questions

1. From reading all the descriptions of roles of CHNs in this chapter, assess which one appeals to you the most in terms of the kind of nursing interventions described.

2. What kind of research would you do before submitting an application to a community health nursing agency?

3. How would you prepare for an interview with your employer of choice?

Table 3.3 also provides a summary of the characteristics of community health nurses practising in other areas besides PHNs and HHNs. See Chapters 12, and 16 to 29 for detailed descriptions of CHNs practising with carried clients and in areas such as school health, long-term care, mental health, correctional nursing, and disaster nursing.

TABLE 3.3
Characteristics of Selected Community Health Nurses in Varied Practice Settings

Characteristic	Forensic Nursing	Nurse Entrepreneurs	Primary Health Care NPs	Community Health Centre/ Outreach Nurse	Outpost or Rural Nurse	Faith Community Nurse	Occupational Health Nurse
Defining Goals	Forensic nurses deal with a range of services to victims of crime and within the prison system. They work with law enforcement and criminal investigations. Sexual assault nurse examiners (SANES) work both autonomously and collaboratively with police to collect physical evidence and to provide care to victims of crime and violence.	Nurse entrepreneurs provide a health service within the private business sector, working in independent practice within the regulatory framework of nurses in each province.	A PHC NP complements the health care team; the PHC NP uses advanced knowledge and skills and formal preparation to work within an expanded scope of practice. This goal may warrant health promotion, preventive, maintenance, and restorative care.	These nurses work in a non-profit organization that provides primary health care and health promotion programs for individuals, families, and communities. Community health centres (CHC) work with individuals, families, and communities to strengthen their capacity to take more responsibility for their health and well-being. CHCs work together with others on health promotion initiatives within schools, in housing developments, and in the workplace. They link families with support and self-help groups that offer peer education, support in coping, or work to address conditions that affect health. As such, the CHC program contributes to the development of healthy communities.	These CHNs or PHNs work exclusively in a rural or outpost setting, generally in isolation from a traditional health care team support. These nurses provide primary health care and make referrals for more in-depth assessments.	Parish nurses are registered nurses with specialized knowledge, who are called to ministry and affirmed by a faith community to promote health, healing, and wholeness. Parish nurses are concerned with the entire person—body, mind, and spirit. They believe there is a strong relationship between faith and health.	Occupational health nurses are registered nurses practising in the specialty of occupational health and safety to deliver integrated occupational health and safety services to individual workers and worker populations. Occupational health nursing encompasses the promotion, maintenance, and restoration of health and the prevention of illness and injury.

TABLE 3.3
continued

Characteristic	Forensic Nursing	Nurse Entrepreneurs	Primary Health Care NPs	Community Health Centre/ Outreach Nurse	Outpost or Rural Nurse	Faith Community Nurse	Occupational Health Nurse
Place of Work	Community health centres, police departments, or ERs. SANEs often are on call and respond to calls as needed.	Centralized office or home, depending on scope of work. May vary from individual counselling in office or client's home to travel worldwide, as in airpatient transport business.	Client's private home, school, public health clinics, street, hospital, community health centre, and collaborative family health practices.	Community health centre building, community location, or the street.	Outpost clinic, clients' homes, or other community location.	Place of worship, client's home.	Workplace.
Work Team/ Colleagues	Physicians, police, mental health counsellors, attorneys, social workers.	Other professional colleagues in community; may employ a contingent of health care providers.	MDs, other nurses (RNs, RPNs/LPNs), supportive care staff, allied professionals (physician, physiotherapist, pharmacist, occupational therapist, etc.).	Multi-disciplinary	Limited to visits from travelling physicians and dental teams, etc. Relies on technology (e.g., phone, email, fax) to keep in touch.	Clergy, parish volunteers	Human resource personnel, physician on consultation.
Role Focus	Primary health care to victims of crime and violence, including health assessment and collection of physical evidence.	Varied from primary health care to specifics, such as foot care, to lactation consultant to private patient transport.	Client as individual/ family. Direct clinical care, case management.	Client as individual, family, group, or population. Direct primary health clinical care.	Client as individual, community, group, or population. Direct primary health care.	Client as individual or group. Holistic primary health care to specific faith community.	Client as individual or group. Primary health care, health education, assessment, and screening.
Minimum Qualifications	RN with specialty certification.	RN	BScN, RN, plus extended practice designation. Some provinces are moving toward master's preparation.	RN	RN	RN	RN with certification in occupational health.

TABLE 3.3
continued

Characteristic	Forensic Nursing	Nurse Entrepreneurs	Primary Health Care NPs	Community Health Centre/ Outreach Nurse	Outpost or Rural Nurse	Faith Community Nurse	Occupational Health Nurse
Unique Characteristics of Nursing Practice	Work with team requires specific technical skills as well as sensitivity.	Requires knowledge of principles of business planning and economics and business insurance.	Work alone and collaboratively with an expanded scope. Practise highly autonomous and independent. Adaptable to client-controlled environment.	Flexibility to follow client/family from clinic to home.	Long travel distances. Adaptability to range of dwellings. Manage broad spectrum of health needs. Work in isolated communities.	Integrates faith-based approach to care. U.S.-based credential available.	Address health, safety, and well-being of employees. May earn specialty credential from CNA COHN.
Funding	Through facility, such as health centre, emergency room, or police.	For-profit business covers salary of nurse and overhead costs.	Provincial government (may be fee-for-service, e.g., Ontario; or global funding, e.g., Regional Health Authority).	Fixed budget from province.	Provincially or federally funded.	Independently funded.	Funded by the employer.
Scope and Standards of Practice	According to two-part certification program.	Within provincial regulatory standards for any service that falls within the practice of nursing.	Framework for advanced practice competencies established (Canadian Nurse Practitioner Initiatives [CNPI], 2006). High requirement for technical clinical skills.	Community health centre or region specific.	In development through Health Canada.	Working on standards of practice.	Standards of practice in place for credentialling purposes.
Relevant Professional Associations (Canada)	Ontario Network of Sexual Assault Care and Treatment Centres (ONSACTC), Canadian Association of Sexual Assault Treatment Centres (CASAC).	CNA, Canadian Nurses Protective Society (CNPS).	CNA, CNPI, provincial NP associations.	Province specific (e.g., Association of Community Health Centres of Ontario) Canadian Alliance of Community Health Centre Associations.	Community Health Nurses Association of Canada (CHNAC).	Canadian Association for Parish Nursing Ministry.	Canadian Association of Occupational Health Nurses.

EXPANDING COMMUNITY HEALTH NURSING PRACTICE

Four nursing specialty areas were chosen to illustrate the expansion of community health nursing practice in Canada. The roles, historical perspectives, and/or scope of each specialty practice are described along with the challenges faced by nurses in those practices—namely, nurse practitioners, nurse entrepreneurs, faith community nurses, and forensic nurses.

Primary Health Care Nurse Practitioners

A **nurse practitioner** (NP) is a registered nurse with additional education preparation and experience who demonstrates the competencies to autonomously diagnose; order and interpret diagnostic tests; prescribe pharmaceuticals; and perform specific procedures within the legislated scope of practice (Canadian Nurse Practitioner Initiative [CNPI], 2006). In an attempt to streamline practice expectations, optimize the contribution of NPs, and develop some consistency in advanced nursing practice across the country, the CNA, through federal funding, established the Canadian Nurse Practitioner Initiative (CNPI). The goal of this initiative was to ensure sustained integration of the NP role in the health system. The mandate was to develop recommendations in five broad areas: legislation and regulation; practice and evaluation; human health resource planning; education; and change management, social marketing, and strategic communication (CNO, 2006).

Major outcomes of the CNPI project revolve around a legislative and regulatory framework that allows for a Canada-wide, consistent, principle-based approach in regulating NP practice, while at the same time giving each provincial and territorial jurisdiction some flexibility in implementation. It also provides a basis for facilitating mobility between jurisdictions and provides clarity for admitting internationally educated NPs (CNPI, 2006). The *Canadian Nurse Practitioner Core Competency Framework* includes the establishment of core competencies as the basis for NP educational programs and a national NP exam as well as a competence assessment framework for ongoing quality assurance of NP practice. It also recommends title protection for the NP so that only nurses with the defined qualifications would be able to use the title NP. In other words, Canadian NPs have a framework of consistent practice expectations and they must demonstrate specific competencies in the expanded scope of their practice. This is defined in provincial regulatory legislation and standards may vary from province to province. As a minimum, NPs can all diagnose a common disease, disorder, or condition; order and interpret prescribed diagnostic and screening tests, such as X-rays or ultrasounds; and prescribe specific medication. The authority to perform these advanced acts is subject to limits and conditions outlined by the regulatory body and the NP's expertise. The NP seeks consultation with a physician when the diagnosis and/or treatment plan is unclear or beyond the scope of the NP to determine.

Historical Perspectives In 2005, there were well over one thousand NPs registered in Canadian jurisdictions, representing approximately 0.5% of RNs in the current workforce, with approximately 95% of licensed NPs employed (Canadian Institute for Health Information [CIHI], 2006a). However, the road to this point was filled with uncertainty. The movement for an advanced nurse position emerged from the 1960s due to perceptions of physician shortages and a trend toward nursing specialization. In 1971 the Boudreau Report made the implementation of the expanded role of the RN a high priority in Canada's health care system. In the 1970s many education programs began graduating NPs, but in the absence of supporting regulatory legislation, these nurses functioned as RNs working under medical directives.

In 1973, the CNA/Canadian Medical Association (CMA) released a joint policy statement on the role of the nurse practitioner, but no formalization of the role in legislation occurred. This was largely due to a lack of public and professional awareness of the valuable role for the NP coupled with a perception of ample physician supply. By the 1980s, most NP initiatives had ceased to exist. A small number of NPs continued to function through the 1980s and early 1990s, working mainly in community health centres and in northern or remote outpost nursing stations, with a variety of educational preparations and responsibilities.

Despite the failure of the first initiative, the NP role was consistently cited by many provincial health care commissions and task forces as valuable in the delivery of health care. During this time, a recognition of the importance of health promotion and the need for more community-based care emerged. Fuelled by limited resources in the 1990s, an enhanced interest and political will to make a shift from a treatment-oriented health care system to a more holistic and upstream approach became a priority. This generated support for a primary health care model of service delivery and ultimately led to the creation of formalized NP roles defined in legislation across Canada.

As indicated in the earlier part of this chapter, *primary health care* includes all services that play a part in health beyond the traditional health care system, including income, housing, education, and environment (Health Canada, 2006). **Primary care** is the element within primary health care that focuses on health care services, including health promotion, illness and injury prevention, and the diagnosis and treatment of illness and injury (Health Canada, 2006). **Primary health care nurse practitioners (PHC NPs)** are registered nurses who are specialists in primary health care and who provide accessible, comprehensive, and effective care to clients of all ages. They are experienced nurses with additional nursing education and have demonstrated competence to perform additional controlled acts by earning the designation Extended Class or RN(EC) (Nurse Practitioners' Association of Ontario [NPAO], 2006). Most PHC NPs have education in NP programs or speciality certificates that enable them to provide individuals, families, groups, and communities with health services in health promotion, disease and injury prevention, cure, rehabilitation, and support (College of Nurses of Ontario [CNO], 2006; CNPI, 2006). A *nurse* *practitioner* (NP) is an advanced-practice nurse, functioning within the full scope of nursing practice, and as such is not a second-level physician nor a doctor's assistant. Physicians traditionally provide primary care to clients, while *PHC NPs* provide a much more holistic level of service. NPs complement the roles of other health professionals with their advanced level of clinical skills, in-depth knowledge of nursing theory, and regulatory autonomy (CNO; CNPI).

Practice Sites

Community Health Centres   Generally, **community health centres** (CHCs) are established to meet the health promotion and treatment needs of a specific population (e.g., geographical area, specific culture or age group). Working in collaboration with physicians, and within a team of health professionals and allied workers and volunteers, the PHC NP plays a pivotal role in delivering a holistic and comprehensive primary health care service to individuals and families. This includes health assessment and diagnosis, therapeutic intervention, education, and community referrals to social agencies, physician specialists such as obstetrics and gynaecology, dermatologists, ear/eye/throat specialists, endocrinologists, urologists, and psychiatrists, and to other services such as social work, speech therapy, audiology, and occupational therapy.

Mental Health Clinics   People with chronic mental health conditions often have unique treatment needs because of their psychiatric diagnoses but also because of their medication side effects. Although part of the role does involve monitoring response to medications for psychiatric conditions, the main focus of the PHC NP working in an outpatient mental health clinic is to attend to the primary health care needs for preventive health care, health maintenance, disease prevention, and management of chronic medical conditions. Complementing the existing skills of a collaborative community team, which can involve family, friends, and medical and service providers, PHC NPs strengthen the individual's natural support system by addressing a broader range of factors, such as mental health promotion, education, prevention of mental illness, and treatment and rehabilitation efforts. Referrals may originate from the PHC NP to the physician or psychiatrist and likewise may return to the PHC NP from the physician and psychiatrist for continued follow-up and management after diagnosis and initial determination of therapy, including monitoring of weight gain and blood glucose levels along with health teaching for meal plans and exercise.

Community and Home Health/Palliative Care   NPs can work within a community and home health nursing agencies to assess and manage the health needs of stable clients with chronic conditions or those in the recovery phase of surgery or an acute illness. With advanced skills for assessment, they can also provide analgesic monitoring and care to palliative clients in the home and provide accessibility of care and support for family members. Working with RNs, LPNs/RPNs, PHNs, dietitians, and other allied health professionals, NPs can provide care to maintain optimum health and decrease transfers and admissions to hospitals. They can be a resource to HHNs and help to establish quality assurance protocols for monitoring long-term and palliative clients.

Public Health Clinics   Along with PHNs, NPs can meet most of the health care needs, preventive interventions, and health maintenance and treatment for individuals, families, and communities through different public health clinics (e.g., prenatal clinics, well baby clinics, sexual health clinics, etc.). NPs working in public health can assess, diagnose, treat, counsel, and provide holistic care that reflects the broad determinants of health according to the PHC model. Referrals to appropriate health and social support agencies and specialists are a large part of the public health NP's practice.

Family Health Teams or Collaborative Networks   Similar to community health centres, family health teams were established to address health service accessibility problems. Family health teams often employ several NPs who work under the direction of a physician to provide a scope of services comparable to a family physician practice.

Challenges and Solutions

The full integration of PHC NPs into the primary health care system is an evolving process that has achieved some success in recent years. However, some challenges still exist. There is a lack of a long-term plan to ensure that education of NPs is sufficient to meet the needs of Canadians if NPs are to assume their full scope and appropriate role in Canada's health system (CNPI, 2006). Currently, 23% of NPs have a graduate degree (CIHI, 2006a). The CNPI has recommended that master's degree preparation be required by 2010 or no later than 2015. However, there is a scarcity of data on the use of PHC NPs due to their relatively small numbers and diverse practice areas, and it is therefore difficult to justify with hard evidence requests for more educational opportunities or additional funding for more positions. Bridging programs for practising NPs without graduate education is being created, and the need for clinical preceptors and supervised clinical practice for all NP education would have to be met.

Underserviced communities would benefit from NP and physician collaborative practices, but there is a need for more permanent funding mechanisms to allow this to happen. More permanent, needs-based funding mechanisms through which communities can apply for NP positions must be in place. Ontario has made some positive growth in this area over the recent years with grants for NP services in areas with a physician shortage. Recruitment for these positions is a challenge because of the salaries that are required to retain qualified NPs.

NPs must be remunerated according to their level of accountability and responsibility. Currently there is a discrepancy in NP salary and benefits across jurisdictions; standardization according to established criteria would help ensure recruitment and retention of qualified NPs. Provincial underserviced-area programs should be expanded to permanently provide assistance to both physicians and NPs to ensure the provision of primary health care in underserviced communities through the development of permanent and sustainable funding mechanisms.

Increased public awareness of the NP role and their ability to assist with health care renewal and access to primary health care is essential to create the policy initiatives to support education and funding needs for a sustained NP workforce. Research on public opinion conducted in conjunction with the CNPI showed that only 60% of Canadians are aware of NPs but a strong majority (88%) support the integration of NPs into the health care system once the role is explained (Decima Research, 2005). The CNPI has recommended a social marketing plan to promote the NP as part of the solution to the wait time problem in the Canadian health care system. If NPs are to practise at their full scope as effective and efficient providers of primary health care, all members of the health care team, the public, and policy makers must work collaboratively with the NPs.

Further evaluation of outcomes and the evaluation of processes/practices that lead to positive outcomes will be required. A systematic review found that care delivered by NPs in various primary care settings resulted in higher patient satisfaction and quality of care compared with physician care, with no difference in health outcomes (Horrocks, Anderson, & Salisbury, 2002).

Despite the uncertainties that accompany the integration of any new player into the community health field, it appears that the future of the NP is bright, with numbers increasing by at least 18% in each jurisdiction (CIHI, 2006a). NPs are a valuable resource that can help provide improved and timely access to quality health care for Canadians.

The Nurse Entrepreneur

Nurse entrepreneurs are owners and operators of businesses that offer nursing services to the public. Directly accountable to the client, these nurses may provide the nursing services themselves, form partnerships, or employ others. They are self-employed professionals who organize, manage, and assume the risks of a business enterprise. As congruent with most CHN practice areas, they work independently and are self-directed and goal-focused. The roles of a nurse entrepreneur include both clinical and non-clinical services involving advocacy, health promotion, direct care, education, research, administration, or consultation. Clinical roles include working in advanced practice, such as nurse practitioners, clinical nurse specialists, or nurse therapists. Non-clinical roles include consultation, education, or research.

Being in independent practice requires that the nurse develop business expertise in addition to professional knowledge and skills. The Canada Health Act of 1984 requires provinces to provide universal coverage only for medically necessary hospital and physicians' services. This means that nurses in independent practice receive private payment for the health care services they provide. Private payment systems limit access to those who can afford to pay or have additional health care coverage. Charging a fee for nursing services is an issue that many nurses, including nurse entrepreneurs, struggle to reconcile. A public health insurance system that includes coverage for nursing services provided by nurses in independent practice would remove the financial barrier, but no such coverage exists at this time.

Nurse entrepreneurs may develop their personal practices to focus on patient care delivery and offer cost-effective treatment options such as foot care, therapeutic touch, and counselling. Clients who purchase these services are not limited to individuals but can include a wide range of people, groups, and organizations. Businesses such as large patient air-transfer corporations have been successfully launched and managed by nurse entrepreneurs (www.foxflight.com, 2006). Businesses that do cosmetic procedures such as skin lasering or injectable cosmetic fillers or Botox injections are owned and managed by nurses working under an external medical directive

Case Study

Linda graduated from a Canadian university with a BScN degree in 1995. Following graduation, she worked in a variety of clinical settings as a registered nurse, primarily in part-time and casual appointments. In the early years of her nursing career, Linda experienced employment insecurity. This required her to juggle several jobs to make the equivalent of a full-time paycheque. Linda became frustrated with her chaotic work schedule and was tempted many times to move out of a nursing career and pursue her other interest of being a teacher. Reluctant to do so, however, Linda made what she called her "last attempt to make it in nursing" and moved to a large urban centre in 2004. She found a full-time position working as a public health nurse in maternal–child health. The full-time position provided her with enough money to support herself while working in a clinical nursing specialty that she enjoyed. Linda also discovered that she has a particular skill in coaching new mothers about breastfeeding. Other nurses often seek her expertise, patience, and skill with challenging cases. A more organized work schedule makes it possible for Linda to pursue an MScN degree part time. Her career path includes becoming a lactation consultant with her own business.

Discussion Questions

1. Has Linda chosen the best path of education and clinical experience in her journey to become a lactation consultant? Are there any other credentials she will need?

2. What should Linda investigate prior to leaving her current position at the health unit to pursue her independent practice as a lactation consultant?

(S. Weiland, personal communication, November 3, 2006). The range and scope of opportunities are endless.

Historical Perspectives Nurses in independent practice are not a new phenomenon. Prior to the Second World War, as many as 60% of all registered nurses in Canada were self-employed in private duty settings for people in their homes (CNA, 1996). Following the war, the demand for hospital nurses escalated with the arrival of universal hospital insurance in the late 1950s. By 1989, very few nurses were still working in private duty as almost 85% of all registered nurses found employment in hospital settings. The 1990s, however, saw a resurgence of interest in private practice as nurses became increasingly frustrated with the bureaucracy of large health care institutions. While employment opportunities for Canadian nurses have often been cyclical, the employment climate changed dramatically in the 1990s, particularly in hospital settings. In 1995, the federal government made major reductions in federal cash transfers to the provinces for health care, education, and social services. Nurses in many provinces found themselves unemployed due to the major cuts in provincial health spending that resulted in layoffs and loss of full-time positions. Going into independent practice generated a great deal of interest for unemployed, underemployed, or retired nurses. Some nurses viewed independent practice as a way to exert control over an often chaotic and complex environment.

Professional Issues More nurses are becoming entrepreneurs as new opportunities for independent practice emerge. In all cases, nurse entrepreneurs are guided by legislation, provincial/territorial standards of nursing practice, and the CNA Code of Ethics for Nursing (CNA, 2002). Most authorities agree that having passion for your chosen area is essential for success as an entrepreneur (Cooper, 2005; Shirey, 2006). (See the case study on previous page.)

The nursing regulatory bodies of each province and territory permit self-employed nurses to offer any service that falls within the defined scope of practice of nursing and does not infringe on the legislated responsibility or the exclusive practice or controlled acts of another health discipline. A nurse who is considering independent practice should begin by reflecting on the competencies required, including personal knowledge, skills, experience, education, and a commitment to continuing education. It is also imperative that the nurse be familiar with the legislated and legal parameters of the profession, both federally and provincially.

Faith Community Nursing

A **faith community nurse** (FCN) is a registered nurse hired or recognized by a faith community to carry out an intentional health promotion ministry. Historically, faith community nurses have been referred to as parish nurses. The Canadian Association for Parish Nursing Ministry (CAPNM, 2004a) defines a **parish nurse** as a registered nurse with specialized knowledge who is called to the faith community to promote health, healing, and wholeness for its members. The term "faith community nurse" is used to convey the broad nature of the concept and to include the rich diversity of faith traditions existing in our multicultural Canadian society.

Faith community refers to a community of people who share similar history, values, and beliefs around their relationship with a higher power and with others in the world. They often gather for purposes of worship and to support one another. **Ministry** refers to the work of a person who represents the mission and purposes of a particular faith community, carries out his or her role in accordance with established standards, and is accountable to the public served rather than working in isolation or carrying out a personal agenda.

Historical Perspectives Faith community nursing developed from what is also known as parish nursing. Granger Westberg is considered the founder of parish nursing. The idea originated in Chicago, Illinois, in the mid-1980s but rapidly grew throughout the United States. Westberg (1999) noticed that the professional knowledge and skills of registered nurses made a significant contribution to the health of people within faith communities. FCNs were prepared to address physical, psychosocial, and spiritual needs, and often served as translators between the faith community and the health care system.

The idea of parish nursing began to develop in Canada in the early 1990s; by 1996, the first Canadian parish nursing practices were established. Since that time, interest in faith community nursing has spread across Canada. In 1998, the Canadian Association for Parish Nursing Ministry was established to bring together Canadians interested and/or working in faith community nursing. This organization establishes core competencies that include spiritual maturity and theological reflection and specific standards of practice for parish nursing and guidelines for the parish nursing education in Canada. The CAPNM standards were released in 2004 and are similar to the CCHN standards but encompass more of the spiritual elements of holist nursing to include facilitation of spiritual care as a separate standard (CAPNM, 2004a, 2004b).

Faith Community Nursing as a Subset of Community Health Nursing Faith community nursing is viewed as a subspecialty of community health nursing. Its practice adheres to the core standards of practice for community health nursing as follows:

- *Promoting Health* FCNs focus on promoting the health of individuals, families, and communities within and beyond faith communities to develop and maintain their personal and communal resources. They address the socio-political and spiritual issues that influence the health of the populations.

- *Building Individual and Community Capacity* FCNs strive to build individual and community capacity with in-depth community, group, and individual assessments. Community development principles are used to address health-related issues that arise in the lives of individuals and families and within the faith community as a whole. Evaluation of the impact of change on individuals and communities is ongoing.

- *Building Relationships* FCNs maintain professional boundaries within a setting where social and professional relationships could become confused.

Termination of professional relationships when appropriate is addressed in this standard. They conduct reflective practice and take clinical pastoral education and/or enrol in courses on theological reflection.

- *Facilitating Access and Equity* FCNs embrace the philosophy of primary health care, work toward universality and equitable access to available services, and act to influence the determinants of health. They often work with groups within and beyond the faith community to promote social justice, a faith community term for ideas similar to universality and equitable access.

- *Demonstrating Professional Responsibility and Accountability* FCNs work with a high degree of independence. They are accountable to their clients, to the faith community, and to the professional body that regulates nursing practice in their province. Professional nursing practice that includes appropriate educational preparation, continuing education, and adherence to professional standards of practice is of utmost importance in this complex and autonomous nursing practice.

Role and Functions of FCNs The client situations are often complex and require the FCN to carry out interconnected functions simultaneously These functions include integrator of faith and health, health educator, personal health counsellor, referral agent, trainer of volunteers, developer of support groups, and health advocate. Each of these functions is discussed below:

- *Integrator of Faith and Health* FCNs work to promote dialogue between faith and health, thus assisting people and groups to realize the interconnection. They work with people who are not currently experiencing difficulty to remind them that strengthening their spiritual dimension assists them to remain whole and healthy. A faith community nurse needs to be knowledgeable about the human spirit, spirituality, the spiritual dimension, and the commonalities and differences between spirituality and religion. This requires reflection on one's own spiritual development and continuous growth related to spiritual health. FCNs need skills in spiritual assessment and spiritual intervention, which may include appropriate referral to spiritual resources such as prayer, music, spiritual literature, worship, sacraments, healing touch, healing services, or meditation.

- *Health Educator* FCNs use every opportunity to carry out health education in formal, planned ways through group work and seminars. At other times, health education occurs spontaneously on an individual basis.

- *Personal Health Counsellor* At times, specific individuals and families within a faith community require intense, short-term interaction with a faith community nurse. FCNs act as personal health counsellors, meeting regularly with the individuals or families around a specific health-related issue in home or hospital visits. They encourage individuals to express feelings, identify their own health issues, explore possible solutions, and appraise the effectiveness of each solution.

- *Referral Agent* FCNs build relationships within the faith community and partner with agencies in the larger community. They link various community resources beyond the faith community to meet the needs of individuals, families, and groups as they arise.

- *Trainer of Volunteers* FCNs recruit, educate, and support volunteers from within the faith community to assist with the health ministry. They value the volunteers' contributions to the health and well-being of others.

- *Developer of Support Groups* The FCNs work to strengthen the existing social networks of the faith community to provide social support for individuals and families. **Social networks** are the relationships that people have with relatives, peers, co-workers, friends, and others within the faith community. **Social support** is derived from ongoing interactions within social networks. The results of being socially supported include feelings of belonging and acceptance, being loved, and being valued for oneself.

- *Health Advocate* Health advocacy involves supporting an individual, family, or group to take action when they are able and stepping in to assist with the action when they are unable or feel they have no voice. FCNs often assist clients to navigate through the health care system or other social systems.

Challenges in Practice Education and Research Faith community nursing is relatively new within Canada. Therefore, many challenges face this evolving type of community health nursing practice. One of the main challenges in practice is the lack of knowledge about the role both within and beyond faith communities. This challenge involves the development of a set of standards for nursing practice that are unique to this role while recognizing that some denominations may require certain theological preparation in addition to sound nursing education. In the area of research, a challenge is to demonstrate outcomes of faith community nursing practice when many of the benefits are difficult to measure. In Alberta, British Columbia, Manitoba, New Brunswick, Ontario, and Saskatchewan, faith community nursing is becoming well established. Early successes have been largely due to continuing education courses for nurses preparing for these roles, various faith groups embracing the idea of nurses on ministry teams, and health care organizations partnering to provide start-up funding for beginning faith community nursing programs.

Forensic Nursing

Forensic nursing is a small but growing field in nursing. Generally speaking **forensic nurses** provide care to victims of crime, collect evidence, and provide health care services within the prison system. It has many sub-specialty areas that are more formally recognized in continuing education nursing courses in the United States than in Canada. They include forensic nurse specialist, forensic nurse investigator, nurse coroner/death investigator, sexual assault nurse examiner, legal nurse consultant, forensic gerontology specialist, forensic

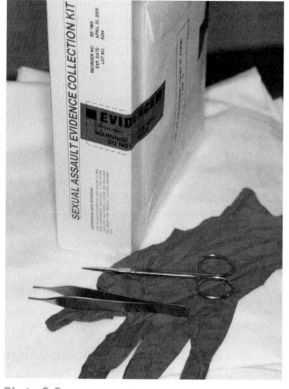

Photo 3.2

Sexual assault evidence collection kit.

Credit: PHOTOTAKE Inc./Alamy

psychiatric nurse, and correctional nurse specialist. Forensic nurses play an important role in the care of survivors of violence including sexual assault. **Sexual assault nurse examiners** (SANEs) are forensic nurses who are registered nurses educated in the nursing field of forensics. They respond specifically to calls relating to sexual assault or domestic violence in the emergency room setting and provide comprehensive care to sexual assault victims.

Sexual assault refers to any unwanted sexual act inflicted by a person. It is closely linked with family violence. (See Chapter 26.) SANEs provide primary health care to a variety of victims of sexual assault. Most sexual assaults involve an assailant known by the survivor (Statistics Canada, 2005). Johnson and Au Coin (2003) noted that 25% of all reported violent crimes were related to spousal violence, and 85% of the victims were female. Of all sexual offences reported to the police, 60% of the victims were children under 18 years of age; of the 2553 reported family-related sexual assaults, 79% of the victims were girls. While all women are at risk, women with disabilities have a much greater risk compared with those without disabilities and of a similar age. Although the number of sexual assaults has remained stable following six years of decline (Statistics Canada), CHNs must understand that sexual assault is an important public health problem in Canada. Sexual assault or violence is preventable. It is also a women's health and gender issue.

Emergence of Forensic Nursing in Sexual Assault Investigations
In the 1970s, a number of hospitals began to implement certification programs for sexual assault response teams and sexual assault nurse examiners (SANEs) as a result of unnecessary delays and repetitive questioning of sexual assault victims in local emergency departments. The sexual assault response team can consist of a SANE, a law enforcement investigator, and a rape crisis advocate. The SANE certification programs are offered in many community colleges or postsecondary education institutes. They provide specialized training to experienced nurses with an aim to increase their sensitivity and specialization in caring for sexual assault victims and to improve quality of forensic evidence collection. The training involves sensitization to issues surrounding sexual assault and domestic violence, recognition of the prevalence of violence in society, services offered by local agencies, the roles of police, history taking, documentation, correct use of the sexual assault kit, physical assessment, documentation in cases of violence, preparation for and appearance in court, the roles of legal and police forensics experts, prophylaxis for infection and pregnancy, and follow-up requirements. This educational path allows SANEs to work to the full scope of their role.

Role of Sexual Assault Nurse Examiners In the past, because the survivors were often medically stable with no visible injuries, they had to wait many hours before being seen by emergency room physicians because other, more urgent, clients had priority status. This added unnecessary emotional trauma to the survivors of violence. The SANE teams were formed to address the specific needs of those survivors of sexual assault and domestic violence at the emergency room immediately following an act of violence. Members of SANE teams are on call around the clock on a daily basis, and they respond quickly to calls from the emergency room for survivors triaged as clinically stable but needing assessment, treatment, and possible referral for matters relating to sexual assault or domestic violence. Response time is usually under one hour, often much less.

Forensic data collection is done for legal purposes. It is neither a prerequisite to nor a replacement for health care. The goals of forensic nurses are to provide for health care needs and to collect evidence for police in a way that respects clients' dignity, right to choice, and self-determination. The SANE therefore aims to return control to survivors very early in the assessment phase of the interaction and strives to maintain a client-led approach throughout the intervention. (See Photo 3.2.)

The SANE needs to be aware that survivors often have very little, if any, visible injury following sexual assault. Some injuries, particularly those to the posterior fourchette area, are very subtle and require careful examination in order to be detected. The examiner must provide empathy and be aware that survivors often feel guilty or not credible if no injuries are present and must take the time to explain the normalcy of this. Also, sensitivity to multicultural issues that may affect reaction to or reporting of sexual assault should be considered (Ontario Network of Sexual Assault Care and Treatment Centres [ONSACTC], 2002). Stereotypes relating to sexual assault must also be recognized and rejected by the SANE; these can taint the survivor–client encounter by closing doors to communication and by compounding survivor guilt and embarrassment relating to the assault.

Case Study

Jana, a sexual assault nurse examiner, receives a pager call from her local emergency room. Calling in for details, she learns that police have arrived with a 23-year-old female survivor of sexual assault that occurred 24 hours ago. Jana arrives to the emergency room 20 minutes later, obtains demographic and triage information from hospital staff, and prepares the examination room. She also ensures that the survivor has been triaged appropriately and is not in need of urgent medical attention. She then greets the survivor and directs her to a confidential room while police wait outside. Jana describes her role and what will occur in the coming hours they will spend together, and obtains informed consent for completion of the sexual assault evidence kit. She approaches the survivor in a non-heterosexist, non-judgmental manner and is sensitive to cultural influences.

Jana proceeds to collect a brief health history and detailed history of the sexual assault. She obtains a urine specimen and splits it into two containers: one for the evidence kit and one for immediate pregnancy testing. Jana establishes that the survivor has been immunized against hepatitis B and does not want HIV prophylaxis. With the survivor, Jana completes the sexual assault evidence kit and physical examination procedures with the assistance of another nurse. She also tests for HIV, syphilis, chlamydia, gonorrhea, trichomonas, and hepatitis B and C. At no time does Jana leave the kit unattended. She again ensures that the survivor is stable and not in need of immediate physician attention.

Once Jana learns that the survivor is not pregnant and has no known allergies, prophylaxis for pregnancy and sexually transmitted infections is offered with counselling related to side effects, risks, benefits, and correct use. She discusses her plan of care with the emergency room physician, following established protocol. Jana and the survivor proceed to safety and follow-up planning. The sealed sexual assault evidence kit is given to the police with copies of the documentation kept for Jana and for the hospital.

Jana files her report for her team supervisor then goes home three hours after being called in. She is aware that she may be called to testify in court about this case and feels confident that her documentation is precise, detailed, and clear enough to help her should this occur. She is also satisfied that she has made a difference in this survivor's life by quickly allowing her to regain control of her situation through facilitation of informed choice and self-determination.

Discussion Questions

1. What is Jana's main priority in this case?

2. Why can't Jana leave the sexual assault nurse examiner kit unattended?

3. What are the advantages of having a SANE collect forensic evidence instead of having a police officer do so?

Domestic violence and sexual assault occur in all cultural, ethnic, and socioeconomic groups at any stage of life. The incidence of domestic violence and sexual assault is not limited to male–female dyads; it can and does occur between same-sex persons and is often harder to disclose because of heterosexist attitudes in society. SANEs need to ensure that their vocabulary and approach do not convey heterosexist messages. The SANE must be non-judgmental and able to explain to survivors the implications of reporting sexual assault or violence as this is frequently a concern of survivors. Candid discussion about factors within and outside a survivor's control and possible consequences of reporting and not reporting incidents can assist the survivor in making informed decisions. The nurse also needs to understand reporting and court procedures in case prosecution does proceed, because nurse testimony may be required. Care must be taken to protect evidence, and documentation of assessment findings must be relevant, clear, objective, and, for the physical assessment, detailed.

FCNs must understand their scope of practice as well as that of collaborators, such as physicians, emergency room staff, police, attorneys, social workers, and crisis intervention workers, in order to utilize resources effectively. Knowledge of community resources, including referral requirements, costs, and specific services, is also required as the nurse acts as an initial liaison between survivors and these agencies. The forensic nursing role requires confidence, knowledge, and valuing of one's skills and limitations, as well as expert communication and assessment skills. Forensic nursing also requires knowledge relating not only to health assessment and treatment but also to legal procedures. (See the adjacent case study.)

ATTRIBUTES OF QUALITY PRACTICE SETTINGS FOR COMMUNITY HEALTH NURSES

As described by the preceding text, CHN practice is complex, diverse, and demanding. As in all nursing sectors, the degree to which community health nurses are able to realize their practice goals and aspirations is significantly influenced by the practice settings they work within and, more specifically, the supports provided in the setting. Practice setting attributes are also important factors in nursing recruitment and retention—as much an issue for community health nursing as for other nursing sectors. Recent literature has clearly identified attributes of quality practice settings and healthy workplaces that apply to both hospital and community-based settings and that promote nursing recruitment and retention (Cameron & Armstrong-Stassen, 2006).

The degree of influence CHNs exert over their practice environments is a key measure of a quality practice setting. Such influence is achieved through designated nursing leadership roles that contribute to senior decision making. For example, the appointment of a Chief Nursing Officer (CNO) for each public health unit has been a goal of Ontario's PHNs and has been achieved in some of the province's health units. There is little uniformity among home health nursing organizations in designating CNO positions, and if such positions are in place, they often lack visibility or legitimate influence on financial and management decision making.

Control over practice, or autonomy, is another attribute of a quality practice environment. Since PHNs focus on empowerment of clients rather than direct client care, they require an empowered work environment as a prerequisite. Similarly, working in isolation, in uncontrolled environments, HHNs also require support for their autonomous practice. These supports include access by CHNs to clinical experts for consultation and/or assistance in managing challenging clinical situations.

As community practice is usually provided by a nurse working alone in a client-controlled environment, personal safety is an important measure of the practice setting. Some employers provide staff with safety training by community police and some provide an environmental safety assessment tool for nurses to use on their first visit. Education regarding driving in urban, rural, and adverse weather conditions, as well as avoidance of injuries from needles or client lifting/transfer activities, is pivotal to workplace safety for CHNs.

Similarly, control over scheduling has also been associated with satisfying practice settings. Most community health employers provide flexible work environments where nurses adjust their own hours within the workweek to meet the demands for their service. This level of autonomy lends itself to nurses who can plan and organize their time effectively. The balance between "effort and reward" as measured by remuneration, recognition, and reward also requires attention by employers. For CHNs, strategies to address the balance between effort and reward include wage parity between nursing sectors, long-term contracts, payment or provision for communication devices such as cell phones, recognition for specialty knowledge and education, and opportunities for socialization as well as the provision of benefits such as sick leave and pension and minimizing unpaid work. Workload is another key influence on practice settings. Where staff shortages exist, CHNs and their colleagues in other sectors are particularly vulnerable to workloads that contribute to burnout and high turnover. It is clear that the establishment of quality practice settings for CHNs is pivotal to ensuring an adequate supply of CHNs to meet the health needs of the public.

TRENDS IN COMMUNITY HEALTH NURSING

Established and emerging trends in health care and nursing will continue to challenge CHNs to evolve their practice in order to continue to play a central role in the health care system and provide effective and relevant care to their clients. Several such trends are described below.

Multiculturalism

Changes in Canadian immigration patterns mean nurses are providing services within increasingly multicultural communities and to a more diversified clientele. (See Chapter 20.)

Sensitivity to cultural care needs is an essential competency. Communication challenges within a diverse community are prompting innovation in health teaching strategies, such as the use of multilingual health literature and pictograms in health classes or counselling sessions.

An Aging Society

Demographic changes and the increase in aging baby boomers will make geriatric care and health promotion for seniors more critical issues for nurses in the community. There is a stronger focus on prevention of chronic diseases as the lifespan increases.

Technological Advances

Technological innovation continues to advance and nurses need to be ready to embrace the resulting changes. (See Chapter 15.) In the community, technology such as voice mail, email, and wireless devices has enhanced connectivity. In some settings, nurses document in the client health record by way of laptop or handheld devices. For nurses working in the far North or rural outposts, it is now possible to send test results electronically and receive a diagnosis and treatment order without having to transport a client to a remote medical centre. The emergence of telehealth applications has reduced travel for clients in rural and northern regions by enabling medical and nursing specialists to provide assessment, diagnosis, and treatment protocols via distance technology. Tele-monitoring applications are providing new opportunities for remote assessments of wound healing, cardiac and respiratory status, or other health indicators, thus making optimal use of scarce nursing and medical resources. Telephone nursing services are now available in many regions of Canada, and nurses are identifying and evolving telehealth nursing competencies that continue to support a therapeutic nurse–client relationship.

Ethics

Increasing attention to identifying, analyzing, and resolving ethical dilemmas will continue to characterize nursing and health care, particularly in an era of cost constraint and limited resources. The nature of the community nurse's relationship with the client gives rise to unique ethical issues in such areas as nurse–client boundaries, access to health services, and risk and vulnerability of the infant, child, or isolated elder. Nurses need to know both their employer's policies and procedures related to ethical dilemmas and their regulatory college standards and mobilize assistance as appropriate. Nurses practising in public health often have to balance harm/risk and benefit in assessing appropriateness of outcomes to the community when making decisions regarding resource allocations between health protection and health promotion programs. (See Chapter 6.) For example, a communicable disease outbreak can take resources away from traditional parenting programs because of the need to respond quickly. Over time, these reallocations can erode the programs with the long-term benefits.

Changing Educational Requirements for Nurses

In many regions of Canada, the educational requirements for both RNs and LPNs/RPNs are changing. A comprehensive understanding of scope of practice for RNs and LPNs/RPNs will be increasingly important, as will collaboration that contributes to optimal client outcomes in all practice settings.

Evidence-Informed Practice

There is a growing emphasis on an evidence-informed approach to health care. Accordingly, best practice guidelines, critical pathways, and care maps will increasingly provide important foundations from which to individualize nursing care and promote consistency and optimal client health outcomes. (See Chapter 14.)

Nursing-Sensitive Outcomes and National Home Care Indicators

The ability to identify, measure, and benchmark the nursing contribution to health outcomes is emerging as an essential competency for all nurses. **Nursing-sensitive outcomes** are "those that are relevant, based on nurses' scope and domain of practice, and for which there is empirical evidence linking nursing inputs and interventions to the outcomes" (Doran, 2003, p. vii). Research has demonstrated that data collection on four nursing-sensitive outcomes (patient's functional status; pressure ulcers; falls; and symptoms of pain, nausea, fatigue, and dyspnea) is feasible by home health nurses, either electronically or manually (Doran et al., 2004).

It is anticipated that data collection by nurses related to their home care clients' clinical care needs, progress, and outcomes will soon be a routine component of practice.

At the organizational and system levels of home care, standardized data collection is also being implemented. The Canadian Institute for Health Information (CIHI) has recently developed a standard data set of home care indicators. These "Roadmap Indicators" include access to home care services, waiting times, health and functional status measures, clinical outcomes, and utilization and informal support. The indicator data will be submitted to CIHI's Home Care Reporting System (HCRS). The HCRS is a national, bilingual database of standardized clinical, demographic, and administrative and resource information for home care clients that supports quality improvement and accountability (CIHI, 2006b). The HCRS accommodates data from the Resident Assessment Instrument–Home Care (RAI–HC), a clinical assessment tool now widely used in Canada and around the world (Kwan et al., 2000) to assess the care needs of clients expected to require long-term home care. It is expected that these indicators will eventually be collected by every jurisdiction in Canada, thereby creating a national home care database about access, outcomes, and service utilization in home care (CIHI, 2006b).

SARS and Emerging Public Health Threats

The 2003 SARS outbreaks galvanized political will to address significant gaps in our public health infrastructure. There were 438 probable and suspected SARS cases in Canada and 44 deaths. More than 100 health care workers became ill and 3 died. In his comprehensive and compelling report, David Naylor referenced Benjamin Disraeli, whose words of 1875 were still as important in 2003 in reminding us that public health was the foundation "for the happiness of the people and the power of the country [and that] the care of the public health is the first duty of a statesman" (Health Canada, 2003). Naylor's report was followed by several others, creating an imperative for government action that responded to the many recommendations to strengthen the public health system in Canada. Table 3.4 illustrates the dramatic changes in public health supports before and after SARS. It provides evidence of the national awareness that now exists of the need to be responsive to potential public health threats ranging from bioterrorism threats to pandemic H5N1 avian flu planning. Nurses are now taking part in emergency preparedness planning education so that they can be leaders in supporting the community in the event of environmental disasters or pandemics. (See Chapter 24.)

Career Planning and Management

A fundamental requirement of a strong nursing profession is the engagement and retention of nurses throughout a long career. The vast scope of nursing roles and settings presents unlimited opportunities for nurses to thrive in roles that offer both challenge and reward. Cultivating the competency of career reflection, planning, and management will contribute to career growth and satisfaction and demonstrate nursing as a profession of choice.

Evolving Roles of Nursing Regulatory and Professional Associations

In most provinces and territories in Canada, a single nurses' association or college fulfills the functions of regulatory body and professional association. Regulatory functions include setting standards of nursing practice; identifying and monitoring educational requirements for the profession; assessing eligibility for registration as a nurse; receiving and investigating complaints about nursing care and determining appropriate discipline; and maintaining the register of nurses for that province/territory. Professional association functions include articulating and publicizing the role and contributions of nurses; advocating on behalf of public access to nursing services and a strong publicly funded, universal health care system; promoting excellence in nursing practice; and providing services to nurses such as educational courses and conferences, nursing position statements, discussion papers or other documents, recognition awards, and career counselling. All of the

TABLE 3.4
Before and After SARS

Before SARS	After SARS
Public Health protection in decline	Minister of State for Public Health appointed Public Health Agency of Canada First-ever Canadian Chief Public Health Officer appointed
No pandemic influenza plan	National, provincial, and local pandemic planning initiatives
No provincial disease control centre in Ontario	Ontario Centre for Health Promotion and Protection
Cost sharing for public health split 50/50 province and municipalities (Ontario)	Cost sharing 75/25 province–municipalities in Ontario
No HHR planning in public health	National public health HHR strategy
No national standards of practice for public health professions	National development of public health competencies for all groups of professionals
Community health nursing not recognized as a specialty and no national certification program	Specialty recognition for community health nursing and national certification program in place

Source: © Mildon, B. (2006). Used with permission.

provincial/territorial associations, with the exception of Quebec, are members of the Canadian Nurses Association (CNA), and CNA is the voice of nursing at the federal level in Canada. Every nurse practising in Canada must pay an annual registration fee and belong to their provincial or territorial regulatory nursing association, and in all jurisdictions except for Ontario the nursing regulatory and professional functions are fulfilled by a single organization. The College of Nurses of Ontario (CNO), the regulatory body for all nurses in that province, is completely separate from the professional organizations to ensure the perception of public protection over advancement of the profession. However, both provincially and nationally, there are also many nursing associations that nurses join on a voluntary basis and pay a membership fee.

On a national basis, these voluntary nursing associations include all of the groups associated with the CNA, such as the Community Health Nurses Association of Canada, the Canadian Orthopedic Nurses Association, and many others. These voluntary nursing associations exist for the purpose of linking nurses who are working in the same specialty area (e.g., strengthening the specific practice area through standards development, educational programs, or information sharing, and supporting members through benefits such as scholarships, newsletters, and research). Through these activities, voluntary nursing associations influence nursing, government, and practice-setting decision makers; create provincial, national, and international connections among nurses working in the same practice area; and provide leadership and professional development opportunities. Choosing membership in a voluntary nursing association is an important way to demonstrate professionalism, contribute to practice excellence, and positively influence the overall health care system.

Summary

This chapter has described the roles and practice settings of Canada's CHNs, with an emphasis on the areas of public health and home health nursing, and highlighted four more focused practice examples. It is clear that CHNs are key players in promoting the health of individuals, groups, communities, and populations across Canada. They have a unique role within nursing in Canada, epitomizing empowerment at all levels of their varied practice areas. (See Canadian Research Box 3.1.)

Canadian Research Box 3.1

VON Canada. (2005–2008). *Issues related to healthy workplaces and recruitment and retention of home and community care nurses: A synthesis paper*. Ottawa: Author. (Available from http://www.von.ca/pdf/special_projects/Healthy_Workplaces/Synthesis_paper_english.pdf).

Funded by Health Canada, VON Canada launched this project in conjunction with a National Advisory Committee in 2005 to explore how best to recruit and retain nurses in home and community care settings. The first part of the project was a literature review to examine the workplace environment for home and community care nurses and volunteers. This resulted in a synthesis paper that identified workplace satisfiers and dissatisfiers for home care nurses and differentiated them from those identified by hospital nurses.

The project found that the current nursing shortage in the Canadian health care system is a product of various

→

factors, including an aging population, fewer younger workers entering the nursing profession, an aging nursing workforce, increased job opportunities for women, and increased job dissatisfaction due to stress, burnout, and longstanding work cutbacks. Job satisfaction for home care nurses was related to their independent practice and one-on-one direct patient care such as teaching patients and their families within the home setting. There was dissatisfaction with the amount of paperwork and documentation, overtime, low salary, inclement weather, need to provide own transportation, isolation, and lack of professional peer support.

Community nurses were significantly older than hospital nurses; 46% of community nurses vs. 19% of hospital nurses had a baccalaureate degree, and community nurses were often paid less than their hospital colleagues. Nurses working in rural and remote Canada have a comparatively lower level of formal education than do nurses working in the urban settings. They had fewer professional supports and fewer opportunities to upgrade their academic qualifications.

The realization of successful recruitment and retention of nurses called for a new vision of health human resources. Nurses must be valued as assets rather than being manipulated to control costs. There must be policies for adequate and stable long-term funding; development of comprehensive strategies to address recruitment and retention; quality leadership, involvement of employees in healthy stable environments, quality care and positive outcomes for patients and their families; and a commitment to research, evaluation, and documentation to ensure that best practices form the foundation of enhancing existing workplace models and to develop new models.

Discussion Questions:

1. Discuss the reasons why innovative retention and recruitment initiatives are important for home and community care.

2. What are the key features of community health nursing that make the role satisfying to nurses?

3. What are the barriers and advantages to recruiting nurses into home care versus public health?

KEY TERMS

primary prevention
secondary prevention
tertiary prevention
health promotion
primary health care
public health nurse
social marketing
product
price

place
promotion
community mobilization
community development
home health nursing
home health nurse
palliative care
nurse practitioner
primary care
primary health care nurse practitioners (PHC NPs)
community health centres
nurse entrepreneur
faith community nurse
parish nurse
faith community
ministry
social networks
social support
forensic nurses
sexual assault nurse examiners (SANEs)
sexual assault
nursing-sensitive outcomes

STUDY QUESTIONS

1. Describe the variety of practice settings for CHNs.

2. List the multiplicity of roles a CHN may perform in all of the practice areas discussed in this chapter.

3. What are effective strategies a PHN may use to encourage healthy lifestyle behaviours in individuals, groups, or communities?

4. How do the HHN, SANE, FCN, and PHC NP incorporate primary health care strategies into their practice?

5. What are five key attributes of quality practice settings for CHNs?

6. Apply practice examples from any of the six CHN practice areas discussed in this chapter to the five community health nursing standards.

INDIVIDUAL CRITICAL THINKING EXERCISES

1. Identify five key roles that are unique to public health as opposed to home health care nursing, and explain how each meets the objective of achieving a healthier community.

2. Describe some examples from your own community where public health has empowered groups to achieve a healthier community.

3. What personal characteristics would draw nurses toward community nursing as opposed to institutional nursing?

4. Describe some attributes for a quality practice setting in the community and explain why they would ultimately enhance nursing outcomes.

5. Describe how you could apply theories and practices from other disciplines and sectors to any of the areas of community health nursing.

GROUP CRITICAL THINKING EXERCISES

1. Outline a comprehensive plan that a PHN may implement for reducing tobacco use among a school-age population in your community. Include the micro and macro strategies your team would employ and describe the collaboration you would have with community partners.

2. Identify strategies to promote an understanding of community health nursing roles among nurses in other sectors.

3. Debate the merits of legislation similar to the Canada Health Act that would provide standardized community care services across Canada.

4. What questions would you ask of a community health nursing organization before accepting employment in that setting?

5. In what ways are the diverse roles of CHNs described in this chapter similar?

REFERENCES

Alligood, R. A., & Tomey, A. M. (Eds.). (2006). *Nursing theory utilization and application* (6th ed.). St. Louis: Mosby.

Barbara, L., Paszat, L., & Chartier, C. (2006). Indicators of poor quality end of life cancer care in Ontario. *Journal of Palliative Care, 2*(12–19). Retrieved November 4, 2006, from ProQuest Nursing &Allied Health database.

Barstable, S. B. (2003). *Nurse as educator: Principles of teaching and learning fornursing practice* (2nd ed.). Boston: Jones and Barlet.

Cameron, S. & Armstrong-Stassen, M. (2006, October). *Factors affecting the work and career of nurses working in different sectors of community health nursing.* Presented at the Practice to Policy: Global Perspective in Nursing Conference. Hamilton, ON.

Canadian Association for Parish Nursing Ministry. (2004a). *Guide for parish nursing core competencies for basic parish nursing education programs.* Retrieved November 5, 2006, from http://www.capnm.ca.

Canadian Association of Parish Nursing. (2004b). *Standards of practice for parish nursingministry.* Retrieved November 5, 2006, from http://www.capnm.ca.

Canadian Institute for Health Information. (2006a). *The regulation and supply of nurse practitioners in Canada.* Ottawa: Author.

Canadian Institute for Health Information. (2006b). *Home care reporting system (HCRS).* Retrieved February 2, 2006, from http://secure.cihi.ca/cihiweb/printPage.jso?toPrintPage=services_hcrs_e&url=/en/services.

Canadian Nurses Association. (1996). *Commitment required: Making the right changes to improve the health of Canadians.* Ottawa: Author.

Canadian Nurses Association. (2002). *Code of ethics for registered nurses.* Ottawa: Author.

Canadian Nurses Association. (2003). *The value of nurses in the community.* Ottawa: Author.

Canadian Nurses Association. (2005a). *Workforce profile of registered nurses in Canada.* Retrieved July 5, 2007, from http://www.cna-nurses.ca/CNA/nursing/statistics/2002highlights/default_e.aspx.

Canadian Nurses Association. (2005b). *List of competencies for the community health nursing certification examination.* Ottawa: Author.

Canadian Nurse Practitioner Initiative. (2006). *Technical report: Nurse practitioners: The time is now.* Retrieved November 1, 2006, from http://www.cpni.ca/cnpe/index.asp.

College of Nurses of Ontario. (2006). *Acute care nurse practitioners.* Toronto: Author.

Community Health Nurses Association of Canada. (2003). *Canadian community health nursing standards of practice.* Ottawa: Author.

Community Health Nurses Association of Canada and the Public Health Agency of Canada. (2007). *Canadian Community Health Nursing Standards of Practice Toolkit.* Ottawa: Author.

Cooper, M. (2005). Becoming an entrepreneur. *The Canadian Nurse, 101*(4), 14–16.

Decima Research. (2005). *Public opinion research for the Canadian nurse practitioner initiative.* Retrieved July 5, 2007, from http://www.cnpi.ca/about_the_cnpi/np_final/index.asp?lang=e&.

Doran, D. M. (Ed.) (2003). *Nursing-sensitive outcomes: State of the science.* Boston: Jones and Bartlett Publishers.

Doran, D., Harrison, M. B., Laschinger, H., Hirdes, J., Rukholm, E., Sidani, S. et al. (2004). *Collecting data on nursing-sensitive outcomes in different care settings: Can it be done? What are the benefits? Report of the nursing and health outcomes feasibility study.* Retrieved December 8, 2006, from http://www.health.gov.on.ca/english/providers/project/nursing/eval_feasibility/report.pdf.

Government of Ontario, Child Development Branch Integrated Services for Children. (2002). *Evaluation of the healthy babies program project report Windsor Essex County 2001–2002.* Toronto: Applied Research Consultants. (NG265).

Health Canada. (2003). *Learning from SARS: Renewal of public health in Canada.* Retrieved December 8, 2006, from http://www.phac-aspc.gc.ca/publicat/sars-sras/naylor/

Health Canada. (2006). *About primary health care.* Retrieved October 27, 2006, from http://www.hc-sc.gc.ca/hcs-ss/prim/about-apropos/index_e.html.

Horrocks, S., Anderson, E., & Salisbury, C. (2002). Systematic review of whether nurse practitioners working in primary care can provide equivalent care to doctors. *BMJ, 324*(7341), 819–823.

Johnson, H., & Au Coin, K. (Eds.). (2003). *Family violence in Canada: A statistical profile, 2003.* Cat. No., 85-224-XIE. Ottawa, Statistics Canada: Canadian Centre for Justice Statistics.

Kwan, C., Chi, I., Lam, T., Lam, K., & Chou, K. (2000). Validation of minimum data set for home care assessment instrument (MDS-HC) for Hong Kong Chinese elders. *Clinical Gerontologist, 21*(4), 35–48.

Nurse Practitioners' Association of Ontario. (2006). *Primary health care nurse practitioner: RN (EC) designation.* Retrieved November 27, 2006, from http://www.npao.org/phcnp.aspx.

Ontario Network of Sexual Assault Care and Treatment Centres. (2002). *Sexual assault nurse examiner program*

(SANE). Retrieved November 26, 2006, from http://www.satcontario.com/.

Patry, L. A. (2006). Certification: Building on what you know. *Canadian Nurse, 102*(2), 17–21.

Public Health Agency of Canada. (2007). *Core competencies for public health in Canada.* Retrieved September 25, 2007, from http://www.phac-aspc.gc.ca/ccph-cesp/pdfs/cc-manual-eng090407.pdf.

Rew, L., Fouladi, R. T., & Yockey, R.D. (2002). Sexual health practices of homeless youth. *Journal of Nursing Scholarship, 34(2),* 139–145.

Shirey, M. (2006). Entrepreneurship: Turning your intellectual capital into tangible results. *Clinical Nurse Specialist, 20*(4), 179–182.

Statistics Canada. (2005). *Canadian crime statistics 2005.* Canadian Centre for Justice Statistics. Retrieved November 5, 2006, from statcan.ca/English/freepub/85-224-xie.2005.

Weinrich, N. (2003). *What is social marketing?* Retrieved November 5, 2006, from http://www.social marketing.com/whatis.html.

Westberg, G. (1999). A personal historical perspective of whole person health and the congregation. In P. A. Solari-Twadell & M. A. McDermott (Eds.), *Parish nursing: Promoting whole person health within faith communities* (pp. 35–41). Thousand Oaks, CA: Sage.

Windsor Essex County Health Unit. (2006). *Campaigns.* Retrieved November 24, 2006, from http://www.wechealthunit.org/campaigns.

World Health Organization. (1984). *Health promotion: A discussion document on the concepts and principles.* Copenhagen: WHO Regional Office for Europe.

ADDITIONAL RESOURCES

Websites

Association of Nursing Directors and Supervisors in Official Health Agencies in Ontario
www.andsooha.org

Association of Ontario Health Centres
www.aohc.org

Canadian Association for Pastoral Practice and Education
www.cappe.org

Canadian Association of Advanced Practice Nurses
www.caapn.com

Canadian Association of Sexual Assault Treatment Centres (CASAC)
www.casac.ca

Canadian Nurses Association
www.cna-nurses.ca

Canadian Nurses Protective Society
www.cnps.ca

Community Health Nurses Association of Canada
www.communityhealthnursescanada.org

Community Health Nurses' Initiatives Group
www.chnig.org

International Association of Forensic Nurses
www.forensicnurse.org

International Council of Nurses (ICN)
www.icn.ch

Metropolitan Action Committee on Violence Against Women and Children: Frequently Asked Questions About Sexual Assault
www.metrac.org/new/faq_sex.htm

National Association of Independent Nurses
www.independentrn.com

Ontario Network of Sexual Assault Care/Domestic Violence Treatment Centres
www.satcontario.com

Ontario Women's Directorate: Sexual Assault: Dispelling the Myths
www.citizenship.gov.on.ca/owd/english/publications/sexual-assault/myths.htm

Sigma Theta Tau International Honor Society of Nursing
www.nursingsociety.org

Women in Technology International
www.witi.com

Readings

Canadian Nurses Association. (2006). *Towards 2020—Visions for nursing.* Ottawa: Author.

Carson, V., & Koenig, H. G. (2002). *Parish nursing: Stories of service and care.* Radnor, PA: Templeton Foundation Press.

Ontario Women's Directorate. (2002). *Sexual assault: Dispelling the myths.* http://www.gov.on.ca:80/MCZCR/owd/english/publications/sexual-assault/myths.htm.

Registered Nurses' Association of Ontario. (2002). *What do I get for my membership?* Retrieved December 29, 2003, from http://www.rnao.org/html/id_mb_01.htm.

About the Authors

Liz Haugh, RN, BA, MScN, is the Director of Health Promotion at the Windsor-Essex County Health Unit in Windsor, Ontario, and is also an adjunct professor at the Faculty of Nursing, University of Windsor. She has more than 35 years of experience in public health nursing, is a past president of the College of Nurses of Ontario, and a current member of the provincial boards of the Ontario Public Health Association and the Association of Local Public Health Agencies.

Barb Mildon, RN, MN, CHE, is the Chief Nurse Executive and VP Professional Practice and Integration at Fraser Health Authority in Surrey, B.C. While President of CHNAC (2000–2004), Barb led the development of national standards of practice for community health nurses. The standards provided the foundation for the designation of community health nursing as a specialty practice and its inclusion in the CNA national certification program.

The authors gratefully acknowledge the original contributions of Linda Patrick, Lynn J. Anderson, Joanne K. Olson, and Sue LeBeau to the first edition of this content.

Advocacy, Ethical, and Legal Considerations

Elizabeth Peter, Louise Sweatman, and Kathleen Carlin

OBJECTIVES

After studying this chapter, you should be able to:

1. Describe the central values of Canadian nursing and how they relate to community health nursing.
2. Understand the relevance of feminist ethics and social justice for community health nursing.
3. Articulate and reflect upon the central ethical and legal issues in community health nursing.
4. Understand the political nature of ethical problems in the community.

INTRODUCTION

Community health nurses (CHNs) encounter ethical issues in all facets of their everyday nursing lives. Ethical nursing practice requires CHNs to be able to reflect upon critically their practice, make sound ethical decisions, and take appropriate action. These capacities must reflect the central values of Canadian nursing expressed in the CNA's (2002) *Code of Ethics for Registered Nurses*. These values are listed in Table 4.1.

The term *ethics* has been defined and used in numerous ways. For the purposes of this chapter, **ethics** refers to those values, norms, moral principles, virtues, and traditions that guide human conduct. Often, ideas that reflect what is right and good and what we ought, and ought not, to do are associated with ethics. Ethics is also a specialized area of philosophy. Moral philosophers study and reflect upon ethics and have developed formal ethical theories. These theories can be helpful in identifying, articulating, and analyzing ethical issues. The term **bioethics**, also defined as *health care ethics,*

TABLE 4.1
CNA Nursing Values
Safe, competent, and ethical care
Health and well-being
Choice
Dignity
Confidentiality
Justice
Accountability
Quality practice environments

refers to the study of ethical issues that are related to health and health care. Nursing ethics examines ethical issues in health care "from the perspective of nursing theory and practice" (Johnstone, 1999, p. 46). Bioethics and nursing ethics have made use of a range of ethical theories and approaches, including deontology, utilitarianism, casuistry, principlism, virtue ethics, and feminist ethics. It is beyond the scope of this chapter to describe all of these in a meaningful and comprehensive fashion. Instead, feminist ethics, along with several Canadian nursing documents that articulate the central ethical values and concepts used in community health nursing, will be used to frame the chapter, including the Canadian Nurses Association's (CNA) *Code of Ethics for Registered Nurses* (2002), *Social Justice ... A Means to an End, an End in Itself* (CNA 2006a), and the Community Health Nurses Association of Canada's (CHNAC) Canadian Community Health Nursing Standards of Practice (2003). Occasionally, insights from other perspectives will be identified and drawn in to add to the understanding of the complex issues CHNs face. Ultimately, this chapter, with its emphasis upon social justice and everyday ethical and legal concerns, will help nurses and nursing students to gain the capacity to reflect upon critically the multiplicity of ethical and legal dimensions inherent in community health nursing.

FEMINIST BIOETHICS

Feminist bioethics brings feminist perspectives and methods to bear on ethical issues that arise in health and health care (Sherwin, 1998). It is important to note that although feminism began as a response to the oppression of women, many feminist perspectives, such as feminist bioethics, address not only gender oppression but also other abuses of power, such as forms of oppression that are associated with race, class, ethnicity, age, disability, sexuality, and professional status within the health care hierarchy. As such, feminist bioethics is not a perspective only for or about women, nor is it anti-male. It addresses inequities that both women and men experience and it seeks to make visible and valuable caring practices, such as those of nursing (Liaschenko & Peter, 2003).

Feminist bioethics can be characterized by a number of generally common features. First, feminist bioethics is concerned with the ethical use of power in health care. It examines the broad political and structural dimensions of problems in health care and also the day-to-day use of power by health professionals. Power, in itself, is ethically neutral. How power is used, however, is of ethical significance. Worthley (1997) defines professional **power** as "the influence stemming from the professional position we hold. It is the ability to have an impact on the state of being of a person—physically, mentally, emotionally, psychologically, spiritually—in the context of the professional role" (p. 62). Nurses, and other health professionals, can use their professional influence to improve the health and well-being of individuals, but they can also use this professional power to deny individuals the right to make choices regarding their health.

Second, feminist bioethics tends to suggest that the ethic of care is a necessary perspective for bioethics, but it is not sufficient. The ethic of justice must also play a role. Gilligan (1982) identified these contrasting ethics in her research that compared the moral reasoning of men and women. She describes an **ethic of care** as reflecting the moral reasoning of women. It embraces the following moral considerations: the care and nurturing of self and others, the alleviation of hurt and suffering, the maintenance of relationships, and the emphasis upon contextual details of concrete situations. In contrast, the **ethic of justice**, which has been associated with the moral reasoning of men, is characterized by the following moral considerations: abstract rules and principles, fairness and reciprocity, and duties and obligations for self and society. Attention tends to be given in these perspectives to differing types of human relationships. The ethic of care tends to focus on close, personal relationships to others while the ethic of justice tends to focus on impersonal relationships or abstract issues involving groups or a society as a whole. It is important to note that although women tend to use care-focused moral reasoning more frequently than do men, both men and women generally use both justice and care considerations in their moral reasoning. Jaffee and Hyde (2000) conducted a meta-analysis to review the work on gender differences in moral orientation. They concluded that the care and justice orientations are more strongly related to context and content of moral dilemma than gender, emphasizing that both orientations are needed to represent moral life fully.

Third, feminist bioethics tends to view persons as unique, connected to others, independent, vulnerable and unequal in power (Sherwin, 1998). It focuses upon how persons are situated or positioned in society, that is, the entire context of their lives, including culture, history, politics, and socioeconomic status. This relational definition of persons is appropriate for community health nursing because CHNs often work with vulnerable individuals and groups who are socially disadvantaged. In working with clients, CHNs also emphasize the importance of their relationships with the clients they serve as a means of caring and empowerment.

Fourth, feminist bioethics tends to concern itself not primarily with crisis issues, such as euthanasia, but with issues of everyday life (Warren, 1989). Not all ethical issues or problems are ethical/moral dilemmas. **Ethical dilemmas** are "situations and issues that arise where equally compelling ethical reasons both for and against a particular course of action are recognized and a decision must be made, for example, caring for a young teenager who is refusing treatment" (CNA, 2002, p. 5). In this situation, a nurse would be compelled not only

to honour the choice of the teenager but also to protect his/her health and well-being. **Everyday ethics** in nursing is "the way nurses approach their practice and reflect on their ethical commitment to the people they serve. It involves the nurses' attention to the minor ethical events of the day such as protecting the person's physical privacy" (CNA, 2002, p. 5). These everyday ethical concerns also can include those related to advocating for clients, working with limited resources, the competence of fellow caregivers, and relieving human suffering. Feminist bioethics expands the agenda of bioethics by examining broad health care issues that have an impact on everyday practice, such as the need to examine the implications of the dominance of the medical model within the health care system and the broader Canadian society. It also recognizes that some perspectives, such as those of clients and nurses, have not been adequately brought into the dialogue and debate on ethical issues; nor have they been drawn upon fully in the development of bioethical theory.

FEMINIST BIOETHICS AND SOCIAL JUSTICE

Leipert (2001) suggests that community health nursing could benefit from a feminist perspective because this perspective facilitates critical thinking about power, gender, and socioeconomic structures, all of which impact significantly upon health. Fundamental to community health nursing is an understanding of the socio-environmental context of health that recognizes that basic resources and prerequisite conditions are necessary to achieve health (CHNAC, 2003). Gebbie (2001) also has discussed how feminism promotes collaboration with oppressed groups to create social change in a way that is consistent with health promotion strategies. Underlying these strategies is a view of health that goes beyond the narrow individual and disease orientation of the medical model.

Feminist bioethics also has the capacity to focus on not only individuals but also entire groups, because it goes beyond traditional individual-focused caring to include considerations of **social justice**. The descriptor "social" places emphasis upon the application of justice to social groups, such as the need to address population health and unjust social institutions and relationships. The experiences of individuals, from this perspective, are embedded within larger political, economic, cultural, and social contexts (Reimer & Browne, 2006). Social justice has been defined by the CNA (2006a) as "the fair distribution of society's benefits, responsibilities and their consequences. It focuses on the relative position of one social group in relationship to others in society as well as on the root causes of disparities and what can be done to eliminate them" (p. 7). It assumes that all societies experience broad, systematic oppression and inequities, such as racism, classism, sexism, and heterosexism, which affect some people more than others. Every individual contributes to this inequitable distribution of oppression and inequity, even if unintentionally, and therefore is responsible for contributing to the achievement of social, political, and economic parity. In this way, we are responsible not only for recognizing inequities and oppression but also for taking responsible action (CNA, 2006a).

Social justice is also important when situating the ethical dimensions of health care policy, such as home care policy, within a broad, political understanding of the role of health care services within societal structures. Currently Canadian home care services, because they are not covered by the Canada Health Act (1985), are often not adequately funded, leaving many vulnerable individuals without services. While most home care recipients are frail and elderly, increasingly children with complex medical problems are cared for in the home. This cost-shifting to the home and family has led to excessive demands being placed on unpaid caregivers, especially women (Peter, Spalding, Kenny, Conrad, McKeever, & Macfarlane, 2007).

Social justice is not just a means to an end or an approach to evaluate current circumstances. It has attributes as a desired result or end. Ten such attributes have been identified. (See Table 4.2.) They include equity (including health equity), human rights (including the right to health), democracy and civil rights, capacity building, just institutions, enabling environments, poverty reduction, ethical practice, advocacy, and partnerships (CNA, 2006a). When recognizing and acting on

problems of inequity in Canadian society, CHNs strive to achieve these attributes in their communities.

ETHICAL AND LEGAL ISSUES ARISING IN COMMUNITY HEALTH NURSING PRACTICE

A number of specific ethical and legal issues can arise in community health nursing practice. These will be identified and addressed by using the CHNAC's (2003) Standards of Practice to structure the discussion.

The CHNAC (2003) has identified five interrelated standards of practice that form the foundation of CHN practice. (See Table 4.3.) Standards of practice are broad descriptions of desired and achievable levels of performance. They are expressions of the minimum knowledge, skills, judgments, and attitudes expected of nurses. As such, they are considered authoritative statements that set out the ethical, legal, and professional basis of nursing practice (CNO, 2002). Failure to maintain these standards can lead to findings of professional misconduct and incompetence, termination of employment, and exposure to civil and criminal liability.

TABLE 4.2 Social Justice: Ten Defining Attributes	
Equity (including health equity)	Equity is founded on the just or fair treatment of all individuals, including equitable access and opportunity for all people to meet health needs and potential (CNA, 2003).
Human rights (including the right to health)	The *United Nations Universal Declaration of Human Rights* and the *Canadian Charter of Rights and Freedoms* defines these rights.
Democracy and civil rights	Democracy and civil rights define a social state in which all have equal rights and where sovereign power resides in the people, without hereditary or arbitrary differences in rank or privilege (Oxford University Press, 2004). Canadian civil rights are outlined in the *Canadian Bill of Rights*.
Capacity building	Capacity building refers to the strengthening of individual and institutional core skills, capabilities, insight, knowledge and experience through means such as coaching, training, technical support and resource networking (The California Wellness Foundation, 2001).
Just institutions	Just institutions engage in fair institutional practices as well as the just treatment of all individuals in institutions and institutional systems.
Enabling environments	Physical, social and political spaces and situations form enabling environments that support positive, sector-wide change, policy development and community empowerment.
Poverty reduction	Projects, programs and/or structural reforms of an economic, political or social nature that reduce poverty, increase the overall standard of living and/or increase the participation of the poor in social and political life (Weidnitzer, 1996).
Ethical practice	Ethic review boards and the CNA *Code of Ethics for Registered Nurses* (2002) define ethical practice for nurses.
Advocacy	This means the active pursuit of support for the rights of a person, including oneself, or a cause by means such as policy or system change (Adapted from Thompson, 2004).
Partnership	Partnerships are based on the equitable sharing of rights, roles and responsibilities among institutions and individuals in private, public, government, education, community or the non-governmental organization sectors (Canadian International Development Agency, 2002).

Source: Reprinted with permission from the Canadian Nurses Association.

TABLE 4.3
CHNAC's Five Standards of Practice

1. Promoting health
   - Health promotion
   - Prevention and health protection
   - Health maintenance, restoration, and palliation
2. Building individual/community capacity
3. Building relationships
4. Facilitating access and equity
5. Demonstrating professional responsibility and accountability

Standard 1: Promoting Health

CHNs promote health through (a) health promotion; (b) prevention and health protection; and (c) health maintenance, restoration, and palliation (CHNAC, 2003). These strategies can each raise specific ethical and legal concerns that require awareness on behalf of CHNs.

Health Promotion CHNs focus on the health promotion of individuals and communities in a variety of ways. The CHNAC (2003) Standards state, "Health promotion is a mediating strategy between people and their environments—a positive, dynamic, empowering, and unifying concept that is based in the socio-environmental approach to health... Community Health Nurses consider socio-political issues that may be underlying individual/community problems" (p. 10). Interventions can include facilitating community action, assisting in the development of skills, and increasing client knowledge and control over the determinants of health (CHNAC, 2003).

Liaschenko (2002) comments that much of the health promotion work that nurses have engaged in has not focused upon the material and socio-political conditions necessary for health. Instead there has been an overemphasis upon individual behaviour patterns. She explains that this may be the result of nurses working within a biomedical system that primarily values repairing diseased or injured bodies and not the social fabric in which bodies live. CHNs are also not always in a position to directly influence those socio-political factors, such as poverty, that they have identified as moral concerns in their work. There is a collective moral responsibility that goes beyond individual CHNs to bring about broad social and political change.

There are also potential moral harms in health promoting activities that need to be discussed. First, because health is a value-laden concept, CHNs can influence individuals to conform to social norms through health promotion strategies (Liaschenko, 2002). In other words, CHNs can unwittingly become agents of social control and medicalization. **Social control** is "usually conceptualized as the means by which society secures adherence to social norms; specifically, how it minimizes, eliminates, or normalizes deviant behaviour" (Conrad & Schneider, 1985, p. 7). The concept of **medicalization**, introduced by Zola (1972), refers to the social process whereby more and more aspects of daily life are understood in terms of health and illness. Many activities, such as madness, child abuse, and

alcoholism, were once considered immoral or criminal but now have been frequently redefined in medical terms. As a consequence, these behaviours now fall into the realm of medical treatment and control (Verweij, 1999).

Second, a possible moral harm of health promotion is its potential to create adversarial relationships between those who actively strive to improve their health and those who do not (Liaschenko, 2002). A danger exists that those who are not always trying to enhance their health through such things as diet, exercise, meditation, and so on may be viewed as morally weak and inferior. Taken to an extreme, this type of adversarial relationship, if it existed between CHNs and their clients, could compromise nurses' respect for clients' dignity. The ethical requirement for nurses to respect the inherent worth of the persons they serve is a fundamental ethical responsibility of Canadian nurses (CNA, 2002). Ultimately, health promotion activities are powerful tools that must be used with careful reflection as to their consequences for the health and well-being of individuals and communities. CHNs must be mindful of the social and professional power they possess as respected and trusted health professionals. An ethical responsibility exists to reflect upon whose good and whose conception of health is being promoted and why.

Prevention and Health Protection CHNs engage in a variety of strategies that minimize the occurrence of diseases and injuries and their consequences. These activities are often prescribed and regulated by mandated programs and laws, and can include education and services regarding such things as birth control and breastfeeding, disease surveillance, immunization, risk reduction, outbreak management, and education about communicable diseases. Social marketing techniques such as media releases and radio interviews may be used to deliver key information to the public (CHNAC, 2003).

While preventive and health protective measures can greatly improve the well-being of populations, they also are not without their potential moral harms. Some of these harms have similarities to those associated with health promotion in that they can further medicalization. Prevention and health protection information can weaken people's confidence and security in their health. Constant surveillance of one's body can be anxiety provoking and could possibly lead to an excess of diagnostic testing as well. These iatrogenic risks are of ethical concern because they can erode a person's sense of well-being (Verweij, 1999). CHNs must strive to find the right balance of providing information to protect their clients without unduly alarming them.

It is important to recognize that efforts to prevent disease and injury restrict the liberty of individuals, thereby limiting their choice and autonomy. For example, seatbelt laws and speed limits restrict the liberty of individuals, but they are needed to protect health. Other strategies such as communicable disease surveillance and reporting not only can restrict liberty but also can go against the ideals of confidentiality and privacy. Sound ethical reasons and legal authority must exist to impose these liberty-limiting strategies upon clients. In some instances, interventions are targeted to one group of people to protect another group's health, such as mandatory reporting of some communicable diseases. These interventions can be ethically justified if they fairly distribute benefits and burdens and limit burdens to the greatest extent possible.

The CNA (2006b) has adopted four principles developed by Upshur (2002) for ethical decision making about public health interventions that are a form of social control. These are the **harm principle, least restrictive or coercive means, reciprocity,** and **transparency**. (See Table 4.4.)

The first principle, *harm,* establishes the initial justification for restricting the liberty of people in a democratic society. It was developed by John Stuart Mill (1974), a utilitarian; he states, "The only purpose for which power can be rightfully exercised over any member of a civilized community, against his will, is to prevent harm to others. His own good, either physical or moral, is not a sufficient warrant" (p. 68). For example, CHNs would be justified quarantining individuals only if they had a harmful communicable disease, such as severe acute respiratory syndrome (SARS).

The second principle, *least restrictive or coercive means,* stipulates that the full force of governmental authority and power should not be used unless less coercive methods are unavailable or have failed. Education, negotiation, and discussion should come before regulation and incarceration (Upshur, 2002). The CHN, therefore, would not incarcerate cooperative individuals exposed to SARS, but instead would provide instructions to them regarding quarantining themselves safely at home.

The third principle, *reciprocity,* indicates that if a public action is warranted, social entities, such as a public health department, are obligated to assist individuals in meeting their ethical responsibilities. In addition, because complying with the requests of the public health department may impose burdens, such as time and money, on individuals, the reciprocity principle demands that compensation be given (Upshur, 2002). Quarantined individuals, therefore, should be compensated with money for lost income and additional expenses, such as childcare, and be assisted with things such as food while quarantined.

The fourth principle, *transparency,* refers to the way in which decisions are made. All relevant stakeholders should participate in decision making in an accountable and equitable fashion that is free of political interference or coercion (Upshur, 2002). For example, this principle indicates that policy development for controlling infectious diseases, such as SARS, requires that all potentially involved people—such as members of the public, health care professionals, hospital representatives, and public health and government officials—be involved in the process.

How the prevalence of disease is understood and explained by CHNs also has ethical implications. Krieger and Zierler (1996) describe two distinct theories that explain the interplay between social and biological factors that shape disease susceptibility and the public's health—the lifestyle and social production of disease frameworks. The lifestyle theory suggests that individuals choose ways of living that have health consequences. For example, promiscuity, prostitution, and shared and unclean injection drug use have been posited as lifestyle factors that explain the distribution of HIV/AIDS in a population. In contrast, a framework of social production of

TABLE 4.4
Four Ethical Principles for Public Health Interventions
1. Harm principle
2. Least restrictive or coercive means
3. Reciprocity
4. Transparency

Source: Upshur, 2002.

disease conceptualizes disease determinants to be economic, social, and political. The relative social and economic positioning of people shapes their behaviours and exposure to disease. With respect to HIV/AIDS, groups that are economically deprived and experience racial discrimination are at increased risk for infection. Gender-based economic inequities, for example, influence a woman's ability to determine the sexual use of her body. Prostitution may offer a woman a strategy for economic survival for herself, and possibly also her children, as opposed to being a lifestyle choice per se.

Without a conscious awareness of these differing perspectives, it is possible that CHNs could too easily place blame on persons who do not heed health information and acquire a disease. Alternatively, CHNs could view these persons as powerless victims of their socio-political and economic positioning, thereby absolving them from any responsibility for their health and absolving CHNs from any responsibility to provide information or other support to assist them in making health choices. Either extreme would not respect the dignity of these persons and would not promote social justice.

A more helpful perspective would put together these explanatory frameworks in a way that does not eliminate the possibility of choice, but situates it. Sherwin's (1998) notion of relational autonomy is helpful here. She describes how individuals are inherently social and relational beings who are significantly shaped by interpersonal and political relationships. Individuals exercise autonomy and choice within this web of interconnected and sometimes conflicting relationships. Options available to individuals are constrained by circumstances and the availability of resources. Pressure from significant others and social forces can also greatly influence decision making. For example, a young woman with limited financial means may engage in unprotected sexual intercourse with her male partner who refuses to wear a condom. She may understand the risk of unprotected sex, but "chooses" to have intercourse with him because she is financially dependent upon him and finds it difficult to say no to his requests for sex. Though she makes a choice, this choice is limited by her economic dependency and perhaps also by societal expectations upon women to sexually satisfy their male partners. Nevertheless, it is possible that future partners will be more receptive to her request and/or her economic situation may improve. Having health information regarding disease prevention in the latter instance could assist her in making choices that protect her health.

Health Maintenance, Restoration, and Palliation CHNs also provide clinical nursing, palliative care, health teaching, and counselling to individuals and families as they experience illness and life crises, such as the birth or death of a family member. In doing so, CHNs engage in a process of mutual participation with their clients in planning, implementing, and evaluating nursing care while maximizing the capacity of individuals and families to take responsibility for and manage their own care. Nursing interventions are wide ranging and can involve health promotion, disease prevention, and direct clinical care strategies (CHNAC, 2003).

This section of the chapter will address the ethical dimensions of several aspects of this multi-faceted CHN role, including community settings as sites of care, informed consent, family caregiving, and palliative care.

Community Settings as Sites of Care Providing care in the community can be challenging, because unlike hospitals, many community settings were not designed primarily for the purposes of caregiving. Because of the variability of settings, CHNs must often adapt their approaches and procedures and they must often travel significant distances to reach their clients. For example, CHNs working for the AIDS Prevention Street Nurse Program in Vancouver go where their clients are to give care. Not only do these nurses have established sites such as jails, detoxification centres, clinics, and drop-in centres, but they also go door-to-door in single-room occupancy hotels and make contacts on the street either by foot or by mobile van (Hilton, Thompson, & Moore-Dempsey, 2000). In a program in rural British Columbia, a street nurse also reaches out to marginalized people who would otherwise not have access to adequate health services. Many barriers in accessing services can exist for these people: homelessness, mental health problems, addictions, involvement in criminal activities, and the discrimination these conditions can bring. Using a truck as a mobile treatment centre and an office, the street nurse tests for sexually transmitted infections, helps clients fill out forms for financial assistance, and provides chlamydia treatment, pregnancy testing, and emergency contraception (Self & Peters, 2005). The practices of these nurses are working toward social justice because their goals reveal a concern for health equity, the right to health, the development of enabling environments, and advocacy.

However, CHNs and other community health workers often face a number of potential threats to their health and safety because of the diverse settings in which they practice. Potential hazards include violence from clients and others, tobacco smoke, pets, ergonomic issues (e.g., lifting patients), and physical conditions (e.g., poor lighting, temperature, broken stairs, snow and ice on walkways, etc.). Travelling from place to place also poses risks (Health & Safety Association of Ontario [HCHSA] and Workplace Safety & Insurance Board [WSIB], 2003). Here again, nurses have an ethical responsibility, one that is expressed in the CNA (2002) *Code of Ethics*. It requires nurses to value and advocate for quality practice environments that have the organizational structures and resources necessary to ensure safety, support, and respect for all persons in the work setting.

Understanding the meaning and impact of various places or settings is central to community health nursing because CHNs deliver nursing services where clients live, work, learn, worship, and play (CHNAC, 2003), not in hospitals. It is also consistent with feminist ethics, which attends to the importance of context and place in everyday moral life (Peter, 2002). MacPhail (1996), whose research explored the ethical concerns of Canadian CHNs, concluded that, "The most obvious and significant factor influencing ethical issues in community-based practice is the setting, the location or environment in which the nurses practice" (p. 50). This conclusion is not surprising, because different places/settings accomplish different kinds of work; have different values, operational codes, and philosophies; and are influenced and structured by different kinds of knowledge and power. These factors combine to influence a person's agency within a particular place or environment (Liaschenko, 1994). Thus, the experience of receiving and providing health care services cannot be overtly detached from the place in which it is received or provided (Andrews, 2002). Bioethics, including nursing ethics, has generally assumed that the hospital, not the community, is the setting of health care delivery, resulting in the neglect of many issues facing CHNs that are strongly shaped by the uniqueness of the settings/places in which they arise.

Special ethical considerations arise when care is provided in the home, because the home is a highly significant place that is imbued with multiple meanings, including personal identity, security, and privacy (Williams, 2002). As nursing services increasingly are offered in homes as opposed to hospitals, it is necessary for nurses to become mindful of the social and ethical implications of this change. McKeever (2001) aptly states:

> The devolution of healthcare to the home setting is changing the meanings, material conditions, spatio-temporal orderings, and social relations of both domestic life and healthcare work. Unlike institutional settings such as hospitals, homes are idiosyncratic places with aesthetic, physical, and moral dimensions that reflect their occupants' gendered, socio-economic, and ethnic characteristics. Little is known about the suitability of contemporary homes for providing and receiving extraordinary care, or about the effects of superimposing one major institutional order (healthcare) over another (the family) in light of the changes in structure and function that both have undergone in recent decades. (p. 4)

The potential lack of suitability of homes for the provision and receipt of care raises ethical concerns. Anderson (2001) suggests that assumptions have been made in health policy that we all have homes with family and friends readily available to provide care and that the necessary resources for care are there, such as bedding, laundry facilities, and so on. The privileged middle class may possess these things, but many others do not. Poverty and homelessness are increasing in Canada, thereby limiting the access to needed health services for large segments of our population. This potential barrier to the receipt of health services is of serious ethical concern. Nurses have a moral responsibility to promote social justice to ensure that all persons receive their share of health services and resources in proportion to their needs (CNA, 2002).

Informed Consent   As in all areas of nursing practice, CHNs must support and respect the informed choices of their clients (CHNAC, 2003). In order for CHNs to assist clients in making informed choices, at least two elements must be considered: the exchange of information between the client and CHN, and respect for the client's autonomy. These two elements are often subsumed in the concept of **informed consent**. Consent is a basic principle underlying the provision of care, such that without it a case for negligence and professional misconduct can be made against the nurse. The process of consent includes CHNs disclosing, unasked, whatever a reasonable person would want to know if they were in the position of the client. In other words, the nurse must give the information that the average prudent person in the client's particular position would want to know. CHNs must provide information about the nature of the treatment/procedures they are offering, including benefits and risks, alternative treatments, and consequences if the treatment is not given. The presentation of this information must consider the client's education, language, age, values, culture, disease state, and mental capacity. When clients provide their consent, it must be done voluntarily (i.e., without being coerced) and they must have the capacity (i.e., mental competence) to do so. Exceptions exist in which consent for treatment is not needed, such as in emergency situations and as required by law.

Family Caregiving   The family's role in caregiving, or informal care, has greatly expanded as responsibility for the provision of health care services has progressively shifted from the state to the family or individual. Like formal (i.e., paid) caregiving in the home, women also provide most informal care in the home (Canadian Policy Research Network [CPRN], 2005). The level of care provision is extraordinary, encompassing both personal and high-tech care. It can include assistance with activities of daily living, for example bathing, eating, cooking, laundry, cleaning, and transportation, and also the provision and management of medications, injections, IVs, catheterizations, dialysis, tube feeding, and respiratory care. These informal caregivers are often responsible for 24-hour care with little available public support and often with inadequate training for the responsibilities they have been expected to assume (Canadian Association of Retired Persons [CARP], 1999; CPRN, 2005). They have been reported to have an increased rate of morbidity and mortality (Shultz & Beach, 1999).

The transfer of caregiving responsibilities to family caregivers raises a number of ethical concerns. CHNs have a responsibility to promote and preserve the health and well-being of their clients. Because persons are relational in nature, nurses also have a similar responsibility to a client's family. At times, it may be somewhat difficult to determine who is or should be the focus of care. The evidence cited above illustrates that the health and well-being of clients may be threatened when caregivers are stressed and inadequately educated for their role. Moreover, CHNs, when delegating responsibilities to family caregivers, may be compromising safe, competent, and ethical care in situations where these caregivers do not have adequate support or resources. Choice is also limited because clients may have no other options than to provide and receive care at home. Ultimately, however, the source of these

ethical problems lies outside of the nurse–client relationship. It is important to recognize that the situations of both CHNs and their clients are the result of broader political forces and agendas that have limited the availability of resources in order to reduce costs. The CNA (2002) *Code of Ethics* addresses the importance of nurses to uphold principles of justice and equity to ensure that persons gain access to a fair share of health services and resources that is of their choosing. Advocacy for clients is one way for CHNs to promote justice. Advocating change for clients would also improve the health and well-being of CHNs because it would lessen the frequency of nurses practising in a way that compromises their ethical ideals.

Canadian Research Box 4.1

Carnevale, F. A., Alexander, E., Davis, M., Rennick, J., & Troini, R. (2006). Daily living with distress and enrichment: The moral experience of families with ventilator-assisted children at home. *Pediatrics, 117*(1), e48–e60.

This Canadian study explored the moral dimensions of family experiences of life with children who require assisted ventilation at home. Twelve families in Quebec were recruited into this qualitative study. Four of the children received ventilation via tracheotomies, while the remaining eight received ventilation via face masks. Seven of these latter children received ventilation only at night. Six principal themes were identified: (1) Confronting parental responsibility: the responsibility for the child's care was experienced as stressful and occasionally overwhelming. (2) Seeking normality: families made significant efforts toward normalizing their lives to resemble those of "normal" families. (3) Conflicting social values: families were offended by reactions they received in their communities that made them believe their child's life was devalued and not worth sustaining. (4) Living in isolation: needs for respite could not be met by extended family or the health care system because of the complexity of their child's medical needs. (5) What about the voice of the child? The children were generally silent when asked to describe their experience with the exception that some described their ventilators as good things that helped them breathe better. (6) Questioning the moral order: parents described their lives as unfair, questioning how good and bad things are determined in the world. Despite the difficulties experienced by these families, the parents also described the deep enrichments and rewards they experienced living with their children. Institutionalizing, or "disconnecting" them from ventilation, which would result in the child's death, would eliminate the distress but also the enrichment.

Discussion Questions:

1. What ethical concerns are raised by the findings of this research?

2. How could advocacy play a role, both at home and prior to hospital discharge, in supporting families with children who require ventilation?

Palliative Care A very special and increasingly frequent part of a CHN's practice is palliative care. Although most deaths occur in institutions, many people are now spending the last days of their lives at home. In fact, the *First Ministers' Accord on Health Care Renewal* (First Ministers of Canada, 2003) has identified palliative home care as a priority area. Though performing palliative care is extremely rewarding, it can also be stressful for the CHN, the client, and the family. This intimate area of practice is one in which respecting a client's dignity and right to choice may be difficult for some CHNs. The philosophy of palliative care is holistic and client-centred. Each CHN may hold his or her own values regarding end-of-life care practices, such as withholding cardiopulmonary resuscitation (DNR) and other treatments, artificial nutrition and hydration, pain control, and assisted suicide or euthanasia (both illegal in Canada). When these do not accord with the choices made by clients or their families, ethical dilemmas may arise. Clients often have cultural and religious practices or rituals that are important to them around the time of death. For example, a Catholic client may ask for a priest to administer the Sacrament of the Sick, and some religions have restrictions on who may care for the body after death. Respecting and facilitating these customs are part of the CHN's care.

One of the most important aspects of palliative care is relief of pain. Promoting the client's health and well-being includes the imperative to provide for the client's comfort. Some CHNs may have moral reservations about advocating for or administering adequate amounts of pain medication. They may worry that they are causing the client's death. Yet, ethically, giving comfort at the end of life is part of effective, dignity-preserving care. The Canadian Senate in its report *Quality End-of-Life Care: The Right of Every Canadian* (2000) recognizes that providing pain control may also shorten life and recommends the clarification of the Criminal Code so that both the public and health professionals can learn that this is an acceptable and legal practice. The Senate also recommends increased training for health care professionals in pain control. It is up to CHNs working in this area of practice to keep up to date. Adequate pain control means not only giving an appropriate dosage of medication but also having a plan in place so that the clients gets the medication when it is needed, that is, without having to wait for a doctor's order or pharmacy delivery at the last minute.

Though clients have the right to make informed choices about their care, as their illnesses progress they often become unable to make decisions (incapable). When a client cannot understand and appreciate the consequences of his or her choices, a substitute decision maker, usually the next of kin, steps in to make decisions for the person. CHNs need to be aware of the laws in their province or territory regarding the process for substitute decision makers. When clients and their families or substitute decision makers have discussed the client's preferences for treatment or withholding treatment, the substitute decision maker is able to make decisions based on what the client has wished. One of the ways that clients can communicate their wishes for care is by means of an **advance directive** (living will). An advance directive contains a person's wishes regarding future health care decisions. Advance directives are not only for people who are terminally ill. Anyone may stipulate what medical treatments they will accept or reject in certain situations. It is used only if the person becomes incapable of making choices. The advantage of an advance directive is that it gives a person an opportunity to express wishes about treatments such as cardiopulmonary resuscitation (CPR), artificial feeding, and pain control while he or she is capable of doing so. Advance directives, however, cannot substitute for communication among patients, their families, and their caregivers.

An advance directive contains two sections. The instructional directive sets out wishes for treatment. For example, a person may state that if she becomes terminally ill, she does not want antibiotics for an infection. Another person may stipulate that he does not want to be transferred to hospital in a crisis. The second section, the proxy directive, is a power of attorney for personal care. This means that a person may designate one or more substitute decision makers for health care. This could be a family member or a friend but should be someone who knows the person well and is comfortable carrying out his or her wishes. Each section of an advance directive may exist separately; wishes concerning treatment may be set down without naming a proxy, or a proxy may be named without making any stipulations about treatment.

Standard 2: Building Individual/ Community Capacity

CHNs work collaboratively with individuals/communities when building individual and community capacity. CHNs begin where individuals and communities are, helping them to identify relevant health issues and to assess their strengths and resources. CHNs use strategies that involve advocacy and empowerment (CHNAC, 2003). The CHNAC (2003) has described **empowerment** in the following way: "Community Health Nurses recognize that empowerment is an active, involved process where people, groups, and communities move towards increased individual and community control, political efficacy, improved quality of community life, and social justice" (p. 6).

Schroeder and Gadow (1996) propose an **advocacy** approach to ethics and community health that embraces the character of the CHNAC's (2003) perspective on empowerment. Their ethic of advocacy calls for the development of partnerships between CHNs, other professionals, and community members to enhance community self-determination. In these relationships, CHNs can help a community to discern its values, needs, and strengths in the form of a unique and encompassing health narrative. The goal of the relationship is "improved community health as defined by the members of the community rather than as defined by the professional" (p. 79). Communities are experts regarding their own health. They are not deviants in need of the normalizing efforts of professionals. Advocacy also requires that all persons within a community are heard and represented, not just those with power or authority (Schroeder & Gadow, 1996).

Actions based on empowerment and advocacy foster the everyday ethical practice of CHNs. Empowerment and advocacy enhance the choices and health and well-being of communities because they draw on a community's fundamental strengths and needs without the values of others being imposed upon them. CHNs can exercise their professional power ethically in a manner that promotes, rather than restricts, the expression of community choices.

For example, CHNs designed the Elderly In Need (EIN) Project, an action research project conducted in a predominantly French-speaking urban community in the Ottawa region. Over a three-year period, CHNs linked with community groups and agencies to make contact with frail and isolated older persons living at home. At an individual level, the CHNs and the older persons developed contractual relationships through which self-care was promoted and supportive ties were fostered. At a community level, the CHNs worked with community groups, such as churches, social committees, clubs, and home support agencies, to strengthen outreach to these older persons and to create initiatives that would strengthen community support for older persons more generally. Together these interventions reduced the social isolation and dependency of these older persons and built community capacity (Moyer, Coristine, MacLean, & Meyer, 1999).

Standard 3: Building Relationships

The CHNAC's (2003) standards describe how CHNs establish and nurture caring relationships with individuals and communities that promote maximum participation and self-determination. They state, "Caring involves the development of empowering relationships, which preserve, protect, and enhance human dignity. CHNs build caring relationships based on mutual respect and on an understanding of the power inherent in their position and its potential to impact on relationships and practice" (CHNAC, 2003, p. 12). CHNs must build a network of relationships with many others, including clients, groups, communities, and organizations.

In building relationships, CHNs must recognize the uniqueness of their own attitudes, beliefs, and values regarding health and also those of their clients. They must also maintain professional boundaries while involving and trusting clients as full partners in the caring relationship. Maintaining professional boundaries can become particularly challenging in the home environment, where nurse and clients often spend sustained periods of time together in relative isolation (CHNAC, 2003). A **professional boundary** in the nurse–client relationship has been defined as, "the point at which the relationship changes from professional and therapeutic to non-professional and personal. Crossing a boundary means the care provider is misusing the power in the relationship to meet his/her own personal needs, rather than the needs of the client, or behaving in an unprofessional manner with the client" (CNO, 2006, p. 4). In other words, the CHN must be cautious that the focus of the relationship remains on

meeting the needs of the client and not on the CHN's own needs. Nevertheless, relationships need not be distant and entirely clinical in nature, given they are often developed in familial settings within home and community.

The caring aspects of the CHN's work reflect some of the fundamental elements of nursing ethics. In recent years, much emphasis has been placed upon the caring nurse–client relationship as foundational to nursing ethics. A caring approach has merit in that it emphasizes the moral importance of reducing human suffering and the relational aspect of nursing practice. Nevertheless, an approach based solely on caring has limitations in that without moral obligation, social justice, and attention to political structures, caring relationships can be exploitative or unfairly partial (Peter & Morgan, 2001). In other words, CHNs require other elements in their moral repertoire beyond caring, such as the promotion of social justice through advocacy, that can assist them in focusing not only upon the health needs of those immediately connected to them, but also upon those who are more distant.

The AIDS Prevention Street Nurse Program in Vancouver exemplifies the importance of building relationships that involve both caring and advocacy in the work of CHNs. These street nurses work with diverse populations, including hard-to-reach and high-risk street-involved adults and youth, to prevent HIV and STI within a broader mandate of harm reduction and health promotion. At the core of their work is their capacity to reach marginalized populations and form trusting relationships with them. These connections are fostered through the nurses' accessibility, consistency, and flexibility and through their non-threatening, nonjudgmental approach. Without these nursing relationships, these nurses' roles in promoting health and reducing harm would not be possible. These roles involve a wide range of activities, from the provision of condoms, bleach, and clean needles to counselling, crisis intervention, and wound care. Through these relationships, these CHNs also help clients gain access to mainstream services and STI and HIV testing (Hilton, et al., 2000).

Standard 4: Facilitating Access and Equity

CHNs collaboratively identify and facilitate universal and equitable access to available health care services and the socioeconomic, social, and physical environmental determinants of health. A number of strategies are employed by CHNs, including advocating for appropriate resource allocation; ensuring access for vulnerable populations, such as the poor, elderly, isolated, and illiterate, through such strategies as home visits, outreach, and case finding; advocating for healthy public policy by participating in legislative and policy making activities; and taking action on identified service gaps and accessibility problems (CHNAC, 2003).

It is through the activities of facilitating access and equity that CHNs strive for social justice. CHNs must take into consideration that social factors such as age, sexual orientation, and socioeconomic status restrict equitable access and distribution of health services and determinants of health. Their activities can be at the local or global level and can entail promoting awareness and action regarding human rights, homelessness, poverty, unemployment, stigma, and so on.

Achieving social justice is extremely difficult. Bayer (2000) describes how the ultimate causes of human suffering and premature death are poverty, inequality, and disregard for fundamental human rights. Therefore, he argues, improvements in health status often can come only with radical social change. Bayer also states, however, that because "public health officials rarely wield the requisite instruments of power, they can only fulfill their mission as advocates for social transformation" (p. 1838). Bayer has termed this perspective "public health nihilism" because public health officials can do so little to alter existing patterns of morbidity and mortality in the absence of social change. Bayer's perspective illustrates well the link between ethics and power. It is important to recognize that small change is nevertheless important in working toward social justice. Two examples of community health professionals facilitating access and equity will be described below to illustrate this possibility.

Lisa Brown, a mental health nurse, is the founder and executive director of Workman Arts (WA) at the Centre for Addiction and Mental Health in Toronto. She was inspired and challenged by the talents of her clients and began to promote their creative expression through theatre. WA employs both professional actors and people who receive mental health services. The mission statement of Workman Arts states, "Workman Arts will promote individuals' well being, expand public awareness of mental health issues and enhance the quality of life in the Province of Ontario by providing to people who receive mental health and addiction services, to artists and to others, opportunities for creative expression through professional theatre and other arts activities" (Workman Arts, 2006). The activities of the WA foster social justice because they promote health equity by helping and advocating for people with mental illnesses, an often marginalized group, to access some of the determinants of health such as employment and income. In doing so, they reduce poverty and build the capacity of vulnerable people.

The Public Health Alliance for Lesbian, Gay, Bisexual, Transsexual, Transgender, Two Spirit, Intersex, Queer and Questioning Equity (PHA for LGBTIQ Equity), a subcommittee of the Ontario Public Health Association (OPHA), is another example of CHNs promoting social justice. The oppression of gay men, lesbians, and bisexual, transsexual, and transgender persons can lead to significant health impacts, such as depression, suicide, homelessness, substance abuse, the transmission of life-threatening infections, and violence. Many public health professionals offer care; however, they are often inexperienced, uninformed, or uncomfortable with the diverse experiences and situations of these individuals. In addition, the lack of acknowledgement of the holistic nature of LGBT issues across the lifespan limits the possibility of consistently providing accessible and appropriate services. The goals of the PHA include the elimination of heterosexism and homophobia in Ontario health units and community agencies, the formation of accessible and inclu-

sive health services, and the development of communities and organizations that will support and celebrate sexual orientations and diversity. Specific activities include creating opportunities for social support, and providing education, research, and programming. In doing so, the PHA recognizes that oppression related to sexual identity is a determinant of health and strives to promote access and equity (Duncan, et al., 2000).

Standard 5: Demonstrating Professional Responsibility and Accountability

CHNs work with a high degree of independence and, like all nurses, they are accountable for the quality of their own practice and at times are also accountable for the care and services others provide. In demonstrating accountability, CHNs must adhere to regulatory standards, federal and provincial/territorial professional standards, laws, and codes of ethics. They have a responsibility to be knowledgeable and competent and must also help others around them, such as colleagues and students, to develop and maintain competence (CNA, 2002; CHNAC, 2003).

Increasingly, there has been attention given to the legal and ethical responsibility of nurses and other health care professionals to keep personal health information private and confidential. At both the federal and provincial/territorial levels privacy legislation has been developed, or is in the process of being developed. Because there are some variations across the country in terms of both the specifics of this legislation and its implementation within organizations, readers are urged to examine privacy regulations within their province/territory and employing organization.

A framework has been developed by Health Canada (2005) that provides CHNs with some guidelines. It summarizes a key principle underlying its provisions in the following way:

> The collection, use and disclosure of health information is to be carried out in the most limited manner, on a need-to-know basis and with the highest degree of anonymity possible in the circumstances. The Framework also recognizes that privacy is a consent-based right and, unless otherwise stated in legislation, the individual's consent must be obtained for any collection, use and disclosure of personal health information. In keeping with current practices within the health care sector, an implied knowledgeable consent model is proposed for the collection, use and disclosure of personal health information within the circle of care. (p. 2)

In terms of community nursing practice, CHNs must ensure that utmost care be exercised when disclosing health information. Under usual circumstances, CHNs share this information with other team members within their organization only when needed, and they must gain the consent of clients to share this information elsewhere.

There are, however, exceptions in which information can be disclosed without consent, including court order or subpoena and to prevent serious harm or reduce significant risk to a person or a group of persons, such as in an emergency situation (Health Canada, 2005). The most common exception in the practice of CHNs is the legal requirement to report child abuse and some infectious diseases. There are also less common situations in which CHNs could encounter individuals who disclose information that reveals a client is a threat to others. In a well-known California case, a psychologist did not warn the intended victim that one of his clients was repeatedly threatening to kill his girlfriend (the intended victim). The court held that the psychologist ought to have warned the girlfriend because he had reasonable grounds to believe that she would be harmed (*Tarasoff* v. *Regents of the University of California*, 1976). In a Canadian case, Mr. Trikha (*Wendan v. Trikha*, 1992), a voluntarily admitted psychiatric patient, eloped from hospital. He drove a car at high speed through a red light, crashing into Ms. Wendan, who suffered severe injuries. In this case, however, the psychiatrist was under no obligation to warn, because there was no way to foresee that Mr. Trikha would pose a threat to himself or others. The general principle is that when nurses are aware that a client represents serious and probable danger to the well-being of another, they owe a duty of care to take reasonable steps to protect such persons—that is, to warn the third party. This principle is supported by the CNA (2002) *Code of Ethics*, which indicates that nurses may disclose information if there is substantial risk of serious harm to the person or to other persons.

Professional Competence When CHNs do not practise competently there may be allegations of negligence made against them. These situations are very stressful for nurses, and it is important to know what negligence comprises in Canadian law. There are four key elements that must be proven to make a finding of negligence: (a) that there was a relationship between the person bringing the claim (i.e., plaintiff, e.g., client, family) and the person being sued (i.e., defendant, e.g., nurse), (b) that the defendant breached the standard of care, (c) that the plaintiff suffered a harm, and (d) that the harm suffered was caused by the defendant's breach of the standard of care.

A nurse–client relationship is usually established from the instant the nurse offers assistance and the client accepts it (Grant & Ashman, 1997). A duty of care is established when a nurse owes a duty to another—the nature and extent will depend on the circumstances. The standard of care has been legally defined as bringing a reasonable degree of skill and knowledge and exercising a degree of care that could reasonably be expected of a normal prudent practitioner of the same experience and standing (*Crits* v. *Sylvester*, 1956). The determination of the standard of care is often based on professional standards, such as those set by regulatory bodies and professional associations, for example CHNAC. Breaches of standard of care often stem from an action the nurse should have done (i.e., omission) or an action that the nurse did negligently (i.e., commission). The mere breach of the standard of care, however, is insufficient to support a negligence claim. There must be harm suffered that was reasonably foreseeable from the breach and there must be a causal connection between the harm suffered and the nurse's conduct.

CHNs, either individually or in partnership with others, also have the responsibility to take preventive and/or correc-

Canadian Research Box 4.2

Oberle, K., & Tenove, S. (2000). Ethical issues in public health nursing. *Nursing Ethics, 7*(5), 425–438.

The purpose of this study was to identify ethical issues experienced by Canadian CHNs. This study incorporated an exploratory descriptive design involving 22 CHNs, 11 in rural and 11 in urban settings. Nurses were asked to describe a frequently recurring ethical problem. Additional questions were focused on determining what support nurses received when they encountered ethical problems and how they resolved those problems.

Five major themes were identified. The first was relationships with health care professionals. Both intraprofessionally and interprofessionally, CHNs struggled with giving the best information and optimal practice when the practices of colleagues were suboptimal or when they were not providing the best information to clients. In short, it was difficult for these nurses to balance the responsibility to maintain standards and to preserve important working relationships. The second major theme concerned system issues. CHNs expressed moral concerns related to their ability to optimize client welfare in a system that both supported and constrained them. Specific concerns included diminishing resources, and policies and laws that were occasionally restrictive. The third theme was related to the character of relationships with clients. CHNs described challenges in being guests in their clients' homes, establishing trust, maintaining confidentiality, and preserving relationships. They also described concern with boundaries and fostering too much dependency in clients. The fourth major theme was respect for persons. Respecting autonomy through advocacy and informed choice was central to these CHNs who expressed their mandate as a responsibility to support clients in making decisions for themselves concerning their needs. The fifth theme concerned putting the self at risk. This included the CHNs' physical danger and value conflicts.

The authors concluded that the ethical issues that CHNs face are contextual and relational in nature, where seldom a clear right or wrong existed, suggesting that CHNs require an exquisite sense of sensitivity in defining what is good and determining whose good should be promoted.

Discussion Questions:

1. How are the ethical concerns of CHNs related to accountability?

2. Why do the authors conclude that the ethical concerns of CHNs are relational or contextual in nature?

3. What political changes would diminish the ethical concerns of CHNs?

tive action to protect clients from unsafe or unethical practice or circumstances. This action may entail reporting to appropriate authorities instances of unsafe or unethical care

Case Study

Jane was recently hired by a visiting nurses agency. She is providing overnight nursing care for five-year-old Anthony, who is ventilator-dependent. Anthony lives with his mother, Susan, and two siblings, ages six months and three years. Susan asks Jane if she could care for all three children while Susan goes to buy groceries at a 24-hour grocery store. Although the children are all sleeping, Jane is reluctant to assume care for Anthony's siblings. She explains to Susan that she cannot. Susan then becomes upset, stating that she cannot afford to pay for a babysitter and that the other nurses have no problem looking after all of the children for short periods of time. Jane does not know what to do.

Discussion Questions

1. What ethical and legal issues are raised by this situation?

2. What socio-political factors situate these issues?

3. How could Jane help Susan in ways that do not violate professional and ethical standards?

provided by family or others to children or vulnerable adults (CNA, 2002; CHNAC, 2003). Every Canadian jurisdiction has statutory laws that require nurses to report instances of physical or sexual abuse of persons, situations where a child's welfare is at risk, and information related to communicable and sexually transmitted diseases. These circumstances are supported by a legislated duty to report, as the protection of the individual and community take priority over the confidentiality of the client.

Summary

In this chapter, common ethical and legal considerations in community health nursing were discussed. Feminist bioethics, the CNA (2006a) framework on social justice, the CNA (2002) *Code of Ethics,* and the CHNAC (2003) standards were introduced as relevant ethical perspectives and standards to articulate and address these considerations. The unique responsibilities of CHNs and the variable settings in which they work raise particular ethical concerns that must be understood socio-politically. Health promotion and protection activities can enhance the well-being of clients, but they also can be means of social control that can compromise client choice and confidentiality. Legislation can often provide guidance to CHNs in these instances, for example, legislative requirements regarding the reporting of some communicable diseases. In many instances, CHNs are in a position to advocate for social justice so that the health and well-being of their clients can be protected. Although

Canada is a developed nation, many Canadians do not have access to the determinants of health.

The health and well-being of CHNs and clients may be threatened when community settings are not suitable for the provision of care and when informal caregivers do not have the necessary resources to assume responsibility for caregiving. CHNs providing palliative care to clients in their homes must possess an excellent knowledge of the ethical and legal considerations regarding end-of-life care, such as advanced directives, pain control, and DNR. Like nurses in all settings, CHNs are required ethically to develop caring relationships with their clients that remain within the limits of professional boundaries. They must also be accountable for their work, and often for the work of others, and must adhere to provincial/territorial and national ethical, legal, and professional standards.

KEY TERMS

ethics
bioethics
power
ethic of care
ethic of justice
ethical dilemmas
everyday ethics
social justice
social control
medicalization
harm principle
least restrictive or coercive means
reciprocity
transparency
informed consent
advance directive
empowerment
advocacy
professional boundary

STUDY QUESTIONS

1. Identify and define the eight central ethical values of Canadian nurses.

2. What are the 10 defining attributes of social justice?

3. What are CHNAC's five standards of practice?

4. List and define the four principles for a public health intervention.

5. What does the process of informed consent involve? What information must the CHN provide and what factors must he/she take into consideration?

6. What are the four key elements that must be proven to make a finding of negligence?

INDIVIDUAL CRITICAL THINKING EXERCISES

1. How are power and ethics related in community health nursing?

2. What aspects of community health nursing bring about social control? Can these be ethically justified? How?

3. How are nurse–client relationships in the community different from those in hospitals? What are the ethical implications of these differences?

4. Why are the working conditions of many CHNs of ethical concern?

5. How can the CHN promote the health and well-being of family caregivers?

GROUP CRITICAL THINKING EXERCISES

1. Identify a group in your community that experiences inequities that constrain its ability to meet health needs. Discuss strategies that would promote social justice.

2. Ask each group member to write down their definition of health and then share these with the group. How are these definitions similar and different? How do they reflect different values?

3. Identify a nursing leader in your community who is promoting social justice. How is the person accomplishing this?

REFERENCES

Anderson, J. M. (2001). The politics of home care: Where is "home"? *Canadian Journal of Nursing Research, 33*(2), 5–10.

Andrews, G. J. (2002). Towards a more place-sensitive nursing research: An invitation to medical and health geography. *Nursing Inquiry, 9*(4), 221–238.

Bayer, R. (2000). Editor's note: public health nihilism revisited. *American Journal of Public Health, 90*(12), 1838.

The California Wellness Foundation. (2001). *Reflections on capacity building – Definition of capacity building.* Retrieved on October 17, 2007, http://www.tcwf.org/pdf_docs/reflections/april2001.pdf.

Canada Health Act. 1985, C.6, s.1.

Canadian Association of Retired Persons. (CARP). (1999). *Putting a face on home care.* Kingston: Queen's Health Policy Research Unit.

Canadian International Development Agency. (2002). *Canada making a difference in the world: A policy statement on strengthening aid effectiveness.* Hull, QC: Author.

Canadian Nurses Association. (2002). *Code of ethics for Registered Nurses.* Ottawa: Author.

Canadian Nurses Assocation. (2003). *Global health and equity* [Position statement]. Ottawa: Author.

Canadian Nurses Association. (2006a). *Social justice... a means to an end, an end in itself.* Ottawa: Author.

Canadian Nurses Association. (2006b). *Public health nursing practice and ethical challenges.* Ottawa: Author.

Canadian Policy Research Network (CPRN). (2005). *A healthy balance: Caregiving policy in Canada.* Ottawa: Author.

Canadian Senate Subcommittee to Update *Of Life and Death.* (2000). *Quality of end-of-life care: the right of every Canadian.* Retrieved April 23, 2007, from http://www.parl.gc.ca/36/2/parlbus/commbus/senate/com-e/upda-e/rep-e/repfinjun00-e.htm.

Carnevale, F. A., Alexander, E., Davis, M., Rennick, J., & Troini, R. (2006). Daily living with distress and enrichment: The moral experience of families with ventilator-assisted children at home. *Pediatrics, 117*(1), e48–e60.

College of Nurses of Ontario (CNO). (2002). *Professional standards (revised 2002) for Registered Nurses and Registered Practice Nurses in Ontario.* Toronto: Author.

College of Nurses of Ontario (CNO). (2006). *Practice standard: The therapeutic nurse–client relationship, revised 2006.* Toronto: Author.

Community Health Nurses Association (CHNAC). (2003). *Canadian community health nursing standards of practice.* Retrieved September 27, 2007, from http://www.chnac.ca/index.php?option=com_content&task=view&id=20&Itemid=38

Conrad, P., & Schneider, J. W. (1985). *Deviance and medicalization: From badness to sickness.* Columbus, OH: Merrill Publishing Company.

Crits v. *Sylvester et al.* (1956) 1 D.L.R. (2d) 502 (Ont.C.A.), affd (1956) S.C.R. 991, (1956) 5 D.L.R. (2d) 601 (S.C.C.).

Duncan, K., Clipsham, J., Hampson, E., Krieger, C., MacDonnell, J., Roedding, D., Chow, K., & Milne, D. (2000). *Improving the access to and quality of public health services for lesbians and gay men.* Toronto: Ontario Public Health Association.

First Ministers of Canada. (2003). 2003 *First Ministers' accord on health care renewal.* Ottawa: Author.

Gebbie, K. M. (2001). Response to "feminism in public health nursing: partners for health." *Scholarly Inquiry for Nursing Practice: An International Journal, 15*(1), 63–66.

Gilligan, C. (1982). *In a different voice: Psychological theory and women's development.* Cambridge: Harvard University Press.

Grant, A., & Ashman, A. (1997). *A nurse's practical guide to the law.* Aurora, ON: Canada Law Book Inc.

Health Canada. (2005). Pan Canadian health information privacy and confidentiality framework. Retrieved August 11, 2006, from http://www.hc-sc.gc.ca.

Health Care Health & Safety Association of Ontario (HCHSA), & Workplace Safety & Insurance Board (WSIB). (2003). *Health and safety in the home care environment* (2nd ed). Retrieved August 17, 2006, from http://www.wsib.on.ca/wsib.

Hilton, B. A., Thompson, R., & Moore-Dempsey, L. (2000). Evaluation of the AIDS Prevention Street Nurse Program: One step at a time. *Canadian Journal of Nursing Research, 32*(1), 17–38.

Jaffee, S., & Hyde, J. S. (2000). Gender differences in moral orientation: A meta-analysis. *Psychological Bulletin, 126*(5), 703–726.

Johnstone, M.-J. (1999). *Bioethics: A nursing perspective.* Sydney: Harcourt Saunders.

Krieger, N., & Zierler, S. (1996). What explains the public's health? A call for epidemiological theory. *Epidemiology, 7,* 107–109.

Leipert, B. D. (2001). Feminism and public health nursing: Partners for health. *Scholarly Inquiry for Nursing Practice: An International Journal, 15*(1), 49–61.

Liaschenko, J. (1994). The moral geography of home care. *Advances in Nursing Science, 17*(2), 16–26.

Liaschenko, J. (2002). Health promotion, moral harm, and the moral aims of nursing. In L. E. Young and V. E. Hayes (Eds.), *Transforming health promotion practice: Concepts, issues and applications* (pp. 136–147). Philadelphia, PA: F.A. Davis Company.

Liaschenko, J., & Peter, E. (2003). Feminist ethics. In V. Tschudin (ed.), *Approaches to ethics: Nursing beyond boundaries* (pp. 33–43). Oxford: Butterworth, Heinemann.

MacPhail, S. A. (1996). *Ethical issues in community nursing.* Unpublished master's thesis, University of Alberta, Edmonton.

McKeever, P. (2001). Home care in Canada: Housing matters. *Canadian Journal of Nursing Research, 33*(2), 3–5.

Mill, J. S. (1974). *On liberty.* London: Penguin Books. (Original work published 1859).

Moyer, A., Coristine, M., MacLean, L., & Meyer, M. (1999). A model for building collective capacity in community-based programs: The Elderly in Need Project. *Public Health Nursing, 16*(3), 205–214.

Oberle, K., & Tenove, S. (2000). Ethical issues in public health nursing. *Nursing Ethics, 7*(5), 425–438.

Oxford University Press. (2004). *Oxford English Dictionary Online.* Retrieved by subscription from http://dictionary.oed.com.

Peter, E. (2002). The history of nursing in the home: Revealing the significance of place in the expression of moral agency. *Nursing Inquiry, 9*(2): 65–72.

Peter, E., & Morgan, K. (2001). Explorations of a trust approach for nursing ethics. *Nursing Inquiry, 8,* 3–10.

Peter, E., Spalding, K., Kenny, N., Conrad, P., McKeever, P., & Macfarlane, A. (2007). Neither seen nor heard: Children and home care policy in Canada. *Social Science & Medicine, 64,* 1624–1635.

Reimer Kirkham, S., & Browne, A. J. (2006). Toward a critical theoretical interpretation of social justice discourse in nursing. *Advances in Nursing Science, 29*(4), 324–339.

Self, B., & Peters, H. (2005). Street outreach with no streets. *Canadian Nurse, 101*(1), 20–24.

Schulz, R., & Beach, S. R. (1999). Caregiving as a risk factor for mortality: The caregiver health effects study. *Journal of the American Medical Association, 282*(23), 2215–2219.

Schroeder, C., & Gadow, S. (1996). An advocacy approach to ethics and community health. In E. T. Anderson & J. McFarlane (Eds.), *Community as partner: Theory and practice in nursing* (pp. 78–91). Philadelphia, PA: Lippincott.

Sherwin, S. (1998). A relational approach to autonomy in health care. In S. Sherwin (Ed.), *The politics of women's health: Exploring agency and autonomy* (pp. 19–47). Philadelphia, PA: Temple University Press.

Tarasoff v. *Regents of the University of California*, California Supreme Court, 17 California Reports, 3rd Series, 425, decided July 1, 1976.

Thompson, J. A. (2004). *Making advocacy work in your community: Definitions and terminology.* Retrieved on June 1, 2005, from http://www.rohan.sdsu.edu/~thompso/defterms.html.

Upshur, R. E. G. (2002). Principles for the justification of public health intervention. *Canadian Journal of Public Health, 93*(2), 101–103.

Verweij, M. (1999). Medicalization as a moral problem for preventative medicine. *Bioethics, 13*(2), 89–113.

Warren, V. (1989). Feminist directions in medical ethics. *Hypatia, 4*(2), 73–87.

Weidnitzer, E. (1996). German aid for poverty reduction. Berlin: Deutsches Institut für Entwicklungspolitik.

Wendan v. Trikha. (1992), 124 AR 1 (QB) affd (1993), 135 AR 382 (CA), leave to appeal denied (1993), 149 AR 160n, (1993) SCCA 126.

Williams, A. (2002). Changing geographies of care: Employing the concept of therapeutic landscapes as a framework in examining home space. *Social Science & Medicine, 55,* 141–154.

Workman Arts (WA). (2006). *About us.* Retrieved August 17, 2006, from http://www.workmantheatre.com.

Worthley, J. A. (Ed.). (1997). *The ethics of the ordinary in healthcare: Concepts and cases.* Chicago: Health Administration Press.

Zola, I. K. (1972). Medicine as an institution of social control. *Sociological Review, 20,* 487–504.

ADDITIONAL RESOURCES

Websites

Canadian Bioethics Society
www.bioethics.ca

Canadian Nurses Association
www.cna-nurses.ca/cna

Community Health Nurses Association (CHNAC)
www.communityhealthnursescanada.org

Dalhousie University, Department of Bioethics
http://bioethics.dal.ca

McGill University, Biomedical Ethics
www.mcgill.ca/biomedicalethicsunit/

NursingEthics.ca
www.nursingethics.ca

Programmes de Bioéthique, University of Montreal
www.bioethique.umontreal.ca/

Quality End-of-Life Care Coalition of Canada
www.cpca.net/qelccc.htm

University of Alberta, John Dossetor Health Ethics Centre
www.ualberta.ca/BIOETHICS/

University of Toronto, Joint Centre for Bioethics
www.utoronto.ca/jcb

The W. Maurice Young Centre for Applied Ethics, UBC
www.ethics.ubc.ca

About the Authors

Elizabeth Peter, RN, BScN (Windsor), BA (York), MScN (Toronto), PhD (Toronto), is Associate Professor and Associate Dean, Academic Programs, in the Lawrence S. Bloomberg Faculty of Nursing, University of Toronto. She is also Member, Joint Centre for Bioethics and the current chair of the Canadian Nurses Association Ethics Advisory Committee. During her studies, she worked for many years at the Queen Street Mental Health Centre in Toronto as both a staff nurse and a nursing coordinator. Her research focuses on the examination of ethical issues in home and community care. She has also has written widely in the field of nursing ethics.

Louise Sweatman, RN, BScN, LLB, MSc (ethics), is a nurse lawyer. She received her bachelor of nursing and master of science—with a focus on ethics—from the Faculty of Nursing, University of Toronto. She worked as a psychiatric nurse and then went back to school for a law degree from Osgood Hall Law School, York University in Toronto. She has worked in various provincial, national, and international organizations, such as the Ontario Nurses Association, Canadian Medical Association, and International Council of Nurses. She currently is the Chief Operating Officer of Assessment Strategies Inc., Canada's Testing Company. She is also Director, Testing Services for the Canadian Nurses Association and the Chair of the Canadian Network of National Associations of Regulators, and sits on the Board of Directors of the Federation of Associations of Regulatory Boards.

Kathleen Carlin, RN, MSc (University of Toronto), PhD (University of Toronto), specializes in health care ethics. Her graduate degrees had specializations in bioethics. She is currently Assistant Professor in the Department of Philosophy at Ryerson University. She is also the consultant to the Ethics Committee, St. Joseph's Healthcare, Centre for Mountain Health Services (formerly Hamilton Psychiatric Hospital) in Hamilton, Ontario, and has consulted to community and long-term care agencies. In 1997, with Louise Sweatman, she co-founded an annual community health ethics workshop day at Victoria College at the University of Toronto. She was the lead author of the chapter on ethics in *A Guide to End-of-Life Care for Seniors.* In addition to numerous presentations on ethics, she has written a continuing "Ethics Corner" column for a palliative care newsletter.

This work was supported through the funding of the Social Sciences and Humanities Research Council.

Concepts of Health

Lynne E. Young and Joan Wharf Higgins

CHAPTER 5

OBJECTIVES

After studying this chapter, you should be able to:

1. Understand health as discourse, the systems view of health, social determinants of health, and lay perspectives on health.
2. Examine how these often conflicting yet parallel perspectives on health influence the practice of community health nursing.

INTRODUCTION

> I know people who have such low self-esteem that they have allowed themselves to become infected with HIV, and yet they are people visually who would be seen by society and treated by society as very healthy people. They compensate for such low images that they're in the gym four or five days a week so they see themselves as healthy. I have come to know some of them to be very unhappy or very shy socially, they feel inadequate. So to me they are not healthy.—Glen (pseudonym), a mid-life man. (Maxwell, 1997, p. 112)

Health is a ubiquitous but confusing term, as Glen so thoughtfully observed in the above quote. We drink to our health, but some people drink themselves to death. We run for our health, but some people are injured running. Health professionals promote health, but patients/clients may choose to live unhealthfully in spite of these urgings. (In this chapter, "client" is defined as an individual, a family, a community, or a population.) As nurses, we hold to a belief that health is wholeness, but then speak of "heart health" or "breast health." There are health acts, health care systems, health management organizations, health fairs, and so on. Health is at the heart of the language of daily living, as expressed when we clink glasses with companions as well as front and centre in the policy, program, and practice arenas that affect nursing (Rootman & Raeburn, 1994). Thus, the term "health," often used in everyday life as well as in circumstances that shape our nursing world, is a term for which we generally assume a shared meaning. But can we? Should we?

DEFINING HEALTH

Definitions of health abound, derived from medicine, nursing, psychology, anthropology, sociology, politics, holism, and lay perspectives (Dubos, 1961; Rootman & Raeburn, 1994). Such definitions portray health as objective and subjective, a state and a process, naturalist and normative. A phenomenon such as health that is portrayed dichotomously is understandably confusing when one attempts to "pin it down." Dubos (1959) captures the nature of health by likening perceptions of health to a receding mirage: from a distance, the health concept is clear, but it is slippery and elusive as one approaches its meaning. What is consistent across definitions is that health is desirable because it encompasses positive qualities such as physical strength and emotional stability.

Health emerged as a central concept for nursing in the writings of Florence Nightingale. In spite of its elusive nature, health as a guiding concept is increasingly embraced by the nursing profession (Meleis, 1991, 2007). Because nursing activities compose a large portion of health expenditures in Canada, the health-related actions of nurses need to be designed to achieve the overall health-related goals of the wider society. With the multitude of definitions of health, what is the relationship between definitions of health and nursing actions?

Reflecting on this in light of numerous scholarly writings on health, what is most important and most interesting to us as chapter authors about the concept of health is not how health is defined, but rather what it means to speak of health in a particular way. Thus, exploring health as discourse, or a patterned way of speaking of something for some purpose, has the potential to clear up some of the confusions that nurses face when trying to think about the meaning of the term "health" relative to their nursing work.

Defining Discourse

Discourse, the noun, can be defined as formal, orderly, and usually extended expression of thought on a subject. Lupton (1992), a nurse theorist, notes that **discourse** is "a patterned system of texts, messages, talk, dialogue, or conversations which can be identified in these communications and located in social structures" (p. 145). In the philosophical literature (e.g., Foucault, 1972; Habermas, 1973), discourses are commonly understood to play major roles in shaping relations of power—what is valued in society—and subsequently receive attention and resources. Borgman (1992) argues that discourses of prediction and control are characteristic of traditional quantitative science and research, whereas the universal principle of qualitative and naturalistic research in health is to "let everyone speak in the first person, singular and plural" (p. 144). Since traditional science has dominated Western thought from the seventeenth century, with critiques of this approach emerging in the late twentieth century (Borgman, 1992), current discourses of health will have elements of both the traditional and naturalistic ways of thinking.

Discourses of Health

Health is desirable, a social good, and therein lies its power to shape action. What is considered healthy and unhealthy is influenced by cultural context (Capra, 1982). In North America, health is currently conceptualized within two major discourses: the medical model and the systems view. In the medical model, health is conceptualized as the absence of disease, whereas in the systems view, health is understood to be constructed through the interrelatedness and interdependence of all phenomena (Capra, 1982). In addition, an emerging sub-discourse on health within the systems view, particularly in Canada, is the **social determinants of health**, wherein health is held to be constructed primarily by social conditions. Finally, lay definitions of health are apparent in scholarly and lay literature.

Medical Model of Health

Health, according to the medical model, is the absence of disease. This definition of health has dominated our culture for the past three centuries (Capra, 1982) and is therefore a deeply entrenched perspective on health. As the dominant health discourse in Western societies (Fox, 1999), the medical model of health has the power to influence massive individual and collective activities and expenditures (Green & Kreuter, 1999; Rachlis & Kushner, 1994).

Current perspectives on medicine can be traced to the seminal work of scholars of the Intellectual Revolution, for example, William Harvey (1578–1657) and Vesalius (1514–1564) (Donahue, 1985). By charting anatomy through investigational procedures with animal and human cadavers, Harvey and Vesalius advanced the view of the body as machine (Donahue, 1985). From these early beginnings, the goal of medicine emerged as primarily to diagnose malfunctioning of the "human machine" and to "fix" it. This legacy pervades modern medicine. Here, achieving and maintaining health is a mechanistic, technical process in which physicians play the role of experts on body functioning (Capra, 1982; Ehrenreich & English, 1978). Thus, the body is conceptualized as a machine disconnected from mind, soul, and social and environmental contexts or settings. Health is the state of a perfectly

functioning, decontextualized mechanical entity. Health professionals, including nurses, who adopt this view of health are technical experts and, by association, guardians of a "social order" that build capacities to predict and control health.

Systems View of Health

A competing discourse to the medical model of health is the systems view of health, a shift in understanding health initiated by the World Health Organization (WHO) in 1948. Here, health is "a state of complete physical, mental, and social well-being, not merely the absence of disease and infirmity" (WHO, 1948, p. 100). Health, then, is more than a physical, mechanistic state; rather, health is conceptualized in terms of dynamic interrelatedness and integration. The systems view of health is embraced by diverse stakeholders: public, population, and community health; health psychology; holism (Larson, 1999); health promotion from an ecological perspective (Green & Ottoson, 1999); holistic nursing models; and proponents of primary health care, to name a few.

This discourse on health began to gain currency in Canada in the mid-1970s with the release of the 1974 report *A New Perspective on the Health of Canadians* (hereafter called the Lalonde Report) (Lalonde, 1974). Signalling the beginning of the current vision for health care in Canada, this report reintroduced lifestyle and environment as key determinants of health, positing that health is tied to overall conditions of living, a long-standing position of the public health tradition (Lalonde, 1974; Raeburn, 1992). The central argument of this report is that health is not achievable solely as a result of medical care, but rather from the interplay of determinants from four health-field elements: human biology, lifestyles, the environment, and health care systems (Labonte, 1994). The Lalonde Report shifted the focus of a vision for the health of a population from illness care to health care and advanced health promotion as a science. Lalonde called this perspective the health-field concept of health.

The Ottawa Charter of Health Promotion (WHO, 1986), written to expand on the 1948 WHO definition of health, stated that, "Health is...a resource for everyday living, not the objective of living" (p. 426). The Charter also proposed five major strategies for promoting health: building healthy public policy, creating supportive environments, strengthening community action, developing personal skills, and reorienting health services. Advocating, enabling, and mediating were identified as central strategies for health promotion practice. It also articulated prerequisites for health: peace, shelter, education, food, income, a stable ecosystem, sustainable resources, social justice, and equity, thereby entrenching specific determinants of health into this discourse on health in Canada.

In the same year, the Epp Report, *Achieving Health for All* (Epp, 1986), was introduced by the Canadian government. It built on the Lalonde Report by identifying specific challenges to achieving health for all Canadians: reducing inequities, increasing prevention, and enhancing coping. In addition, the Epp Report postulated that these challenges could be addressed by the health promotion mechanisms of self-care, mutual aid, and healthy environments, and that central implementation strategies are fostering public participation, strengthening community health services, and coordinating public policy.

In these documents, family plays second fiddle to community as a unit of concern for health professionals, yet the family unit is of particular importance to the development and maintenance of the health of its members (Young, 2002). An **ecological perspective** on health promotion reflects a systems view and does much to highlight broad contextual factors (such as family) that influence health (Green & Ottoson, 1999; Green, Richard, & Potvin, 1996; Richard, Potvin, Kishchuk, Prlic, & Green, 1996). Ecology is concerned with the relationships between organisms and their environment (Kleffel, 1991), and social ecology is concerned with the nature of the relationships between humans and their social, institutional, and cultural worlds (Stokols, 1992). Health here is the consequence of the interdependence between the individual and the family, community, culture, and the physical and social environments (Green & Kreuter, 1999; Moos, 1979).

The next wave of thinking in this systems view of health was disseminated in the report entitled *Strategies for Population Health: Investing in the Health of Canadians,* prepared by the Federal, Provincial, and Territorial Advisory Committee on Population Health (FPTACPH, 1994). This report further clarified key factors that influence health: the social and economic environment, the physical environment, personal health practices and coping skills, biology and genetic endowment, and health services. According to the population health approach, health is the capacity of people to adapt to, respond to, or control life's challenges and changes (Frankish, Green, Ratner, Chomik, & Larsen, 1996). The population health movement in Canada, in collaboration with Health Canada, set out a template to guide action to achieve population health. Key elements of the Population Health Template are depicted in Figure 5.1. (For further explanation, see Appendix 11A, Chapter 11.)

The Canadian Nurses Association led an impressive effort to incorporate these new ideas, beginning with the document *Putting Health into Health Care* (Rodger & Gallagher, 1995). Subsequently, provincial nursing associations across Canada produced position statements and discussion documents that captured these ideas (McDonald, 2002). For example, the Registered Nurses' Association of British Columbia (RNABC) incorporated strategies from the Ottawa Charter (WHO, 1986) in their New Directions for Health Care policies and programs. As well, these ideas were incorporated into a document entitled *Determinants of Health: Empowering Strategies for Nursing Practice* that was a socio-environmental framework for health promoting nursing practice. It directed nurses' attention to concerns of not only individuals, but also families, small groups, communities, and society (McDonald, 2002). In keeping with the evolution of thinking within the systems view of health, the RNABC has recently published a position statement on primary health care (RNABC, 2002).

According to the systems view, health is envisioned as a dynamic process embedded in a web of relations within which, and as a result of, capacities for living are constructed. In Canada, the systems view of health has been entrenched in

FIGURE 5.1 Population Health Key Elements

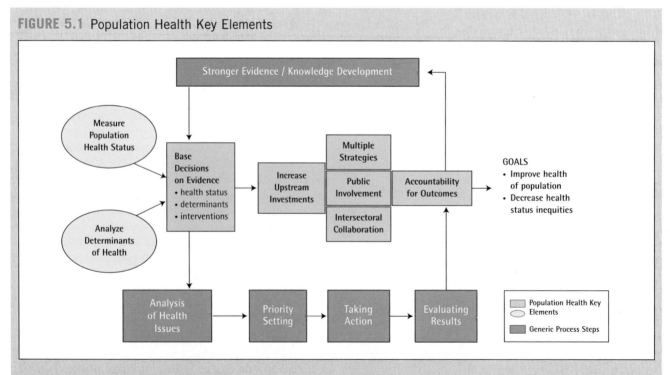

Source: Population health template: Key elements and actions that define a population health approach. Accessed September 27, 2007, from www.phac-aspc.gc.ca/ph-sp/phdd/pdf/overview_handout_colour.pdf, Public Health Agency of Canada, (2001). Reproduced with the permission of the Minister of Public Works and Government Services Canada, 2007.

our thinking over the past three decades through a series of government documents, frameworks, and blueprints and their related professional practices. Health professionals, including nurses, who practise from a systems, process-oriented perspective hold to a view that attends carefully to a multitude of capacity-building social and economic relationships, including the relationship between practitioner and client.

Medical Discourse versus Systems Discourse

Following the Second World War and the discovery of penicillin, the medical model of health irrefutably eclipsed other discourses of health. The near-miraculous discoveries emerging from medical science (e.g., the control of and near-eradication of some communicable diseases, such procedures as heart transplantation, and more recently genetic engineering) have captured our money and imagination. Anyone who has witnessed the recovery of a loved one from a near-death traumatic experience because of innovative surgical procedures, or the prolongation and improved quality of life of an aging parent because of newly developed cardiac medications, stands in awe of medical science and practice. While these successes are real and tangible, they are not the whole story.

Critics of the medical model make strong arguments that such an approach to health does not make for a healthy society (Batt, 1994; Evans & Stoddard, 1990; Illich, 1975; Rachlis & Kushner, 1994; Raphael, 2001). In a seminal work, *Medical Nemesis,* published more than 25 years ago, Illich attacked the value of the medical model in producing healthy societies. He opens the book with: "The medical establishment has become a major threat to health" (p. 11) and goes on to argue that a medicalized health care system is a monopoly that serves the interests of medical and paramedical personnel. To this end, he posits that such a health care system obscures the political conditions that render society unhealthy, while seizing the power of individuals to heal themselves.

Heartened by such arguments, consumers have taken steps to regain control over their own health and ensure that medical care and medical science truly serve their interests rather than those of health professionals (Batt, 1994; Porter-O'Grady, 1995). Such consumers understand their health to be embedded in a web of social relations. The breast cancer movement is a consumer movement that exemplifies a challenge to the medical model as a dominant discourse on health. Batt, an award-winning Canadian journalist, charts the journey of breast cancer activism in her book *Patient No More.* The idea for the book emerged from her need as a breast cancer survivor to better understand why breast cancer treatments were regarded widely as a medical success when thousands of women die each year in spite of those treatments. At first she was hesitant to take on the experts, but her investigative work revealed themes that pointed to the detrimental influence of vested interests and world views on the medical care of women with breast cancer. She writes, "Our [breast cancer survivors'] central task is precisely to develop and advance a perspective of our own. Our voice must be a counterweight to the medical point of view that dominates discussions of the disease" (Batt,

p. xiii). Thus, women began to ask why it is difficult to access accurate information about breast cancer and its treatments and moved on to explore how funding decisions are made. Batt writes, "Many now question the premises of past policies, such as the emphasis on treatment rather than prevention, and the strictly biomedical model of cancer" (p. xiv). Batt notes that the activists have inspired breast cancer specialists to examine the world view that guides their research. She writes, "A new order is forming..." (p. xiv).

While the medical view of health as discourse can silence voices and distinguish ideas that do not fit, there are those, such as breast cancer activists, who take issue with the dominance of the medical model and, by their actions, open minds to new ways of thinking about health.

Social Determinants of Health: An Emerging Sub-discourse

As mentioned earlier, Canadian governments prioritize the funding of health care based on the medical model but fund interventions aimed at discouraging unhealthy lifestyles to a much lesser extent, a perspective that reflects the health-field concept of health. (This fact exemplifies the power of a dominant discourse to shape social and political action.) However, it is estimated that only 5 of the 30 years added to life expectancies during the past century can be attributed to clinical medicine (Bunker, Frazier, & Mosteller, 1994). This is in spite of the fact that about 95% of health expenditures in Canada are spent on medical treatment and 5%, at most, are devoted to prevention (Brown, Corea, Luce, Elixhauser, & Sheingold, 1992). Thus, researchers have begun to explore what constellations of factors that determine health status lie "upstream" of medical treatment (McKinlay & Marceau, 2000). An emerging body of research on the social determinants of health provides compelling evidence that challenges the dominance of the medical model as a key perspective. Such research indicates that factors with the greatest impact on the development of life-threatening diseases are usually out of an individual's personal control, factors tied to culture and socioeconomic status (Wilkinson & Marmot, 1998).

Indeed, large-scale studies conducted in recent years point to poverty, income, place of residence, and education levels, rather than medical and lifestyle factors, as better predictors of individuals' health (Colhoun, Rubens, Underwood, & Fuller, 2000; Diez Roux et al., 2001; Feldman, Makuc, Kleinman, & Cornoni-Huntley, 1989; Lantz, House, Lepkowski, Williams, Mero, & Chen, 1998). For example, Lynch et al. (1997) found that poor adult health behaviours and psychosocial characteristics (sense of hopelessness, depression, or lack of coherence or meaning in life) were more prevalent among men whose parents were poor, regardless of their own socioeconomic standing as adults. The authors suggested that the environmental influences in childhood play themselves out later in adulthood. As such, the "free choice" associated with lifestyle behaviours may not be totally under an individual's control.

Rather than focusing on health practices as rational behaviours that one chooses to do at random, the notion of lifestyle is more useful once we understand the determinants of lifestyle choice, that is, what factors and conditions influence our lifestyle habits (Gillies, 1998). With this definition in mind, Lyons and Langille (2000) offered the following determinants of lifestyle choice:

1. Personal life skills are those abilities for adaptive and positive behaviours that enable people to deal effectively with the demands of everyday life. Personal life skills include literacy, numeracy, decision making and problem solving, creative and critical thinking, empathy, mutual support, self-help and advocacy, communication, and coping. These are not necessarily linked to specific health practices, but all contribute to helping people increase control over their lives and health.

2. Perceived stress in life influences the choices people make about their lifestyle. To cope with the time pressures they face, Canadians report watching television, eating comfort foods, smoking cigarettes, or consuming alcohol. In fact, "health enhancing" activities such as exercise are perceived as even more stressful when time is limited (Heart and Stroke Foundation of Canada, 1999).

3. The influence of community norms and culture both reflect and limit lifestyle choices.

4. Control over one's life and a sense of coherence about the world enhance one's ability to choose healthy behaviours over unhealthy ones.

5. A sense of belonging is critical to health. To a large extent, connectedness and belonging may overcome the traditional epidemiological risk factors of smoking, physical inactivity, obesity, and poor nutrition (Putnam, 2000), risks that are more prevalent among those with lower incomes (FPTACPH, 1999).

6. Healthy choices in life are not always the most pleasurable, and the benefits of healthy living are not always immediately reaped or apparent. To make matters worse, persons living with low incomes are more likely to engage in risk behaviours as they provide respite from difficult and painful life situations (Stewart et al., 1996).

7. Personality traits such as learned helplessness or individuals who are "other" directed (believe that luck/fate is responsible for their lot in life) can discourage uptake of healthy behaviours.

8. Overabundance of choice and information about what is the "right" thing to do can confuse and paralyze people rather than galvanize them into action.

Shaping environments in support of healthful living and healthy lifestyles and addressing the social determinants of health require a new way of thinking. The **primary health care** model offers such a way and has gained some currency in the discourse on health care in Canada. Primary health care (PHC) is perceived to be the key to reforming a health care system dominated by the medical model (Green & Ottoson, 1999). PHC was conceived by participants representing 134 nations at the WHO Alma Ata Conference in 1978. They pledged their support for a worldwide effort to shift the emphasis from hospital-based medical treatment to a community-based, participatory model of care (Green & Ottoson, 1999). The catchphrase that emerged from this conference

was "Health for All by the Year 2000." Many influential Canadians who believe that the tenets of PHC will indeed improve the health of Canadians have been in a prolonged, difficult, and often embittered battle to expand the vision for health care in Canada beyond the medical model. Such tensions speak to the power of the medical discourse on health to shape political will. Recently, social and health researchers, policy experts, and professionals gathered in Toronto to network and discuss the health of Canadians. On the final day, delegates composed *Strengthening the Social Determinants of Health: The Toronto Charter for a Healthy Canada* (Social Determinants of Health Across the Life-Span Conference, 2002). This document outlines ten social determinants of health, which include early life experiences, education, food security, housing, and income distribution.

In the U.S., the 1990s were a decade of failed health care reform (Oberlander, 2002). The Clinton plan for universal insurance failed but nonetheless spawned the spread of managed care, which, for a time, controlled the costs of health care. Now, however, medical care costs are rising again, and 40 million Americans lack health insurance (Oberlander, 2002). In Canada, each day brings a new challenge to the universal, single-payer health care system. The Romanow report *Building of Values: The future of health care in Canada* (Romanow, 2002) indicated widespread support for health care policy consistent with a public system with key aspects of primary health care embedded in its principles. However, unlike the report *The Health of Canadians: The Federal Role,* released by Senator Michael Kirby early in 2002, Romanow mentioned the importance of the social determinants of health only briefly, instead emphasizing the role of governments in supporting Canadians to make healthy lifestyle choices to prevent or delay chronic disease (Raphael, 2003). Moreover, power and money interests have a foothold in private clinics and ever-more effective technologies that promise quick and effective diagnoses and cures, a direction consistent with a medical model view.

Canadian Research Box 5.1

Thurston, W. E., Rutherford, E., Meadows, L. M., & Vollman, A. R. (2005). The role of the media in public participation: Framing and leading? *Women and Health, 41*(4), 101–122.

These researchers were interested in finding out how the media shaped and framed public discourse related to the women's health services that were impacted during a health care reorganization in Calgary. Through examination of newspaper archives and key organizational documents, it was possible to track the public discourse during this time.

During the creation of the health region, health agencies that had previously been under other organizations such as the Salvation Army were brought under the organization and mandate of the new health region. The examination revealed that it was through the highly visible Salvation Army presence, and public presentation of its philosophy of holistic health care, that the media were influenced to keep women's health part of the public discourse. Through this process, the holistic delivery philosophy of the agency remained, even after the organizational change was complete.

The researchers concluded that for women's health to remain an issue within the public discourse, women from many arenas must be willing to use the media to get their message across to the general public, thus influencing future health care delivery for women.

Discussion Questions:

1. How is women's health represented in the media in your community?

2. Why do you think women's health is represented in this way? What are the sources for the media reports on women's health in your area? Do these sources represent your own beliefs?

Social Determinants of Health: Heart Health, a Case Example

Low-income lone mothers are a particular cohort in which operates a constellation of factors detrimental to health. Such women are more likely to live in poverty, to achieve low levels of education, and to be on social assistance than are partnered mothers (Young, Cunningham, & Buist, 2005; Young, James, & Cunningham, 2004). Overall health status is poorer among lone mothers (Perez & Beaudet, 1999), as are health behaviours. In particular, Canadian lone mothers are three to four times more likely to be smokers than partnered mothers of any income (Young et al., 2004). In a U.S. study, women who had experienced a cardiovascular disease event were 3.28 times more likely to be a lone mother than a partnered mother (Young et al., 2005). In a qualitative study designed to augment the findings of the related quantitative studies, Wharf-Higgins, Young, Naylor, & Cunningham (2006) found that low-income lone mothers attribute policies and practices that shape their lives as foundational to their lifestyle patterns. Thus, female-headed households are associated with a higher risk for heart disease among women (LeClere, Rogers, & Peters, 1998).

The established approach to promote heart health and prevent heart disease has been, and continues to be, individually focused and behaviourally oriented (Raphael, 2003) despite findings that suggest that only a portion of inter-individual variability in CVD incidence can be explained by the major risk factors (Marmot, 1996; Nettleton, 1997). Indeed, Raphael (2001) estimates that 23% of all premature years of life lost prior to age 75 in Canada can be attributed to income differences. Of these premature deaths related to income differences, heart disease and stroke cause the greatest proportion of these years lost: 22%. As such, health policy makers have been encouraged to address issues of poverty, powerlessness, and a lack of social support in addition to the usual care of risk reduction (Marmot & Wilkinson, 1999; Petrasovits, 1992).

Gender is also a critical determinant of heart health. The social determinants of health do not affect women and men in the same way: women are relatively disadvantaged compared with men (Spitzer, 2005). Marked differences exist between men's and women's ability to access, and gender role expectations of accessing, health promoting opportunities (e.g., recreation, continued education, satisfying work). Moreover, the gendered effects of reduced funding to health and social services include fewer jobs for women, more unpaid care work, and reduced access to health care (Kaufert, 1996). As a result, low income is especially concentrated among women. In 1998, 56% of Canadian sole-support mothers lived below the low-income cut-off (Townson, 2000).

Gender needs to be treated as an important explanatory variable in determining health. As well, more focused efforts are required to ensure that policies and programs take into account existing and new knowledge about women's health. Thus, while the "determinants" model is receiving (deserved) increasing attention for situating lifestyle behaviours and risk factors in their proper social, cultural, and economic contexts, women, in various degrees, continue to bear an unfair burden of poor health related to gender roles, economic disparities, and other related factors (Spitzer, 2005). A further challenge to the epidemiological tradition of studying heart disease is its ignorance of the lived experience of women (Raphael, 2001).

Lay Definitions of Health: Giving Voice to Our Clients

Before we move on, let's return to the opening scenario in which Glen points to the tension between what "society" defines as healthy and what he observes in his friends. In pointing to what society says about health, Glen refers to society's dominant discourse on health. Reflect on how health is portrayed by society in Canada as a discourse on health. Now, reflect on the difference between what society says is health and how Glen defines health. Reflect on what this difference means to Glen.

Lay perspectives on health are diverse, ranging from popular Western definitions that reflect the medical perspective—health as the absence of disease—to a perspective evident in many non-Western cultures—health as living in harmony with nature (Calnan, 1987; Spector, 1985). In our view, lay perspectives orient nurses to the views on health of those in their care. In this section, an overview of the findings of a qualitative study designed to reveal lay perspectives on health (Maxwell, 1997) is presented and then discussed relative to research in the field. Participants in the study were male and female, ranged in age from 7 to 81, and lived in urban and rural settings. The researcher met with families in their own homes for 1–2 research interviews that lasted for 1.5–2 hours.

Health was perceived by most to be fundamental to living a functional, meaningful life. As one middle-aged woman put it, "This sounds very cliché but being healthy is…if you don't have your health, obviously you don't have anything." Another female participant, a financially strained, married mother of three, elaborates:

> You need your health to have energy to raise your family and everyone wants to raise healthy, happy kids, you know, for the future. (p. 112)

For several people, having energy was an indicator of health. One man observed:

> Healthy is a mental attitude, physically feeling well, and having an energy level to get through the day, and, it's a lifestyle. (p. 111)

Health emerges as an energized state that has physical, mental, and social dimensions, and health is a lifestyle. A health care professional male in his 60s provides a well-thought-through position on his lived experience of health:

> I feel healthy if my back isn't sore or if things don't hurt or my throat is not sore. To me personally, on any given day, whether I feel healthy that day or not is an absence of complaints. But, what does health count as a year? What is a healthy year? Or, what is a healthy decade? Then, we get into that more holistic definition of health. You know the background thing...we're comfortable, we have a nice home, we have adequate money and live with it well, and we're not living in fear and this sort of thing. So that background is okay and so that you can sit around and worry about whether or not you've got a sore throat. If you lived in a war-torn country, you really wouldn't give a damn if you had a sore throat or not.
>
> Researcher: So if you had a healthy year, what would that have been like?
>
> Man: I guess free from relatively, well number one, good physical health, free from sort of major worries, free from family worries, that there weren't a lot of things pressing down and adequate rest so that I am not overtired. (p. 113)

This man evaluates his state of health by noting his physical state and the context within which his physical health is experienced, including his family, socioeconomic circumstance, and the political climate of the country. His idea of health counting "as a year" or "decade" is unique.

Not all participants found it easy to speak of health, however. One woman, married, with three children under age six, and employed full time, observed:

> I've never thought of "I feel healthy." It's either you feel tired or you don't feel tired. I've never said, "Oh I feel healthy today." I wouldn't even know where to start with that one. (p. 115)

A single mother coping with the aftermath of breast cancer treatment and living meagrely with two early teens views health in the following way:

> Gee, I just can't answer that. Isn't that amazing? I don't know. I'm not grasping what health is, being healthy? [pause] Being fit? Is there more? (p. 115)

While most participants openly discussed their views on health, not all found it an easy term to define. Some partici-pants offered thoughtful definitions of, or personal theories about, health. From these interviews, health emerged as an energized, balanced, dynamic, multidimensional state related to self-perception, interpersonal processes, and socioeconomic context, a perspective aligned with a systems view of health but with unique and individualized twists and variations.

A systematic review of 112 qualitative studies that was conducted to develop theory regarding an individual's experience of health and disease was revealing (Jensen & Allen, 1994). These studies involved informants with disease or chronic illness as well as those who considered themselves to be "healthy." Participants ranged in age from early adulthood to very old. The authors identified the following themes to describe the lived experience of health and disease:

- **abiding vitality**, the idea that when one is healthy there is sparkle and animation;
- **transitional harmony**, the idea that, when healthy, one has a sense of harmony and balance, a notion that resonates with the words of participants in the Maxwell (1997) study;
- **rhythmical connectedness**, the idea that, when healthy, one experiences wholeness and an accompanying attachment to the world and that these social connections provide a positive sense of personal contribution or effectiveness as well as positive identity;
- **unfolding fulfillment**, the notion that engaging with life's challenges is meaningful; and
- **active optimism**, the idea that one can cope with life and meet its challenges; that is, one has the attitude and resources to do so.

Two recent qualitative studies revealed meanings of health similar to but also different from those claimed by the above authors. Maddox's (1999) study of older women and the meaning of health reported that the primary themes arising from research interviews were interactions with a being greater than themselves, acceptance of self, humour, flexibility, and being other-centred. Mexican-American women view health as a compilation of good physical health, sound mental health, and a socially and spiritually satisfying life (Mendelson, 2002). Health for these women exceeded more than these component parts, an embodied experience that transcends illness and is grounded in relationships with family and supported by their spirituality.

The lay perspectives on health presented here mirror each other and resonate with both the medical and systems models of health. A study in Alberta found that survey respondents recognized their health is broadly influenced by social and environmental variables, including issues of social support, supportive environments, and income (Reutter, Dennis, & Wilson, 2001). In an attempt to understand how people arrive at a subjective evaluation of their health, Kaplan and Baron-Epel (2003) surveyed people in three broad age groups (20–40, 41–60, and 61+). When they probed respondents about what factors may have influenced their rating, they found that:

[H]ealth is a social construction and our beliefs and conceptions of it are rooted in wider socio-cultural contexts. People's perceptions of health are also found to be influenced by biomedicine and by prevailing social and medical ideologies.... People's perceptions and judgements about their own health are at once individual and social. (pp. 6–7)

As health professionals, our practice is enriched if we listen carefully for our clients' definitions of health and choose this as a starting point.

DISCOURSES ON HEALTH AND THE ROLE OF THE COMMUNITY HEALTH NURSE

In the previous sections, we discussed health in terms of medical and systems discourses and lay perspectives on health. These are "lenses" on health that community health nurses can draw on as they perform their roles. Used in this way, "lens" refers to a particular way of understanding a concept, in this case *health*. One of the primary challenges nurses face is to sort out how each lens on health can be applied to or incorporated into their practice. However, the first step in addressing this dilemma is to understand how and why a particular lens on health shapes health care practice, be it nursing, medicine, or another health care discipline such as physiotherapy, family therapy, or community health promotion.

Canadian Research Box 5.2

King, K. M., Thomlinson, E., Sanguins, J., & LeBlanc, P. (2006). Men and women managing coronary artery disease risks: Urban–rural contrasts. *Social Science and Medicine, 62,* 1091–1102.

This study is one of a series of studies examining the role of gender and ethnocultural background on the perceptions of individuals making lifestyle changes associated with coronary artery disease (CAD) risks. Purposive sampling contributed to the participation of 42 Euro-Celtic men and women with varying ages, time since diagnosis, and degree of disease involvement, and their audiotaped interviews were transcribed to form the data. In this particular study, a rural–urban variation among participants was also sought.

The researchers indicated that the core variable was "meeting the challenge" of managing the risks associated with the diagnosis of CAD. The influence of intrapersonal, interpersonal, and extrapersonal factors was directly or indirectly swayed by the elements of knowledge of the disease process, and their perceptions of the amount of lifestyle change required. There were three distinct phases of the disease—prediagnosis, the changing person, and living with CAD.

In addition to these factors, the researchers noted that gender and rural or urban residency contributed to the participant's perceived ability to manage their disease. Rural residents tended to view their situation as more healthy than urban living—although stressors were still present. For instance, even though rural residents lived farther away from neighbours, they reported greater perceived social support than some of the urban dwellers. Conversely, they also reported high turnover of health care providers, particularly physicians, as a negative factor. Women reported initial symptoms that were not classic and therefore ignored by the women and their physicians alike.

The researchers concluded that rural-living persons, and especially rural-living women, were the most vulnerable. They noted that continuing research was needed with varying cultural groups including both genders and urban and rural residents.

Discussion Questions:

1. How would you as a community health nurse use this research to plan and provide care to an urban environment? a rural environment?

2. How might this research affect how you think about your own health?

For purposes of stimulating thinking, discussion, and debate, we suggest that the medical model of health, with its focus on prediction and control, has the potential to engender nurses who enact their role as experts who can predict the causes of, and intervene to control, the health of those in their care. Nurses who fall within this genre take on the role of the expert in identifying problems and catalyzing solutions. When functioning in this role nurses may seem heroic, charging in to instigate a "fix" or solution, or they may act to guard the social order to ensure health: superhero nurses. Society needs nurses who can detect health problems and offer effective solutions, for example, when a community experiences the outbreak of a communicable disease.

In contrast, nurses who practise from a systems view, in which health is wholeness, carry out a relational practice in which relationships with clients are paramount to the clients' constructions of health and experiences of wholeness. In such a nursing practice, the nurse builds trusting relationships, collaborates with clients to identify and address their health-related issues, fosters clients' strengths, promotes and protects clients' rights, practises in an intersectoral manner to address the determinants of health, and strives for a respectful, integrated, accessible system of health care delivery. A metaphor for such a nurse might be nurse as dancer, in which the nurse and client strive to connect across life space—a delicate, gentle act, beautiful in its execution but nonetheless precarious.

Community health nurses may find themselves caught between the roles of the nurse as superhero and the nurse as dancer, roles that may at times feel untenable. Nurses in British Columbia experienced such tensions and took action to change their practice (Griffiths, 2002). The Public Health Nursing Practice Advisory Committee (PHNPAC), in the

South Fraser area of the Fraser Health Authority, received a referral from nursing colleagues concerning dissatisfaction with the problem-oriented recording system (POR). The POR was incongruent with the philosophy of nursing that the nurses shared. The PHNPAC initiated a series of consultations to assist them in addressing this concern. A presentation by a nursing professor on "The Power of the Text" raised the nurses' awareness of the incompatibility between the way the documentation system was shaping their practice and their philosophy of nursing. More specifically, the POR documentation system, as a problem-oriented practice, shaped their practices to emphasize detecting problems rather than fostering family strengths. Yet, the act of acknowledging and fostering family strengths was what these nurses held to be fundamental to health promotion practice with families.

Tackling this issue head on, the PHNPAC created its own model for working with high-risk families through a brainstorming process. Key themes that emerged to inform the development of the model included strengths-based practice, collaboration with clients, and taking steps to increase choices and control for families. As one participant noted, "As nurses, we support people to live in ways that are productive for them" (Griffiths, 2002, p. 16). They linked their work to a systems view of health, citing the Ottawa Charter definition of health promotion, "the process of enabling people to increase control over and improve their own health" (WHO, 1986), as a conceptual and philosophical guide for their newly conceived practice standards.

A **population health** model, offered by McKinlay and Marceau (2000), is a useful framework for thinking about where one's nursing practice fits within the discourses of health. This model suggests that there are three streams to promoting population health:

1. **downstream**, an individual-focused orientation to treatment and cure (e.g., pharmacology, surgery, and rehabilitation);

2. **mid-stream**, support at the community and organization level for creating environments conducive to living healthfully (e.g., opportunities for physical activity, prenatal care programs); and

3. **upstream**, in which healthy public policies, programs, and services deal with macro-level issues of employment, education, and reimbursement mechanisms that affect all in a community (e.g., universal health care).

"Downstream" practice falls within a biomedical view of health, whereas "mid-stream" and "upstream" practices fit within a systems view of health. Where does your usual practice fit?

Summary

In this chapter, we discussed discourses of health, suggesting that there are two primary discourses of health in Canada, the medical model and the systems view on health. Health, a concept of primary importance to community health nurses, is not a concrete entity, but rather a concept that has a range of meanings to various groups of health care professionals. What is important about the concept of health for community health nurses is to clearly grasp by whom and how health is defined, and for what purposes. Understanding health as a discourse is a first step in grasping who is defining health and for what purposes. Community health nurses can engage in client-centred care when they can link a particular definition of health to whoever is making claims on the definition, and then determine how well a particular definition aligns with clients' definitions of health in addition to clients' health care needs. Community health nurses, because of their location in the community, are well positioned to work in intersectoral relationships to address the social determinants of health, factors that are increasingly held to be the key to health.

Case Study

The Saanich Peninsula Diabetes Prevention Project explores how community recreation programs and services can prevent or delay the onset of type 2 diabetes in "at-risk" populations. Rather than adhering to a medical model orientation and relying on biomedical variables, such as glucose intolerance, as identifying risk factors, the definition of "at-risk" used in this project is consistent with Health Canada's population health framework and a social determinants view and includes low-income citizens, isolated seniors, persons living with disabilities, and Aboriginal populations. Working with recreation professionals, community nutritionists, diabetes educators, social workers, and public health nurses, project staff work to dismantle the barriers to a diabetes-healthy lifestyle for these at-risk groups, as well as create a supportive community environment. In response to an identified need from these populations, a Diabetes Education and Awareness Fair was held in the fall of 2002. The goal of the fair was to increase the at-risk groups' education and awareness of type 2 diabetes, as well as provide information about, and access to, the resources and supports available in the community for healthy living. The overall focus was to facilitate a change to a diabetes-healthy life while acknowledging the social, economic, and cultural contexts within which lifestyle behaviours occur.

The fair consisted of brief seminars on risk factors and conditions, healthy eating, meal preparation, physical activity, and stress management. As well, on-site booths provided information concerning community resources and supports for healthy and active living and access to dietitians, community nurses, kinesiologists, and other health professionals. Participants could also visit booths to have their heart rate, blood pressure, body-mass index, and blood glucose levels measured. The fair was held in the local recreation centre, thought to be a more welcoming and non-threatening environment than a health department or hospital.

Despite an emphasis on the broader social determinants of health to the project, the nursing staff at the fair found it difficult to communicate the importance of such factors to visitors, whose questions and search for information reflected a medical model understanding of diabetes. Although the design of the fair and its staff acknowledged and appreciated the population health systems approach, fair participants were mired in the medical model and intent on gathering information concerning physiological and behavioural risks and solutions.

Discussion Questions

1. How might you, as a community health nurse, think about why the nursing staff reported difficulty communicating the importance of the social determinants of health to fair visitors?

2. Is it necessary to emphasize one understanding or discourse of health over the other?

3. How might the fair be reorganized/restructured to encourage a systems understanding of health over a medical one? What different activities, resources, staff, and so on would be important to include?

KEY TERMS

discourse
social determinants of health
ecological perspective
primary health care
abiding vitality
transitional harmony
rhythmical connectedness
unfolding fulfillment
active optimism
population health
downstream
mid-stream
upstream

STUDY QUESTIONS

1. Define "discourse."
2. What are the principles of primary health care?
3. What is the difference between the medical model and the systems view of health?
4. What is the challenge to nurses working within these two views of health?
5. Why was the Lalonde Report important?
6. Why does the ecological perspective on health fit within a systems view of health?
7. What is a relational nursing practice?

8. Where do the traditional and non-traditional articles presented in Canadian Research Box 5.1 fit into the discourses of health as discussed in this chapter?

9. What has been Canada's role in shaping discourses of health?

10. What are your responses to the metaphors of nursing offered by the authors of this chapter?

INDIVIDUAL CRITICAL THINKING EXERCISES

1. How do you define your own health?

2. Within which view or discourse of health did you frame your response to the previous question?

3. When you assess clients, what questions would you include to help you understand their perspectives on health?

4. Locate the majority of your nursing work on the McKinlay and Marceau (2000) model and identify distinct tasks that fit on the stream continuum.

5. If you were to move your work more "upstream," what would that look like so that you achieved similar outcomes to your present work?

GROUP CRITICAL THINKING EXERCISES

1. What are the sources of stress for you as a student? How might you balance study, work, and family to "let go" of stress?

2. Relative to the above discussions about discourses of health, what does it mean to frame school-related stress as a problem that requires an individual-level solution?

3. How do you as students and the nursing faculty honour the idea of the determinants of health in the everyday life of your school? Brainstorm factors that could be addressed in your school community to make your school a healthier place to be.

REFERENCES

Batt, S. (1994). *Patient no more: The politics of breast cancer.* Charlottetown: Synergy.

Borgman, A. (1992). *Crossing the post-modern divide.* Chicago: University of Chicago Press.

Brown, R., Corea, J., Luce, B., Elixhauser, A., & Sheingold, S. (1992). Effectiveness in disease and injury prevention: Estimated national spending on prevention—United States 1988. *MMWR: Morbidity and Mortality Weekly, 41*(29), 529–531.

Bunker, J. P., Frazier, H. S., & Mosteller, F. (1994). Improving health: Measuring effects of medical care. *Millbank Quarterly, 72,* 225–258.

Calnan, M. (1987). *Health and illness: A lay perspective.* London: Tavistock.

Capra, F. (1982). *The turning point: Science, society, and the rising culture.* New York: Simon and Schuster.

Colhoun, H. M., Rubens, M. B., Underwood, S. R., & Fuller, J. H. (2000). Cross-sectional study of differences in coronary artery calcification by socioeconomic status. *British Medical Journal, 18,* 1262–1263.

Diez Roux, A. V., Stein Merkin, S., Arnett, D., Chambless, L., Massing, M., Nieto, F. J. et al. (2001). Neighborhood of residence and incidence of coronary heart disease. *New England Journal of Medicine, 345,* 99–106.

Donahue, P. (1985). *Nursing: The finest art.* Toronto: C.V. Mosby.

Dubos, R. (1959). *Mirage of health, utopias, progress, and biological change.* New York: Anchor Books.

Dubos, R. (1961). *Mirage of health.* New York: Doubleday.

Ehrenreich, B., & English, D. (1978). *For her own good.* Toronto: Doubleday.

Epp, J. (1986). *Achieving health for all: A framework for health promotion.* Ottawa: Health and Welfare Canada.

Evans, R. G., & Stoddard, G. L. (1990). Producing health, consuming health care. *Social Science & Medicine, 31,* 1347–1363.

Federal, Provincial, and Territorial Advisory Committee on Population Health. (1994). *Strategies for population health: Investing in the health of Canadians.* Ottawa: Minister of Supply and Services.

Federal, Provincial, and Territorial Advisory Committee on Population Health. (1999). *Toward a healthy future: The 2nd report on the health of Canadians.* Ottawa: Health Canada.

Feldman, J. J., Makuc, D. M., Kleinman, J. C., & Cornoni-Huntley, J. (1989). National trends in educational differentials in mortality. *American Journal of Epidemiology, 129,* 919–933.

Foucault, M. (1972). *The archaeology of knowledge and the discourse on language.* New York: Pantheon Books.

Fox, N. (1999). *Beyond health: Postmodernism and embodiment.* London: Free Association Books.

Frankish, C. J., Green, L. W., Ratner, P. A., Chomik, T., & Larsen, C. (1996). *Health impact assessment as a tool for population health promotion and public policy.* Vancouver: University of British Columbia, Institute of Health Promotion Research.

Gillies, P. (1998). Effectiveness of alliances and partnerships for health promotion. *Health Promotion International, 13,* 99–120.

Green, L., & Ottoson, J. (1999). *Community health and population health.* Toronto: McGraw-Hill.

Green, L. W., & Kreuter, M. W. (1999). *Health promotion planning: An educational and ecological approach* (3rd ed.). Mountain View, CA: Mayfield.

Green, L. W., Richard, L., & Potvin, L. (1996). Ecological foundations of health promotion. *American Journal of Health Promotion, 10,* 270–281.

Griffiths, H. (2002). Participatory action research. *Nursing BC, 34,* 15–17.

Habermas, J. (1973). *Theory and practice* (J. Viertel, Trans.). Boston: Beacon Press.

Heart and Stroke Foundation of Canada. (1999). *The changing face of heart disease and stroke in Canada 2000.* Ottawa: Author.

Illich, I. (1975). *Medical nemesis: The expropriation of health.* Toronto: McClelland & Stewart.

Jensen, L., & Allen, M. N. (1994). A synthesis of qualitative research on wellness-illness. *Qualitative Health Research, 4,* 349–369.

Kaplan, G., & Baron-Epel, O. (2003). What lies behind the subjective evaluation of health status? *Social Science and Medicine, 56*(8), 1669–1676.

Kaufert, P. (1996, August). *Gender as a determinant of health.* Paper presented at the Canada–US Forum on Women's Health, Ottawa. Abstract retrieved April 20, 2007, from http://www.hc-sc.gc.ca/hl-vs/pubs/women-femmes/can-usa/can-back-promo_12_e.html.

Kleffel, D. (1991). Rethinking the environment as a domain of nursing knowledge. *Advances in Nursing Science, 14,* 40–51.

Labonte, R. (1994). Death of a program, birth of a metaphor. In A. Pederson, M. O'Neill, & I. Rootman (Eds.), *Health promotion in Canada* (pp. 72–90). Toronto: W.B. Saunders.

Lalonde, M. A. (1974). *A new perspective on the health of Canadians.* Ottawa: Health and Welfare Canada.

Lantz, P. M., House, J. S., Lepkowski, J. M., Williams, D. R., Mero, R. P., & Chen, J. J. (1998). Socioeconomic factors, health behaviors, and mortality. *Journal of the American Medical Association, 279,* 1703–1708.

Larson, J. S. (1999). The conceptualization of health. *Medical Care and Review, 56,* 123–136.

LeClere, F. B., Rogers, R. G., & Peters, K. (1998). Neighbourhood social context and racial differences in women's heart disease mortality. *Journal of Health and Social Behavior, 39,* 91–107.

Lupton, D. (1992). Discourse analysis: A new methodology for understanding the ideologies of health and illness. *Australian Journal of Public Health, 16,* 145–150.

Lynch, J. W., Kaplan, G. A., & Salonen, J. T. (1997). Why do poor people behave poorly? Variation in adult health behaviours and psychosocial characteristics by stages of the socioeconomic life course. *Social Science and Medicine, 44,* 809–819.

Lyons, R., & Langille, L. (2000). *Healthy lifestyle: Strengthening the effectiveness of lifestyle approaches to improve health.* Ottawa: Health Canada, Population and Public Health Branch.

Maddox, M. (1999). Older women and the meaning of health. *Journal of Gerontological Nursing, 25,* 26–33.

Marmot, B. G. (1996). Socio-economic factors in cardiovascular disease. *Journal of Hypertension, 14*(5), S201–S205.

Marmot, M., & Wilkinson, R. G. (1999). *Social determinants of health.* Oxford, UK: Oxford University Press.

Maxwell, L. (1997). *Family influences on individual health-related decisions in response to heart-health initiatives.* Unpublished dissertation, University of British Columbia, Vancouver.

McDonald, M. (2002). Health promotion: Historical, philosophical and theoretical perspectives. In L. E. Young & V. E. Hayes (Eds.), *Transforming health promotion practice: Concepts, issues, and applications* (pp. 25–42). Philadelphia, PA: F.A. Davis.

McKinlay, J., & Marceau, L. (2000). US public health and the 21st century: Diabetes mellitus. *The Lancet, 356,* 757–761.

Meleis, A. I. (1991). *Theoretical development in nursing: Development and progress.* New York: J. B. Lippincott.

Meleis, A. I. (2007). *Theoretical nursing: Development and progress* (4th ed.). Philadelphia: Lippincott Williams & Wilkins.

Mendelson, C. (2002). Health perceptions of Mexican American women. *Journal of Transcultural Nursing, 13,* 210–217.

Moos, R. H. (1979). Social ecological perspectives on health. In G. Stone & F. Cohen (Eds.), *Health psychology: A handbook* (pp. 523–547). San Francisco: Jossey-Bass.

Nettleton, S. (1997). Surveillance, health promotion and the formation of a risk identity. In M. Sidell, L. Jones, J. Katz, & A. Peberdy (Eds.), *Debates and dilemmas in promoting health* (pp. 314–324). London: Open University Press.

Oberlander, J. (2002). The US health care system: On the road to nowhere? *Canadian Medical Association Journal, 167,* 163–168.

Perez, C., & Beaudet, M. P. (1999). The health of lone mothers. *Health Reports, 11*(2), 21–31.

Petrasovits, A. (1992). *Promoting heart health in Canada: A focus on heart health inequities.* Ottawa: Minister of Supply & Services.

Porter-O'Grady, T. (1995). Consumer ownership of health. *Advances in Practical Nursing Quarterly, 1,* 87–88.

Public Health Agency of Canada. (2005). *The population health template: Key elements and actions that define a population health approach.* Retrieved October 2, 2007, from http://www.phac-aspc.gc.ca/ph-sp/phdd/pdf/overview_handout_colour.pdf.

Putnam, R. D. (2000). *Bowling alone, the collapse and revival of American community.* New York: Simon & Schuster.

Rachlis, M., & Kushner, C. (1994). *Strong medicine: How to save Canada's health care system.* Toronto: HarperCollins.

Raeburn, J. (1992). Health promotion with heart: Keeping a people perspective. *Canadian Journal of Health Promotion, 1,* 3–5.

Raphael, D. (2001). *Inequality is bad for our hearts: Why low income and social exclusion are major causes of heart disease in Canada.* Toronto: North York Heart Health Network.

Raphael, D. (2003). Bridging the gap between knowledge and action on the societal determinants of cardiovascular disease: How one Canadian community effort hit—and hurdled—the lifestyle wall. *Health Education, 103*(3), 177–189.

Registered Nurses' Association of British Columbia. (2002). Primary health care. *Nursing BC, 34*(4), 13.

Reutter, L., Dennis, D., & Wilson, D. (2001). Young parents' understanding and actions related to the determinants of health. *Canadian Journal of Public Health, 92,* 335–339.

Richard, L., Potvin, L., Kishchuk, N., Prlic, H., & Green, L. (1996). Assessment of the integration of the ecological approach in health promotion programs. *American Journal of Health Promotion, 10,* 318–328.

Rodger, G., & Gallagher, S. (1995). The move toward primary health care in Canada: Community health nursing 1985–1995. In M. Stewart (Ed.), *Community nursing: Promoting Canadian's health* (pp. 2–36). Toronto: W.B. Saunders.

Romanow, R. (2002). *Building on values: The future of health care in Canada.* Retrieved October 4, 2007, from http://www.hc-sc.gc.ca/english/pdf/romanow/pdfs/HCC_Final_Report.pdf.

Rootman, I., & Raeburn, J. (1994). The concept of health. In A. Pederson, M. O'Neill, & I. Rootman (Eds.), *Health promotion in Canada* (pp. 139–151). Toronto: W.B. Saunders.

Social Determinants of Health Across the Life-Span Conference. (2002). *Strengthening the social determinants of health: The Toronto Charter for a healthy Canada.* Retrieved April 20, 2007, from http://www.socialjustice.org/subsites/conference/torontoCharter.PDF.

Spector, R. E. (1985). *Cultural diversity in health and illness.* Norwalk, CT: Appleton-Century-Crofts.

Spitzer, D. L. (2005). Engendering health disparities. *Canadian Journal of Public Health, 96,* S2, S78–96.

Stewart, M. J., Brosky, G., Gillis, A., Jackson, S., Johnston, G., Kirkland, S. et al. (1996). Disadvantaged women and smoking. *Canadian Journal of Public Health, 87,* 257–260.

Stokols, D. (1992). Establishing and maintaining healthy environments: Toward a social ecology of health promotion. *American Psychologist, 47,* 6–22.

Townson, M. (2000). A report card on women and poverty. *Canadian Centre for Policy Alternatives.* Retrieved April 25, 2007, from http://policyalternatives.ca/documents/National_Office_Pubs/women_poverty.pdf.

Wharf-Higgins, J., Young, L. E., Naylor, P. J., & Cunningham, S. (2006). Out of the mainstream: Low-income lone mothers' life experiences and perspectives on heart health. *Health Promotion Practice, 7*(2), 221–233.

Wilkinson, R., & Marmot, M. (1998). *Social determinants of health: The solid facts.* Geneva, Switzerland: World Health Organization, Centre for Urban Health.

World Health Organization. (1948). *Constitution of the World Health Organization as adopted by the International Health Conference* (Official Records of the World Health Organization, No. 2). Geneva, Switzerland: Author.

World Health Organization, Canadian Public Health Association, & Health and Welfare Canada. (1986). *Ottawa Charter for health promotion.* Ottawa: Health and Welfare Canada.

Young, L. E. (2002). Transforming health promotion practice: Moving toward holistic care. In L. E. Young & V. E. Hayes (Eds.), *Transforming health promotion practice: Concepts, issues, and applications* (pp. 1–25). Philadelphia, PA: F.A. Davis.

Young, L. E., Cunningham, S., & Buist, D. (2005). Lone mothers are at higher risk for cardiovascular disease compared to partnered mothers. Data from the National Health and Nutrition Examination Survey III (NHANES III). *Health Care for Women International, 26,* 604–621.

Young, L. E., James, A. & Cunningham, S. (2004). Lone motherhood and risk for cardiovascular disease: The National Population Health Survey, 1998–99. *Canadian Journal of Public Health, 95,* 329–335.

ADDITIONAL RESOURCES

Websites

B.C. Centre of Excellence for Women's Health
www.bccewh.bc.ca/index.htm

Health Canada Publications
www.hc-sc.gc.ca/ahc-asc/pubs/index_e.html

No Easy Task—A General Health Resource Website
www.noeasytask.com

Social Determinants Approach to HIV/AIDS
www.healthplanning.gov.bc.ca/hiv/determinants.html

Women's Breast Cancer Resource Center of Murrieta and Temecula Valley
www.michellesplace.org

World Health Organization Publications
www.who.int/pub/en/

Readings

Douglas, P. (Ed.). (2002). *Cardiovascular health and disease in women.* Toronto, ON: W.B. Saunders.

Keating, D., & Hertzman, C. (1999). *Developmental health and the wealth of nation: Social biological and educational dynamics.* New York: Guilford Press.

Morrow, M., Hankivsky, O., & Varcoe, C. (eds) (2007). *Women's health in Canada: Critical theory, policy and practice.* Toronto: University of Toronto Press.

Pederson, A., O'Neill, M., & Rootman, I. (1994). *Health promotion in Canada: Provincial, national and international perspectives.* Toronto, ON: W.B. Saunders.

About the Authors

Lynne Young, RN, PhD (University of British Columbia), is an Associate Professor in the School of Nursing, University of Victoria. Her research focuses on health promotion and families in the context of cardiovascular care.

Joan Wharf Higgins, PhD (University of British Columbia), is an Associate Professor in the School of Physical Education, University of Victoria. Her research and teaching interests include the social determinants of health and physical activity and social marketing.

Population Health Promotion Models and Strategies

Benita Cohen

CHAPTER 6

OBJECTIVES

After studying this chapter, you should be able to:

1. Compare and contrast the three approaches to health promotion that have been dominant since the early twentieth century and give examples of how each approach may be utilized by community health nurses.

2. Identify the milestones in the development of health promotion as a multidisciplinary field of policy and practice since the 1970s.

3. Discuss how the concepts of (a) "empowering" strategies for health promotion and (b) a microscopic ("downstream") versus macroscopic ("upstream") approach to health promotion can be applied to community health nursing practice.

4. Describe the population health promotion model and apply it to a typical community health nursing scenario.

5. Discuss guiding principles for a health-promoting community health nursing practice.

INTRODUCTION

Before reading any further, take a minute to think about the following question: "What does the term *health promotion* mean to you?" If you asked five people that question, you would probably get five different answers. Though one might expect differences in the interpretation of the concept of health promotion between nursing and other disciplines, it might surprise you to know that there is considerable diversity *within* nursing as well (Maben & MacLeod Clark, 1995). This phenomenon is reflected in the responses of a group of Canadian nursing students in a third-year course on community health promotion, who were asked what the term *health promotion* meant to them:

■ "Health promotion means educating people to make healthy lifestyle choices."

■ "Health promotion is a way of being with clients. It's more a philosophy of practice than something specific you do."

■ "Health promotion means taking action on the determinants of health—things like poverty, discrimination, marginalization, and so on. It means getting politically active."

■ "Everything nurses do is about promoting health. There isn't something specific that is health promotion." (MacDonald, 2002, p. 22)

Is your own description of health promotion similar to one of these responses? Whether it is or not, you may be wondering if there is one interpretation of health promotion that is the *correct* one. The short answer is, no. The purpose of this chapter is to explore the different ways of thinking about the concept of health promotion. The goal is not to provide a step-by-step guide on how to "do" health promotion, but rather to help the reader think critically about the various conceptual and philosophical approaches to health promotion and their implications for community health nursing practice. We will begin by tracing the historical development of health promotion as a multidisciplinary field, including major approaches and key milestones, then explore the historical role of health promotion in community health nursing, and finally end with a few general principles that may guide community health nurses' (CHNs') health promotion practice. It should be noted that although the discussion in this chapter relates primarily to the Canadian context, many of the concepts can be applied to global health promotion issues.

HISTORICAL DEVELOPMENTS IN THE APPROACH TO HEALTH PROMOTION

Labonte (1993) provides a useful way of organizing the discussion by suggesting that there have been three major approaches to health enhancement since the beginning of the twentieth century: biomedical, behavioural (lifestyle), and socio-environmental. In the following sections, each of these approaches will be discussed, highlighting the key concepts, documents, and strategies associated with them—but, even more importantly, highlighting the dominant theories and values that underlie them. Please note that although these approaches emerged at different points in time, they are all still present to varying degrees in the health field, depending on one's area of practice. Labonte (1993) suggests that all three approaches are useful and that health professionals may find themselves alternating among them at different times and for different purposes. Let's explore these approaches in more detail.

Dominance of the Biomedical Approach

Beginning with the discovery of disease-causing pathogens in the eighteenth and nineteenth centuries, and gaining momentum with the immense expansion of scientific knowledge during the twentieth century, the **biomedical approach** to health enhancement has dominated mainstream thinking in Western society.[1] The key features of this perspective are outlined in the second column of Table 6.1. Essentially, you can think of this approach as synonymous with preventive health care. It is focused on preventing disease or disability in individuals by decreasing their **physiological risk factors** (hypertension, hypercholesterolemia, lack of immunity, etc.). Although the biomedical approach was never the *only* way that people understood the concept of health, and there have always been areas of overlap with the next approach that we will discuss, this conceptualization of health and health promotion still remains a powerful perspective in our society today. Biomedical strategies, such as immunization and screening tests for early detection and treatment of disease, remain an important part of public health practice.

TABLE 6.1
Summary of Different Approaches to Health Enhancement

	Biomedical	Behavioural	Socio-environmental
Health concept	• absence of disease or disability	• physical-functional ability; physical-emotional well-being	• goes beyond physical-emotional well-being to include social well-being at individual and community levels; may be viewed as a resource for daily living rather than a "state" that one aspires to
Health determinant	• physiological risk factors (e.g., hypertension)	• behavioural risk factors (e.g., smoking); lifestyle	• psychosocial risk factors (e.g., low self-esteem) • socio-environmental risk conditions (e.g., poverty)
Target	• primarily high-risk individuals (because of above risk factors)	• primarily high-risk groups (because of above risk factors)	• high-risk conditions and environments
Principal strategies	• screening for risk factors • patient education and compliance for behaviour change (e.g., dietary counselling) • immunization	• health education • social marketing • regulatory measures and public policies supporting healthy lifestyle choices (e.g., smoking ban)	• *Ottawa Charter* strategies (strengthening community action, creating supportive environments, developing healthy public policy, developing personal skills, reorienting health systems) • empowerment strategies (personal empowerment, small-group development, community organization/ development, advocacy for healthy public policy, political action)
Program development	• professionally managed	• professionally managed, or may be community-based[1]	• community development[2]
Success criteria	• decrease in morbidity and mortality rates • decrease in prevalence of physiological risk factors	• decrease in behavioural risk factors; improved lifestyles • enactment of healthy public policies related to health behaviours	• improved personal perception of health • improved social networks, quality of social support • improved community group actions to create more equitable social distribution of power/resources • enactment of healthy public policies related to social equity and environmental sustainability

1. Community-based programming: the process of health professionals and/or health agencies defining the health problem, developing strategies to remedy the problem, involving local community members and groups to assist in solving the problem, and working to transfer major responsibility for ongoing programs to local community members and groups.

2. Community-development programming: the process of supporting community groups in their identification of important concerns and issues and in their ability to plan and implement strategies to mitigate their concerns and resolve their issues.

Source: Adapted with permission from Labonte, R. (1993). Health promotion and empowerment: Practice frameworks. *Toronto, ON: University of Toronto, Centre for Health Promotion.*

The Behavioural/Lifestyle Approach

It is generally agreed that the birth of the modern era of health promotion as an organized and distinct multidisciplinary field in health policy and practice occurred in the 1970s. The major turning point in thinking about the concept of health promotion occurred in 1974 with the publication of a discussion paper by the Canadian Department of Health and Welfare entitled *A New Perspective on the Health of Canadians* (Lalonde, 1974). The **Lalonde Report** (as it is commonly referred to) noted that, in spite of a massive expansion of spending on health services during the previous two decades, the health of Canadians was not improving. In fact, morbidity and premature mortality rates for certain chronic or degenerative diseases (such as heart disease, cancer, respiratory disease, sexually transmitted infections) and injuries (especially motor vehicle related) were steadily increasing. Instead of pouring more and more money into services for the sick, the Lalonde Report argued for a "new perspective"—one that paid more attention to the promotion of health.

The Lalonde Report was important for several reasons, one of them being that this was the first time a national government had made such a statement regarding the importance of health promotion as a key strategy for improving the health of a population. Another contribution of the Lalonde Report was that, although the concept of health was still defined in its most basic form as "freedom from disease and disability" (Lalonde, 1974, p. 8), the added reference to promoting "a state of well-being sufficient to perform at adequate levels of physical, mental and social activity" (p. 8) did allow for a slightly expanded interpretation of health that included the idea of increased functional "ability" and a sense of "wellness" (Labonte, 1993). Perhaps the most important contribution was that the document challenged the dominant thinking of the time, which viewed access to health services as the key to population health. Instead, it suggested that the organization and availability of health services was one of four main categories of factors (or "health fields") that influenced the health of Canadians, the others being human biology, the environment, and lifestyle.

While the Lalonde framework appeared to place equal weight on each of the four fields, a central argument was that a large proportion of the premature mortality and morbidity occurring among the population at the time appeared to be due to individual behaviours or lifestyles that could be modified (smoking and other addictions, poor nutrition, lack of physical activity, risky sexual behaviour, etc.). Therefore, it was argued, the focus of health promotion efforts should be on the use of strategies that encourage the adoption of behaviours or lifestyles that promote functional ability and well-being. This perspective on health and health promotion has come to be known as the **behavioural** or **lifestyle approach** (both terms are commonly used in the literature). The key characteristics of this approach are outlined in the third column of Table 6.1. Essentially, the behavioural approach focuses on the prevention of disease and disability (often expressed in terms of promoting "wellness") in people who are at risk because of their lifestyle or behavioural risk factors such as a high-fat diet, lack of exercise, unsafe sexual practices, or use of tobacco, alcohol, or other drugs. A brief description of strategies that focus on changing behaviour can be found in Table 6.2.

The common thread in each of these strategies is the underlying belief that the main determinant of health is individual behaviour or lifestyle, and that information, persuasion, or any other method (including legal coercion) that encourages people to adopt healthier behaviours or lifestyles is the key to health promotion.[2] The behavioural approach to health promotion continues to be very popular. National and provincial governments frequently rely on health communication campaigns to deliver "healthy lifestyle" messages, social marketing techniques have been used in HIV/AIDS prevention initiatives, health education programs based on various

---

TABLE 6.2
Strategies that Focus on Changing Behaviour/Lifestyle

Health education	Usually refers to activities associated with formal education, including use of audiovisual materials, printed educational materials, teaching strategies for the classroom (e.g., lecture/discussion, case studies, brainstorming), teaching strategies outside the classroom (e.g., health fair). May also refer to one-on-one teaching.
Health communication	Usually refers to the use of the mass media, direct mail, product labels, pamphlets, and posters to communicate a health message to the public. May also refer to health professional–client interaction.
Social marketing	Refers to "the application of commercial marketing technologies to the analysis, planning, execution and evaluation of programs designed to influence the voluntary behaviour of target audiences in order to improve their personal welfare and that of society" (Andreasen, 1995, cited in Nutbeam & Harris, 1998, p. 49). Usually involves health communication techniques mentioned above; may include sponsorship, participation events, direct selling, and competitions.
Behaviour modification	Refers to a systematic procedure for changing a specific behaviour by changing the events that precede or result in modification from the behaviour that is to be modified. Most often used to alter smoking, eating, or exercise patterns.
Regulatory measures	Refers to mandated activities (laws, policies, regulations). Examples include laws requiring the use of seatbelts or motorcycle helmets and banning smoking in public places.

theories of behaviour change are commonly used within the school system, and health teaching remains a major part of health care professionals' practice.

The Socio-environmental Approach to Health Promotion

A number of factors contributed to a new way of thinking about health promotion in the 1980s. The first factor relates to ideological responses to the behavioural approach. Labonte (1993) notes that the 1980s were a time when many of the social movements that emerged in North America in the 1960s and 1970s were maturing. Within these social movements, such concepts as **social justice** (the belief that all persons are entitled equally to key ends such as health protection and minimum standards of income) and the **common good** (where the needs of the many have priority over the needs of the individual) (Beauchamp, 1976) were central principles. Many of the activists who took part in these social movements later moved into professional jobs, including those in the health and social services fields. These individuals were critical of the focus on individual behaviour that had come to dominate the field of health promotion in the early 1980s. They argued that health and illness are the result of broad factors such as the socioeconomic and physical environment, the level of social support and social cohesion among individuals and communities, the level of education, working conditions, and so on. They viewed **social change** (as opposed to individual behaviour change) as the most important goal of health promotion, and **social responsibility for health** as paramount. From this perspective, approaches that focus solely on individual behaviour change and individual responsibility for health were viewed as a form of **victim-blaming**, whereby individuals end up being implicitly blamed for being sick because they have "chosen" unhealthy lifestyles or they have unhealthy coping styles when, in fact, their social and economic circumstances have often left them with limited options (Crawford, 1977; Labonte & Penfold, 1981).

At the same time that this ideological critique of the behavioural approach was being articulated, a theoretical perspective emerged from the field of social ecology, which is referred to as an **ecological** or **socio-ecological perspective** on health promotion. The central premise of this perspective is that health is a product of the *interdependence* between the individual and subsystems of the ecosystem (family, community, culture, and physical and social environment). From an ecological perspective, both individual behaviour change and environmental or system change are required elements of health promotion initiatives—neither one on its own is sufficient. This perspective had a major influence on the approach to health promotion that emerged in the mid-1980s.[3]

In addition to the ideological and theoretical critiques of the behavioural approach to health promotion outlined above, two other factors influenced the development of a new way of thinking about health promotion. In the 1980s, several high-profile, population-wide, disease-prevention initiatives to reduce the behaviours that were viewed as major

contributors to coronary heart disease (such as smoking, high intake of dietary fat, low levels of physical activity) failed to achieve their intended results (Syme, 1997). Even in cases where disease prevention initiatives *did* result in reductions in high-risk behaviours, it was primarily the better educated, middle-class members of society who benefited. Many of these programs failed to reach individuals from lower socio-economic groups who suffered from the poorest social and physical health (Labonte, 1993). As a result, it has been suggested that "effective" health promotion programs that focus on lifestyle change can actually contribute to the *increase* of social inequalities in health (Makara, 1997).

The final contributing factor to a new way of thinking about health promotion in the 1980s was the epidemiological evidence that could not be ignored. Beginning in the 1970s and escalating in the 1980s and beyond, a substantial body of research emerged suggesting that the distribution of disease in any given society is *not* the result of individual behaviours, but *is* the result of the economic, political, and social relationship between individuals and groups in society. In particular, there is now a powerful body of evidence indicating that social and economic inequality is one of the major determinants—some would argue, *the* major determinant—for disease (Wilkinson & Pickett, 2006). There is also a robust body of evidence suggesting that social support is a major influence on the well-being of individuals (Heaney & Israel, 2002). At the community level, *social stress* (as evidenced by economic deprivation, crowding, family instability, and crime) or *social cohesion* (the flip side of social breakdown) are important determinants of health and disease (Patrick & Wickizer, 1995; Sampson, 2003; Stansfeld, 2003). Together, the various bodies of research suggest that health promotion approaches that focus on individual behaviour change are insufficient to address the key determinants of population health.

Key Milestones in the Development of the Socio-environmental Approach In addition to the factors previously discussed, several pivotal events and policy statements mark the formal development of a new approach to health promotion. First, it has been noted that the seeds of a social definition of health promotion were sown as early as 1977 when the World Health Organization (WHO) proposed its vision for *Health for All by the Year 2000,* and in 1978 when the WHO released the *Alma Ata Declaration on Primary Health Care* (MacDonald, 2002). Primary health care (PHC) was anticipated to be the means of achieving the goals outlined in the *Health for All* document, and several principles of PHC—especially the importance of community participation and the need for intersectoral collaboration in order to address the broad social and environmental determinants of population health—emerged as key principles in the new approach to health promotion (a more detailed discussion of PHC is available in Chapter 7).

Several Canadian conferences in the early 1980s had an influence on the shift in thinking about health promotion, both in this country and internationally. For example, at the 1984 "Beyond Health Care" conference in Toronto, the concept of healthy cities and the need for healthy public policies that focus on environmental determinants of health such as housing (and other factors contributing to the health of cities) was raised for the first time. This concept challenged the notion of health as an individual characteristic and focused very much on its social and environmental dimensions. The conference is widely recognized as having given birth to a worldwide movement to establish **healthy cities/communities** (Raeburn & Rootman, 1998).

At the international level, 1984 was the year that the WHO released a discussion document that identified five key principles of health promotion:

- Health promotion involves the population as a whole and the context of their everyday life, rather than focusing on people at risk for specific diseases.

- Health promotion is directed toward action on the determinants or causes of health.

- Health promotion combines diverse, but complementary, methods or approaches.

- Health promotion aims particularly at effective and concrete public participation.

- Health professionals, particularly in primary health care, have an important role in nurturing and enabling health promotion. (World Health Organization, 1984, p. 3)

This idea was elaborated on a couple of years later, when two key events occurred that have contributed to the popular identification of 1986 as the birth date of the "new health promotion." First, the Canadian Minister of National Health and Welfare at the time, Jake Epp, released a document entitled *Achieving Health for All: A Framework for Health Promotion* (Epp, 1986), which clearly distanced itself from the behavioural/lifestyle approach to health promotion. In acknowledgment of the growing body of evidence regarding the social and economic determinants of population health, the Epp Report argued that health promotion was as much a societal responsibility as an individual responsibility. It identified three leading health challenges facing Canadians: the need to reduce inequities in the health of low- versus high-income groups; the need to find new and more effective ways of preventing the occurrence of injuries, illnesses, chronic conditions, and their resulting disabilities; and the need to enhance people's ability to manage and cope with chronic conditions, disabilities, and mental health problems. In order to meet these challenges, three mechanisms for health promotion were identified: *self-care*, referring to the decisions taken and practices adopted by an individual specifically for the preservation of their health; *mutual aid*, referring to people's efforts to deal with their health concerns by working together (either through informal social support networks, voluntary organizations, or self-help groups); and the *creation of healthy environments* at home, school, work, or wherever else Canadians may be. Lastly, three main health promotion strategies were identified as the basis for putting these mechanisms into action: *fostering public participation*, by helping people assert control over the factors that affect their health; *strengthening community health services*, by allocating a greater share of resources to those services that have an orientation to health promotion and disease prevention; and *coordinating*

health public policies between sectors (such as income security, employment, education, housing, etc.) that make it easier for people to make healthy choices. It is important to note that the Epp Report clearly stated that a focus on one strategy or mechanism from the framework on its own would be of little significance; it was only by putting the pieces of the framework together that health promotion would be meaningful.

Epp's framework was presented later in 1986 at the first International Health Promotion Conference in Ottawa, where it influenced the development of the **Ottawa Charter for Health Promotion** (World Health Organization, 1986)—a document that was signed by delegates from 38 countries, including Canada. The *Ottawa Charter* defined health promotion as "the process of enabling people to increase control over, and improve, their health"[4] (p. 5), and it emphasized that achieving **equity in health** was considered to be the main focus of health promotion. A number of essential prerequisites for health were identified (peace, shelter, education, food, income, a stable ecosystem, sustainable resources, social justice, and equity), and the importance of coordinated intersectoral action to ensure these prerequisites for health was underlined. The *Ottawa Charter* proposed five key strategies for health promotion:

- **Strengthening community action**—Involves supporting those activities that encourage community members to participate in, and take action on, issues that affect their health and the health of others. Community development or community empowerment is viewed as both the means and the end result of this process. Priority is given to those individuals and communities whose living and working conditions place them at greatest risk for poor health.

- **Building healthy public policy**—Involves advocacy for any health, income, environmental, or social policy that fosters greater equity, creates a setting for health, or increases options/resources for health.

- **Creating supportive environments**—Involves generating living, working, and playing conditions that are safe, stimulating, satisfying, and enjoyable and by ensuring that the protection of the natural environment is addressed in any health promotion strategy.

- **Developing personal skills**—Involves supporting personal and social development through the provision of information—education for health and enhancing life skills—in order to increase the options available to people to exercise more control over their own health and environments and to make choices conducive to health.

- **Reorienting health services**—Involves moving beyond the health sector's responsibility for providing clinical and curative services in a health promotion direction that is sensitive to the needs of the community. (World Health Organization, 1986)

An important feature of the new health promotion perspective found in the *Ottawa Charter* is the link made between the concept of **empowerment** and the promotion of health. Empowerment refers to "an active, involved process where people, groups, and communities move toward increased individual and community control, political efficacy, improved quality of community life, and social justice" (Community Health Nurses Association of Canada [CHNAC], 2003, p. 6). It also refers to the outcome of that process (Vollman, Anderson, & McFarlane, 2004). Wallerstein (1992) distinguishes between individual psychological empowerment, which involves self-efficacy and motivation to act, and community empowerment, which involves increased local action, stronger social networks, resource access/equity, transformed conditions, and community competence. While health care professionals cannot directly empower others— empowerment is something that cannot be given; it must be taken (Vanderplaat, 2002)—they can help people and communities develop, secure, and/or use the resources and skills that promote a sense of control and self-efficacy (Gibson, 1991).

The publication of the *Ottawa Charter* is widely recognized as marking the transition, at least in theory, from an "old" health promotion practice that focused on medical and behavioural health determinants to a "new" health promotion practice that defined health determinants in psychological, social, environmental, and political terms. See column 4 of Table 6.1 for a summary of the key features of this **socio-environmental approach** to health promotion. Canadian Research Box 6.1 describes a community health problem in which each of the three approaches to health promotion that we have discussed might be applicable.

Canadian Research Box 6.1

Broughton, M. A., Janssen, P. S., Hertzman, C., Innis, S. M., & Frankish, C. J. (2006). Predictors and outcomes of household food insecurity among inner city families with preschool children in Vancouver. *Canadian Journal of Public Health, 97*(3), 214–216.

The purposes of this study were to measure household food security and to determine its association with potential predictor variables related to household and community environments, as well as the relationship between household food insecurity and preschool children's nutritional status. Household food insecurity was measured by using the 18-item United States Department of Agriculture's Food Security Survey Module. In this survey, household food insecurity is defined as anxiety about a household's food supply or reduced quality or quantity of food consumed. The study sample included 142 households in low-income neighbourhoods in Vancouver, each with a child between the ages of 2 and 5.

The prevalence of food insecurity was five times higher in the study sample compared with the Vancouver population. One-third of the children sampled were overweight or obese, and preschoolers in food-insecure households had more than twice the odds of a body mass index indicating overweight/obesity compared with those in food-secure households. Low income was the primary risk factor for food insecurity, but factors apart from household income, in household and community environments, were potential barriers to food security. For example, parents with less

access to food of reasonable quality (e.g., convenience stores offering foods of lower quality with less nutritional value, often the only option for mothers with small children and without access to a vehicle), fewer kitchen appliances, and a lower rating of their cooking skills had greater odds of experiencing household food insecurity.

The authors note that evidence indicates food insecurity has adverse consequences on children's ability to participate in learning experiences due to difficulty concentrating, poorer health status, more disruptive behaviour, and aggression. They suggest that collaborative efforts among government, social planners, and public health practitioners to remove barriers to food security for families are required.

Discussion Questions:

1. What roles/activities could CHNs engage in as part of a comprehensive health promotion initiative aimed at improving food security and healthy child development among families in low-income neighbourhoods?

2. How would your answer to question 1 differ if you applied each of the approaches to health promotion?

Population Health Promotion

In 1994, the Federal, Provincial, Territorial Advisory Committee on Population Health published a document entitled *Strategies for Population Health: Investing in the Health of Canadians,* which described an approach to public policy that focuses on taking action on the interrelated conditions that influence population health status. These interrelated conditions were identified as income and social status, social support networks, education, employment and working conditions, safe and clean physical environments, biology and genetic makeup, personal health practices and coping skills, early childhood development, and health services. Since that time, the population health perspective has been adopted at the policy level by the federal government, several provincial governments, and some regional health authorities.[5] However, there are a number of characteristics of a population health approach that differ from those of the socio-environmental approach to health promotion outlined earlier. For example, the socio-environmental approach focuses on addressing inequities in health experienced by disadvantaged and marginalized groups; it defines health in its broadest sense as a resource for daily living; and it identifies a wide range of strategies for change that emphasize individual and community empowerment. In contrast, population health is mostly concerned with gradients in health status across all socioeconomic levels; health is defined in terms of traditional epidemiological "sickness" indicators; and the focus is on identifying determinants of disease and death rather than strategies for change.

In an effort to bridge the gap between population health and health promotion a **population health promotion**

model (PHPM) was developed by Health Canada (Hamilton & Bhatti, 1996), which attempts to integrate concepts from both perspectives. (See Figure 6.1.) This three-dimensional model combines the strategies for health promotion outlined in the 1986 *Ottawa Charter* on one side, the determinants of population health on another side, and various levels of potential intervention on a third side. This model can be used from different entry points. One can begin with the health determinant that one intends to influence, the action strategy to be used, or the level at which action is to be taken. Or, alternatively, the model can be used to plan a comprehensive range of actions on emerging health issues or issues related to the health of a particular priority group (Hamilton & Bhatti, 1996). Figure 6.2 shows examples of how the model can be used to identify possibilities for influencing various determinants of health. The model can also be used to address the health concerns of groups who are at risk for poor health. The PHPM reflects the socio-environmental perspective. From this perspective we are primarily concerned with social and environmental risk conditions and psychosocial risk factors that are known to affect health status, either directly or indirectly via behaviours. An example of risk conditions would be a deprived neighbourhood where the housing is substandard, there are few recreational facilities, community spirit is weak, and there are feelings of danger and insecurity (Hamilton & Bhatti, 1996).

The positive contribution of the PHPM is that it addresses one of the main criticisms of the population health perspective—that is, that it doesn't provide a model for change (Cohen, 2006a; Labonte, 1995; Raphael & Bryant, 2000).

Rather than simply identifying the broad determinants of health, the PHPM proposes strategies for acting on them. Limitations of the PHPM (like the *Ottawa Charter* itself) include the fact that it does not provide an explanatory model regarding the exact pathways between the determinants of health and health status; the population health determinants don't necessarily include all of the prerequisites for health that may be important, and there are few concrete details of how to carry out the PHPM strategies or indicators or tools for evaluating them (leaving each one open to wide interpretation).

SOCIETAL DETERMINANTS OF HEALTH

One of the limitations of the PHPM (and the population health approach in general) is that the list of population health determinants appears to give equal weight to behavioural and socio-environmental determinants, yet there is now

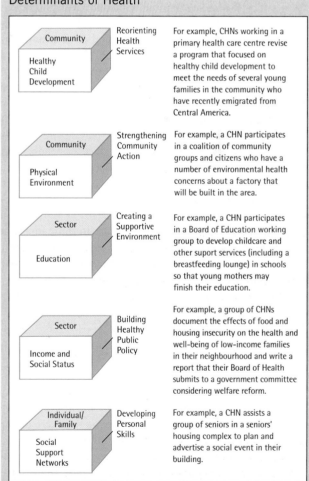

FIGURE 6.2 Using the PHPM to Influence Determinants of Health

Community / Healthy Child Development	Reorienting Health Services	For example, CHNs working in a primary health care centre revise a program that focused on healthy child development to meet the needs of several young families in the community who have recently emigrated from Central America.
Community / Physical Environment	Strengthening Community Action	For example, a CHN participates in a coalition of community groups and citizens who have a number of environmental health concerns about a factory that will be built in the area.
Sector / Education	Creating a Supportive Environment	For example, a CHN participates in a Board of Education working group to develop childcare and other suport services (including a breastfeeding lounge) in schools so that young mothers may finish their education.
Sector / Income and Social Status	Building Healthy Public Policy	For example, a group of CHNs document the effects of food and housing insecurity on the health and well-being of low-income families in their neighbourhood and write a report that their Board of Health submits to a government committee considering welfare reform.
Individual/ Family / Social Support Networks	Developing Personal Skills	For example, a CHN assists a group of seniors in a seniors' housing complex to plan and advertise a social event in their building.

Sources: Adapted from Hamilton & Bhatti, 1996, Population health promotion: An integrated model of population health and health promotion. Ottawa: Health Canada, Health Promotion and Development Division. Reproduced with the permission of the Minister of Public Works and Government Services Canada, 2007.

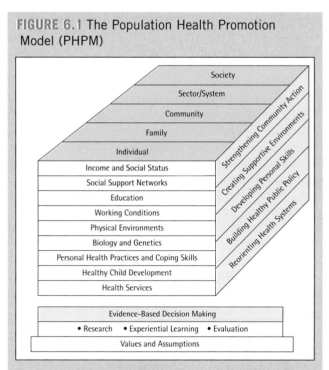

FIGURE 6.1 The Population Health Promotion Model (PHPM)

Society
Sector/System
Community
Family
Individual

Strengthening Community Action
Creating Supportive Environments
Developing Personal Skills
Building Healthy Public Policy
Reorienting Health Systems

Income and Social Status
Social Support Networks
Education
Working Conditions
Physical Environments
Biology and Genetics
Personal Health Practices and Coping Skills
Healthy Child Development
Health Services

Evidence-Based Decision Making
• Research   • Experiential Learning   • Evaluation
Values and Assumptions

Sources: Hamilton & Bhatti, Population health promotion: An integrated model of population health and health promotion, (1996) © Adapted and Reproduced with the permission of the Minister of Public Works and Government Services Canada, 2006.

Social Determinants of Health:
The Toronto Charter for a Healthy Canada,
2002 (Raphael, 2004)

Early child development

Education

Employment and working conditions

Food security

Health care services

Housing shortages

Income and its equitable distribution

Social exclusion

Social safety nets

Unemployment

substantial evidence that social and economic conditions are the most influential determinants of health (Raphael, 2004). In 2002, a conference of more than 400 Canadian social and health policy experts, community representatives, and health researchers took place at York University in Toronto to consider the state of ten key **social or societal determinants of health** (SDOH) across Canada (see the box "Social Determinants of Health: The *Toronto Charter for a Healthy Canada, 2002*") and to outline policy directions to improve the health of Canadians by influencing the quality of these SDOH (Raphael, 2004). The immediate outcome of the conference was the drafting by conference participants of *The Toronto Charter for a Healthy Canada.* (See Appendix 1 in Raphael, 2004.) The *Toronto Charter* resolved that staff of all health care agencies should be knowledgeable about the SDOH and called for specific immediate and long-term actions to address them. If you look at the list of SDOH, you will see that some of them are very similar to those found in the PHPM, but some are not (e.g., food security, social safety net). If you are interested in addressing one or more of these determinants, they could easily be inserted into the PHPM.

Health Promotion in Community Health Nursing

Now that we have explored the major theoretical developments in the multidisciplinary field of health promotion, let's take a look at the role of health promotion in community health nursing. The idea that nurses are at the heart of the practice of health promotion, are in a position to play a strong leadership role in health promotion, and are the most strategically placed health professionals to accomplish health promotion goals with clients is not uncommon in the nursing literature (Dallaire, Hagan, & O'Neill, 2000; MacDonald, 2002). The question is, does everyone use the term "health promotion" in the same way? MacDonald (2002) notes that many nursing authors seem to assume there is a widely shared

understanding of the term health promotion, whereas in reality there is considerable diversity in the interpretation and underlying ideologies of health promotion within the nursing profession. In one review of the nursing practice and health promotion literature, the authors identified six different understandings of health promotion: (i) as an umbrella term referring to any activity designed to foster health; (ii) as a synonym to health education; (iii) as the marketing or selling of health; (iv) as a strategy concerned with lifestyle behaviour change; (v) as health education plus environmental and legislative measures designed to facilitate the achievement of health and prevention of disease; and (vi) as an approach that encompasses a set of values including concepts of empowerment, equity, and collaboration (Maben & MacLeod Clark, 1995). The authors note that the first four understandings are in line with a traditional behavioural approach to health promotion, whereas the latter two are synonymous with the socio-environmental approach as outlined in the *Ottawa Charter* (WHO, 1986). Which understanding of health promotion is the most influential among nurses? This is the question that will be explored in the following sections.

The Behavioural Approach in Nursing

In the early 1980s, Brubaker (1983) found that the primary emphasis of health promotion in the nursing literature of the time was on personal responsibility, lifestyle behaviour change, and high-level wellness. In the 1990s, in spite of the emergence of the socio-environmental perspective in the broader health promotion movement and among certain nursing theorists, the behavioural conceptualization of health promotion remained predominant in nursing *practice,* including community health nursing practice (Benson & Latter, 1998). In the 2000s, there is evidence that this still remains the case (Whitehead, 2003).

Why have nurses adopted the lifestyle approach to health promotion? It could be argued that this is simply an extension of what they have been doing for years. Healthy lifestyles and behaviours have long been of concern to nurses, and health education has always been a central focus of nursing practice. This is true in the hospital, where nurses provide health teaching to patients and their families, but it has been even more so for nurses working in the community. In the late nineteenth century, Florence Nightingale—widely considered the founder of modern nursing—wrote about the importance of teaching mothers proper sanitation methods and childcare under the supervision of district nurses; by the early twentieth century, advising and instructing people on how to avoid illness through personal hygiene and how to promote healthy child development was a primary duty of public health nurses (Novak, 1988). Providing information related to healthy child development and health promoting behaviours remains a central role of CHNs to this day.

Another reason why the behavioural approach remains influential in nursing practice may have to do with the fact that many of the nursing models used in nursing education and practice since the 1970s have been strongly influenced by concepts and theories from the behavioural sciences, where individual behaviour change is the outcome of interest. For example, Pender's (1996) **Health Promotion Model (HPM)** was the first nursing model to focus *explicitly* on health promotion, and it remains an influential model in community health nursing education and practice (Stewart & Leipert, 2000). Strongly influenced by the Health Belief Model, which was developed to explain why individuals do or do not take action to prevent disease, the HPM suggests that (a) cognitive factors such as perceived benefits and barriers to action and perceived self-efficacy combine with (b) individual biological, psychological, and socio-cultural characteristics and experience (e.g., prior related behaviour, age, gender, socioeconomic status) and (c) intrapersonal and situational influences (e.g., family, peers, health care providers, environmental cues) to (d) lead the individual to commit to a plan of action that will (e) result in health-promoting behaviour. One of the limitations of this type of health promotion model is that attempting to change someone's health behaviour may be futile if the individual does not have the material or social resources to support the desired behaviour change. Although Pender's revised HPM (Pender, Murdaugh, & Parsons, 2005) acknowledges the need for social and environmental change, the nurse's role remains primarily to change perceptions and attitudes that are viewed as non-health-enhancing and to assist the client to develop, carry out, and evaluate a behaviour-change plan.[6]

The Socio-environmental Approach in Nursing

MacDonald (2002) notes that a critique of the lifestyle/behavioural approach to health promotion (which was consistent with the concepts and ideas that were central to the socio-environmental perspective on health promotion) emerged in the mid-1980s, but it never represented more than a marginal position in nursing until the late 1990s. Since that time, many of the foundational concepts in nursing (client, environment, etc.) have expanded to be more congruent with the socio-environmental perspective. For example, "environment" has been challenged to expand from a traditional, narrow focus on the psychosocial environment of the individual to a broader focus on the socio-political context that affects the health of individuals, groups, and communities (MacDonald, 2002). Others have explored the relevance of concepts inherent in the WHO's statements on PHC and the *Ottawa Charter*—such as empowerment, community participation, community development, and partnerships—to nursing theory and practice in particular settings or with particular client groups (MacDonald, 2002).

One of the most well known critiques of traditional nursing practice was articulated by Butterfield (1997). Using McKinlay's (1979) famous "upstream–downstream" analogy of people (read: health care providers) being so caught up with rescuing victims (patients) from a swiftly flowing river (representing illness) they have no time to look upstream and see who is pushing these people into the water (the root cause of illness). Butterfield suggested that CHNs needed to adopt a **macroscopic approach** in their practice—more commonly referred to as **thinking upstream**—as opposed to the traditional "downstream" or **microscopic approach**. (See Table 6.3.) An important aspect of the macroscopic approach in community health nursing is that it is not usually carried out by one nurse alone but often involves the cooperative efforts of nurses and other service providers from school, occupational, and other community settings (Butterfield, 1997).

The concept of thinking upstream is a valuable contribution to community health nursing practice because it encourages CHNs to address the root causes of health issues in individuals, families, and communities. However, two of the central features of the socio-environmental approach to health promotion—the idea of health promotion as a process of empowerment and the belief that reducing social and economic inequalities in health is a central goal—are not immediately apparent in the macroscopic approach outlined by Butterfield. In contrast, other critiques of traditional approaches to nursing—sometimes referred to as **emancipatory nursing** or **critical social nursing**—have focused specifically on the nurse's role in addressing inequalities in health, and they address the issue of empowerment as well (Reutter, 2000; Vanderplaat, 2002).

Reutter (2000), a Canadian promoter of a critical social approach to community health nursing, notes that this approach includes asking critical questions to expose inequities, facilitating community involvement by listening to community needs, and assisting in bringing about changes. Rather than presenting solutions and directing lifestyle changes, the nurse's role is facilitative: assisting individuals and groups to reflect on the social and political factors that influence health, sharing expertise, and providing support. More specifically, Reutter suggests that a critical social approach to reducing inequities in health would include empowering strategies at the personal, interpersonal (small group), community, and policy levels. (See Figure 7.2 in Chapter 7.) At the personal or individual level, Reutter suggests that an empowering nursing strategy would involve not only understanding the psychosocial and socio-environmental context of the individual's concerns and problems and acknowledging these constraints, but also focusing on increasing the capacity of individuals to act upon the roots of their distress and advocating for and with clients to access the resources that they require to change their situation. This level of empowering strategy is similar to the *Ottawa Charter* strategy of *developing personal skills*. It may involve the provision of information and advice, but it goes beyond that to building individual capacity for problem solving, decision making, and other life skills. At the interpersonal level, Reutter points out that CHNs can be involved in empowering strategies through facilitating the development of small groups that can decrease the social isolation that often accompanies poverty and providing affirmational, informational, and emotional support. Small groups, therefore, can increase personal empowerment and may foster community action. Small-group development also fits with the *Ottawa Charter* strategy of *creating a*

TABLE 6.3
"Thinking Upstream": Macroscopic vs. Microscopic Approaches in Community Health Nursing

"Downstream" (Microscopic) Approach	"Upstream" (Macroscopic) Approach
• Assessment focuses on individual (and family) responses to health and illness; often emphasizes an individual's behavioural and coping responses to illness or lifestyle patterns	• Assessment focuses on interfamily and intercommunity themes in health and illness • Identifies social, economic, and environmental factors in the community and population that perpetuate the development of illness or foster the development of health
• Nursing interventions are often aimed at modifying an individual's behaviour (including coping behaviours) through changing their perceptions or belief system or providing information	• Nursing interventions may include modifying social or environmental variables (in other words, working to remove barriers to care or improving sanitation or living conditions); this may include social or political action

Source: Community Health Nursing: Promoting the Health of Aggregate, *1997, Butterfield. W. B. Saunders Company, Mosby Churchill Livingstone, Elsevier Science.*

supportive environment. At the community level, Reutter suggests that CHNs can use a community development approach to support community groups in identifying important issues related to poverty and in organizing collectively to plan and implement strategies to resolve these issues. This approach fits nicely with the *Ottawa Charter* strategy of *strengthening community action.* At the policy level, Reutter notes that CHNs can play an active role in advocating for structural changes that mitigate the effects of or reduce poverty, and/or they can support community groups in their own advocacy efforts to do the same—an approach that Labonte (1993) referred to as "advocacy with." For example, CHNs can serve on inter-sectoral boards and committees that influence public policy in such areas as housing, unemployment, income security, childcare, and environmental health, or they may get involved with neighbourhood associations, citizens' groups, and advocacy groups such as anti-poverty organizations. This approach is similar to the *Ottawa Charter* strategy of *advocacy for healthy public policy.*

One traditional nursing concept that has been given a socio-environmental twist is that of "caring." A Canadian educator and researcher (Falk-Rafael, 2005a) has developed a **critical caring theory** for public health nursing that aims to reincorporate the social justice agenda (characteristic of early public health nursing practice), which has not featured prominently in contemporary nursing theories. One of the core carative processes of PHNs' practice Falk-Rafael identifies is contributing to the creation of supportive and sustainable physical, social, political, and economic environments. The idea that CHNs have a critical role to play in addressing social inequities in health such as poverty and social exclusion through advocacy and action for social change is now more common in the literature (Ballou, 2000; Cohen & Reutter, 2007; Falk-Rafael, 2005b; Spenceley, Reutter, & Allen, 2006; Williamson & Drummond, 2000).

Relatively little has been written about family health promotion compared with individual-level and community-level

health promotion (Young, 2002). In Canada, several models have been developed that focus on the family as the unit of nurses' health promoting interactions (Feeley & Gottlieb, 2000; Hartrick, 2000; Wright & Leahey, 2005). However, only Hartrick's (2000) model of family health promotion is specifically based on an emancipatory approach to nurses' family health promotion practice. Developed at the University of Victoria School of Nursing, this health-promoting family nursing assessment framework suggests that the focus of family assessment is on identifying and resourcing family potential, and facilitating the promotion of client autonomy and empowerment as the family itself identifies courses of action for positive change.

The Socio-environmental Approach in Canadian Nursing Practice Between 1987 and 1993 in Canada, position statements and discussion documents from national and provincial nurses' associations and the community health nursing section of the Canadian Public Health Association (CPHA) identified health promotion—as defined in the *Ottawa Charter* (WHO, 1986) and *Achieving Health for All* (Epp, 1986)—as the primary goal of nursing practice (Canadian Nurses Association, 1992; Canadian Public Health Association, 1990; MacDonald, 2002). In Manitoba, a document entitled *The Role of the Public Health Nurse within the Regional Health Authority* (Manitoba Health, 1998) framed its discussion within the context of the *Ottawa* Charter strategies for health promotion. (See Figure 6.3.) At the national level, the Community Health Nurses Association of Canada (2003) developed a new set of standards for practice that identifies the socio-environmental approach to health promotion as the basis for CHNs' practice. The role of the CHN, as outlined in these standards, includes seeking to address root causes of illness and disease and facilitating planned change through the application of Hamilton and Bhatti's (1996) PHPM. The case study on p. 104 gives an example of applying the PHPM to a community health nursing scenario.

FIGURE 6.3 Role of the PHN within the Regional Health Authority

Build Healthy Public Policy

Goal

Public policy is developed consistent with improvements in the determinants of health.

Services

- Encourage and support community-based advocacy for healthy public policy at all levels and in all sectors (e.g., justice, education, housing, social services, recreation).
- Direct advocacy for healthy public policy.
- Educate and encourage decision makers in all sectors and at all levels to participate in the development of healthy public policy.
- Foster partnership with community decision makers to evaluate public policy.

An Example of Service

PHNs work with communities to advocate for smoke-free public buildings.

Outcome: Ninety percent of public buildings are smoke free.

Create Supportive Environments

Goal

Community members live in healthy social, emotional, spiritual, physical and ecological environments.

Services

- Assess and directly act on the factors affecting health in the community's social, emotional, spiritual, physical and ecological environment.
- Encourage and participate in health promoting initiatives with other communities and sectors.
- Increase awareness of the ecological and social environments affecting the health of individuals, families, groups, or communities. Encourage and support related action.

An Example of Service

PHNs work with communities to develop strategies to promote safe environments for children.

Outcome: The number of latch-key children under 12 is reduced by 10 percent.

Reorient Health Services

Goal

Responsibility for the determinants of health is shared among individuals, community groups, health professionals, health service institutions, all levels of government, and all sectors, including justice, health, education, business, housing, social services and recreation.

Services

- Primary role in community assessment. Provide consultation with decision makers (e.g., RHA management and board) regarding community strengths and needs as a foundation for health care decisions.
- Promote responsible and effective use of the health care system and community resources.
- Refer individuals, families, groups, and communities for appropriate service.
- Engage other sectors in addressing the determinants of health.

An Example of Service

PHNs work with a community to reorient speech and language services from a facility to accessible community locations based on a partnership among health, education, and community members.

Outcome: A 5 percent increase in early identification and intervention for preschool children with speech and language problems.

Strenghten Community Action

Goal

Community members are actively involved in achieving health.

Services

- Mobilize individuals, families, groups, and communities to take individual and collective action on the determinants of health in the contexts in which they live, learn, work, and play (e.g., schools, workplaces, homes, economic, and social environments).
- Develop and support community-based and self-care services in which community members have ownership and an active role.
- Increase awareness of the ecological and social environments affecting the health of individuals, families, groups or communities. Encourage and support related action.

An Example of Service

PHNs work with a community to identify their assets and needs, determine priority issues, develop strategies, and take action.

Outcome: An active "Healthy Community" network is established.

Develop Personal Skills

Goal

Community members will make effective choices to attain an optimal level of physical, emotional, spiritual, and social development.

Services

- Mobilize individuals to take individual and collective action on the determinants of health.
- Provide information regarding choices.
- Counsel and facilitate healthy choices.

An Example of Service

PHNs facilitate "Nobody's Perfect" parenting sessions for teen mothers and fathers.

Outcome: All parents involved in the parenting program have identified an improved understanding of early childhood development.

Source: Reprinted with permission of Manitoba Health. Prepared by the public health staff of Manitoba Health and Regional Health Authorities.

Case Study

One of the key roles of the CHN working in a public health setting is to support the family in the first year of the life of a new child. This includes assisting parents in their new role(s), promoting optimal child development, and connecting the family with appropriate community resources.

Imagine that you are a CHN who has been given a postpartum referral from the local hospital. The referral contains the following information: first-time mother, 17 years old; newborn male born at 36 weeks' gestation, weighing six pounds; unclear if infant's father is involved; very little contact with the health care system prior to giving birth; receiving social assistance; has no phone. You arrive at the address, which is located in a low-income neighbourhood, and find the mother alone with her infant in a tiny one-bedroom apartment on the third floor of a poorly maintained building without an elevator. You observe that the apartment has very few furnishings, dirty dishes piled in the sink, empty junk food wrappers and containers everywhere, and a strong smell of cigarette smoke. The mother quickly becomes tearful, stating that she doesn't have enough money to pay the rent, and she has no family and few friends in the community.

Using the population health promotion model as a guide, answer the following.

Discussion Questions

1. What information do you already know and what additional information do you need to obtain about the determinants of health affecting this family?

2. Give specific examples of one or more health promotion strategies that you as the CHN could use at the individual/family or community level to address each of the following determinants of health affecting this family. Consider other health professionals or workers in other disciplines/sectors with whom you might collaborate in these strategies:

   a) income and social status
   b) social support networks
   c) personal health practices/coping
   d) healthy child development
   e) access to health services

3. What knowledge/skills/attitudes does the CHN require in order to effectively engage in the strategies identified in question 2?

Recently, the Canadian Nurses Association (CNA) has released two discussion papers that provide strong support for a socio-environmental approach in nursing. *Social*

Determinants of Health and Nursing: A Summary of the Issues (Canadian Nurses Association, 2005) summarizes the impact of social and economic factors (such as poverty and economic inequality, low social status, social exclusion, job and food insecurity) on population health. The CNA suggests that nurses can play an important role in addressing these social determinants of health by working on their individual practices (e.g., including SDOH in client assessments and treatment and follow-up plans), helping to reorient the health care system (e.g., ensuring that health promotion programs go beyond lifestyle and behaviour to include SDOH), and advocating for healthy public policies (e.g., using stories from patients to help advocate for policies that address SDOH, making decision makers aware of the research on the links between socioeconomic factors and health). In *Social Justice: A Means to an End, an End in Itself* (Canadian Nurses Association, 2006), it is proposed that to put social justice into practice, the nursing profession must work toward ten specific attributes, including "projects, programs and/or structural reforms of an economic, political or social nature that reduce poverty, increase the overall standard of living and/or increase the participation of the poor in social and political life" (p. 14).

Challenges of Implementing the Socio-environmental Approach in Community Health Nursing While the socio-environmental approach to health promotion has been officially adopted by many community health nursing professional associations at the policy level, barriers to putting this approach into action have been identified (Benson & Latter, 1998; Chalmers & Bramadat, 1996; Cohen, 2006b; Reutter & Ford, 1998; Shuster, Ross, Bhagat, & Johnson, 2001). Some of these barriers originate at the level of the individual CHN (e.g., feeling that they don't have well-developed "upstream" skills or having difficulty in giving up control over the agenda and direction of nurse–client interactions); some originate at the level of the organizations that CHNs are employed in (e.g., lack of organizational culture/policies that value and support this type of approach in CHNs' practice settings). Other barriers originate from the communities where CHNs work (e.g., lack of recognition from the public that this approach is a legitimate part of a CHN's role). In spite of these challenges, there are some excellent examples in Canadian settings of the application of the socio-environmental approach to health promotion in which CHNs have played an active role. See the box "Examples of the Socio-environmental Approach to Health Promotion" for a description of a few of these initiatives.

Guidelines for Health Promoting Community Health Nursing Practice

What conclusions can we draw from the preceding discussion? First, it is clear that there can never be one universally accepted definition of health promotion. How one views health promotion will depend on a variety of factors including one's professional and educational background, the

Examples of the Socio-environmental Approach to Health Promotion

Example 1:

It was obvious from the heavy utilization of a number of school-based services in a low-income neighbourhood that a larger community service centre would be desirable. CHNs participated in a coalition of agencies to plan for a centre that would meet the needs of the community. Local residents were hired to do a door-to-door survey asking people to list their skills and the strengths of the community and what they would like to see in a neighbourhood centre. A plan was developed that would build upon these strengths and respond to the dreams of the community. A phased-in plan for local staffing and governance was strictly adhered to. This centre has been functioning very well for many years and is well respected by the community. The role of the CHNs in its development is no longer remembered, but the important thing is that people in this neighbourhood have a place where they can meet and join with others in addressing their needs.

Example 2:

When working in a program intended to follow individuals with sexually transmitted infections, CHNs noticed that clients who were receiving social assistance payments could not afford to purchase condoms. Though many drugs were paid for by social assistance when they were given by prescription, condoms were not. The CHNs successfully worked with their managers to lobby for a change in policy to make condoms available by prescription.

Example 3:

A disadvantaged neighbourhood has an annual "Take Pride Week" that is run primarily by residents but is supported in several ways by local community service providers. "Take Pride Week" provides opportunities for area residents (especially people who are new to the area) to meet their neighbours and become involved in ongoing local activities. CHNs support this community-building event in different ways every year, sometimes helping to plan activities and usually being there to staff some events.

Example 4:

Based on data gathered in the community on postpartum visits, district CHNs noticed a high level of isolation among young moms, whether it was their first or subsequent child. The CHNs partnered with the local child and family services agency, which was able to secure funding for a one-year pilot of a moms' group, and with the local church, which provided space and other resources. Personal contact was made with all postpartum moms, inviting them to participate in a planning meeting. The moms, not the CHNs, decided that they wanted the group and determined how they wanted it to function and the weekly agenda. The group has been meeting twice weekly for the past two years and now has plans to expand to an evening session to accommodate working parents. (They have successfully secured additional funding.) The group periodically invites the CHNs to facilitate discussion on topics chosen by the group, but the members now run the group.

Example 5:

A CHN is a member of a neighbourhood network that developed in response to several community meetings that identified community needs. The meetings were initiated by a local citizens' group whose original concern was lack of local services and employment opportunities for developmentally delayed students once they became adults. The initial network has expanded to include accessible services related to all areas identified in earlier visioning exercises. The CHN's role is one of consultation, advocacy, and facilitation.

Example 6:

The "Families First" program is funded by Healthy Child Manitoba and offered through Public Health. Public health nurses work collaboratively with home visitors, who offer regular home visiting during the first three years of life to families who are identified as requiring assistance to ensure healthy early child development—one of the key determinants of population health. The focus of the program is on building and enhancing family strengths.

dominant ideology of the time, and one's personal world view. At the level of nursing practice, health promotion appears to be most widely viewed as a set of specific actions or strategies aimed at changing individual behaviours and with a focus on disease prevention and functional ability. This is in contrast to nursing at the policy and academic levels, where an increasing number of policy and discussion statements and nursing theorists have adopted a broader view of health promotion—one that is based upon specific values and principles such as social justice, equity, and participation—and focused on modifying the social, political, and economic environment that shapes behaviour (either through direct action or by enabling others to do it for themselves). Second, although a certain percentage of the gap between the rhetoric and reality of nurses' health promotion practice may be due to organizational or societal factors over which they have little control, there is no doubt that much of this gap can be explained by the way that nurses have been socialized—beginning with their educational experiences and continuing in the workplace. How can CHNs narrow the gap between the rhetoric and reality of health promotion in their practice? The following guidelines are offered as a starting point.

Focus on Health and Building Capacity for Health In spite of the fact that nursing theorists have conceptualized health in positive terms, such as "self-actualization," "positive adaptation," and "optimal functioning" (Novak, 1988), the truth is that CHNs' health promotion practice has often focused on the negative. For example, most individual, family, and community health assessment models used by nurses focus on the identification of needs, deficits, and problems. If CHNs want to truly help to shift the focus of their services to the promotion of *health,* then we need to utilize a range of assessment tools and empowering strategies that start by identifying the strengths of individuals, families, and communities, and work with them to build their capacity for health. A focus on capacity building means that the CHN must strive to form collaborative relationships with clients (whether at the individual, family, or community level) and to maximize their involvement in planning, implementing, and evaluating health promotion actions. Remember—*every* individual, family, or community has some strength that can be capitalized on—your job is to find it and build on it!

Think Upstream It is true that the practice situations of the majority of CHNs involve a lot of work with individuals and families. However, these individuals and families live in communities and societies in which the broader ecological, socioeconomic, political, and cultural environment influences their daily lives. "Thinking upstream" means that, in addition to meeting the immediate needs of individual clients or families (which may involve helping them to cope with their immediate situation or providing information that will assist them to make health-enhancing choices), the CHN should always be (a) assessing the broader socio-environmental determinants of health, (b) thinking about possible strategies that can influence those determinants in a positive manner, and (c) identifying potential partners with whom you might collaborate for maximum effectiveness. (See discussion below.) While the majority of CHNs' health promoting practice may be "downstream" at the level of personal and small-group empowerment, it is essential to identify all possible opportunities for involvement "upstream" in community empowerment and healthy public policy initiatives. Having said that, whether one works upstream or downstream may not be as important as *how* one engages in health promotion. That is to say, it is possible to be involved in "upstream" strategies that are disempowering (e.g., taking the initiative to mobilize community action around an issue that the community has not identified as a priority) and "downstream" strategies that are empowering (e.g., working with a single, teenage mother to identify the specific skills she feels are important to improve her chances for success in parenting and finding gainful employment).

Look for Partnership Opportunities One of the most challenging aspects of a socio-environmental approach to health promotion for community health practitioners is the recognition that the main determinants of population health—especially social and economic inequalities—lie outside the usual scope of the health system. This has led many CHNs to feel power-less and has no doubt contributed to a focus in community health nursing practice on helping clients cope with their circumstances, rather than on changing those circumstances. It is imperative that for maximum impact on individual, family, or community health, CHNs identify potential partners with whom they might collaborate. The partners may be from other disciplines within the health sector (e.g., community nutritionists, public health physicians) or they may be from other sectors (e.g., social workers, educators, recreation workers). The key is to leave one's sense of ownership of the issue at the door and to find ways in which each partner can make a unique but complementary contribution to the ultimate goal. It is even more imperative that the partnership includes members from the community who are directly impacted by the initiative. A partnership made up only of service providers can easily lose track of grassroots concerns and will not result in an empowerment process that benefits those who need it most.

Be Patient Perhaps the most challenging aspect of a socio-environmental approach to health promotion is the fact that, unlike many nursing activities, it may take a long time to see positive results. In the case of community development initiatives, this could mean several years. Patience is a virtue in the field of community health nursing. Having to work with multiple partners, follow their lead, and endure frequent delays can leave nurses impatient with the community development process and make them retreat into "safer" direct service work. Constantly sharing and evaluating one's experiences with colleagues and receiving support and encouragement from one's managers may help to alleviate this problem. Ultimately, keep in mind that the empowerment process—as painfully slow and awkward as it may sometimes be—is the most likely way to achieve long-term positive health outcomes.

Summary

We began by exploring the historical development, underlying assumptions, and key characteristics of the three approaches to health promotion—biomedical, behavioural/lifestyle, and socio-environmental—that have been dominant in the twentieth and early twenty-first centuries. While all three of these approaches may be used by health professionals at different times, the biomedical and behavioural/lifestyle approaches have tended to dominate the health promotion practice of nurses and other health professionals. However, the socio-environmental approach has gained momentum within the field of community health nursing in recent years and, in Canada, it has now been formally adopted as the basis for CHNs' practice. Decreasing social and economic inequalities in health, and increasing personal and community empowerment, are at the heart of the socio-environmental approach to health promotion. Educating people regarding healthy behaviours is insufficient to achieve health from this perspective and may actually increase inequities in health. While CHNs who would like to practice from a socio-environmental perspective face a number of challenges, a few guidelines have been provided that may assist in this process.

KEY TERMS

biomedical approach
physiological risk factors
Lalonde Report
behavioural or lifestyle approach
social justice
common good
social change
social responsibility for health
victim-blaming
ecological or socio-ecological perspective
healthy cities/communities
Ottawa Charter for Health Promotion
equity in health
strengthening community action
building healthy public policy
creating supportive environments
developing personal skills
reorienting health services
empowerment
socio-environmental approach
population health promotion model (PHPM)
social or societal determinants of health
Health Promotion Model (HPM)
macroscopic approach
thinking upstream
microscopic approach
emancipatory nursing
critical social nursing
critical caring theory

STUDY QUESTIONS

1. What are the main differences between the three approaches to health promotion in terms of (i) type of health determinant most concerned with; (ii) target of the initiative; (iii) program management (including the difference between community-based and community development programs); and (iv) criteria for success?

2. Identify the six different interpretations of the concept of health promotion found in the literature. Which ones reflect the behavioural approach to health promotion? Which ones reflect the socio-environmental approach to health promotion?

3. What were the main strengths and weaknesses of the Lalonde Report?

4. Give a brief description of each of the five key strategies that focus on changing behaviour/lifestyle. Which one of these strategies is also used in a socio-environmental approach to health promotion?

5. What are the limitations of using an approach to health promotion that focuses exclusively on behaviour change?

6. What are the four main factors that contributed to the emergence of the socio-environmental approach to health promotion?

7. What is the central concept that lies at the heart of the socio-environmental approach to health promotion? How would you define this concept and how does it link with health promotion?

8. What are the five key principles of health promotion from a socio-environmental perspective?

9. What are three ways that nurses can play an important role in addressing social determinants of health?

10. What are four guidelines for health promoting CHN practice?

INDIVIDUAL CRITICAL THINKING EXERCISES

1. Prior to reading this chapter, what did the term "health promotion" mean to you? Has your initial interpretation changed? If so, how?

2. Analyze your personal level of comfort with using the three main approaches to health promotion outlined in this chapter. What factors would increase your comfort in using each one?

3. Think about the community you live in. What are the main issues affecting your community's health or quality of life? Which approach to health promotion would be the most appropriate to deal with these issues? (There may be more than one.) What role could a CHN play in a health promotion initiative that addressed each issue?

4. For each of the examples listed in the box on page 105, identify which of the *Ottawa Charter* strategies are being implemented. (More than one may apply.)

5. You are a CHN in a community where there appears to be an increasing number of obese children in the elementary school that you visit. Describe a microscopic ("downstream") versus a macroscopic ("upstream") approach to community health promotion in this situation.

GROUP CRITICAL THINKING EXERCISES

1. Discuss your answers to Individual Critical Thinking Exercise 1 with one or more partners. How do your responses compare? What factors influenced your original understanding of health promotion?

2. With a partner, interview a CHN in your community. Ask the following questions: What does the term *health promotion* mean to you? What are the main health promotion issues in your area? Describe some of the health promotion activities in your practice. What are the barriers to engaging in health promotion activities? Analyze the responses with your partner. How would you summarize this CHN's approach to health promotion?

3. With one or more partners, identify examples of each of the behavioural/lifestyle strategies (listed in Table 6.2) that are in use in Canada and/or your region of the country today. Critically assess the strengths and weaknesses of these strategies.

4. With one or more partners, read the *Toronto Charter for a Healthy Canada* (Raphael, 2004), and identify specific strategies that CHNs could use to address all or some of the SDOH in their practice.

NOTES

1. Of course, other perspectives on health and disease have always existed, both within certain populations in Western societies and among non-Western societies. However, it is beyond the scope of this chapter to explore those perspectives and the approaches to health enhancement that they have generated.

2. Not surprisingly, many of these strategies are based on theories and models—e.g., the health belief model (HBM), the transtheoretical (stages of change) model, social learning/cognitive theory—that were developed in the field of psychology to explain, predict, and change health behaviours. For a comprehensive discussion of these models, and other theories and models used in the behavioural approach to health promotion, see Glanz, Lewis, & Rimer, (2002).

3. One of the most popular frameworks for health promotion program planning in use today—the "PRECEDE–PROCEED" model (Green & Kreuter, 1999)—is based on the ecological perspective. For further discussion of this and other ecological models, see chapters in Glanz et al. (2002).

4. This original WHO definition is still very popular. However, in recent years it has been expanded as "the process of enabling individuals and communities to increase control over the determinants of health" (Nutbeam, cited in Green, Poland, & Rootman, 2000, p. 6).

5. See discussion in Chapter 2.

6. This is not to say that there has been no discussion of concepts or models related to the socio-environmental perspective on health promotion in nursing curricula since the 1980s. In fact, a recent study (Canadian Association of Schools of Nursing Task Force on Public Health Education, 2006) indicates that the vast majority of nursing programs in Canada have done so. The problem may be that discussion of these concepts/models tends to occur in one particular course or in one semester that focuses on population health promotion (often in the final year of the program), rather than being integrated throughout the program (L. L. Stamler, CASN Sub-Committee on Public Health Education, personal communication, April 9, 2007).

REFERENCES

Andreasen, A. R. (1995). *Marketing social change: Changing behaviour to promote health, social development, and the environment.* San Francisco, CA: Jossey-Bass.

Ballou, K. (2000). A historical-philosophical analysis of the professional nurse obligation to participate in sociopolitical activities. *Politics, Policy, & Nursing Practice, 1*(3), 172–184.

Beauchamp, D. (1976). Public health as social justice. *Inquiry, 13,* 3–14.

Benson, A., & Latter, S. (1998). Implementing health promoting nursing: The integration of interpersonal skills and health promotion. *Journal of Advanced Nursing, 27,* 100–107.

Brubaker, B. (1983, April). Health promotion: A linguistic analysis. *Advances in Nursing Science,* 1–14.

Butterfield, P. (1997). Thinking upstream: Conceptualizing health from a population perspective. In J. Swanson & M. Nies (Eds.), *Community health nursing: Promoting the health of aggregate* (pp. 69–82). Philadelphia, PA: W.B. Saunders Company.

Canadian Association of Schools of Nursing Task Force on Public Health Education. (2006). *Shaping the future of public health and community health nursing education in Canada.* Presentation to the Pan-Canadian Symposium on Public Health Education, Toronto, Canada, April 11, 2006.

Canadian Nurses Association. (1992). *Policy statement on health promotion.* Ottawa: Author.

Canadian Nurses Association. (2005). *Social determinants of health and nursing: A summary of the issues.* Retrieved April 5, 2006, from http://cna-aiic.ca/CNA/documents/pdf/publications /BG8_ Social_Determinants_e.pdf.

Canadian Nurses Association. (2006). *Social justice: A means to an end, an end in itself.* Retrieved April 5, 2006, from http://cna-aiic.ca/CNA/documents/pdf/publications/Social_ Justice_e.pdf.

Canadian Public Health Association. (1990). *Community health/public health nursing in Canada: Preparation and practice.* Ottawa: Author.

Chalmers, K., & Bramadat, I. (1996). Community development: Theoretical and practical issues for community health nursing in Canada. *Journal of Advanced Nursing, 24,* 719–726.

Cohen, B. (2006a). Population health as a framework for public health practice: A Canadian perspective. *American Journal of Public Health, 96*(9), 1574–1576.

Cohen, B. (2006b). Barriers to population-focused health promotion: The experience of public health nurses in the province of Manitoba. *Canadian Journal of Nursing Research, 38*(3), 52–67.

Cohen, B., & Reutter, L. (2007). Development of the role of public health nurses in addressing child and family poverty: A framework for action. *Journal of Advanced Nursing 60*(1), 96–107.

Community Health Nurses Association of Canada. (2003). *Canadian community health nursing standards of practice.* Retrieved December 3, 2003, from www.communityhealthnursescanada.org/StandardsofPractice.pdf.

Crawford, R. (1977). You are dangerous to your health: The ideology and politics of victim blaming. *International Journal of Health Services, 7*(4), 663–680.

Dallaire, C., Hagan, L., & O'Neill, M. (2000). Linking health promotion and community health nursing. In M.

Stewart (Ed.), *Community nursing: Promoting Canadians' health* (pp. 317–332). Toronto: W.B. Saunders Company.

Epp, J. (1986). *Achieving health for all: A framework for health promotion.* Ottawa: Health and Welfare Canada.

Falk-Rafael, A. (2005a). Advancing nursing theory through theory-guided practice: The emergence of a critical caring perspective. *Advances in Nursing Science* 28(1), 38–49.

Falk-Rafael, A. (2005b). Speaking truth to power: Nursing's legacy and moral imperative. *Advances in Nursing Science, 28*(3), 212–223.

Federal, Provincial, Territorial Advisory Committee on Population Health. (1994). *Strategies for population health: Investing in the health of Canadians.* Ottawa: Ministry of Supply and Services.

Feeley, N., & Gottlieb, L. (2000). Nursing approaches for working with family strengths and resources. *Journal of Family Nursing, 6*(1), 9–24.

Gibson, C. (1991). A concept analysis of empowerment. *Journal of Advanced Nursing, 16,* 354–361.

Glanz, K., Lewis, F., & Rimer, B. (2002). *Health behaviour and health education* (3rd ed.). San Francisco: Jossey-Bass.

Green, L., & Kreuter, M. (1999). *Health promotion planning: An educational and environmental approach* (3rd ed.). Mountain View, CA: Mayfield.

Green, L. W., Poland, B. D., & Rootman, I. (2000). The settings approach to health promotion. In B. D. Poland, L. W. Green, & I. Rootman (Eds.), *Settings for health promotion: linking theory and practice* (pp. 1–43). Thousand Oaks, CA: Sage Publications.

Hamilton, N., & Bhatti, T. (1996). *Population health promotion: An integrated model of population health and health promotion.* Ottawa: Health Canada, Health Promotion and Development Division.

Hartrick, G. (2000). Developing health-promoting practice with families: One pedagogical experience. *Journal of Advanced Nursing, 31*(1), 27–34. doi:10.1046/j.1365-2648.2000.01263.x.

Heaney, C., & Israel, B. (2002). Social networks and social support. In K. Glanz, F. Lewis, & B. Rimer (Eds.), *Health behavior and health education: Theory research and practice* (3rd ed., pp. 179–205). San Francisco: Jossey-Bass.

Labonte, R. (1993). *Health promotion and empowerment: Practice frameworks.* Toronto: University of Toronto, Centre for Health Promotion & ParticipACTION.

Labonte, R. (1995). Population health and health promotion: What do they have to say to each other? *Canadian Journal of Public Health, 86*(3), 165–188.

Labonte, R., & Penfold, S. (1981). Canadian perspectives in health promotion: A critique. *Health Education, 19*(3/4), 4–9.

Lalonde, M. (1974). *A new perspective on the health of Canadians.* Ottawa: Department of National Health and Welfare.

Maben, J., & MacLeod Clark, J. (1995). Health promotion: A concept analysis. *Journal of Advanced Nursing, 22,* 1158–1165.

MacDonald, M. (2002). Health promotion: historical, philosophical, and theoretical perspectives. In L. Young & V. Hayes (Eds.), *Transforming health promotion practice: Concepts, issues, and applications* (pp. 22–45). Philadelphia, PA: F.A. Davis Company.

Makara, P. (1997). Can we promote equity when we promote health? *Health Promotion International, 12*(2), 97–98.

Manitoba Health. (1998). *The role of the public health nurse within the regional health authority.* Winnipeg: Author.

McKinlay, J. (1979). A case for refocusing upstream: The political economy of illness. In E. Jaco (Ed.), *Patients, physicians, and illness* (pp. 9–25). New York: The Free Press.

Novak, J. (1988). The social mandate and historical basis for nursing's role in health promotion. *Journal of Professional Nursing Practice, 4*(2), 80–87.

Nutbeam, D., & Harris, E. (1998). *Theory in a nutshell: A practitioner's guide to commonly used theories and models in health promotion.* National Centre for Health Promotion, Department of Public Health and Community Medicine. University of Sydney, NSW, Australia.

Patrick, D., & Wickizer, T. (1995). Community and health. In B. Amick, S. Levine, A. Tarlov, & D. Chapman Walsh (Eds.), *Society & health* (pp. 46–92). New York: Oxford University Press.

Pender, N. (1996). *Health promotion in nursing practice* (3rd ed.). Stamford, CT: Appleton & Lange.

Pender, N., Murdaugh, C., & Parsons, M. (2005). Health promotion in nursing practice (5th ed). Ann Arbour, MI: Pearson Education.

Raeburn, J., & Rootman, I. (1998). *People-centred health promotion.* Chichester, UK: John Wiley & Sons.

Raphael, D. (Ed.). (2004). *Social determinants of health: Canadian perspectives.* Toronto: Canadian Scholars Press Inc.

Raphael, D., & Bryant, T. (2000). Putting the population into population health. *Canadian Journal of Public Health, 91*(1), 9–12.

Reutter, L. (2000). Socioeconomic determinants of health. In M. Stewart (Ed.), *Community health nursing: Promoting Canadians' health* (2nd ed., pp. 174–193). Toronto: W.B. Saunders Company.

Reutter, L., & Ford, J. (1998). Perceptions of changes in public health nursing practice: A Canadian perspective. *International Journal of Nursing Studies, 35,* 85–94.

Rush, K. (1997). Health promotion ideology and nursing education. *Journal of Advanced Nursing, 25,* 1292–1298.

Sampson, R. (2003). Neighbourhood-level context and health: Lessons from sociology. In I. Kawachi & L. Berkman (Eds.) *Neighbourhoods & health* (pp. 132–146). Oxford: Oxford University Press.

Shuster, S., Ross, S., Bhagat, R., & Johnson, J. (2001). Using community development approaches. *Canadian Nurse, 97*(6), 18–22.

Spenceley, S., Reutter, L., & Allen, M. (2006). The road less traveled: Nursing advocacy at the policy level. *Policy, Politics, & Nursing Practice, 7*(3): 180–194.

Stansfeld, S. (2003). Social support and social cohesion. In M. Marmot & R. Wilkinson (Eds.), *Social determinants of health* (pp. 155–178). Oxford: Oxford University Press.

Stewart, M., & Leipert, B. (2000). Community health nursing in the future. In M. Stewart (Ed.), *Community Nursing:*

Promoting Canadians' Health (pp. 602–631). Toronto, ON: W. B. Saunders Company.

Syme, S. L. (1997). Individual vs. community interventions in public health practice: Some thoughts about a new approach. *VicHealth, 2*, 2–9.

Vanderplaat, M. (2002). Emancipatory politics and health promotion practice: The health professional as social activist. In L. Young & V. Hayes (Eds.), *Transforming health promotion practice: Concepts, issues and applications* (pp. 87–98). Philadelphia, PA: F.A. Davis Company.

Vollman, A.R., Anderson, E.T., & McFarlane, J.M. (2004). *Canadian community as partner: Theory and practice in nursing.* Philadelphia and New York: Lippincott.

Wallerstein, N. (1992). Powerlessness, empowerment, and health: Implications for health promotion programs. *American Journal of Health Promotion, 6*(3), 197–205.

Whitehead, D. (2003). Incorporating socio-political health promotion activities in clinical practice. *Journal of Clinical Nursing, 12*(5), 668–677.

Wilkinson, R., & Pickett, K. (2006). Income inequality and population health: A review and explanation of the evidence. *Social Science & Medicine, 62*, 1768–1784.

Williamson, D., & Drummond, J. (2000). Enhancing low-income parents' capacities to promote their children's health: Education is not enough. *Public Health Nursing, 17*(2), 121–131.

World Health Organization. (1977). *Health for all by the year 2000.* Geneva: Author.

World Health Organization. (1978). *Declaration of Alma Ata.* Retrieved September 4, 2002, from www.who.int/hpr/archive/docs/almata.html

World Health Organization. (1984). *Health promotion: A discussion document on the concepts and principles.* Copenhagen: WHO Regional Office for Europe.

World Health Organization. (1986). *Ottawa Charter for health promotion.* Ottawa: Canadian Public Health Association and Health and Welfare Canada.

Wright, L., & Leahey, M. (2005). *Nurses and families: A guide to family assessment and intervention* (4th ed.). Philadelphia, PA: F.A. Davis Company.

Young, L. (2002). Transforming health promotion practice: Moving toward holistic care. In L. Young & V. Hayes (Eds.), *Transforming health promotion practice: Concepts, issues and applications* (pp. 3–21). Philadelphia, PA: F.A. Davis Company.

ADDITIONAL RESOURCES

Websites

Annotated Bibliography of Selected Health Promotion Titles
www.utoronto.ca/chp/who/hpbib.htm
Minnesota Public Health Department: Interventions Manual
www.health.state.mn.us/divs/cfh/ophp/resources/docs/phinterventions_manual2001.pdf

Dr. Dennis Raphael, York University
Quartz.atkinson.yorku.ca/QuickPlace/draphael/Main.nsf
Health Promotion: Capacity Checklists
www.usask.ca/healthsci/che/prhprc/programs/finalworkbook.pdf
World Health Organization: Health Promotion Glossary
www.who.int/hpr/NPH/docs/hp_glossary_en.pdf

Readings

Naidoo, J., & Wills, J. (2000). *Health promotion: Foundations for practice.* London: Bailliere Tindall.

Poland, B., Green, L., & Rootman, I. (2000). *Settings for health promotion: Linking theory and practice.* Newbury Park, CA: Sage Publications.

Stewart, M. (Ed.). (2000). *Community nursing: Promoting Canadians' health* (2nd ed.). Toronto: W.B. Saunders Canada.

Young, L. E., & Hayes, V. (2002). *Transforming health promotion practice: Concepts, issues, and applications.* Philadelphia, PA: F.A. Davis Company.

The following periodicals are good sources of theoretical and practice-based research articles related to community health nursing and health promotion in the community:

Community Health Promotion
Health Education Quarterly
Health Promotion International
Journal of Advanced Nursing
Public Health Nursing

About the Author

Benita Cohen, RN, PhD (University of Manitoba), is an Assistant Professor in the Faculty of Nursing at the University of Manitoba, where she teaches courses in the undergraduate, graduate, and post-RN programs related to prevention of illness and health promotion in the community. She previously worked as a Public Health Nurse in the Toronto area and in the Baffin region of Nunavut. She is currently a member of the Canadian Association of Schools of Nursing Sub-Committee on Public Health Education.

The author would like to thank Horst Backe, Bluma Levine, Susan Permut, and Lynda Tjaden—nurses at the Winnipeg Regional Health Authority—for their input into the development of the case study and provision of examples of population health promotion strategies used in their own practice.

Primary Health Care

Dawn Smith, Lori Jacobson, and Lucia Yiu

OBJECTIVES

After studying this chapter, you should be able to:

1. Describe the concept of primary health care.

2. Define primary health care and describe its values, principles, and elements.

3. Describe differences and similarities between primary health care, primary care, health promotion, and population health.

4. Describe community development and empowerment strategies to implement primary health care, including personal care, small group development, coalition formation, and policy advocacy.

5. Understand the concepts of international and global health, and organizations and projects involved in primary health care in international settings.

6. Describe primary health care reform and related community health nursing involvement as well as its future directions.

INTRODUCTION

The primary health care approach was first described in the landmark document *The Declaration of Alma Ata,* produced at the WHO-UNICEF conference in Alma Ata, Kazakstan in the former Soviet Union in 1978. In 1977, the World Health Assembly recognized the unsatisfactory state of health of the world's population and adopted the goal to achieve "Health for All by the Year 2000." The approach required to meet this goal was dubbed "primary health care." **Primary health care** was defined as "essential health care based on practical, scientifically sound and acceptable methods and technology made universally accessible to individuals and families in the community through their full participation and at a cost that the community and country can afford to maintain at every stage of their development in the spirit of self-reliance and self-determination" (World Health Organization [WHO], 1978, p. 2).

More specifically, primary health care can be summarized as:

- evidence-based;
- universally accessible;
- the first level of contact, providing for essential health needs;
- providing a full spectrum of needs, including health promotion, prevention, treatment, and rehabilitation;

- addressing the main determinants of health;
- affordable to community and country;
- relevant to the social, cultural, economic, and political context;
- addressing community priorities;
- multi-sectoral and integral to overall social and economic development;
- requiring and promoting individual and community self-reliance and participation;
- sustained by an effective health information system; and
- relying on a diverse team of appropriately trained and responsive health workers.

The *Declaration of Alma Ata* explicitly outlines the inter-sectoral and community-driven nature of the approaches to improving health and reducing inequities in health. Primary health care is based on an ecological understanding of health (Smedley & Syme, 2000). However, the *Declaration of Alma Ata*'s explicit attention to the importance of changing structures and policy and enabling socially just values and beliefs is often missed.

The *Declaration of Alma Ata* marked its 30-year anniversary in 2008. How successful has the PHC approach been in achieving "health for all"? What has been accomplished, and what remains to be done? The *Declaration of Alma Ata* has had a tremendous influence on improving health, providing health services, and developing national health systems. "It has drawn attention to the needs of the many, and has been a powerful instrument for making governments and their partners recognize that the provision of health care cannot be left to the professionals alone..." (WHO, 2006a, p. 4). Overall improvements in diet, sanitation, disease prevention, and health care are resulting in increased life expectancy and a general aging of the population, with the gap in life expectancy between industrialized and developing countries continuing to close. Regretfully, in some countries those overall improvements in life expectancy and the health gains of past decades are being reversed by the impact of communicable diseases such as HIV/AIDS.

However worthy the "health for all" target, in reality it was not met. Some scholars (Hall & Taylor, 2003; Hope, 2005) claim that emerging health problems such as childhood obesity are beyond the scope of the initial principles of primary health care. For example, the increasing economic gap between the rich and the poor is associated with inequitable access to health care services in both developing and more developed countries. There is evidence that the implementation of PHC is incomplete or is not delivering the expected results envisioned decades ago. This may be attributable to the complexity of the policy environment in which decisions have to be made. However, health policy makers agree that the principles of PHC, penned close to 30 years ago, still have lasting relevance in our complex world and must evolve in response to changing demographic and societal needs (WHO, 2002).

PRIMARY HEALTH CARE: VALUES, PRINCIPLES, AND ELEMENTS

Primary health care principles describe the nature and scope of action to enact the values. These values shape the "elements," which describe more concrete actions fundamental to achieving health and well-being.

Primary Health Care Values

Achieving "health for all" is a fundamental value of primary health care. Primary health care values are comparable to those of the Canadian Nurses Association's *Code of Ethics for Registered Nurses* (Canadian Nurses Association [CNA], 2002) and the *Standards for Community Health Nursing in Canada* (Community Health Nurses Association of Canada [CHNAC], 2003). Social justice and equity are two distinctive primary health care values.

Principles of Primary Health Care

Accessibility means that the five types of health care are universally available to all clients regardless of geographic location. In many cases, the principle of accessibility can best be operationalized by having communities define and manage necessary health care services. Distribution of health professionals in rural, remote and urban communities is key to the principle of accessibility. Accessibility means that clients will receive appropriate care from the appropriate health care professional, within a time frame that is appropriate.

Public participation means clients are encouraged to participate in making decisions about their own health, in identifying the health needs of their community, and in considering the merits of alternative approaches to addressing those needs. Adoption of the principle of public participation ensures respect for diversity. It also means that the design and delivery of health care is flexible and responsive. Participation ensures effective and strategic planning for, and the evaluation of, health care services in a community.

Health promotion involves health education, nutrition, sanitation, maternal and child health care, immunization, prevention and control of endemic disease. The goal of health promotion is to reduce the demands for curative and rehabilitative care. Through health promotion, individuals and

families build an understanding of the determinants of health.[1] Individuals and families thereby develop skills to improve and maintain their health and well-being. School health programs are an important method of promoting health and self-esteem.

Appropriate technology means that the modes of care are appropriately adapted to the community's social, economic and cultural development. The adoption of the principle of appropriate technology highlights the importance of improved knowledge and of on-going capacity building to the design and delivery of health care services. It means consideration of alternatives to high-cost, high-tech services. The principle of appropriate technology recognizes the importance of developing and testing innovative models of health care and of disseminating the results of research related to health care.

Intersectoral cooperation recognizes that health and well-being is linked to both economic and social policy. Intersectoral cooperation is needed to establish national and local health goals, healthy public policy, and the planning and evaluation of health services. The adoption of the principle of intersectoral cooperation will ensure the providers from different disciplines collaborate and function interdependently to meet the needs of health care consumers and their families. It also means that health professionals will participate in government policy formulation and evaluation, as well as in the design and delivery of health care services. It also means that services must be delivered and evaluated in an integrated and congruent fashion.

[1]*Ottawa Charter for Health Promotion, WHO, (1989). Strategies for Population Health – Investing in the Health of Canadians, ACPH, (1994).*

Source: Reprinted with permission from the Canadian Nurses Association.

Social justice refers to the degree of equality of opportunity for health made available by the political, social, and economic structures and values of a society. The extent to which a society provides opportunities for its citizens to develop socially and economically productive roles influences the well-being of individuals as well as the healthfulness of the whole population (Wilkinson, 1996). One example is the inequities that exist in health status, where the rich are healthier than the poor. It is important that community health nurses (CHNs) consider how the concept of social justice is enacted in their practice and by the health care organization that employs them.

Equity in health is "the absence of systematic and potentially remediable differences in one or more aspects of health status across socially, demographically, or geographically defined populations or population subgroups" (Macinko & Starfield, 2002, p. 3). Equity is a political concept; it has "normative ethical values that entails fair distribution of resources and access within and among various population groups.... Equity efforts include reducing any discrimination in access to the benefits of health initiatives" (WHO, 2005, p. 44). An example would be strategies to improve access of rural/remote clients to specialized health services offered only in urban centres. This may require financial support for transportation and housing costs to facilitate equitable and timely access.

The emerging socioeconomic inequity is perhaps the biggest factor affecting the health of the population (Public Health Agency of Canada [PHAC], 2003; Raphael, 2002). Moreover, relationships also exist between inequality in macro-level social structures, meso-level social processes, and micro-level health effects (Bezruchka, 2002). Usually the term **macro** refers to the "big picture" levels of influence such as policy, and **micro** refers to the very smallest levels of influence or impacts such as the individual person or even cells. The **meso** level is the "in between," such as family, group, community, and organization. Planning and implementing interventions that take action on causes of poor health at all levels is fundamental to the primary health care approach.

Principles of Primary Health Care

The CNA (2000) formulated its position on primary health care based on the five principles embodied in the WHO's (1978) original definition, with an emphasis on structural and political reform necessary to reduce inequities in health. These principles include accessibility, public participation, health promotion, appropriate technology, and inter-sectoral cooperation. The five types of health care include promotive, preventive, curative, rehabilitative, and supportive/palliative care. (See box on Principles of Primary Health Care.)

The Elements of Primary Health Care

The *Declaration of Alma Ata* (WHO, 1978, p. 2) outlined the following eight essential elements to achieve "health for all":

- education concerning prevailing health problems and the methods of preventing and controlling them;
- promotion of food supply and proper nutrition;
- an adequate supply of safe water and basic sanitation;
- maternal and child health care, including family planning;

- immunization against the major infectious diseases;
- prevention and control of locally endemic diseases;
- appropriate treatment of common diseases and injuries; and
- provision of essential drugs.

These elements have been used extensively to guide health programs and policy development in developing countries. Although it was the emphasis on these elements that initially stamped primary health care as a developing country approach, the inherent political, social, and economic messages of the PHC philosophy have not been applied to the same degree in more developed countries due to the strong biomedical and behavioural approach to health care that predominated during the 1970s and 1980s. The strong biomedical and behavioural approach to thinking about health during the 1970s and 1980s in developed nations contributed to the fact that the political, social, and economic messages in the *Declaration of Alma Ata* were overlooked. More recently, the growing emphasis on the determinants of health underscores the relevance of these elements across the globe regardless of a nation's level of wealth or development. Canadian and provincial governments are now emphasizing PHC and moving toward a more health promotive socio-environmental perspective on health. For example, the increase in homelessness in Canada demonstrates the relevance of these elements. (See case study below.)

PRIMARY HEALTH CARE: WHAT IT IS AND WHAT IT IS NOT

Primary health care, primary care, health promotion, and population health: what do these terms mean and how are they related, if at all? There has been considerable confusion, and often fairly heated debate, about the meanings of and relationships among these terms. CHNs can make a significant contribution to primary health care by understanding differing perspectives and developing clear and simple definitions of terms. Table 7.1 compares the focus, the principal actors, and the level and primary emphasis of action commonly associated with each of these terms.

Case Study

Toronto's 2003 Report Card on Housing and Homelessness reported that despite a strong economy, many people in need of affordable housing are being left behind (City of Toronto, 2003). The Report Card found that 552 000 Toronto households had incomes below the poverty line; 71 000 households were on the waiting list for affordable social housing; and about 160 000 people per month used food banks. In 1995 food bank clients used food banks an average of 6 times per year as compared with the average of 17 times per year in 2002. During 2002, 31 985 homeless

individuals (including 4779 children) stayed in a Toronto shelter at least once, an increase of 21% since 1990.

Discussion Questions

1. Using your textbook and relevant literature, describe health issues that a CHN might encounter when working with homeless populations.

2. Based on Figures 7.1 and 7.2, describe an example of how you could implement the five principles of PHC and its elements to promote the health of the homeless population described in the case study or in your own community.

TABLE 7.1
Comparison of Terms

Term	Focus	Principal Actors	Level and Primary Emphasis for Action
Primary care	Disease	Health professionals	• Micro level • Provision of essential care to individuals with health problems
Primary health care	System-wide (e.g., from provision of care to individuals to action on the determinants of health)	Inter-sectoral partners, community members	• Micro, meso, and macro levels • Multifaceted: from provision of essential care to individuals to changing social and economic policy
Health promotion	Determinants of health	Community members, health professionals, government and non-governmental organizations	• Micro level (e.g., individuals and small groups) • Meso level (e.g., organizations and community coalitions) • Bottom-up development of capacity of individuals and groups to change the things that affect health in the community
Population health	Determinants of health	Government and non-governmental organizations	• Macro level (e.g., government policy and legislative change) • Meso level (e.g., organizational change) • Top-down strategies to influence broad social and economic factors

The difference between primary care and primary health care is often unclear. Primary care is narrower in scope than primary health care and often is biomedical in focus (Starfield, 1998). However, access to primary care is an essential component of primary health care. The distinctions between primary health care, health promotion, and population health are less clear. As Lavis (2002) points out, "The language used to discuss ideas about non-medical determinants of health has changed with each passing decade." Canadian policy makers and researchers talked about "health fields" in the 1970s, "health promotion" in the 1980s, and "population health" in the 1990s. There is a close relationship between health promotion and primary health care in both philosophy and methods. However, primary health care also involves curative, rehabilitative, and palliative care methods as a part of provision of first-line contact with the community.

Population health focuses on maintaining and improving the health of entire populations and reducing inequities in health status among population groups (PHAC, 2003). It is often associated with a "top down" approach to reducing inequities in health, such as developing healthy public policy (Lavis, 2002). This approach to population health is congruent with the original thinking of primary health care outlined in the *Declaration of Alma Ata* (WHO, 1978); and also it has a strong orientation to evidence-based interventions.

COMMUNITY DEVELOPMENT AND EMPOWERMENT STRATEGIES

Though PHC is often equated with community-based nursing, it is an approach to health care engagement that can be applied across many areas of health care, such as acute care of adults, children, and the elderly. PHC "reflects the values and principles that have always guided registered nurses in their practice: promoting health, preventing disease and working with other members of the multidisciplinary team" (College and Association of Registered Nurses of Alberta [CARNA], 2005, p. 3). CHNs practise PHC in a variety of roles with individual, family, and population-level clients. The *process* inherent in PHC values and philosophy has been described as community development (shown in Figure 7.1). In this section we describe in greater detail community development as a process for enacting PHC. Community development is "the planned evolution of all aspects of community well-being (economic, social, environment, and cultural). It is a process whereby community members come together to take collective action and generate solutions to common problems" (Frank & Smith, 1999, p. 6). Community development requires an understanding and careful handling of community history, resources, and key players.

While the process shown in Figure 7.1 resembles the nursing process of assessment, planning, implementation, and evaluation, there are several key differences. Foremost is the CHN's role as facilitator, rather than as definer or controller of the process. In a community development approach, CHNs engage with citizens to develop a mutual understanding of issues and priorities, resources, and challenges. Their essential ability to actively listen to and understand the experiences of people and organizations in a community enables them to effectively promote dialogue and synthesize similarities and differences among community members. Creating a climate of trust and curiosity, along with exploratory dialogue, facilitates others to question the

FIGURE 7.1 The Process of Achieving a Healthy Community

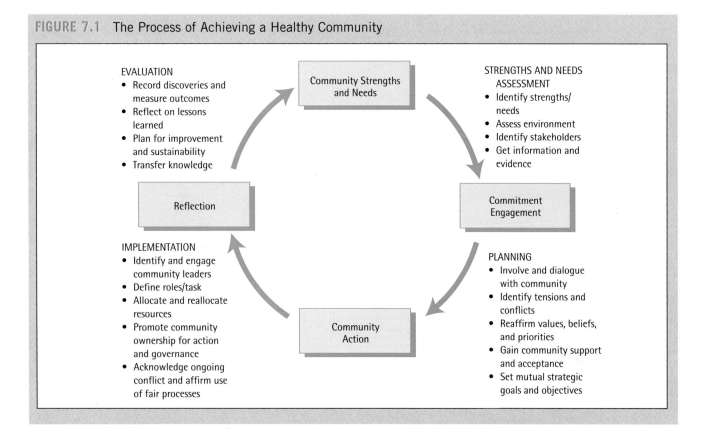

status quo and is important to a shared envisioning and creation of plans for action.

Primary health care values and principles are respected in a community-owned and -driven process, from entry right through to intervention and evaluation. This approach builds the skills and capacity of those involved in the process, contributing to sustainability. Community development requires considerable patience, humility, and learning. CHNs using this philosophical and practical approach would include themselves as part of the community being "developed," rather than as external controllers of the process.

Essential to CHNs' work in community development is the notion of empowerment. Empowerment is a concept closely related to social justice. "Empowerment is an active, involved process where people, groups, and communities move toward increased individual and community control, political efficacy, improved quality of community life, and social justice" (CHNAC, 2003, p. 10). CHNs use empowerment in their work with all levels of clients, whether they be individuals, families, small groups, or whole communities.

Labonte's (1993) "empowerment holosphere" (Figure 7.2) shows the overlap in CHNs' work with individual clients (personal care), families, or small groups as client, or whole communities as client (community organization, coalition advocacy, and political action). CHNs practise all five roles to implement the principles of primary health care. For example, in their "individual and family as client" work during postnatal visits, CHNs develop an intimate understanding of the joys and challenges unique to each new mother's experiences. In rapidly growing suburbs, some new mothers may be at home alone with their babies and not yet socially integrated into their new community. Individual and family health promotion is a critical part of supporting the woman and her family, helping them develop their capacity to manage the challenges of new parenthood in a new community setting. CHNs also use their understanding of the issue, the relationships they develop through one-on-one interactions with many new mothers during postnatal visits, and their knowledge of community organizations in order to facilitate "women-owned" education, support, and activity groups. This health promotion strategy builds the capacity of the individuals who choose to get involved and develops linkages between the women who have a variety of strengths and challenges but who just happen to be new to the community. Facilitating development of small groups in response to community priorities builds linkages, shares resources, encourages mutual aid and social support between women of similar experiences, and improves access to resources and opportunities from a variety of sectors.

Canadian Research Box 7.1

Smith, D., & Davies, B. (2006). Creating a new dynamic in Aboriginal health. *Canadian Nurse, 102*(4), 36–39.

In 2004, an evidence-based prenatal care workshop was held for 81 community health nurses working in First Nations communities in British Columbia. These nurses discussed the use of evidence to improve prenatal care in

→

the Aboriginal communities. Of the 52 respondents to the workshop questionnaire, 73% of the nurses reported that a participatory model of knowledge transfer was important. They acknowledged the lack of evidence regarding health care interventions for Aboriginal people, identified the importance of working with the stakeholders as a knowledge transfer strategy, and stressed the need to create informal dialogue among these groups to stimulate participatory transfer and exchange of knowledge to improve prenatal care in their communities.

Discussion Questions:

1. Why would stimulating stakeholder dialogue to improve care for other populations be relevant in your community? Propose how you would engage communities to do this.

2. Examine the range of health care services offered by an Aboriginal health care organization in or near your community. If possible, arrange to interview a provider regarding similarities and differences in their role and that of community or public health services offered to the mainstream population with respect to the five principles of PHC.

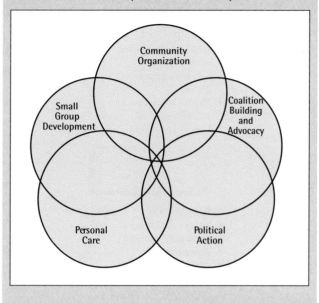

FIGURE 7.2 The Empowerment Holosphere

Sources: Labonte, R. (1993). A holosphere of healthy and sustainable communities. Australian Journal of Public Health, 17, 4–12.

Definitions

Primary health care: "essential health care based on practical, scientifically sound, and acceptable methods and technology made universally accessible to individuals and families in the community through their full participation and at a cost that the community and country can afford to maintain at every stage of their development in the spirit of self-reliance and self-determination" (WHO, 1978, p. 2).

Social justice: equal opportunity for health (e.g., socially and economically productive lives) made available by the political, social, and economic structures and values of a society.

Primary care: the point of first contact with the health care system, generally referring to preventive, curative, and rehabilitative care provided to individuals (Stanhope & Lancaster, 2001).

Primary nursing: a model of nursing care whereby a nurse is primarily responsible for planning and delivering total care for a specific patient. Like primary care, primary nursing is an illness-oriented concept.

Health promotion: "the process of enabling people to increase their control over and improve their health" (WHO, 1986, p. 1).

Population health: "the health of a population as measured by health-status indicators and as influenced by social, economic, and physical environments; personal health practices; individual capacity and coping skills; human biology; early childhood development; and health services. As an approach, population health focuses on the interrelated conditions and factors that influence the health of populations over the life course, identifies systematic variations in their patterns of occurrence, and applies the resulting knowledge to develop and implement policies and actions to improve the health and well-being of those populations" (Federal, Provincial, and Territorial Advisory Committee on Population Health, 1999, p. 7).

Determinants of health: factors and conditions that have been shown to influence health over the life course. They include social, economic, and physical environments; early childhood development; personal health practices; individual capacity and coping skills; human biology; and health services (PHAC, 2003).

Community development: "the planned evolution of all aspects of community well-being (economic, social, environmental, and cultural). It is a process whereby community members come together to take collective action and generate solutions to common problems" (Frank & Smith, 1999, p. 6).

Empowerment: "a social action process in which individuals and groups act to gain mastery over their lives in the context of changing their social and political environment" (Wallerstein & Bernstein, 1994, p. 142).

CHNs can also use their understanding of individual and community issues to mobilize interested citizens and organizations to take action. For example, CHNs have often facilitated the opening of Planned Parenthood Services in their communities in response to poor access to sensitive and relevant reproductive health services. Development of such initiatives often requires full and sensitive engagement in the community development process. CHNs have engaged private- and public-sector partners to participate in environmental change that supports heart health, injury prevention, and tobacco-use reduction Their work demonstrates the primary health care principle of inter-sectoral cooperation. For example, the recreation sector has developed walking trails and other environmental factors that support a more active lifestyle. Private-sector restaurants are increasingly implementing "heart healthy" menu choices. The text box on p. 118 illustrates how CHNs used community development to enact the five principles of primary health care in the development of the Brock Youth Centre.

The primary health care principles of accessibility, health promotion, and public participation are often used in CHNs' community development work, in which the community is the client. For example, political action has been used by CHNs to increase access to adequate housing, change legislation to prevent drunk driving, and make bicycle helmets mandatory. A well-known example is the work of Cathy Crowe, a street nurse, educator, and social activist. She co-founded Nurses for Social Responsibility, the Toronto Coalition Against Homelessness, and the Toronto Disaster Relief Committee. The latter organization seeks to have homelessness declared a national disaster (Ward & Piccolo, 2001).

Identification of health and socioeconomic inequalities and taking action on their root causes are critical components of practising primary health care. The rapid growth of homelessness in Canada provides a contemporary example of CHNs' practise of primary health care to tackle this worsening social-justice issue. Changes in Canada's social, political, and economic structures are widening the gap between the rich and poor and creating inequalities in opportunity for health. Toronto's homeless population, described in the case study (see p. 113), is typical of many communities across Canada. A PHC approach is required that focuses on rectifying those macro-level factors that enable homelessness to flourish.

INTERNATIONAL HEALTH/ GLOBAL HEALTH

Though often used interchangeably, the terms international health and global health have different foci. **International health** refers to issues surrounding health inequities between developing countries and more developed countries—such as differences between health conditions and the state of health care in African nations versus those in Canada, the U.S., or Britain. International health is concerned with development, strengthening of health care systems, and efforts to improve health conditions in developing countries. Primary health care is often the focus of **international development** efforts to

Developed World vs. Developing World

When discussing international and global health issues, CHNs must seek to sensitize and change the notion that the "developed" world is the global standard against which the "developing" world must model its own development. For example, Canadians rank 6th highest in water consumption in the world (approximately 340 litres/day/person, while the global norm is 20–40 litres per day/person) (Environment Canada, 2005). Canadian consumption patterns are not sustainable in Canada and are a poor model for the rest of the world. Canadians can learn important lessons about water conservation from the "developing" world. There are many alternatives to denote the different stages of development of countries that would be more sensitive and reflect CHN values, such as overdeveloped/developing; north/south; or minority/majority worlds. Nurses must keep abreast of growing sensitivity and awareness to issues of language and power.

reduce such inequalities. International health can also refer to health crises and public health emergencies frequently arising in developing countries, such as the tsunami that killed several hundred thousand South East Asians in December 2004.

The term **global health** usually refers to health challenges that span national borders and present global health challenges. Two recent examples of global health issues are severe acute respiratory syndrome (SARS), which originated in China yet posed a global challenge, and the recent and continuing global health risk of avian influenza. These are issues that face all nations and are not necessarily the result of underdevelopment, poverty, and low incomes. Global health issues are increasing in prominence as a result of changing demographics, evolving migration patterns, increasing cultural interactions, and ease of travel. There is clearly a close relationship between the two terms.

Over the past few decades, through international health efforts, the world has made great strides in improving health outcomes. Smallpox has been eliminated, polio and measles are nearing extinction, maternal mortality rates have fallen, child mortality rates have been reduced dramatically and life expectancy across the globe has risen markedly (UNICEF, 2005). However, health indicators in developing countries significantly lag behind those in more developed countries. Every day in the developing world, 28 000 children under the age of 5 die, most from easily treatable and preventable causes; 1440 women do not survive childbirth; and 13 000 people contract HIV. As a result of HIV/AIDS, life expectancy in some countries has fallen more than 20 years, with life expectancy once again under 40 years compared with the average Canadian life expectancy nearing 80 years of age (WHO, 2006b). However, it must also be recognized that inequities in health and social conditions within more developed countries also exist. For example, life expectancy, infant mortality, and percentages of households without clean water in many First Nations communities in Canada are similar to rates in southern nations (Canadian Population Health Initiative [CPHI], 2004).

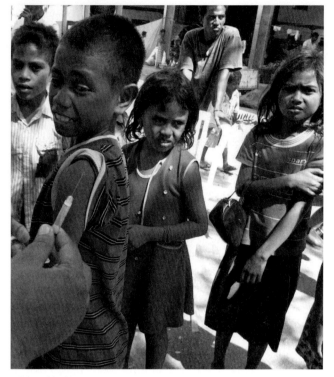

Photo 7.1

Mass immunization in developing country.

Credit: AP/Firdia Lisnawati

Key Global Players

The **World Health Organization** (WHO) is considered the leading international health institution. Related to primary health care and international health, in March 2005 the WHO created the Commission on Social Determinants of Health (CSDH) to support countries and global health partners to address the social factors leading to ill health and focus on health inequities. It seeks to identify, analyze, and draw attention to the social determinants of health that are known to be among the worst causes of poor health and inequalities between and within countries (WHO, 2006c).

The **Pan American Health Organization** (PAHO), of which Canada and the United States are members, has a mission to strengthen national and local health systems and improve the health of the peoples of the Americas. PAHO assists countries in fighting diseases that have re-emerged, such as cholera, dengue fever, and tuberculosis, as well as "new" diseases such as HIV/AIDS. It provides technical cooperation including education and social communications support, promotes work with non-governmental organizations, and supports programs to prevent transmission of communicable diseases. In its efforts to improve health, PAHO targets the most vulnerable groups, including mothers and children, workers, the poor, the elderly, and refugees and displaced persons. It promotes primary health care strategies and addresses issues related to equity for those who lack access to health, and on a Pan-American approach encouraging countries to work together on common issues (PAHO, n.d.).

The Brock Youth Centre: The Enactment of the Five Principles of Primary Health Care

Background

The Brock Youth Centre is a CHN-led community development project that began in 1988 with a series of community-needs assessments implemented by local CHNs, the Brock Township municipal council, and youth service organizations with non-governmental agencies (e.g., the Addiction Research Foundation). This group found that area youth were at risk due to lack of access to services and youth-friendly spaces. Youth also reported feeling that they were negatively perceived by area adults. Planned interventions were to create youth-friendly spaces; increase youth knowledge, leadership, and decision-making skills; and promote self-esteem and a sense of community belonging.

This initially led to creation of Summer Camp 1999, which sought to change the image of youth within the community from negative to positive. The success of this summer camp led to development of a community-supported, youth-created, and youth-led organization. "Youth for Youth" evolved into an incorporated, non-profit, grassroots, community organization. Essential to the program's success was leadership from youth and local community members and in-kind and administrative support from key community organizations. Examples of how the primary health care principles used a community development approach to develop the Brock Youth Centre are described below.

Accessibility

The community-needs assessment identified that youth lacked access to health, social, employment, and recreation services. There was a lack of available health and social services within Brock Township and a generally negative attitude toward youth in the community. Improvements achieved through community development include greater access to supportive adults and peers, more recreation opportunities, enhanced crisis intervention, behaviour management, and health education services through linkages with community partners.

Public Participation

The project aimed to advocate and engage youth and community organizations in genuine rather than token forms of participation. Connecting youth and community members with opportunities to use their creativity and voice in ways that are meaningful to them was critical to capacity building for a more socially just society. CHNs played a major role in facilitating numerous outcomes of youth-led projects through their participation in the Brock Youth Centre programs. Some examples included securing resources for the project and the program logo and centre's name through the Youth Services Canada Project and Youth Participation Study.

→

Health Promotion

Capacity building is key to health promotion and community development (Frank & Smith, 1999). An example of the project's capacity-building approach was the multi-level mentorship initiatives involving youth at various stages of growth and leadership development, strengthening program effectiveness and sustainability. Flexibility and creativity enabled many youth to remain involved in spite of moving on for work and study opportunities. The Brock Youth Centre example demonstrates how balancing small group development, advocacy for inclusion of previously marginalized groups, conflict resolution, community organizing, and political action can achieve sustainable community development.

Appropriate Technology

The resulting activities and interventions at the Brock Youth Centre succeeded at reducing risk-taking behaviours and highlighting youth's positive contributions to their communities. Rather than developing a "high-tech" model of service delivery by health care specialists to manage "troubled youth," the community came up with low-tech, capacity-oriented interventions that matched the youth and community needs with local resources.

Intersectoral Cooperation

Intersectoral linkages and partnerships were developed and continue to be nurtured at the local, regional, and provincial level. Regional engagement and resource sharing occurred through cooperation with various stakeholders such as school councils, employment resource centres, local businesses, service clubs, the North Durham Social Development Council, the Regional Youth Centre Network, the Ontario Healthy Communities Coalition, TeenNet at the University of Toronto, the Town Youth Participation Strategies network, and the Youth Services Network.

Note: Many thanks to community health nurses Tracy Prinzen, Kathy McLaughlin, and Pam Frisby and supporting participants of the Brock Youth Centre for sharing their stories.

Key Canadian Players

The mandate of the **Canadian International Development Agency** (CIDA) is to help developing and poor countries by offering them the support and assistance they need to improve their quality of life. Health is one of five priority sectors identified by CIDA. Within the health sector, Canada assists developing countries to improve health outcomes, particularly among the poorest, through a focus on preventing and controlling communicable, poverty-linked diseases (especially HIV/AIDS), strengthening the capacity of health systems, improving infant and child health and sexual and reproductive health, and improving food security.

Canadian International Development Agency (CIDA) works in partnership with WHO, the United Nations, and UNICEF to promote global health. It also is involved in major international initiatives such as the Global Fund to Fight AIDS, Tuberculosis, and Malaria, and the Global Polio Eradication Initiative. In addition, CIDA collaborates with partner countries to strengthen local health care systems by improving access to basic health services for the most vulnerable groups and by increasing human resources capacity through the use of PHC principles. Examples of these efforts can be seen in provision of vitamin A supplementation, reproductive health, immunization campaigns, the distribution of mosquito nets, tuberculosis clinics, and HIV/AIDS prevention and care (CIDA, 2006).

CIDA also works in partnership with and funds numerous Canadian non-governmental health organizations (NGOs) whose mandates include assisting the world's neediest in achieving optimal health. Two such organizations are the Canadian Public Health Association (CPHA) and the Canadian Nurses Association (CNA). For example, the CPHA has been contracted by CIDA to implement the technical assistance component of the Canadian International Immunization Initiative. This initiative aims to increase the capacity of health care–related staff in infectious disease surveillance and control, and in vaccination safety. CPHA's role involves identifying and recruiting Canadian technical consultants, including nurses, to assist the WHO, PAHO, and UNICEF to establish and maintain successful national childhood immunization systems in developing countries and in Eastern and Central Europe. It also promotes the benefits of global immunization to the Canadian public.

Since 1970, CNA has been working in partnership with national nursing associations to strengthen the capacities of the nursing profession in more than 30 countries. CNA collaborates with the International Council of Nurses and other international nursing and health development organizations to ensure that the expertise of Canadian nurses contributes to the advancement of global health and equity. For example, following the tsunami disaster in South and South East Asia, CNA is now working with the Indonesian National Nurses Association to gain from the experience by identifying what was done right and what could be improved. CNA brings valuable resources and expertise in emergency preparedness, especially when it comes to the role of nurses in a strong, effective response to emergency situations (CNA, 2006). Nurses may become involved in international health, either as volunteers or on a paid basis, working from within Canada or abroad through such organizations as the Canadian Red Cross, Canadian Council for International Co-operation, Canadian Society for International Health, and International Development Research Centre (IDRC). These agencies, as well as international education departments in many Canadian universities, offer nursing students opportunities for international clinical experiences.

Much of the focus in international health efforts is related to primary health care. Given that many of the health issues facing developing countries are poverty related, health systems based on a primary health care approach can reach the greatest number of people and have the greatest impact. Water-borne diseases; malaria prevention and treatment; malnutrition-related conditions; reproductive, maternal, and child health care; immunization; and the care and nurturing of AIDS patients are all appropriately and effectively addressed through a primary health care approach. Governments in many developing countries, facing scarce budgets and technological and human resource capacity challenges within their health care systems, are increasingly recognizing primary health care as the most effective use of their scarce and valued resources (CIDA, 2006). CHNs play a key role in many of these countries' PHC systems.

ACHIEVING A PRIMARY HEALTH CARE SYSTEM IN CANADA

While the World Health Organization's primary health care approach (WHO, 1978) was initially viewed as an approach to address health issues in developing countries, eight years later, the *Ottawa Charter for Health Promotion* (WHO, 1986) was developed. The Ottawa Charter shares many of the key values and principles of primary health care and has been more readily adopted by developed nations. For example, the Canadian government's *Achieving Health for All* framework (Epp, 1986) reflected the rapid and extensive acceptance of the Ottawa Charter in Canada. Despite these endorsements of the charter's values and principles, Canada has been slow in implementing primary health care.

In Canada, a change to different systems such as primary health care is stifled by the structural and ideological legacy of three major policies. First, the BNA Act of 1867 gave responsibility for health care to the provinces, presenting a significant legislative barrier to *national* health care reform. Second, the limitation of compulsory coverage to hospitals and physician services was entrenched by the Hospital and Diagnostic Services Act of 1957, which has resulted in a lingering belief system that equates technology and curative intervention with health care. Third, public payment for private medical practice was established through the Medical Care Act of 1968, further reinforcing the curative focus for the health system. Despite the successful lobbying by the Canadian Nurses Association and other organizations to broaden the scope of providers in the Canada Health Act, the entrenchment of physicians as the point of entry into the health care system remains relatively unchanged.

Achieving PHC in Canada would require several conditions, including greater receptiveness to PHC values, willingness of key stakeholders to overcome existing legislative barriers, and additional funding. There has been a slow but steady development of these PHC-friendly conditions. In the late 1980s and early 1990s, significant interest in health system change was evident in the numerous commissions on health care across the country (Angus, 1995). The conclusions reached by a majority of the commissions reflected a growing recognition for the need to address inequities in health and supported the approach and philosophy of primary health care (Mhatre & Deber, 1992). These resulted in several concerted efforts on behalf of provincial and territorial governments and institutions to advance the primary health care agenda. For example, in Nova Scotia, the provincial

government funded a Task Force on Primary Health Care. From 1994–1999, the federal government sponsored the National Forum on Health, a forum of experts and citizens from across the country. They produced several reports and emphasized the need for action on the determinants of health, the importance of using evidence to inform health system intervention and change, and the need to shift to more upstream approaches. As a result, the Health Transition Fund was created to support initiatives that would test and demonstrate effectiveness of alternative approaches.

Nursing Involvement in Primary Health Care Reform

CHNs have been active in promoting primary health care since its adoption by the World Health Assembly (Labelle, 1986; Maglacas, 1988). The numerous primary health care demonstration projects that have been fought for and initiated by CHNs have made significant contributions to advancing the "health for all" agenda in Canada. CHNs' roles and close relationships with individual and community clients enable them to observe the strengths and gaps in the current health care system. Their expertise with community development has been vital to their success in implementing primary health care demonstration projects. For example, nurses in Newfoundland and Labrador have gained key insights into health care reform based on the Danish–Newfoundland Primary Health Care Project and other primary health care initiatives (Association of Registered Nurses of Newfoundland & Labrador, 2002). In Nova Scotia, nurses were integral to the development and success of the Cheticamp Primary Health Care Project, which focused on cultural awareness, economic development, education, general community development, organizational development, self-help, and social support (Downe-Wamboldt, Roland, LeBlanc, & Arsenault, 1994). The Registered Nurses' Association of Ontario has been closely involved in the formation and ongoing action of the Coalition for Primary Health Care. This organization continues its public education, coalition advocacy, and political action strategies to promote adoption of a primary health care approach (Coalition for Primary Health Care, 2000).

The Registered Nurses' Association of British Columbia (RNABC) was at the forefront of developing models for the application of the primary health care approach in British Columbia. Their New Directions initiative made a significant contribution through the development of a series of background papers, a concerted professional and public education strategy to inform nurses and the public about primary health care, and policy development on nurses' potential to contribute to improved health within a primary health care-based system (RNABC, 1998). The RNABC advocated for and achieved government commitment to launch primary health care demonstration projects and initiated a community-determined process that resulted in establishing a nursing centre in a small rural community on Vancouver Island (Clarke & Mass, 1998). Other provincial nursing associations in Canada have also been active in promoting primary health care.

Future Directions of Primary Health Care Reform in Canada

CHNs have been effective in implementing innovative approaches to primary health care in a number of provinces and settings in Canada. They have been active as care providers, researchers, administrators, and educators in building the capacity needed to implement primary health care in Canadian and international contexts. CHNs have used their organizational base to influence the direction of health policy in Canada and abroad. And they have contributed to the research base needed to inform the design of interventions with special populations and in challenging contexts.

As Labelle (1986) stated more than 20 years ago, CHNs have several sources of power close at hand, including their presence in multiple settings and at all levels in society, direct and continuous contact with the public, access to and control over massive amounts of information, and access to communication channels and linkages between each other through their organizational structures. What Labelle identified then, and what has been validated through research, is that CHNs' fundamental commitment to equity and social justice has made them some of the most trusted members of society (Buresh & Gordon, 2000). Though they have demonstrated that they can use these sources of power effectively, they must do so more consistently and strategically.

At a time of growing inequities in health in Canada and waning political commitment to implementing social and economic interventions to narrow that gap (Raphael, 2002), CHNs must continue to work in multiple roles to create the environments and capacity needed to achieve health for all. Now more than ever, CHNs must expand their participation in community organization, coalition building and advocacy, and political action activities to increase awareness and action on the inequities in health.

CHNs must add their expertise to the growing imperative to address inequities in health between countries (Labonte & Spiegel, 2001). Thus, at various levels, CHNs can contribute to the creation of local and global health care delivery systems that exemplify the values and principles of primary health care. However, similar to the act of recycling to protect the environment, individual CHNs can implement these same values and principles in their practice on a daily basis. One person alone may not make a big impact at a macro level, but if each CHN works toward the same goals, the effort is more likely to impact the entire system.

Summary

This chapter discussed the concept and definition of primary health care and a description of its overall approach. The importance of understanding primary health care based on its original description in the *Declaration of Alma Ata* was highlighted. Its principles and elements as well as the philosophy and values at its heart were identified, and its fit with nursing values explored. Primary health care and related terms were defined and compared. Community health nursing's practice of community development and empowerment to implement primary health care values and principles were discussed.

Concepts of international and global health were explained. The role of primary health care in international and global health was reviewed and examples of Canadian and international organizations working in the field were introduced. Factors influencing the shape and extent of primary health care reform in Canada were summarized. Finally, CHNs were challenged to develop and implement strategies that address these macro- and meso-level root causes of inequities in health.

KEY TERMS

primary health care
accessibility
public participation
health promotion
appropriate technology
intersectoral cooperation
social justice
equity in health
macro, micro, meso levels
primary care
primary nursing
health promotion
population health
determinants of health
community development
empowerment
international health
international development
global health
World Health Organization
The Pan American Health Organization
Canadian International Development Agency

STUDY QUESTIONS

1. Describe the difference between primary health care and primary care.
2. Describe the differences and similarities between primary health care, population health, and health promotion.
3. Define the five principles of primary health care.
4. Describe various interventions to promote the health for homeless people in Canada.
5. Describe the differences between international health and global health, and provide an example of each.

INDIVIDUAL CRITICAL THINKING EXERCISES

1. Why is it important for CHNs to study and understand the *Declaration of Alma Ata*?

2. Visit the website of your provincial/territorial nursing association. Search for policy or position statements on primary health care. Look for description of activities that influence or contribute to health care reform. Discuss the initiative with your peers and colleagues. Identify opportunities for CHNs to participate in the initiative, and reflect on how you can become involved.

3. Relate your own values to the role of CHNs as facilitators of primary health care policy and action at local, regional, provincial, or national levels.

4. Compare your findings on nursing association policy with those of your provincial ministry.

5. Compare and contrast the role of a primary health care nurse working in Canada with a primary health care nurse working in a developing nation such as the Sudan or Sri Lanka.

GROUP CRITICAL THINKING EXERCISES

1. Describe how nursing has and will continue to contribute to reform efforts aimed at the root causes of poor health.

2. As community developers in small communities, how might community health nurses apply the "process of achieving a healthy community" (Figure 7.1)?

3. In small groups, brainstorm various ways nursing students could become involved in international health on campus, in the community, or abroad.

4. How might the practice of community health nursing in Canada differ from that in developing countries?

REFERENCES

Angus, D. (1995). *Health care reform: Revisiting the review of significant health care commissions and task forces.* Ottawa: Canada Community Health Nurses Association.

Association of Registered Nurses of Newfoundland & Labrador. (2002). Sustaining our public health care system. Submission to the Commission on the Future of Health Care in Canada.

Bezruchka, S. (2002). Foreword. In D. Raphael, *Social justice is good for our hearts: Why societal factors—not lifestyles—are major causes of heart disease in Canada and elsewhere.* Toronto: Centre for Social Justice, Foundation for Research and Education. Retrieved July 2002 from www.socialjustice.org/pdfs/JusticeGoodHearts.pdf.

Buresh, B., & Gordon, S. (2000). *From silence to voice: What nurses know and must communicate to the public.* Ottawa: Canadian Nurses Association.

Canadian International Development Agency. (2006). *CIDA's Agenda for Action on Health.* Ottawa. Retrieved November 16, 2006, from www.acdi- cida.gc.ca/CIDAWEB/acdicida. nsf/En/REN-21813536-PN6.

Canadian Nurses Association. (2000). *Fact sheet: The primary health care approach.* Ottawa: Author.

Canadian Nurses Association. (2002). *Code of ethics for registered nurses.* Ottawa: Author.

Canadian Nurses Association. (CNA). (2006). *Partners in health... Nurses working together make a difference.* Retrieved November 14, 2006, from http://www.cna-nurses.ca/CNA/international/involved/default_e.aspx.

Canadian Population Health Initiative. (2004). *Improving the health of Canadians.* Ottawa: Canadian Institute of Health Information.

City of Toronto. (2003). *The Toronto report card on housing and homelessness.* Toronto: Author.

Clarke, H., & Mass, H. (1998). *Comox Valley Nursing Centre: From collaboration to empowerment.* Public Health Nursing, 15(3), 216–224.

Coalition for Primary Health Care. (2000). *Primary health care coalition: Backgrounder.* Toronto: Author.

College and Association of Registered Nurses of Alberta. (2005). *Primary health care.* Edmonton: Author. Retrieved March 28, 2007, from http://www.nurses.ab.ca/pdf/Primary%20Health%20Care.pdf.

Community Health Nurses Association of Canada. (CHNAC). (2003). *Canadian community health nursing standards of practice.* Ottawa: Author.

Downe-Wamboldt, B., Roland, F., LeBlanc, B., & Arsenault, D. (1994). Cheticamp primary health care project. *Nurse to Nurse, 3,* 14–15.

Environment Canada. (2005). *State of the environment infobase.* Retrieved May 18, 2007, from http://www.ec.gc.ca/soer-ree/English/about.cfm.

Epp, J. (1986). *Achieving health for all: A framework for health promotion.* Ottawa: Health and Welfare Canada.

Federal, Provincial, and Territorial Advisory Committee on Population Health. (1999). *Toward a healthy future: Second report on the health of Canadians.* Ottawa: Health Canada.

Frank, F., & Smith, A. (1999). *The community development handbook: A tool to build community capacity.* Ottawa: Human Resources Development Canada.

Hall, J., & Taylor, R. (2003). Health for all beyond 2000. *Medial Journal of Australia, 178*(1), 17–20.

Hope, J. (2005). Health for all by the year 2000: A retrospective look at the ambitious public health initiative. *Promotion and Education, 12*(2), 77.

Labelle, H. (1986). Nurses as a social force. *Journal of Advanced Nursing, 11,* 247–253.

Labonte, R. (1993). A holosphere of healthy and sustainable communities. *Australian Journal of Public Health, 17,* 4–12.

Labonte, R., & Spiegel, G. (2001). *Setting global health priorities for funding Canadian researchers.* Ottawa: Canadian Institutes for Health Research, Institute of Population and Public Health.

Lavis, J. (2002). Ideas at the margin or marginalized ideas? Non-medical determinants of health in Canada. *Health Affairs, 21*(2), 107–112.

Macinko, J., & Starfield, B. (2002). Annotated bibliography on equity and health. *International Journal for Equity and Health, 1*(1), 1–20.

Maglacas, A. (1988). Health for all: Nursing's role. *Nursing Outlook, 36*(2), 666–671.

Mhatre, S., & Deber, R. (1992). From equal access to health care to equitable access to health: A review of Canadian provincial health commissions and reports. *International Journal of Health Services, 22*(4), 645–668.

Pan American Health Organization. (n.d.). *What is PAHO?* Retrieved October 4, 2007, from http://www.paho.org/english/paho/What-PAHO.htm.

Public Health Agency of Canada (PHAC). (2003, March). *What determines health?* Retrieved November 15, 2006, from http://www.phac-aspc.gc.ca/ph-sp/phdd/determinants/index.html.

Raphael, D. (2002). *Social justice is good for our hearts: Why societal factors—not lifestyles—are major causes of heart disease in Canada and elsewhere.* Toronto: Centre for Social Justice, Foundation for Research and Education. Retrieved July 2002 from www.socialjustice.org/pdfs/JusticeGoodHearts.pdf.

Registered Nurses' Association of British Columbia. (1998). *The new health care: A nursing perspective.* Vancouver: Author.

Smedley, B., & Syme, L. (2000). *Promoting health: Intervention strategies from social and behavioral research.* Washington, DC: National Academy Press.

Stanhope, M., & Lancaster, J. (2001). *Foundations of community health nursing: Community oriented practice* (2nd ed.). St. Louis, MO: Mosby.

Starfield, B. (1998). *Primary care: Balancing health needs, services and technology.* New York: Oxford University Press.

United Nations Children's Fund (UNICEF). (2005). *The state of the world's children 2006.* New York. Retrieved November 15, 2006, from http://www.unicef.org/sowc06/.

Wallerstein, N., & Bernstein, E. (1994). Introduction to community empowerment, participatory education, and health. *Health Education Quarterly, 21*(2), 141–148.

Ward, M., & Piccolo, C. (2001, Winter). It's because I am a nurse. *Medhunters,* 1–4. Retrieved January 2003 from www.medhuntersmagazine.com/PDFstories/winter2001/ItsBecauseIAmANurse.pdf.

Wilkinson, R. (1996). *Unhealthy societies: The afflictions of inequality.* New York: Rutledge.

World Health Organization. (WHO). (1978). *The Declaration of Alma Ata.* Geneva, Switzerland: Author. Retrieved November 15, 2006, from www.who.dk/eprise/main/WHO/AboutWHO/Policy/20010827_1.

World Health Organization. (WHO). (1986). *Ottawa Charter for Health Promotion.* Geneva, Switzerland: Author.

World Health Organization. (WHO). (2002). *The world health report—Reducing risk: Promoting healthy life.* Geneva: Author.

World Health Organization. (WHO). (2005). *Health for All Policy Framework for the WHO European Region.* Geneva: WHO. Regional Office for Europe.

World Health Organization. (WHO). (2006a). *Report prepared for the fifty-seventh World Health Assembly, Health systems, including primary health care: Report by the Secretariat.* Geneva.

World Health Organization. (WHO). (2006b). *WHO mortality data.* Geneva. Retrieved November 15, 2006, from www.who.int/who.sis/mort/en.

World Health Organization. (WHO). (2006c). *Working for Health: An introduction to the World Health Organization.* Geneva. Retrieved November 16, 2006, from www.who.int/about/brochure_en.pdf.

ADDITIONAL RESOURCES

Websites

Canadian Council for International Co-operation
www.ccic.ca

Canadian Council on Social Development
www.ccsd.ca

Canadian International Development Agency
www.acdi-cida.gc.ca

Canadian Nurses Association
www.cna-nurses.ca

The Canadian Health Network
www.canadian-health-network.ca

The Canadian Public Health Association
www.cpha.ca

The Canadian Institute for Health Information
www.cihi.ca

Canadian Population Health Initiative
www.cihi.ca/cphi

Canadian Red Cross
www.redcross.ca

Canadian Society for International Health
www.csih.org/en/index.asp

International Development Research Council
www.idrc.ca

International Society for Equity in Health
www.iseqh.org

Network learning (in Primary Health Care)
www.networklearning.org/index.html

Pan American Health Organization
www.paho.org

Books

British Columbia Ministry of Health. (1987). *Healthy communities: The process.* Victoria, BC: Author.

Hachey, Jean-Marc. (2005). *The big guide to working and living overseas.* University of Toronto Press, Toronto, ON: Author.

Wilson, R., Shortt, S. E. D., & Dorland, J. (2004). (Eds.). *Implementing primary care reform—Barriers and Facilitators.* Montreal, QC: McGill-Queen's University Press.

Registered Nurses' Association of British Columbia. (1998). *The new health care: A nursing perspective.* Vancouver, BC: Author.

About the Authors

Dawn Smith, RN, BScN (British Columbia), MN (Community, Dalhousie), PhD (Population Health, University of Ottawa), is an assistant professor at the University of Ottawa, School of Nursing, where she teaches Community Health. She has practised community health nursing in several Canadian provinces as well as overseas.

Lori Jacobson, BA (Psychology/Women's Studies, Carleton), is a fourth-year nursing student at the University of Ottawa. Lori decided to return to school to study health care after working on international health projects in Nepal and Zimbabwe. She plans to work overseas as a community health nurse after graduating in May 2007. Lori would like to thank Dawn Smith, her professor, mentor, and research supervisor, for the opportunity to contribute to this chapter.

Lucia Yiu, RN, BScN, BA (Psychology, Windsor), BSc (Physiology, Toronto), MScN (Administration, Western Ontario), is an Associate Professor in the Faculty of Nursing, University of Windsor, and an Educational and Training Consultant in community nursing. She has published on family and public health nursing. Her practice and research interests include multicultural health, international health, experiential learning, community development, breast health, and program planning and evaluation. She has worked overseas and served on various community and social services committees involving local and district health planning.

Epidemiology

Lynnette Leeseberg Stamler

OBJECTIVES

After studying this chapter, you should be able to:

1. Describe the theoretical underpinnings of the epidemiologic process and its historical and present value to community health nurses.

2. Differentiate between association and causality and explain some of the criteria that, when satisfied, suggest a causal relationship.

3. Identify the various measurements used in epidemiologic research and reports, understand how the measurements were calculated, and identify their meaning for community health nurses.

4. Describe the research study designs commonly used in epidemiologic research and link the research question with the appropriate design.

5. Discuss how epidemiology has expanded to include not only the study of disease but also the factors that promote health.

INTRODUCTION

Throughout history, humans have ascribed different causes for disease. During the religious era, disease was thought to be a consequence of divine intervention. The environment was the next general cause of disease, which was attributed to miasmas (vaporous atmospheres) or other physical forces. It was not until the 1870s that specific bacteria were recognized as causing disease. During the past century, health professionals have come to understand that there are multiple factors or influences on many diseases and health challenges. In addition to learning the many causes of disease, health researchers are working to discover the factors that promote health.

In this chapter, you will learn the basics of the science of epidemiology, understand the types of data used in community health nursing, and begin to acquire the skills to identify and ask questions, using epidemiologic data to find some of the answers.

WHAT IS EPIDEMIOLOGY?

Epidemiology is defined as "the study of the distribution and determinants of health-related states or events in specified populations, and the application of this study to control of health problems" (Last, 2001). Webb, Bain, & Pirozzo, (2005) have

further identified sub-disciplines of epidemiology. While the most well-known of these would be public health epidemiology (or infectious disease epidemiology), these authors go on to note that the sub-disciplines can be divided into two streams: the exposure-oriented sub-disciplines (e.g., nutritional, social, environmental) and the disease-oriented sub-disciplines (e.g., cancer, injury, perinatal). Some sub-disciplines have less clear categorizations, such as occupational epidemiology or molecular epidemiology.

Epidemiologists first seek to describe health-related events by answering the questions who, what, when, and where. Further exploration answers the questions how and why. Though the above definition does not specify health promotion, epidemiology can be used to accomplish that goal as well as that of controlling health problems. The science of epidemiology helps community health nurses (CHNs) to examine and understand the past and to increase the accuracy of future predictions. From that understanding and those predictions CHNs can plan, implement, and evaluate appropriate and timely actions.

Historical Background of Epidemiology

Though large-scale, focused epidemiologic studies are a relatively new phenomenon, the basis of understanding for such studies has been noted throughout history. Hippocrates is credited with being the first to notice and record a possible relationship between the environment and the health or disease of people.

He suggested that physicians study "the mode in which the inhabitants live and what are their pursuits, whether they are fond of eating and drinking to excess, and given to indolence, or are fond of exercise and labour, and not given to excess in eating and drinking" (Hippocrates, 400 BCE).

Though history has recorded the existence and duration of epidemics such as the plague or the Black Death, few large-scale efforts were made to accurately record data that would increase the understanding of these epidemics. By the 1600s, statistics such as numbers of births and deaths were being recorded in London, England, and a haberdasher, John Graunt, was the first to study these statistics. He noted, for instance, gender differences in births (more males than females), seasonal variations in deaths, and high levels of infant deaths.

It was not until 1839 that Dr. William Farr initiated a more complete gathering of statistical data in England. With these data he was able (among other things) to compare death rates between workers in different types of jobs, and between prison inmates and the rest of the population. During a cholera epidemic in the mid-1850s, Dr. John Snow noticed an apparent relationship between the number of cholera deaths in various neighbourhoods and the source of the drinking water. He clearly demonstrated that people who lived in areas/homes served by particular water companies had much higher death rates from cholera than those in neighbourhoods served by other water companies.

Florence Nightingale, a contemporary of Snow and Farr, was also convinced of the effect of the environment on disease and death. When she arrived at Scutari during the Crimean War, she discovered horrendous conditions and a lax method of recording deaths and their causes. She increased the recording of these statistics and used them to explain and publicize the reality of the situation. Her polar diagrams, for instance, clearly demonstrated that in January 1855, 2761 soldiers died from contagious diseases, 83 from wounds, and 324 from other causes. It became clear that without ongoing recruitment, the entire army could have been wiped out from disease alone (Cohen, 1984). It was through her influence and her record-keeping that she was able to persuade authorities to allow her to implement sanitation practices that significantly decreased the death rates during and after the war.

In the 1900s, it became evident that although vital statistics of death and illness were important, following populations for a period of time to ascertain the progression of various diseases and their treatments was also important. As well, new research methodologies were developed to gather and compare data appropriately. As medical scientists discovered and implemented new treatments, the primary causes of death changed over time from predominantly contagious diseases to chronic diseases that were influenced by lifestyle behaviours. For instance, between the 1920s and the 1970s, death rates from health challenges such as cardiovascular and renal diseases rose, while death rates for such diseases as tuberculosis and influenza decreased. (See Figure 8.1.) In 1949, the first cohort study—the Framingham Heart Study—was begun, followed in 1950 by the publication of the first case-control studies of smoking and lung disease. Four years later, the Salk polio vaccine field trial was conducted. Modern epidemiological studies have all been developed from these pioneering works.

Basic Building Blocks in Epidemiology

Several concepts and processes are the basic building blocks of the science of epidemiology. These include the epidemiologic model, the concept of susceptibility, modes of transmission, the natural history/progress of disease, association and causation, and the web of causation. These concepts and processes arose from early epidemiologic observations and analyses and were developed to help scientists understand the hows and whys of disease. Modern CHNs use these same concepts and processes to determine and test appropriate interventions.

FIGURE 8.1 Comparison of the Most Common Causes of Death of Canadians over Time

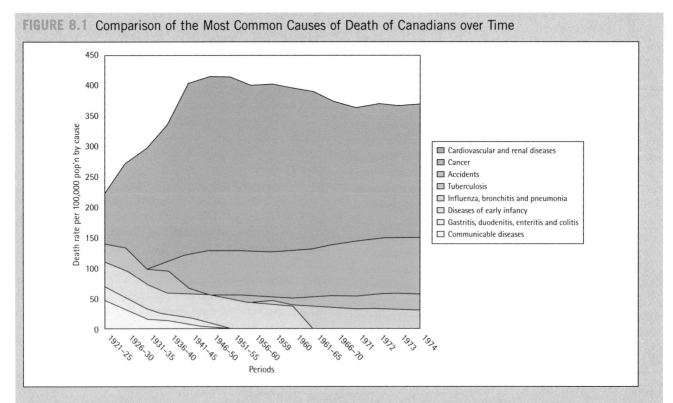

Data Source: Fraser, R. D. (1983). Section B: Vital statistics and health (Table B35-50). In F. H. Leacy (ed.), Historical statistics of Canada. Online at Statistics Canada, retrieved October 2, 2007, from http://www.statcan.ca/english/freepub/11-516-XIE/sectionb/ sectionb.htm#Vital%20Stats.

Epidemiologic Model The classic epidemiologic model contains the elements of host, agent, and environment. The model is frequently presented as a triangle. (See Figure 8.2.) The **host** is the human being in which the disease occurs. The **agent** is the contagious or non-contagious force that can begin or prolong a health problem. Agents include bacteria and viruses, as well as "stimuli" such as smoking or the absence of vitamin C. The **environment** is the context that promotes the **exposure** of the host to the agent. The **epidemiologic model** posits that disease is the result of the interaction among these three elements.

Some authors have included other elements in the epidemiologic model. For example, Gordis (2000) included the vector as an additional concept. He defined **vector** as a factor (such as a deer tick) that moves between the agent and the host, assisting the movement of the disease between the other two elements. Timmreck (1998), on the other hand, added the concept of time to the model. Harkness (1995) noted that using a **Venn diagram** instead of the classic triangle emphasized the interrelatedness within the model. A Venn diagram uses curves and circles to represent relationships. (See Figure 8.3.)

Epidemiologic Variables As noted, epidemiologists answer the questions who, what, when, and where. In order to completely and accurately describe the patterns of health challenges, the descriptive variables of epidemiology are used. These are named person, place, and time (Gerstman, 2003). Within each variable are factors or characteristics that further describe the event. For instance, under the variable of person, one might look at age differences, sex, ethnicity, genetic predisposition, immune status, marital status, place of birth, and immigration. Other environmental influences for the person such as education level, socioeconomic status, and occupation are also important pieces of information. Last, individual lifestyle characteristics such as dietary practices, use of alcohol or tobacco, and physical activity may be helpful.

The variable of time considers such characteristics as cyclic or seasonal variation of a health event, health challenges following specific events (such as postpartum depression), or time trends (increase of chronic disease over time) (Friis & Sellers, 2004). The variable of place can include variation between regions, countries, or continents; population density; rural/urban; or specific geographical characteristics such as working in a particular building or living close to a cataclysmic event such as Chernobyl (Gerstman, 2003). It is evident that

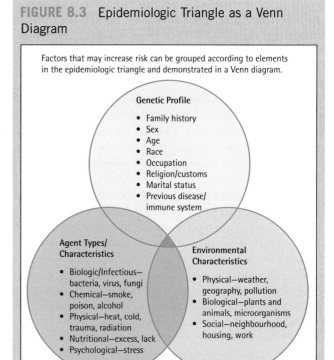

FIGURE 8.3 Epidemiologic Triangle as a Venn Diagram

Factors that may increase risk can be grouped according to elements in the epidemiologic triangle and demonstrated in a Venn diagram.

Genetic Profile
- Family history
- Sex
- Age
- Race
- Occupation
- Religion/customs
- Marital status
- Previous disease/immune system

Agent Types/Characteristics
- Biologic/Infectious—bacteria, virus, fungi
- Chemical—smoke, poison, alcohol
- Physical—heat, cold, trauma, radiation
- Nutritional—excess, lack
- Psychological—stress

Environmental Characteristics
- Physical—weather, geography, pollution
- Biological—plants and animals, microorganisms
- Social—neighbourhood, housing, work

some characteristics (e.g., lifestyle behaviours) can be modified by the individual or group, while others (e.g., age, sex, genetic makeup) are not under the control of the individual. During the beginning identification of AIDS, careful documentation of person, time, and place assisted health professionals to accurately describe the health challenge.

Susceptibility One might think that if a group of people were all exposed in the same manner to the same disease, all would get the disease to the same degree. However, the combination of characteristics of each individual within that host group, interacting with the factors present or absent in the other elements of the epidemiologic triangle, determines the **risk** (or degree of **susceptibility**) of each person to a particular agent. Susceptibility and risk can also be described as vulnerability, which determines the individual host response. The answers to the person/place/time questions, while pointing to group susceptibility, can also point to group protection. For instance, we may discover that one or more of the characteristics studied (such as age or physical activity) may in fact mitigate some of the effects of other characteristics.

Within each element of the epidemiologic triangle are factors or characteristics that may increase or decrease the risk or susceptibility of the host to the disease. Figure 8.3 identifies some of these factors/characteristics.

Modes of Disease Transmission A **mode of transmission** is one way in which a disease moves to a new host. There are two main modes of transmission: direct and indirect. **Direct transmission** involves contact between the person with the disease and another person. This may be accomplished through touching with contaminated hands, skin-to-skin contact, or sexual intercourse. **Indirect transmission**

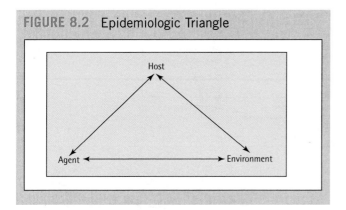

FIGURE 8.2 Epidemiologic Triangle

Host

Agent ⟷ Environment

involves a common vehicle or vector that moves the disease to the new host. An example of a common vehicle is a contaminated water supply or lake. A mosquito can also function as a common vector in disease transmission. Indirect transmission may be airborne (droplets or dust), water-borne, vector-borne, or vehicle-borne (contaminated utensils, hygiene articles, or clothing). Different **pathogens** (microorganisms or other substances that cause disease)are viable under different conditions; therefore, one needs to ascertain the potential mode of transmission for each disease.

Because a given disease may have more than one mode of transmission, understanding those modes is central to controlling the disease. For example, when AIDS first became recognized as a threat to public health, the mode of transmission was greatly misunderstood: it was not known whether the disease could be contracted through everyday contact, such as by using a toilet seat used by someone with AIDS or by shaking that person's hand. It soon became clear that such minimal contact did not result in disease transmission. However, the fear of AIDS greatly increased the use of universal precautions by health professionals—a positive outcome.

Natural History/Progression of a Disease A disease in a human host should be seen as a process rather than as a single incident. In 1965, Leavell and Clark plotted the natural progression of the disease process and identified prevention and health promotion strategies that could be employed at each stage. As illustrated in Figure 8.4, the first stage in the disease process is the **prepathogenesis** period. During prepathogenesis, the human host may be exposed to a variety of agents through several modes of transmission. Depending on the unique characteristics of the prospective host, repeated exposure or a combination of additional stressors may be required for the host to become susceptible to the agent and the disease to begin. **Stressors** are events or situations that cause discomfort to a person, such as chronic fatigue or a poor diet. During the prepathogenesis period (also called the **incubation** period), general health promotion as well as specific health promotion interventions may be employed. General health promotion interventions, such as physical activity and attention to proper diet, optimize health. Specific health promotion activities are directed at particular challenges, such as increased personal hygiene during cold and flu season, or rou-

---

FIGURE 8.4 Natural History of a Disease

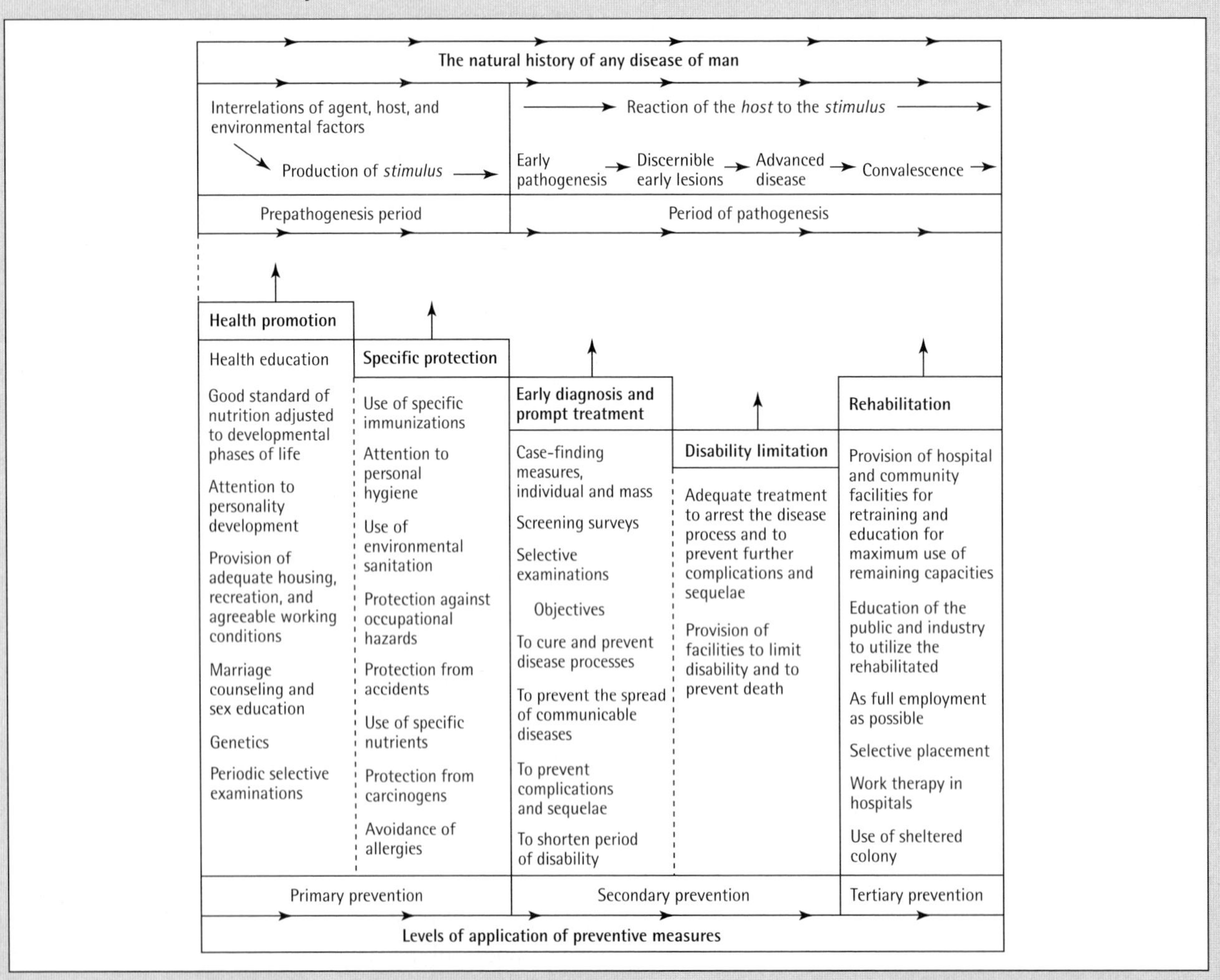

Source: Leavell, H. R., Clark, E. G., Preventive Medicine for the Doctor in His Community, 1965, McGraw-Hill, p. 21. Reproduced with permission of the McGraw-Hill Companies.

tine childhood immunizations. Both general and specific health promotion activities are referred to as **primary prevention**.

When the human host begins to react to the agent (or stimulus), the period of **pathogenesis** begins. Depending on the disease, the host may or may not experience symptoms, but microscopic changes take place that indicate the presence of the disease. Pathogenesis ends with recovery, disability, or death. Two categories of health promotion activities are used during the period of pathogenesis. The first category is early diagnosis and treatment, which occurs early in the pathogenesis period. For instance, screening mammography is used for early detection of breast cancer, and the Pap test screens for cervical cancer. The second category, disability limitation, occurs later in the pathogenesis period, when the disease is active or there are recognizable symptoms. During this period, health promotion activities are aimed at preventing complications, for example, ongoing examination and care of the feet in persons living with diabetes. Early diagnosis and disability limitation may also be called **secondary prevention**. **Screening** is a tool for early diagnosis and is the application of a specific test to detect the presence of a disease.

Tertiary prevention is the term given to the last health promotion category and occurs during the latter phases of the pathogenesis period. At this stage, health promotion activities might include client/family education to understand the chronicity of the disease, to adapt to sequelae of the disease process, or to maximize the health of the individual through use of aids such as a walker or adapted eating utensils. Figure 8.4 identifies this period as rehabilitation, but it may be the time when palliative care and assistance for the individual and family to move toward a dignified death would be appropriate. It is important to recognize that the presence of chronic diseases/health challenges in individuals also increases their vulnerability or susceptibility to additional health challenges. This has become increasingly evident as more and more of our population live longer due to enhanced medical care and health practices. Disease processes that would have ensured a speedy death only a few decades ago are now managed with little ongoing medical care. CHNs can use their knowledge of the progression of a disease and the levels of prevention to plan and implement interventions at the individual, family, aggregate, and population levels.

Association and Causation Before planning interventions that prevent or ameliorate a disease or health problem, one has to clearly understand the how and why of the disease or health problem. Two terms are used to describe the relationship between a stressor and a disease: association and causation. An **association** occurs when there is reasonable evidence that a connection exists between a stressor or environmental factor and a disease or health challenge. For example, a CHN might notice that many patients who exhibit a certain condition spent their childhoods in a particular geographic location. Thus, the relationship is first noticed through observation. Based on these observations, the CHN or epidemiologist

examines the data to see if the relationship or association is strong or weak—is it all patients or just a few? If the association appears strong from the limited data sample, then a larger, more comprehensive exploration might be conducted. Such investigations often generate data from several sources.

When a relationship or association has been confirmed beyond doubt, **causation** (or causality) is said to be present. In other words, causality occurs when one can state that there is a definite, statistical, cause-and-effect relationship between a particular stimulus and the occurrence of a specific disease or health challenge, or that the occurrence could not happen by chance alone.

In some ways, causation was simpler when the majority of diseases were infectious, as they were more likely to have only one cause. For example, streptococcus bacteria produce strep infection. Two important concepts in establishing causality are "necessary" and "sufficient." "Necessary" refers to the notion that a particular stressor *must* be present before a given effect can occur. For example, exposure to *Mycobacterium tuberculosis* is required before a person becomes ill with tuberculosis. "Sufficient" refers to the amount of exposure required to result in the disease. For instance, some people exposed to *Mycobacterium tuberculosis* only once (minimal dose) become ill, and some do not become ill unless exposed several times (larger dose).

In the past 40 years, several authors have identified factors or criteria that researchers and practitioners could use to assess a causal relationship between a stimulus and the occurrence of a disease (Hill, 1965). Timmreck's (1998) criteria of causation were chosen for this text because of their comprehensiveness and clarity. Timmreck's criteria are summarized in Table 8.1. The criteria may be used for individual health challenges as well as population events.

Though strict adherence to these criteria is perhaps the purview of researchers, CHNs can use them as well. When reading research that examines a particular nursing practice or new intervention, it is prudent to examine the presented results/recommendations in light of the ten criteria in Table 8.1. Similarly, when CHNs observe a recurring phenomenon that appears to have a relationship with a human or environmental factor, a close examination of the data in light of the ten criteria may assist them in planning subsequent observations.

Web of Causation Previous chapters have introduced the concept of determinants of health. In contrast to the time when each illness was thought to have a unique and specific cause, it is now recognized that many health problems have multiple causal factors, both direct and indirect. For instance, issues of poverty, education, and environment (e.g., pollution) have been shown to be influential in many health challenges. It is in looking for the causes for today's health challenges and assessing for the presence or absence of particular determinants of health that the CHN is well served by partnering with practitioners from a variety of disciplines. For instance, in addition to other health professionals, the CHN looking at population influences might look to the disciplines of

TABLE 8.1
Illustrations of Causation Criteria

Criterion	Example
Consistency	Everyone who eats food contaminated with a certain bacteria gets sick. If other food at a different time and place is contaminated with the same bacteria, the illness recurs.
Strength	Persons who are most exposed to the contaminated food (e.g., ate the most) are the most ill.
Specificity	The cause is linked to a specific problem: *Mycobacterium tuberculosis* does not cause chickenpox.
Time relationship	A person does not get a disease until after exposure to the cause. Similarly, an intervention designed to decrease complications in diabetes is unlikely to be the cause of an immediate decrease since the development of complications is a lengthy process.
Congruence (coherence)	Since the possibility of contamination of raw meat is quite high, it is more logical to assume that eating raw meat is more likely to expose the person to the disease than eating well-cooked meat.
Sensitivity	A test is used to discriminate between persons who get ill from one source and those who get ill from another source— the greater the discrimination, the stronger the sensitivity.
Biological/medical	If children play with a child who has a disease (cold, measles), they will be more likely to get the disease than if they played with children who were not sick.
Plausibility	People used to think that only vigorous, painful exercise was valuable. Research has demonstrated that sustained moderate exercise may be more helpful for maintenance of cardiovascular health.
Experiments and research	Rigorous, scientific comparisons replicated over time add weight to the evidence that an association is present.
Analogy factors (transfer of knowledge)	Since vaccinations have been found to decrease chances of becoming ill with a viral disease, it was reasonable for early researchers to search for a vaccination for the AIDS virus.

sociology, anthropology, genetics, psychology, geography, and economics. As well, working with experts in social trends and public policy could bring additional understanding to the specific issue at hand.

A model called a **web of causation** can be helpful to CHNs in visualizing the relationships among the many causes or influences of a given health challenge. Within that model, the relationship between the direct and indirect causes can be hypothesized, at which point research studies can be designed to test the hypotheses suggested by the web of causation.

Figure 8.5 illustrates a web of causation for teenage pregnancy. Obviously, the most direct causes of teen pregnancy are sexual activity and lack of use of contraceptives. However, behind those primary causes are several other causal factors possessing various levels of influence. For instance, the causal factor of knowledge can be stratified into knowledge of several topics and the sources of the knowledge. Both are influenced by community attitudes.

At any one time, each individual is subjected to multiple agents delivered through many modes of transmission. If one compared webs of causation for several common health challenges, some specific health promotion activities would appear to serve more than one purpose. Conversely, there may be a health promotion activity that is helpful for one challenge, but contributes to susceptibility for another challenge. CHNs must examine all possible benefits and consequences of an intervention.

MEASUREMENT IN EPIDEMIOLOGY

To determine the extent of a disease process or health challenge and its final effects on a population, data must be collected and analyzed. However, for the resulting measurements to be useful to the CHN, the raw data or crude numbers must be presented in conjunction with other factors, such as population, time frame, or human characteristic (e.g., gender, race, age). These numbers, expressed as fractions, are known as **rates**. The numerator of each fraction is generally the crude count of the disease in question, and the denominator is generally the size of the population in question. In each case, the population or subpopulation of the numerator and denominator of the fraction are the same. For example, a rate of teen pregnancies might look like this:

$$\text{Rate} = \frac{\text{number of live births delivered to teen mothers in the population}}{\text{total number of teen women in the population}}$$

This fraction, or rate, is usually expressed for a set number of the population (e.g., per 100 000 people, per 100 cases, or per 1000 births) so that different-sized populations can be compared. Table 8.2 presents the formulae for commonly used rates, and the following section describes these rates and shows how they are calculated and how they might be used by CHNs.

FIGURE 8.5 Web of Causation for Teen Pregnancy

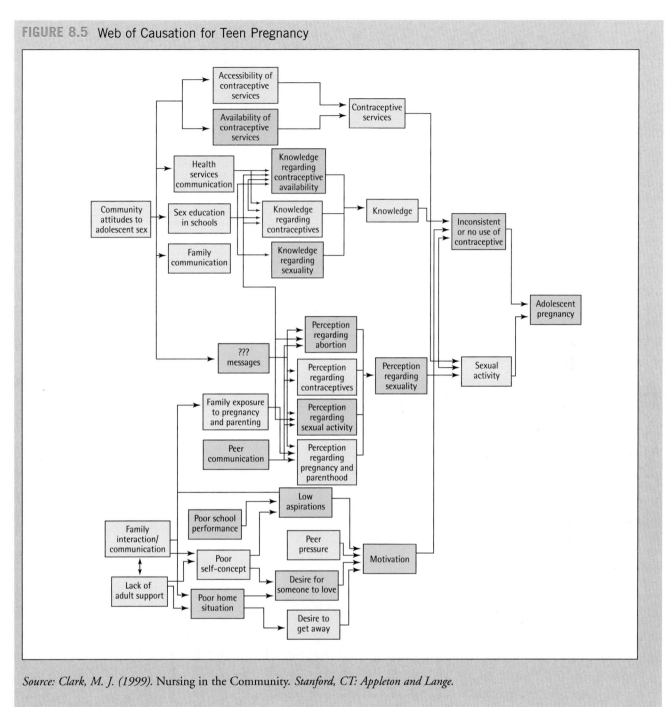

Source: Clark, M. J. (1999). Nursing in the Community. *Stanford, CT: Appleton and Lange.*

Mortality (Death) Rates

Physicians are legally required to complete death certificates for all deaths and file them with the government authorities. Thus, death or **mortality rates** are generally complete and easily obtainable. Mortality rates can be crude or specific in nature. **Crude mortality rates** compare the number of deaths from a specific cause within the entire population, while **specific mortality rates** compare the number of deaths from a specific cause in a particular subgroup with that whole subgroup. For example, if one examined all deaths from motor vehicle collisions and compared them with the total population, one would have a crude mortality rate. However, if one examined only teenage male deaths from motor vehicle collisions, one would compare that with the number of male teens driving at that time, a specific mortality rate. Mortality rates from a specific cause are often different when different subgroups (e.g., teenage males, children aged 4–8, elderly persons) are examined. For example, Figure 8.6 illustrates the age-specific suicide rates for Canada for 2004, stratified (divided) by gender. Note the line that represents the specific total mortality rate for each age group. If only these data were

TABLE 8.2
Commonly Used Rates in Epidemiology

Rate	Formula
Crude mortality rate	$\dfrac{\text{Total deaths from any cause in a given year in a population}}{\text{Average total population for the same year}}$
Specific mortality rate	$\dfrac{\text{Total deaths from a specific cause in a given year in a population (subgroup)}}{\text{Average number of population (subgroup) for the same year}}$
Infant death rate	$\dfrac{\text{Total deaths of infants in given year in population}}{\text{Total number of live births in same year in population}}$
Prevalence rate	$\dfrac{\text{Number of people with given disease in given population at one point in time}}{\text{Total in given population at same point in time}}$
Incidence rate	$\dfrac{\text{Number of new cases of given disease in population in given time (1 year)}}{\text{Average total population in same time}}$
Relative risk	$\dfrac{\text{Incidence rate of disease in exposed population}}{\text{Incidence of disease in unexposed population}}$

FIGURE 8.6 Suicide Rates by Age and Gender, Canada, 2004

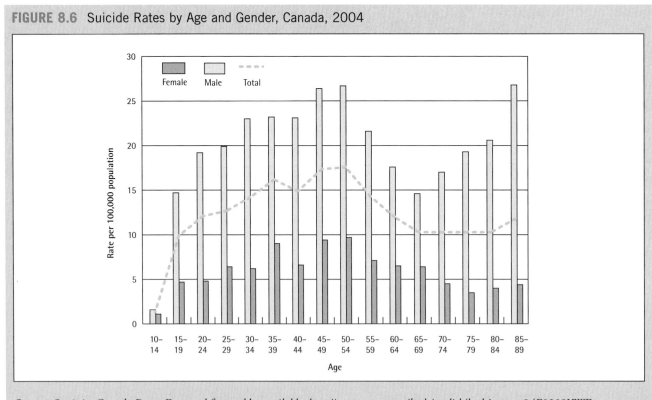

Sources: Statistics Canada Data. Extracted from tables available: http://www.statcan.ca/bsolc/english/bsolc?catno=84F0209XWE.

presented, it would be statistically correct, but would fail to inform the reader that the rate for males is significantly higher than for females in each age group. These stratified data would lead one to conclude that males are more susceptible (or at least more successful) than females to death by suicide.

Proportional mortality rates can be used to stratify crude mortality rates. The number of deaths from a specific cause in a given population for a particular time period is compared with the total number of deaths in that same population and time period. A common use of proportional mortality rates is to state that *x*% of the deaths in a given year were due to breast cancer or motor vehicle collisions. (See Figure 8.7.) Note that two causes of death, cancers and diseases of the heart, account for over half the deaths.

FIGURE 8.7 Selected Leading Causes of Death, Canada, 2004

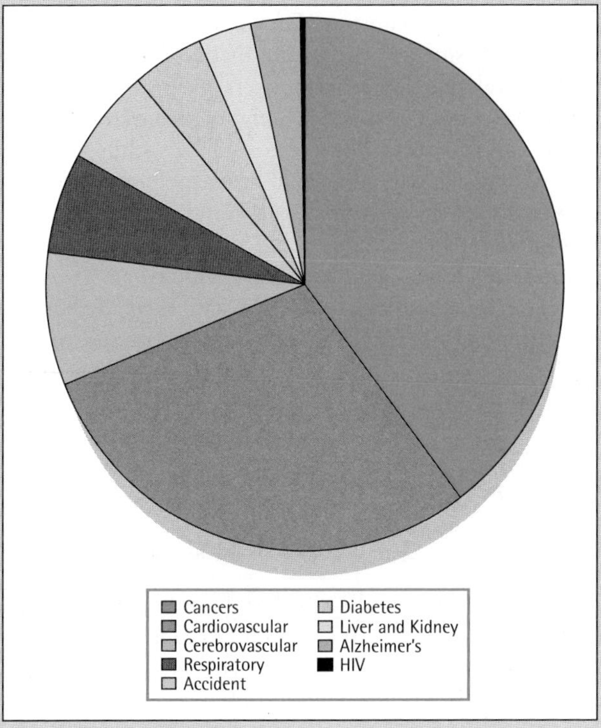

Legend:
- Cancers
- Cardiovascular
- Cerebrovascular
- Respiratory
- Accident
- Diabetes
- Liver and Kidney
- Alzheimer's
- HIV

Sources: Statistics Canada Data. Available: http://www40.statcan.ca/l01/cst01/health30a.htm?sdi=mortality%20rates.

Historically, the health of a population has been exemplified by maternal and infant mortality rates. Families used to have many children, partly because few were expected to live past the first years of life (assuming the mother and child survived the birth and neonatal period). With the advent of better hygiene, as well as prenatal and postnatal care, maternal and infant mortality rates decreased. CHNs often compare infant mortality rates across developing and developed countries, the assumption being that lower maternal and infant mortality rates are indicative of a healthier population. When looking at these statistics, it is particularly important to determine the stage (e.g., perinatal vs. infant) that has been studied so that the comparisons are accurate. The following definitions are used in maternal and infant mortality statistics. In all but the perinatal rate, the denominator is the number of live births in that year in that population.

- Maternal or puerperal death rate: any deaths of the mother resulting from pregnancy-related causes.
- Perinatal death rate: fetal deaths occurring during the last few months of pregnancy and during the first seven days of life. Here the denominator includes both live births and fetal deaths.
- Neonatal death rate: deaths occurring in infants in their first 28 days of life.
- Infant death rate: deaths occurring in the first year of life.

A more recent way of presenting mortality statistics in is terms of potential years of life lost (**PYLL**). This has arisen

from the assumption that a person who dies early in life has lost greater potential than has a person who dies much later in life. PYLL statistics give CHNs additional information on which health challenges or diseases result in the greatest lost potential to the population. While this may raise some ethical issues in terms of where a society or country chooses to place its resources, PYLL statistics are certainly a part of the picture that must be heeded.

Survival (Prognosis) Rates

Survival rates are often used to describe the effect of a given disease (e.g., cancer) and are also referred to as prognosis rates. Survival rates partially answer the common client question "How bad is it?" Survival rates can also be used to compare the efficacy of various treatments for a specific disease. For such diseases as cancer, and its treatments, the prognosis or survival rate most frequently used is the five-year survival rate. This is determined by calculating the percentage of persons with the disease who are alive five years after diagnosis. While five years is a convenient time period to use for comparing the effect of various treatments, it is easy for clients and health professionals alike to fall into the trap of somehow equating five-year survival with a decreased risk of future mortality from that disease. One of the arguments presented in favour of widespread breast screening is early detection of the disease. While it is hoped that early detection coupled with prompt treatment will increase the survival time, there is still conflicting evidence that these actions in fact contribute to decreased mortality rates from breast cancer.

The **case-fatality rate** is calculated by dividing the number of people who die from a disease by the number of people who have the disease, answering the question "How likely is it that I will die from this disease?" For instance, while recent advances have greatly increased the length of time between the diagnosis of a person with a positive HIV test and that person's death, the case-fatality rate for HIV/AIDS remains very high, as most people will die from the complications of the disease. The case-fatality rate for a person with arthritis, for instance, is much lower.

Morbidity (Illness) Rates

Illness or morbidity rates are valuable for the CHN. **Morbidity rates** give a picture of a population and a disease or health challenge over time, suggesting questions about the susceptibility of the population or subpopulation and the effectiveness of either health promotion or treatment strategies. Two types of rate are commonly used to describe morbidity in a population. The first is **prevalence**, which provides a picture of a specific disease process in a population at one given point in time. The second is **incidence**, which describes the identification of new cases of a disease in a population over time. Together with mortality rates and survival rates, they present a fairly complete picture of the population's response to a disease or health challenge.

If the disease is short-lived, such as measles or the flu, the prevalence does not reveal much. However, CHNs might use this rate in epidemic situations to plan for extra staff to deal with increased inquiries or clinic visits from concerned clients and parents. If the disease is short-lived, resulting in few deaths, the incidence and prevalence rates are very similar. If, on the other hand, the health challenge is chronic in nature, the incidence rate (number of new cases) stays fairly static over time, while the prevalence rate increases as more people live with the disease. If the disease is long-term with complications, such as diabetes or multiple sclerosis, the prevalence rate over time informs CHNs about the need for community and institutional support for the future. This is very important in terms of public and community health planning.

The population in question is usually the population at risk for the disease. For instance, when calculating the incidence of prostate cancer, the number of cases is compared with the population of males, rather than with the whole population. Incidence rates, when calculated within the same population over several years, show whether the population seems more or less susceptible to the disease in question. For example, the number of motor vehicle collisions in a given year involving teenage drivers might change over time in response to changes in the legal drinking age.

When CHNs test for a specific cause of a health challenge, they compare the incidence of that health challenge in a population exposed to the identified cause with the incidence of the same health challenge in a population not exposed to the same cause. If the suspected cause was indeed a factor, one would expect the incidence rates to be quite different. For example, one would expect the incidence of lung cancer to be much greater in smokers than in non-smokers. If the cause being examined is not the *only* cause of the disease (e.g., lung cancer), one might find that the incidence rates are more similar than expected. Such results might lead the CHN to explore other factors (e.g., second-hand smoke) to explain the incidence rates.

One frequently asked question is "Are some populations more at risk of or vulnerable to a specific disease than others?" To find the answer to that question, a statistic known as **relative risk** is used. This measure divides the incidence of a given problem or disease in a population exposed to a given risk factor by the incidence of the same problem in a population not exposed to the same risk. For example, CHNs might compare the incidence of childhood asthma in a population exposed to a certain air pollutant with the incidence in a population not exposed to that pollutant. If the resulting number is 1.0, it means that both groups have the same risk of the health problem, and most likely the risk factor in question makes little or no difference. If the resulting number is > 1.0, it indicates that the risk in the exposed group is higher than the risk in the unexposed group, and the risk factor in question is at least one of the significant risk factors for the problem or disease. Should the relative risk ratio be < 1.0, the given risk factor is probably not significant for the problem or disease. However, such results may indicate that the factor in question has a protective effect; for example, a population where the physical activity is high may have a low relative risk for diabetes.

Incidence and prevalence rates can be further stratified to increase the descriptiveness of the statistic. Data are frequently obtained through interviewing members of the population, also known as self-reporting. For instance, the question "Do you currently smoke?" elicits data that could contribute to a **point prevalence** statistic of smokers in the population. This statistic describes the situation only for that particular point in time. The question "Have you smoked within the last six months?" gives us data that could be useful for **period prevalence** statistics. However, asking "Have you ever smoked?" gives the researcher data that could be used for **cumulative** or **lifetime incidence** statistics. This demonstrates why it is important for researchers to clearly state their methods and sources of data in journal articles and reports, and why it is equally important for CHNs reading those articles to critically examine the evidence presented.

RESEARCH IN EPIDEMIOLOGY
Sources of Epidemiologic Data

Surveillance has been described as the ears and eyes of public health (Webb et al., 2005) and is the constant watching or monitoring of diseases to assess patterns and quickly identify events that do not fit the pattern. In the case of infectious diseases, surveillance may also include the monitoring of people with the disease, and their contacts. In the case of diseases with a genetic component, data may be collected to track the disease through extended family relationships.

Surveillance and other epidemiological analyses and research are only as good as the data on which they are based. Thus, CHNs need to ensure that they use consistent and accurate sources of data. One of the largest sources of epidemiologic data is the government. Canada has several sources of government or government-funded data such as the Public Health Agency of Canada, Health Canada, Statistics Canada, and the provincial government health ministries. As birth and death statistics are required by law to be filed with the appropriate government agency, they are generally very accurate. Birth and death statistics can be teamed with the census data reported by Statistics Canada for further detail. Statistics Canada data can be found in their daily newsletter (*The Daily*), which reports on recent data and analysis and often provides a historical trend analysis for the disease (e.g., breast cancer) or issue (e.g., family structure in Canada). Statistics Canada also has a website where more detailed information such as profiles of individual communities and archived newsletters can be found.

In the wake of SARS and other public health events, it was recognized that a stronger emphasis on public health by the government was required. In response, the Public Health Agency of Canada (PHAC) was formed. Many of the reports and statistics previously reported by Health Canada may now be found at the PHAC website. These include information on surveillance of **reportable diseases** (diseases that are required to be reported by law, for example, tuberculosis, sexually transmitted infections, AIDS) as well as surveillance data on cancer, chronic disease, and cardiovascular diseases. Health

Canada remains a source of information on many disease states, including epidemiological data and links to other sites. All provinces also maintain health websites that provide information for the province in question. Specifically, many of the provincial health ministry websites provide birth and infant mortality statistics.

The Canadian Institute for Health Information (CIHI) is also an excellent source for data. A non-governmental organization, CIHI collects and collates information from many sources to provide analyses that can inform policy. The epidemiological data that it reports includes data from hospital sources and from the various provincial health plans. Thus, this organization may provide information on incidence and prevalence of non-reportable diseases.

Both Health Canada and the Public Health Agency of Canada offer statistics on a variety of disease entities. In addition, there are agencies that focus solely on specific disease issues. For example, the Canadian Diabetes Association or the Heart and Stroke Foundation of Canada are sources for statistics relative to those diseases. When using information found on the internet, the CHN needs to examine the source of the data to ensure it is from a reputable organization.

For the CHN wanting to compare data between Canada and the United States, the Centers for Disease Control and Prevention website is a valuable resource. For international data, the World Health Organization's website is very helpful. These and other selected websites are listed at the end of this chapter.

In addition to websites, many organizations produce a variety of reports that are frequently found in university and college libraries or are available for download or purchase in print.

The final source of data is to gather data oneself. Although this can result in accurate data that deal with the specific question being asked, the cost of creating a survey instrument that is clear and understood by all respondents, choosing an appropriate sample (especially a national sample), and gathering the data often is beyond the financial reach of most researchers. If this is the case, researchers may be able to add questions to a survey being conducted by a community health care centre or agency.

Types of Epidemiological Research

Research is one method of finding answers to questions. It is critical that CHNs have a clear understanding of research methodologies in order to understand, participate in, and conduct research. This is because the study design is strongly linked to the research question: if an inappropriate study design is chosen, the results will not provide answers. Basic research designs are presented in this section, illustrated by studies completed by using the designs.

There are two basic categories of research in epidemiology: observational and experimental. Some observational is sometimes also called descriptive research. It is most frequently concerned with the variables of time, person, and place, and answers the basic questions of who, when, and where. Other observational research may be termed analytic research. In these cases, the epidemiologist is attempting to answer the questions how and why. The answers to these questions may be achieved through comparison of variables such as age and gender or application of statistics to determinants of health such as levels of education or employment status. Examples of research questions answered using observational research include "Are mortality rates for cardiac disease higher for men than for women," "Does age at diagnosis or geographic residency affect survival rates for persons with multiple sclerosis?" and "What are the current incidence rates for HIV in young homosexual males compared with 5, 10, or 20 years ago?" In observational research, the epidemiologist does not manipulate or change the variables, but rather observes and reports the reality of the situation. Frequently, the factors that increase risk may be used as a variable of interest; for example, gender may be considered to be a risk factor for heart disease.

In contrast, during experimental research, the epidemiologist assumes greater control over selected variables. These studies are designed to compare two or more groups of people that are statistically similar except for the selected variables. Experimental research can be used to compare a new treatment with one already in existence, to provide support for cause-and-effect relationships, or to compare the results of a public health intervention in a community with the intervention and a similar community without the intervention.

Types of Observational Studies

Observational studies can be cohort, case-control, or cross-sectional. In **cohort studies**, the researcher examines the individual histories of a group of people manifesting a particular disease to find out what common factors they share and what differences can be discerned. (For examples, see Canadian Research Box 8.1 or Borugian, Spinelli, Mezei, Wilkins, Abanto, & McBride, 2005.) In **case-control studies**, the individuals in the cohort with the disease are matched with individuals who are similar in some characteristics (e.g., age, gender, time, geographic residence) but who have not manifested the disease in question. The health histories or characteristics of the individuals in both groups are then obtained. These data are compared and the common factors/differences are identified between the two populations. (For examples, see Canadian Research Box 8.2 or Kasim, Levallous, Abdous, Auger, Johnson, & Canadian Cancer Registries Epidemiology Research Group, 2005.)

A case-control study of children with type 2 diabetes would include children with the disease in one group and children without the disease in the other group. The two groups would be matched for age and geographic location. The epidemiologist might search for common and different factors such as amount of physical activity, obesity, and family history of diabetes. In each case, the researcher would expect to find some similarities and differences between the two groups that could contribute to theories of causality.

The relative risk ratio compares the risk for a particular disease between two populations: one exposed to a stressor and one not exposed to the stressor. (For an example, see

TABLE 8.3
Calculation of Odds Ratio

Risk Factor	Persons with Lung Cancer	Persons without Lung Cancer	Total
Smokers	35 (a)	15 (b)	55
Non-smokers	15 (c)	135 (d)	145
Total	50	150	200

$$\text{Odds ratio} = \frac{\text{Exposed persons with the disease/unexposed persons with the disease}}{\text{Exposed persons without the disease/unexposed persons without the disease}}$$

$$OR = \frac{a/c}{b/d} = \frac{ad}{bc} = \frac{(35)(135)}{(15)(15)} = \frac{4725}{225} = 21$$

The odds ratio for these data is 21. As with the relative risk ratio, a number > 1.0 means that the persons exposed to the risk factor are more likely to develop the disease than those who are not exposed. In this example, male smokers are 21 times as likely to develop lung cancer as men who do not smoke.

Canadian Research Box 8.2.) Case-control studies also involve two groups: one group composed of individuals who have the disease and one of individuals who do not have the disease. Relative risk cannot be calculated here because neither the incidence nor the prevalence is known. The **odds ratio** provides epidemiologists with an estimate of the relative risk factor. To demonstrate the calculation of this statistic, consider the following example. A hypothetical community health centre practice has 200 male patients between the ages of 45 and 65; 50 of them have lung cancer and 150 do not. Thirty-five of the patients with lung cancer are smokers, while 15 patients without lung cancer are smokers. Table 8.3 illustrates the calculation of the odds ratio for this example.

Canadian Research Box 8.1

Davies, H. W., Teschke, K., Kennedy, S. M., Hodgson, M. R., Hertzman, C., & Demers, P. A. (2005). Occupational exposure to noise and mortality from acute myocardial infarction. *Epidemiology, 16*(1), 25–32.

Noise pollution is a common stressor in many occupations. The researchers hypothesized that occupational noise exposure increased mortality from acute myocardial infarction (MI) among workers. This was based on evidence of hypertension increase in workers exposed to high occupational noise. The occupation chosen was blue-collar workers in sawmills in British Columbia. A cohort of 27 464 individuals who worked at least one year between 1950 and 1995 was examined retrospectively. Using a calculation of cumulative noise exposure and data from Canadian Mortality Database, standardized mortality rates were estimated against the general population. The researchers accounted for the effect of hearing protection equipment by examining a subset of workers who already met the inclusion criteria who worked before 1970, before hearing protection was widespread, and comparing them to those who worked after 1970, when the use of hearing

protection was greater. Employment records, motor vehicle and pension records, and linkage to the B.C. medical insurance registration were utilized to ascertain current mortality status of the cohort members. Relative risks for MI were found to be elevated in the full cohort and were additionally elevated in the sub-group not using hearing protection. Highest relative risks were found during the working years of the subjects (2.0–4.0). The researchers concluded that chronic noise pollution found in many modern workplaces had an association with increased risk for MI. The evidence found in this study points to the need for further research in this area.

Discussion Questions:

1. What other occupations could contribute to noise pollution comparable to the levels found for these workers?

2. How could the CHN use this study to plan a campaign encouraging the use of hearing protection at work?

Canadian Research Box 8.2

Friedenreich, C. M., Courneya, K. S., & Bryant, H. E. (2001). Influence of physical activity in different age and life periods on the risk of breast cancer. *Epidemiology, 12*(6), 604–612.

The researchers in this study wanted to move past the current evidence that physical activity reduces the risk of breast cancer and discover if there were specific periods in a woman's life when physical activity was most beneficial. Using the Alberta Cancer Registry, 1239 women with breast cancer completed an in-person interview. Random-digit dialing was used to identify and match by age and residence (urban/rural) 1241 women who were cancer free. These women were also interviewed. Extensive data were gathered about family history, medical history, dietary practices, and lifetime physical activity. Physical activity was measured two ways, both lifetime totals and physical activity completed during five different age periods and four different life periods. The odds ratios were calculated for all the different variations. The authors concluded that the greatest risk reduction occurred with physical activity after menopause and before the reference year. They further concluded that postmenopausal women who participated in lifetime physical activity had 30% less risk for breast cancer. Additionally, the authors concluded that moderate activity produced the greatest risk reduction, while light or heavy activity produced no further risk reduction.

Discussion Questions:

1. How could the CHN use this study to facilitate a group of postmenopausal women to increase their physical activity?

2. What other determinants of health might influence women's choices to be or not to be physically active at different times in their lives?

Cross-sectional studies—snapshots of the present—are also called prevalence studies. These studies are used to suggest relationships between a disease and environmental factors or to provide health professionals with data that assist in planning further interventions. For example, CHNs may be concerned about the age of initiation of smoking behaviours relative to a specific planned health curriculum. The CHNs may work with the community to develop an anonymous survey that asks about smoking behaviours and administer it to students in various grade levels within the school district. The results of the survey may indicate that more than one-third of students in Grade 6 have already tried smoking, suggesting that beginning health education about smoking in Grade 6 is too late. The CHNs and teachers decide to move their initial anti-smoking education to Grades 1 and 2, in which fewer than 3% of the students have tried to smoke. A time series of cross-sectional studies could also be used with a particular group of students to assess the effectiveness of the intervention. After implementing the new curriculum in Grades 1 and 2, Grade 6 classes would be tested in subsequent years. The data would be compared with those from the present Grade 6 students, who did not receive the intervention, to ascertain if the program made a difference in the future smoking behaviours of students.

Cohort studies, which follow a specific group, may be retrospective or prospective. **Retrospective studies** are studies that begin in the present and search the past for information to explain the present. (For an example, see Canadian Research Box 8.3.) **Prospective studies** (or longitudinal studies) begin in the present and follow the subjects into the future or make predictions about the future that can be tested at a later date. These studies focus on individuals exposed to a particular health problem or potential stressor over time. For a prospective study, it is important to measure the incidence of the problem at various times. For instance, a group of people with high exposure to a stressor (e.g., occupational stress) may be matched with a group of people with low exposure to the problem, and both are followed for a period of time. The incidence levels of the health problem being studied (e.g., hypertension or myocardial infarction) in the two groups are compared at each measuring time.

Prospective studies have several problems:

- The sample size must be very large at the beginning to allow for attrition as people move, die, or lose interest.

- It is evident that health problems generally increase with increased age. By its very nature, a longitudinal study follows a group of people who are aging. Thus, a method to control for the effects of aging must be applied to any results.

- Outside factors may affect the different groups differently. For instance, researchers may decide to compare hypertension in Canadian and U.S. executives who live in large cities and experience long commutes to work. The cities chosen are Toronto, Montreal, Chicago, and New York. The time frame is 1990–2010. Might the events of September 11, 2001 have an effect on the data and results?

Ethical Concerns Ethical concerns during observational studies are rare but possible because of the nature of those studies. The researcher is not manipulating the variables but is systematically collecting and analyzing observations to make inferences and predictions. However, CHNs must always remember that most people are interested in participating in any study that they perceive will help someone else with a health problem. If a researcher has no intention of *using* the data (e.g., to plan interventions that are intended to be carried out), it is unethical to collect them. Ethics approval must be sought for any study where data are collected about or from humans. This topic will be expanded in the discussion on experimental studies.

Canadian Research Box 8.3

Pickett, G, E., Campos-Benitez, M., Keller, J. L., & Duggal, N. (2006). Epidemiology of traumatic spinal cord injury in Canada. *Spine, 31*(7), 799–805.

In this retrospective study, researchers examined charts of all patients entering with a traumatic spinal cord injury (SCI) to a specific institution from January 1997 to June 2001. Examination of the charts included such variables as age, gender, length of stay in hospital, type and mechanism of injury, neurologic deficit, and treatment. It was found that the incidence rates were 42.4/million for adults ages 15 to 64 years, and 51.4/million for adults over 65. Thirty-five percent of all the SCI were the result automobile accidents, but, perhaps surprisingly, 63% of the SCI in persons over age 65 were due to falls. Cervical SCI was the most common, especially in the elderly population. Mortality was also higher in the elderly population. The authors concluded that prevention of falls in the elderly population would be a good primary prevention strategy for decreasing the incidence of SCI in this population.

Discussion Questions:

1. This article describes the experience of a single tertiary care institution, albeit supported by other literature. How might the CHN find out if these results are generalizable to other parts of Canada?

2. How could the CHN use this information to augment or plan a falls-prevention program for older adults?

3. What are the implications of the results of this study for health care planning in the community?

Types of Experimental Studies

In experimental studies, the researcher manipulates some of the variables in order to ascertain the effect of the manipulation. **Manipulation** means to change something that is happening to some or all of the subjects within the study, rather than only observing what is present. In health care, the manipulation usually involves a new treatment or the encouragement of a new behaviour. (For examples, see Bettinger, Halperin, De Serres, Scheifele, & Tam, 2007; Carabin, Gyorkos, Soto, Joseph, Payment, & Collet, 1999.) The researcher believes that the new treatment or behaviour will positively affect the health of the subjects and uses the research to test that belief or hypothesis.

The "gold standard" of experimental study design is the **randomized controlled trial** (RCT). In fact, some scientists consider this the only valid form of experimental design. In an RCT design, individuals are assigned randomly either to a group that receives the new treatment or to a group that does not receive the new treatment. The latter is known as the control group. After a period of time, specific variables are measured in each group and compared. Frequently, neither the researchers nor the subjects are aware of which group they are part of until the end of the study. This is known as a blind RCT.

In community nursing and health promotion, the treatment or intervention studied may be a new health education or social marketing protocol (e.g., new advertisements for breast screening) or a change in policy (e.g., adding fluoride to drinking water for a community). In the example of new marketing for screening, the outcome examined could be the increase or decrease in numbers of persons participating in the screening. In the case of adding fluoride to the drinking water, the outcome measured might be the number of dental cavities found in six-year-olds.

In the examples above, randomized control groups would be almost impossible. One variation of this might be that several communities may be compared, with one or more serving as treatment groups and the others serving as control groups. Another variation may be that the community might serve as its own control group—measuring the outcome of interest (e.g., participation in screening) before and after the treatment (e.g., advertising for breast screening clinics).

Ethical Concerns In any experimental study, the competing issues of strong scientific experimental design and ethical considerations must be addressed. The first ethical concern is how the human subjects are approached. Most health care agencies and university research centres have an ethics committee that reviews research proposals to ensure that humans are treated fairly, the information is gathered and used in a confidential manner, and the privacy of the subjects is protected. However, ethical questions also arise about the design of the research. For instance, is it ethical to withhold a treatment that is felt to be beneficial from people who need it because a research design with a control group would be more scientific? Researchers must consider these questions and consult with appropriate sources for advice when designing scientific and ethical research studies.

Case Study

The outbreak of E. coli 0157:H7 due to contaminated drinking water in Walkerton, Ontario, affected more than 2300 people and resulted in seven deaths, with unknown long-term issues. Immediate causes were attributed to human error on the part of officials, complicated by heavy rainfall immediately prior. Ali (2004), however, suggests that the modern epidemiologist will examine a variety of factors that contribute to public health disasters. In this case, Ali describes the outbreak as "not simply an anomalous event limited to one point in time and place, but the emergent product of an extended set of processes that evolved over time and through different geographic scales of involvement at the political-economic, social and biophysical levels" (p. 2602). In the socio-ecological autopsy of the event, Ali combines the work of epidemiology, sociology, political science, agriculture, and human and animal medicine to arrive at a socio-ecological matrix (p. 2603) to describe the causative factors.

TABLE 8A.1

| | Downstream — - — - — - — - — Upstream | | |
	Micro Level	Meso Level	Macro Level
Ecological Dimension	Individual water well Extreme weather event	Regionalized factory farming setting	Evolution of new and (re)emerging diseases Process of global climate change
Social Dimension	Operator failure Individual farmer	Public utilities company Government agencies Private lab testing	International political economy Agribusiness

Discussion Questions

1. Discuss the meaning of each of the items in the matrix in terms of its contribution to the Walkerton disaster.

2. After reading the article, can you think of additional factors that you might add to the matrix?

3. How can the CHN use this method of using epidemiological and other data for health promotion and injury prevention at a population level?

Source: Ali, S. H. (2004). A socio-ecological autopsy for the E. coli 0157:H7 outbreak in Walkerton, Ontario, Canada. Social Science & Medicine, 58, 2601–2612.

Summary

In this chapter, the science of epidemiology, its historical influences, and the evolution of its theoretical underpinnings were examined. The theories have been presented with modern examples, illustrating how the historical continues to have influence in the present. The notions of agent, host, and environment have been discussed, as well as modes of transmission and the natural history of disease.

Measurement is an important concept in epidemiology, and mortality, morbidity, and survival rates were each presented. The notion of risk or susceptibility was examined both theoretically and statistically. The importance of accurate sources for epidemiologic data was noted, as well as sources for Canadian data. Observational and experimental research designs were presented, with the caution that it is very important that the research design fits the research question. Causality as a societal belief as well as a statistical conclusion was noted, and causality criteria that the CHN can use to examine observations as well as published research were included. The notion of the web of causation was presented to coincide with the current belief in multiple direct and indirect causes for most health challenges.

The science of epidemiology is an important one for the CHN. Community health professionals are confronted with increasingly complex health challenges that were unheard of just a few short decades ago, such as type 2 diabetes in children. It is becoming increasingly evident that Hippocrates had it right more than two millennia ago: nurses must look at what the person eats, what the person does, and what the person's habits are. Health practitioners face the task of using the results of epidemiologic research to influence citizens to change or enhance their activities of daily living to actively promote maximum health, while recognizing that the individual and group environment may well influence people in other directions.

Modern CHNs, while facing more complex challenges, also have the advantages of access to strong data, government and societal interest in health, and a better-educated populace. The science of epidemiology is but one of their tools.

KEY TERMS

epidemiology
host
agent
environment
exposure
epidemiologic model
vector
Venn diagram
risk
susceptibility
mode of transmission
direct transmission
indirect transmission
pathogens
prepathogenesis
stressors
incubation
primary prevention
pathogenesis
secondary prevention
screening
tertiary prevention
association
causation
web of causation
rates
mortality rates
crude mortality rates
specific mortality rates
proportional mortality rates
PYLL
survival rates
case-fatality rate
morbidity rate
prevalence
incidence
relative risk
point prevalence
period prevalence
cumulative or lifetime incidence
surveillance
reportable diseases
cohort studies
case-control studies
odds ratio
cross-sectional studies
retrospective studies
prospective studies
manipulation
randomized controlled trial

STUDY QUESTIONS

1. Identify and define five criteria for causality.

2. Differentiate between mortality and morbidity rates. How does each inform the CHN?

3. Name and define three types of observational studies relating to CHN practice. Using different examples from those in the chapter, suggest two research questions that might be answered with each of the types.

4. Identify the three elements of the epidemiologic triangle and define each.

5. Differentiate between incidence and prevalence. What does it mean when the incidence and prevalence rates for a given health problem are very different? What does it mean when they are very similar?

6. Describe prospective and retrospective studies and give two examples of research questions that could be answered with each.

INDIVIDUAL CRITICAL THINKING EXERCISES

1. Select a health problem. Using Figure 8.4 as a guide, suggest five CHN actions for each level of prevention. Include actions for individuals as well as populations. How might CHNs collaborate with other health professionals to implement the actions?

2. Discuss the pros and cons of having national registries for disease process, such as tumours, diabetes, and HIV/AIDS. Did your discussion differ according to the statistics available regarding incidence and prevalence? What about possible social stigma?

3. One of the more recent mortality statistics is PYLL. Suicide is one health problem that is examined in terms of PYLL. Using the data in Figure 8.6, at what age group would you target your prevention interventions? Why? How did the concept of PYLL influence your decision?

4. How might CHNs use their knowledge of surveillance and epidemiological data for their community to influence their practice? How can CHNs be involved in epidemiological research and/or the collection and analysis of epidemiological data?

5. Why are infant and child mortality rates used as a measure of the health of a population? Using the national and provincial infant mortality rates (**www40.statcan.ca/l01/cst01/health 21a.htm**), what do you discern about provincial disparities? Are you surprised? What factors might influence the rates noted? Where might you go to find further evidence?

GROUP CRITICAL THINKING EXERCISES

1. Select a condition that you are familiar with (e.g., type 2 diabetes, asthma, heart disease). From two different provinces' health websites and the Health Canada website, compare the mortality and morbidity rates for that condition. Are they similar or different? What factors might influence the rates in those jurisdictions?

2. As a group, discuss the pros and cons of using an epidemiological approach to planning CHN actions.

3. Physical activity is recognized as protector of health for all humans, regardless of age and current health status. By using the table found at **www40.statcan.ca/l01/cst01/ health46.htm**, consider how you might design a national campaign aimed at increasing physical activity. Which groups would be most important to target? Why?

REFERENCES

Bettinger, J. A., Halperin, S. A., De Serres, G., Scheifele, D. W., & Tam, T. (2007). The effect of changing from whole-cell to acellular pertussis vaccine on the epidemiology of hospitalized children with pertussis in Canada. *Pediatric Infectious Disease Journal, 26*(1), 31–35.

Borugian, M. J., Spinelli, J. J., Mezei, G., Wilkins, R., Abanto, Z., & McBride, M. L. (2005). Childhood leukemia and socioeconomic status in Canada. *Epidemiology, 16*(4), 526–531.

Carabin, H., Gyorkos, T. W., Soto, J. C., Joseph, L., Payment, P., & Collet, J. P. (1999). Effectiveness of a training program in reducing infections in toddlers attending day care centres. *Epidemiology, 10*(3), 219–227.

Cohen, I. B. (1984). Florence Nightingale. *Scientific American, 3,* 128–137.

Friis, R. H., & Sellers, T. A. (2004). *Epidemiology for public health practice* (3rd ed). Sudbury, MA: Jones and Bartlett Publishers.

Gerstman, B. B. (2003). *Epidemiology kept simple: An introduction to traditional and modern epidemiology* (2nd ed.). Hoboken, NJ: Wiley-Liss Inc.

Gordis, L. (2000). *Epidemiology* (2nd ed.). Philadelphia, PA: W. B. Saunders.

Harkness, G. A. (1995). *Epidemiology in nursing practice.* St. Louis, MO: Mosby.

Hill, A. B. (1965). The environment and disease: Association or causation? *Proceedings of the Royal Society of Medicine, 58,* 295–300.

Hippocrates. (400 BCE). *On airs, waters and places.* The Internet Classics Archive. Retrieved November 25, 2006, from http://classics.mit.edu/Hippocrates/airwatpl.1.1.html

Kasim, K., Levallous, P., Abdous, B., Auger, P., Johnson, K. C., & Canadian Cancer Registries Epidemiology Research Group. (2005). Environmental tobacco smoke and the risk of adult leukemia. *Epidemiology, 16*(5), 672–680.

Last, J. M. (Ed.). (2001). *A dictionary of epidemiology* (4th ed.). New York: Oxford University Press.

Leavell, H. F., & Clark, E. G. (1965). *Preventive medicine for the doctor in his community: An epidemiologic approach.* New York: McGraw-Hill.

Timmreck, T. C. (1998). *An introduction to epidemiology* (2nd ed.). Sudbury, MA: Jones and Bartlett.

Webb, P., Bain, C., & Pirozzo, S. (2005) *Essential epidemiology: An introduction for students and health professionals.* New York: Cambridge University Press.

ADDITIONAL RESOURCES

Websites

B.C. Ministry of Health Services
www.vs.gov.bc.ca/stats/

Alberta Health Ministry
www.health.gov.ab.ca

Saskatchewan Ministry of Health
www.health.gov.sk.ca/

Saskatchewan Population Health Branch
www.health.gov.sk.ca/population-health

Manitoba Health, Public Health
www.gov.mb.ca/health/publichealth/

Ontario Ministry of Health and Long-Term Care
www.health.gov.on.ca

Quebec—Santé et services sociaux
www.msss.gouv.qc.ca/en/

New Brunswick Health and Wellness 2000–2001
Performance Indicators
www.gnb.ca/0391/pdf/
HEALTHPerformanceIndicators2002-e.pdf

Nova Scotia, Department of Health
www.gov.ns.ca/health/

Prince Edward Island Health and Social Services
www.gov.pe.ca/hss/index.php3

Newfoundland and Labrador Health Information System
www.nlchi.nf.ca/

Canadian Institute of Health Information
www.cihi.ca

CCDR (Canada Communicable Disease Report)
www.phac-aspc.gc.ca/publicat/ccdr-rmtc/

Centers for Disease Control and Prevention (U.S.)
www.cdc.gov

CDC Morbidity and Mortality Weekly Report
(CDC—U.S.)
www.cdc.gov/mmwr/

CDC National Center for Health Statistics (U.S.)
www.cdc.gov/nchs

Health Canada
www.hc-sc.gc.ca

Public Health Agency of Canada
www.phac-aspc.gc.ca

Public Health Agency of Canada Notifiable Disease Report
www.phac-aspc.gc.ca/bid-bmi/dsd-dsm/ndmr-rmmdo/
index.html

Statistics Canada
www.statcan.ca

World Health Organization Weekly Epidemiological Record
www.who.int/wer

About the Author

Lynnette Leeseberg Stamler, RN, PhD, is Professor and Graduate Chair at the College of Nursing, University of Saskatchewan. She completed her BSN at St. Olaf College, Minnesota; her MEd at the University of Manitoba; and her nursing PhD at the University of Cincinnati. Her research interests include patient/health education, breast health, diabetes education, and nursing education. She was a VON nurse for four years prior to her teaching career and is a researcher with NCE—Auto 21. She is active in national and international nursing organizations including Sigma Theta Tau International, the Nursing Honor Society. She is President Elect of the Canadian Association of Schools of Nursing.

Communicable Diseases

Leeann Whitney, Sheila Marchant-Short, and Lucia Yiu

OBJECTIVES

After studying this chapter, you should be able to:

1. Discuss the changing perspectives on communicable diseases.

2. Explain the nature and types of communicable diseases: vaccine-preventable diseases, foodborne and waterborne infections, vector-borne diseases, zoonotic infections, and parasitic infections.

3. Describe surveillance and contact tracing in the control and management of communicable diseases.

4. Describe the roles of international, national, provincial/territorial, and local authorities in the management of communicable diseases.

5. Describe the role of the community health nurse in the control and management of communicable diseases.

INTRODUCTION

As long as humans have inhabited the earth, communicable diseases have been a part of their lives. Communicable diseases occur in every society, from rural areas to urban cities, from country to country, and without discrimination between rich and poor. With advances in technology and modern medicine, the severity of the illnesses associated with many of these diseases has been reduced. However, with increasing population mobility due to efficient transportation systems, and with lifestyle and environment changes, communicable diseases know no boundaries and are now seen in previously untouched areas across the world. Community health nurses (CHNs) must have a sound knowledge base of communicable diseases in order to prevent or limit the transmission of these diseases and protect the health of the public. This chapter will describe the general concepts of communicable diseases and discuss the role of CHNs in communicable disease control and management in relation to the legislative mandate locally, provincially/territorially, and federally.

CHANGING PERSPECTIVES ON COMMUNICABLE DISEASES

For many centuries, communicable diseases such as tuberculosis, smallpox, leprosy, cholera, scarlet fever, typhoid, diphtheria, and poliomyelitis have caused many casualties and threatened the health of humankind. The first recorded worldwide threat from a communicable disease was bubonic plague, which killed about one-third of the population in Europe in the thirteenth century. More recently, the influenza pandemic (Spanish flu) in 1918–1919 was a major global threat, resulting in at least 20 million deaths worldwide (Heymann, 2004). Many communicable diseases were brought to Canada with the arrival and migration of early settlers in the sixteenth century. Since aboriginals had not had exposure to these diseases, and therefore an opportunity to develop natural immunity, they had little or no resistance to these diseases. Aboriginal people were decimated by the infectious and parasitic diseases carried by the settlers.

Since the mid-1800s, advances in scientific and medical knowledge and public health measures have contributed to the declining mortality and morbidity among Canadians from communicable diseases. The development of microscopes, germ theories, and vaccines, and the improvement of nutrition, sanitation, and living conditions, have been instrumental in this decline (McKay, 2005). Additionally, the 1974 World Health Organization's (WHO) Expanded Program on Immunization initiative led to the vaccination of 85% of the children around the world against measles, mumps, rubella, tetanus, pertussis, diphtheria, and poliomyelitis by 1985, and the eradication of smallpox in 1979 (WHO, 1998). Public health professionals continue their efforts to combat infectious diseases such as malaria, tuberculosis, and parasitic diseases, which can cause life-long disabilities and socioeconomic consequences (WHO, 2003).

As a result of recent developments in vaccine production and disease control, infectious diseases such as TB and influenza now cause less threat and impact on morbidity and mortality in Canada. However, new emerging and re-emerging infectious diseases are increasingly challenging the public health system worldwide. (See Figure 9.1.) The most recently emerging infectious diseases in Canada are Creutzfeldt-Jakob disease (CJD), severe acute respiratory syndrome (SARS), and West Nile virus (WNV). For example, the first case of CJD in Canada was diagnosed in 1994. Between 1994 and 2007 there were 320 deaths in Canada. Mortality from CJD may have peaked in 2004 with 41 deaths (Public Health Agency of Canada [PHAC], 2007a). Increasing public awareness of CJD and reporting by health care professionals through the CJD federal surveillance program is vital in creating disease data to demonstrate the prevalence and incidence of this emerging infection.

When treatment protocols to cure tuberculosis were developed in 1948, it was anticipated that the disease would be eradicated by 2000. Ironically, tuberculosis has now

FIGURE 9.1 Examples of Recent Emerging and Re-emerging Infectious Diseases, 2003–2006

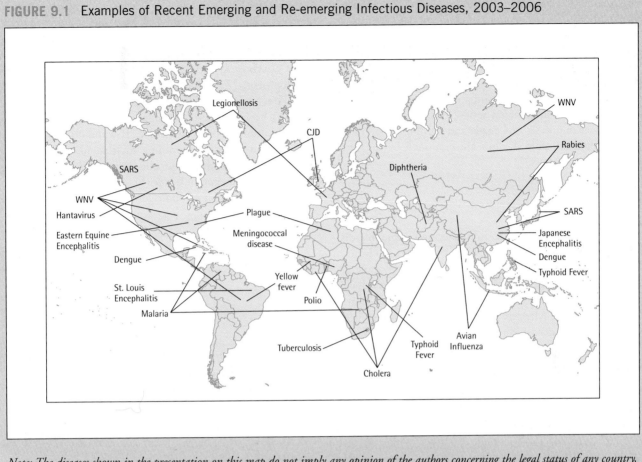

Note: The diseases shown in the presentation on this map do not imply any opinion of the authors concerning the legal status of any country, city, province/territory, or area.

Source: Based on http://www.promedmail.org. Accessed September 8, 2006.

re-emerged as an increased public health threat because of multi-drug-resistant strains and clients non-compliant with chemotherapy. Tuberculosis affects vulnerable populations such as older adults, the poor, or those with immune deficiencies. Today's global travel and trade, climate changes, poverty, inconsistent health care resources, the challenges of vector control programs, overuse of antibiotics, and changing lifestyle practices can lead to rapid transmission of infectious diseases within a very short time (WHO, 2000). Determinants of health such as income, education, and housing have been shown to globally affect the incidence of TB, such as in the First Nations and homeless populations where the incidence of TB is higher than in the general population.

COMMUNICABLE DISEASES

Communicable diseases are illnesses caused by a "specific infectious agent or its toxic products that arise through transmission of that agent or its products from an infected person, animal, or reservoir to a susceptible host, either directly or indirectly through an intermediate plant or animal host, vector, or the inanimate environment" (Health Canada, 2003). There are

four main categories of infectious agents that can cause diseases: bacteria, fungi, parasites, and viruses. Some communicable diseases are passed on by direct or indirect contact with infected hosts or with their excretions. Many diseases are transmitted or spread through contact or close proximity because the causative bacteria or virus is airborne. (See Chapter 8.)

A communicable disease may occur as an individual case or a group of cases, known as an outbreak. An **outbreak** occurs when the cases of a disease exceed the normal occurrence during a given period of time. For example, TB and invasive pneumococcal disease are common outbreaks in underhoused populations in winter/spring seasons in Canada. **Endemic** refers to the steady presence of a disease in a defined geographic area or population group (e.g., tuberculosis among foreign-born Canadians). Occasionally, the occurrence of a disease is higher than what would be expected normally; this is called an **epidemic** (e.g., influenza). More rarely, a **pandemic** occurs when a disease spreads and affects a large number of populations worldwide (e.g., Spanish influenza, SARS, and acquired immune deficiency syndrome [AIDS]).

"Communicable diseases kill more that 14 million people each year mainly in the developing world. In these countries, approximately 46% of all deaths are due to communicable diseases, and 90% of these deaths are attributed to acute diarrhoeal and respiratory infections of children, AIDS, tuberculosis, malaria, and measles" (Heymann, 2004). Preventing transmission is key to controlling the number of people infected with an organism. Understanding the infectious agent's characteristics is paramount to assisting health care personnel diagnose, control, and manage a communicable disease. Table 9.1 summarizes several of the communicable diseases that are present in Canada and preventable by vaccination. Communicable diseases are examined in the categories described below.

Vaccine-Preventable Diseases

Every minute, six children die from vaccine-preventable diseases around the world (WHO, 1998). The purpose of immunization in preventing disease and eradicating it must be noted. Smallpox (globally) and poliomyelitis (in developed countries) have been eradicated through successful immunization programs. Measles, mumps, and rubella have been dramatically reduced in some countries. Diphtheria, haemophilus influenzae type b, hepatitis B, influenza, measles, meningococcal disease, mumps, pertussis, streptococcus pneumoniae (pneumococcus), poliomyelitis, rubella, tetanus, and varicella are vaccine-preventable diseases. An age-specific schedule of immunizations (see Table 9.2) aims at providing optimum protection throughout life. Depending on resources and the burden of illness in the specific province, this schedule, developed by Health Canada, can be modified by the individual provinces.

Across Canada, approximately 4000 to 8000 people die from influenza-related illness each year (PHAC, 2006a). *Human influenza* is a respiratory infection caused by influenza virus and is spread by droplets through coughing or sneezing. Vaccination against influenza lasts four to six months and is routinely given on an annual basis at the onset of the influenza season, typically starting in October in the northern hemisphere. Each year, influenza vaccine consists of three new influenza strains predicted by WHO to be the most common to give protection from circulating viruses. Due to the significant morbidity, mortality, and societal costs associated with influenza, everyone 6 months or older should be vaccinated, especially those with selected chronic illness, people aged 65 and over, residents in chronic care and nursing homes, and essential health care service providers (PHAC). The spread of *avian influenza H5N1* (or bird flu) throughout Southeast Asia and Europe has generated much discussion on the implications for human health. Globally, all nations are on alert for a possible influenza pandemic. This issue has heightened pandemic influenza planning at federal, provincial, and local levels throughout Canada, challenging resource allocation in regard to preparation and acquisition of policies, processes, and supplies.

New vaccines licensed in Canada since August 2006 include the *human papillomavirus (HPV)* vaccine and the rotavirus vaccine. HPV is mainly transmitted by sexual contact, and the vaccine is available to prevent an infection that occurs years before but is associated with the appearance of cervical cancer. The rotavirus vaccine would decrease rotaviruses consistently involved in acute gastrointestinal illnesses in children. Vaccines against avian influenza, West Nile virus (Drebot & Artsob, 2006), and malaria are all in development.

The National Advisory Committee on Immunization (NACI) has developed 17 guidelines for the most desirable immunization practices to assist CHNs and other health care providers in critically examining their standards of practice related to immunization. The guidelines noted in its *Canadian Immunization Guide* (PHAC, 2006b) "are deliberately broad, far-reaching and rigorous" (p. 22), as follows:

1. Immunization services should be readily available.
2. There should be no barriers or unnecessary prerequisites to the receipt of vaccines.
3. Providers should use all clinical opportunities to screen for needed vaccines and, when indicated, vaccinate.
4. Providers should educate parents and adult vaccine recipients in general terms about immunization.
5. Providers should inform patients and parents in specific terms about the risks and benefits of vaccines that they or their child are to receive.
6. Providers should recommend deferral or withholding of vaccines for true contraindications only.
7. Providers should administer all vaccine doses for which a recipient is eligible at the time of each visit.
8. Providers should ensure that all vaccinations are accurately and completely recorded.
9. Providers should maintain easily retrievable summaries of the vaccination records to facilitate age-appropriate vaccination.
10. Providers should report clinically significant adverse events following vaccination—promptly, accurately, and completely.
11. Providers should report all cases of vaccine-preventable diseases as required under provincial and territorial legislation.
12. Providers should adhere to appropriate procedures for vaccine management.
13. Providers should maintain up-to-date, easily retrievable protocols at all locations where vaccines are administered.
14. Providers should be properly trained and maintain ongoing education regarding current immunization recommendations.
15. Immunization errors should be reported by providers to their local jurisdiction.
16. Providers should operate a tracking system.
17. Audits should be conducted in all immunization clinics to assess the quality of immunization records and assess immunization coverage levels.

A number of factors are integral to meeting the guidelines, such as considerations for cold-chain management of vaccines for guideline 12 and mature minor consent for guideline 2. For example, the CHN needs to ensure that all vaccine that is

TABLE 9.1
Selected Communicable Diseases in Canada

Disease	Infectious Agent	Mode of Transmission	Incubation	Clinical Presentation	Period of Communicability	Control Measures
Acquired immuno-deficiency syndrome (AIDS)	Human immuno-deficiency virus (HIV), types 1 and 2 (retrovirus)	Unprotected intercourse with an infected person; inocula-tion with or exposure to infected blood, other body flu-ids, needle stick injuries/ sharing; from infected woman to the fetus during pregnancy or breastfeeding	3 weeks to 20 yrs+ (aver-age 10 years)	Initially, mononucleosis-like illness for a week or two; may then be free of clinical signs or symptoms for months or years before developing Pneumocystis carinii pneumonia, opportunistic infections and cancers Infants and young children pres-ent with failure to thrive, inher-ited immuno-deficiencies and other childhood health problems	From onset of infection and persists for life Infectivity is high during first few months of infection	• Contact tracing and HIV testing. • Public education. • Zidovudine (AZT), dideoxycytidine (DDC), and dideoxyinosine (DDI) treatment including prophylaxis for the opportunistic infectious diseases that result from HIV infection. • AZT treatment to pregnant mother and newborn can reduce risk of perinatal transmission. • Recommendations for HIV postexposure prophylaxis include a basic four-week regimen of two drugs (zidovudine plus lamivudine, stavudine plus lamivudine, or stavudine plus didanosine) for most HIV exposures and an expanded regimen that includes the addition of a third antiretroviral drug for HIV exposures that pose an increased risk of transmission.
Chickenpox/ Herpes Zoster (varicella)	Varicella-zoster Virus	Air-borne through respiratory secretions or direct or indirect contact from vesicle fluid of person with varicella-zoster	10–21 days	Low-grade fever, maculopapular rash in trunk, face, scalp, mucous membrane of mouth then changed to vesicular for 3–4 days Herpes zoster is a local manifes-tation of reactivation of latent varicella infection in the dorsal root ganglia	2–5 days before onset of rash and until skin lesions have crusted	• Exclude from childcare, school, work, and public places at least 5 days until all vesicles become crusted. • Avoid contact with immunosuppressed persons. • Varicella-zoster immunoglobulin (IG) within 96 hours of exposure in susceptible close contacts of cases.
Diphtheria	Corynebacterium diphtheriae	Droplet spread through direct contact with a patient or car-rier or indirect contact with articles soiled with naso-pharyngeal secretions	2–5 days	Greyish spots on tonsils; sore throat, enlarged and tender cer-vical lymph nodes; marked swelling and edema of the neck in severe cases	If untreated, 2 weeks to several months Treated, 2–4 weeks	• Offer needed immunization to contacts, surveillance for 7 days. • Throat culture. • Antitoxin and benzathine penicillin or erythromycin treatment for infected persons. • Isolate until two cultures taken more that 24-48 hours apart are negative after the cessation of antibiotics; or isolate for 14 days if no culture available. • Disinfect contact articles. • Quarantine—adult contacts with food-handling occupations.

TABLE 9.1 *continued*

Disease	Infectious Agent	Mode of Transmission	Incubation	Clinical Presentation	Period of Communicability	Control Measures
Hemophilus influenza type B	*H. influenza* type B (Hib)	Droplet infection and discharges from nasopharyngeal discharges	Unknown, probably short, 2–4 days	Upper respiratory obstruction, vomiting, fever, bulging fontanelle in infants, stiff back and neck in older children, epiglottitis, meningitis, bacteremia, septic arthritis, cellulitis	Most infectious in the week prior to onset of illness and during the illness until treated, usually 24–48 hours after treatment started	• Early surveillance on children under six to prompt early medical treatment as needed. • Provide needed immunization and antibiotic prophylaxis.
Hepatitis A	Hepatitis A virus (HAV)	Direct or indirect contact through fecal-oral route transmission, through contaminated water, or non-cooked food contaminated by infectious food handlers	15–50 days, range is 28–30 days	Non-jaundiced in infants, acute febrile nausea, anorexia, diarrhea, lethargy, abdominal discomfort, jaundice	2 weeks before to 1 week following onset of symptoms	• Exclude from school or work for 1 week following onset of illness. • Health education, immunoglobulin treatment, contact tracing. • Sanitary disposal of feces, urine, and blood.
Hepatitis B	Hepatitis B virus (HBV)	Sexual, perinatal, and percutaneous exposure through blood, serum, and vaginal fluids	Usually 60–90 days, range is 45–180 days	Insidious onset of symptoms, nausea, vomiting, anorexia, lethargy, abdominal discomfort, jaundice	Many weeks before onset of symptoms, may persist for life	• Pre-exposure vaccination to at-risk populations; vaccination to susceptible sexual contacts. • Give HBIG treatment to contacts as needed. • Universal precautions to prevent exposure to blood and blood products.
Hepatitis C	Hepatitis C virus (HCV)	Parenterally; less frequently are sexual and mother to child	6–9 weeks	Insidious, with anorexia, nausea, vomiting, lethargy, abdominal discomfort, jaundice. Progression to jaundice less frequent than Hep B (90% asymptomatic).	From 1 or more weeks before onset of symptoms. Persists in most people indefinitely	• No vaccine is available. • Routinely screen blood products. • Education. • Interferon treatment for active disease.
Influenza	Influenza A and B virus	Airborne spread and direct contact in crowded populations in enclosed spaces	1–3 days	Fever, headache, prostration, coryza, sore throat and cough. Nausea, vomiting and diarrhea are uncommon, but may accompany respiratory phase, usually in children.	From 24 hours before onset of symptoms to 5 days in adults; up to 7 days in children	• Education about basic personal hygiene (hand hygiene). • Yearly immunization for immunocompromised, those with chronic conditions, elderly, and those who might spread infection (health personnel). • Antivirals are available to unimmunized and to residents in institutions. • Cohort ill from well in institutions and at home, if possible.
Measles	Measles virus (morbillivirus)	Airborne by droplet spread or by direct contact with infected nasal or throat secretions	7–18 days	Fever ≥ 38°C, cough, coryza, conjunctivitis, Koplik's spots on buccal mucosa, red blotching rash appearing on 3rd to 7th day, beginning on face then generalizing to body	1/2 day before onset of symptoms to 4 days after appearance of rash	• Exclude from childcare or school for at least 4 days after first appearance of rash. • Check immunization of all close contacts and offer vaccination within 72 hours of contact for non-immune persons.

TABLE 9.1
continued

Disease	Infectious Agent	Mode of Transmission	Incubation	Clinical Presentation	Period of Communicability	Control Measures
Meningo-coccal infections	*Neisseria meningitides*	Direct contact including respiratory droplets from nose and throat of infected persons	2–10 days	Acute onset of meningitis and septicemia with fever, intense headache, nausea, vomiting, stiff neck, purpuric rash on trunk, limbs, and body, joint pain.	Unit 24 hours of effective therapy has been received	• Prompt treatment with parenteral penicillin followed by 24-hour respiratory isolation. • Close surveillance of all close contacts and exclusion from school or work until at least 2 days after chemotherapy.
Mumps	Paramyxovirus	Droplet spread; airborne transmission and contact with saliva of an infected person	14–25 days	Swelling of salivary glands (usually parotid), orchitis, fever	2 days before to 4 days after onset	• Exclude susceptibles from childcare, school, or workplace. • Respiratory isolation for 9 days from onset of parotitis.
Pertussis	*Bordetella pertussis*	Direct contact via airborne or droplet spread from respiratory discharges of infected persons	6–20 days, usually 9–10 days	Whooping cough, slight fever, non-specific respiratory tract infection in infants. Paroxysms frequently end in vomiting with adults.	To three weeks after onset of paroxysms if not treated	• Exclude from childcare or school until at least 5 days after a minimum of the 14-day erythromycin treatment. • Immunize non-immune infants, children, and young adults.
Poliomyelitis	Poliovirus, types 1, 2, and 3 (enterovirus)	Direct contact via fecal-oral route where sanitation is poor; pharyngeal spread more common during epidemics and when sanitation is good	3–21 days	Fever, malaise, headache, nausea and vomiting, muscle pain, stiffness of the neck and back with or without flaccid paralysis	Greatest for 7–10 days after onset of symptoms, and up to 6 weeks or longer	• Isolate. • Exclude from school for at least 14 days after onset of illness. • Disinfect throat discharges and fecal soiled articles. • Vaccinate all non-immunized close contacts.
Rubella	Rubella virus	Droplet or direct spread with infected persons through pharyngeal secretions	14–21 days	Fever ($\leq$ 38.3°C) diffuse, punctate maculopapular skin rash. Malaise, headache, coryza, and conjunctivitis more common in adults.	7 days before to 4 days after onset of rash	• Contact should avoid pregnant women. • Exclude from school and work at least 5 days after onset of rash. • Routine MMR immunization as preventive measure.
Severe Acute Respiratory Syndrome (SARS)	Corona virus	Direct or indirect transmission of respiratory secretions via droplet or airborne through close contact with a symptomatic person	2–10 days	Sudden onset of high fever ($\geq$ 40°C), malaise, headache, cough, shortness of breath, sore throat, diarrhea	Early symptoms up to 10 days after fever subsides	• Wear mask; isolation; hand hygiene. • Active daily surveillance for 10 days. • Quarantine of close contacts for 10 days. • Public education and traveller advisory and screening.
Tetanus	*Clostridium tetani*	Bacterial spores may be introduced through contaminated puncture wounds, lacerations, burns, trivial wounds, or injected contaminated street drugs	2 days– 2 months average 10 days	Painful muscular contractions generalized from site of injury to back muscles; lockjaw; respiratory and laryngeal spasm.	Not transmitted from person to person; spores enter and devitalize tissues in infected wound	• Use IV tetanus immune globulin (TIG) and penicillin in large doses for 14 days. • Adequate wound debridement.

Sources: Heymann, D. L. (2004). Control of communicable diseases manual *(18th ed.). Health Canada, Population Health Branch. (1999). Routine practices and additional precautions for preventing the transmission of infection in health care: Revision of isolation and precaution techniques. Pickering, L. K. (Ed.). (2006). Red book: 2006 report of the Committee on Infectious Diseases (27th ed.). Elk Grove Village, IL. American Academy of Pediatrics. Government of Victoria, Australia. (2005). The blue book: Guidelines for the control of infectious diseases. Retrieved December 9, 2006, from http://www.health.vic.gov.au/ideas/downloads/bluebook.pdf*

TABLE 9.2

Recommended Immunization Schedule for Infants, Children and Youth, 2006

Table 1 Routine Immunization Schedule for Infants and Children

Age at vaccination	DTaP-IPV	Hib	MMR	Var	HB	Pneu-C-7	Men-C	Tdap	Inf
Birth					Infancy 3 doses ★				
2 months	●	✦				⋈	⊙		
4 months	●	✦				⋈	(⊙)		
6 months	●	✦				⋈	⊙ or ⊙		6–23 months
12 months			■	●		⋈ 12–15 months	if not yet given		☣ 1–2 doses
18 months	●	✦	■		or				
4–6 years	●		or ■						
14–15 years					Pre-teen/teen 2–3 doses		⊙ if not yet given	▲	

Table 2 Routine Immunization Schedule for Children < 7 Years of Age Not Immunized in Early Infancy

Timing	DTaP-IPV	Hib	MMR	Var	HB	Pneu-C-7	Men-C	Tdap
First visit	●	✦	■	●	★	⋈	⊙	
2 months later	●	(✦)	■		★	(⋈)	(⊙)	
2 months later	●					(⋈)		
6–12 months later	●	(✦)			★			
4–6 years later	(●)							
14–16 years later								▲

Table 3 Routine Immunization Schedule for Children ≥ 7 Years of Age up to 17 Years of Age Not Immunized in Early Infancy

Timing	Tdap	IPV	MMR	Var	HB	Men-C
First visit	▲	♥	■	●	★	⊙
2 months later	▲	♥	■	(●)	(★)	
6–12 months later	▲	♥			★	
10 years later	▲					

Table 4 Routine Immunization Schedule for Adults ≥ 18 Years of Age Not Immunized in Childhood

Timing	Tdap	Td	MMR	Var	Men-C	Pneu-C-23	Inf
First visit	▲		■	●	⊙		
2 months later		❏	(■)				
6–12 months later		❏				(❏)	(☣)
10 years later		❏					

Source: Immunization schedules: Recommendations from the National Advisory Committee on Immunization (NACI). *Retrieved April 21, 2007, from http://www.phac-aspc.gc.ca/im/is-cv/index.html#a. Public Health Agency of Canada, (2007). Reproduced with the permission of the Minister of Public Works and Government Services Canada, 2007.*

Notes

( ) Symbols with brackets around them imply that these doses may not be required, depending upon the age of the child or adult. Refer to the relevant chapter for that vaccine for further details.

● **Diphtheria, tetanus, acellular pertussis, and inactivated polio virus vaccine (DTaP-IPV):** DTaP-IPV(± Hib) vaccine is the preferred vaccine for all doses in the vaccination series, including completion of the series in children who have received one or more doses of DPT (whole cell) vaccine (e.g., recent immigrants). In Tables 1 and 2, the 4–6 year dose can be omitted if the fourth dose was given after the fourth birthday.

✦ *Haemophilus influenzae* **type b conjugate vaccine (Hib):** the Hib schedule shown is for the Haemophilus b capsular polysaccharide-polyribosylribitol phosphate (PRP) conjugated to tetanus toxoid (PRP-T). For catch up, the number of doses depends on the age at which the schedule is begun. Not usually required past age 5 years.

■ **Measles, mumps and rubella vaccine (MMR):** a second dose of MMR is recommended for children at least 1 month after the first dose for the purpose of better measles protection. For convenience, options include giving it with the next scheduled vaccination at 18 months of age or at school entry (4–6 years) (depending on the provincial/territorial policy) or at any intervening age that is practical. In the catch-up schedule (Table 2), the first dose should not be given until the child is ≥ 12 months old. MMR should be given to all susceptible adolescents and adults.

● **Varicella vaccine (Var):** children aged 12 months to 12 years should receive one dose of varicella vaccine. Susceptible individuals ≥ 13 years of age should receive two doses at least 28 days apart.

★ **Hepatitis B vaccine (HB):** hepatitis B vaccine can be routinely given to infants or pre-adolescents, depending on the provincial/territorial policy. For infants born to chronic carrier mothers, the first dose should be given at birth (with hepatitis B immunoglobulin), otherwise the first dose can be given at 2 months of age to fit more conveniently with other routine infant immunization visits. The second dose should be administered at least 1 month after the first dose, and the third at least 2 months after the second dose, but these may fit more conveniently into the 4 and 6 month immunization visits. A two-dose schedule for adolescents is an option.

⋈ **Pneumococcal conjugate vaccine - 7-valent (Pneu-C-7):** recommended for all children under 2 years of age. The recommended schedule depends on the age of the child when vaccination is begun. (See *Canadian Immunization Guide, Seventh Edition, 2006,* Pneumococcal Vaccine chapter.)

❏ **Pneumococcal polysaccharide - 23-valent (Pneu-P-23):** recommended for all adults ≥ 65 years of age

⊙ **Meningococcal C conjugate vaccine (Men-C):** recommended for children under 5 years of age, adolescents and young adults. The recommended schedule depends on the age of the individual (see the *Canadian Immunization Guide, Seventh Edition, 2006,* Meningococcal Vaccine chapter) and the conjugate vaccine used. At least one dose in the pimary infant series should be given after 5 months of age. If the provincial/territorial policy is to give Men-C to persons ≥ 12 months of age, one dose is sufficient.

▲ **Diphtheria, tetanus, acellular pertussis vaccine - adult/adolescent formulation (Tdap):** a combined adsorbed "adult type" preparation for use in people ≥ 7 years of age, contains less diphtheria toxoid and pertussis antigens than preparations given to younger children and is less likely to cause reactions in older people.

❏ **Diphtheria, tetanus vaccine (Td):** a combined adsorbed "adult type" preparation for use in people ≥ 7 years of age, contains less diphtheria toxoid antigen than preparations given to younger children and is less likely to cause reactions in older people. It is given to adults not immunized in childhood as the second and third doses of their primary series and subsequent booster doses; Tdap is given only once under these circumstances as it is assumed that previously unimmunized adults will have encountered Bordetella pertussis and have some pre-existing immunity.

☣ **Influenza vaccine (Inf):** recommended for all children 6–23 months of age and all persons ≥ 65 years of age. Previously unvaccinated children < 9 years of age require two doses of the current season's vaccine with an interval of at least 4 weeks. The second dose within the same season is not required if the child received one or more doses of influenza vaccine during the previous influenza season.

♥ **IPV Inactivated polio virus**

administered is viable by virtue of having been stored in appropriate environmental conditions. This responsibility also extends to vaccine that is provided to other immunizers, such as physicians. The mature minor consent refers to "a reliable decision to vaccinate…a child can be based exclusively on the information elicited by the recipient or the child's parent, and on the provider's observations and judgement about the health of the potential vaccine recipient at the time" (PHAC, 2006b, p. 23).

CHNs must respond to questions and concerns of those being immunized or parents of children being immunized. For example guidelines 4, 5, and 14 refer to education for recipients/parents, informing of risks and benefits of vaccine, and maintaining ongoing education of current recommendations. They respond in a respectful and supportive manner to educate and alleviate concerns from all clients/parents, including from parents choosing not to immunize their children.

Although many health care providers may rely entirely on providing up-to-date information and education to non-immunizing parents and expect that the evidence will speak for itself, there is an equal responsibility to continue to provide a supportive environment when a decision is made not to immunize. For parents who are seeking information about immunization, accurate information from health care professionals is crucial. The health care provider must be genuinely knowledgeable about immunization, since parents making an immunization decision tend to be well-informed and will not tolerate half-thought-out explanations from health care professionals, including CHNs. In the case of parents who choose not to immunize, they need to be able to trust or believe in the health care professional's expertise based on their demonstration of knowledge and willingness to seek answers or critically question alternative perspectives.

Foodborne Infections

Foodborne infection and **foodborne intoxication** are illnesses acquired through the consumption of contaminated food. Riemann and Cliver (2005) noted that *infections* occur when people consume food containing pathogenic microorganisms, which multiply in the gastrointestinal tract; *intoxications* occur when bacteria multiply in food and produce a toxin that is poisonous to the person ingesting the food. The most common causes of foodborne illnesses include:

- toxins released by bacterial growth in food before consumption (e.g., clostridium botulinum, staphylococcus aureus, and bacillus cereus) or in the intestines (clostridium perfringens);
- bacterial, viral, or parasitic infections (brucellosis, campylobacter enteritis, diarrhea caused by Escherichia coli, hepatitis A, listeriosis, salmonellosis, shigellosis, toxoplasmosis, viral gastroenteritis, trichinosis); and
- toxins produced by harmful algal species (shellfish poisoning).

Foodborne infections can usually be recognized by illness that occurs within a variable but usually short time frame after a meal. **Foodborne outbreaks** are recognized when illness presents among individuals who had consumed common foods. A thorough and prompt collection and testing of implicated foods is essential, as is laboratory testing of stool samples obtained from cases. Many cases are often unreported to health authorities, and outbreaks are often unrecognized.

Foodborne diseases can be prevented and controlled by (a) avoiding food contamination; (b) destroying contaminants (e.g., meat irradiation is one option); and (c) eliminating spread or multiplication of the contaminants. Ultimately, prevention rests on educating food handlers about proper practices in cooking and storage of food and personal hygiene. This includes (a) keeping clean, (b) separating raw and cooked, (c) cooking thoroughly, (d) keeping food at safe temperatures, and (e) using safe water and raw materials (WHO, 2006a).

Waterborne Zoonoses

Waterborne pathogens usually enter water supplies through fecal contamination from animals or humans to cause enteric illnesses (e.g., cholera, typhoid fever, dysentery, some types of salmonella, shigellosis, vibrio, and various coliform bacteria including E. coli 0157:H7). Municipal water systems that have appropriate filtration and chlorination have decreased diseases such as amebic dysentery and giardiasis. Control of protozoa requires effective filtration devices, as they do not respond to traditional chlorine treatment. Recent outbreaks of cryptosporidium in North Battleford, Saskatchewan (PHAC, 2001) and E. coli in Walkerton, Ontario (PHAC, 2000) have raised awareness of the importance of safe municipal water systems across Canada.

An **outbreak of waterborne disease** is usually defined as two cases that are epidemiologically linked that experience similar symptoms after consuming water from a common source. Public health inspectors and public health nurses work closely with the local medical officer of health to investigate, track, and determine linkages between cases. Provincial databases such as the integrated Public Health Information System (iPHIS; explained in more detail later in this chapter) allow tracking of disease occurrence and its source, if known.

Vector-borne Diseases

Vector-borne diseases are illnesses for which the infectious agent is transmitted by a carrier, or vector, which is usually a mosquito, tick, or fly. Climate change has a potential impact on the distribution of various diseases. Vector-borne diseases most commonly seen in Canada include Eastern equine encephalitis, lyme disease, and West Nile virus.

Lyme disease, for example, is transmitted by black-legged ticks carried by migratory birds. Black-legged ticks can be found in all areas of Canada; however, only about 10% are infected with lyme disease. Areas of concern include parts of southern Ontario; Lunenburg County, Nova Scotia; and parts of southern British Columbia. Lyme disease is not a nationally reportable disease in Canada (PHAC, 2006c), although provincial surveillance and reporting is common. Malaria and dengue fever, also vector-borne diseases, are seen in travellers who have contracted these diseases in other countries from the bite of an infected mosquito.

Zoonotic Infections

Zoonotic infections are diseases transmissible between animals and humans; however, they do not need humans to maintain their life cycles. Transmission is by bites, inhalation, ingestion, direct contact, and arthropod intermediaries. Rabies, hantavirus pulmonary syndrome, salmonellosis, listeriosis, and brucellosis are zoonotic diseases.

Rabies has the highest case fatality rate of any known human infection, considered essentially 100%. The major carriers of rabies in Canada include bats, foxes, raccoons, and skunks. The virus is transmitted through a bite, scratch, or pre-existing open wound, and attacks the central nervous system. The best prevention is the vaccination of animals against rabies and pre-exposure vaccination of animal workers. Post-exposure prophylaxis (PEP) is available after an exposure, done in consultation with public health officials. Determination of the need for follow-up by a CHN requires critical assessment of the endemic rates; for example, a bat exposure in Newfoundland and Labrador would not require further investigation, since rabies is not present in the bat population. An exposure in Eastern Ontario, where raccoon rabies is prevalent, would require further investigation. Often CHNs recommend or administer dosages of rabies immune globulin (RIG) based on weight in addition to rabies vaccine. The animal, if located, should be kept in a confined area for a period of 10 days, in order to determine if the animal was infectious with rabies at the time of the exposure. Most infected animals will succumb to rabies within a five-day period, but ten days is used to avoid any possible exceptions. If the animal exhibits signs and symptoms of rabies or dies during the isolation period, the exposed person is started on PEP as soon as possible. If the animal is dead immediately following the exposure, rabies testing of brain tissue is conducted at a national laboratory and the exposed individual is offered PEP based on the findings.

Hantavirus is a viral disease carried by deer mice (in Canada) that can be transmitted through direct or indirect contact. Mice shed the virus in urine, feces, or saliva. Humans can inhale the virus, which may lead to hantavirus pulmonary syndrome. From 1993–2004, 88 cases of hantavirus were identified in Canada (Pan American Health Organization, 2004). The first case was reported in British Columbia in 1994, and although the risk of being infected is low, the mortality rate in humans is high, at approximately 35% (Canadian Food Inspection Agency, 2006). Prevention can be taken especially by those at risk, such as workers in agricultural or rural settings or hikers/campers. Precautions include keeping woodpiles away from dwellings, keeping items off the floor to prevent rodent nesting, trapping rodents, wet-mopping areas with droppings to prevent aerilization of feces, and not camping near rodent-infected areas.

West Nile virus (WNV) is carried and spread by mosquitoes (Drebot & Artsob, 2006). WNV can cause severe neurological complications. Personal protection against this vector and the reduction of areas where mosquitoes breed are important in its control.

Parasitic Diseases

Often found in developing countries, parasites are generally not considered important in Canada, although international travel, immigration, and recent outbreaks remind us that we are not immune. *Pinworm infections* are seen most often in children and are common in crowded and institutional settings. Another common parasite is *giardia*. Control of both parasites is available with effective drug treatment. Unlike *cryptosporidium*, which is another intestinal protozoa that can cause diarrheal illness and is transmitted by fecal–oral contact, there is no treatment other than rehydration. Correct identification of parasites is essential to providing appropriate treatment and prevention education. Diagnosis is dependent on an accurate travel history, clinical signs and symptoms, and appropriate specimen and laboratory testing. Safe sexual practices, effective sanitation, and personal hygiene practices, including hand hygiene, are paramount in controlling parasitic disease.

Diseases in Travellers

Travellers may be exposed to a number of communicable diseases, depending on the country and location within the country being visited. The risk of infection is directly related to the purpose of the trip (business or pleasure), the standard of accommodations (backpacking or staying in a resort), as well as the risk tolerance and recreational activities of the traveller. Some diseases can be prevented by vaccine, while others, often the most dangerous, require personal protection measures.

Malaria is the most prevalent vector-borne disease in the world and occurs in more than 100 countries. More than 40% of the world's population is considered to be at risk, with 90% of the cases presenting in sub-Saharan Africa (Kakkilaya, 2006). There is no vaccine for this disease, and drug resistance is an increasing problem in prevention. Decisions about prophylaxis must be made individually with the traveller based on the travel arrangements. Antimalarials are taken before travel and are continued after travel to be effective. Avoiding insect bites is crucial where infestation is likely to be present. Examples of vector-borne diseases include malaria, yellow fever, dengue, and tick-borne encephalitis. Sleeping under mosquito nets, using insect repellent, wearing recommended clothing, and avoiding areas of infestation are strongly recommended.

The CHN may work in settings that provide travel counselling advice, education, and administration of the recommended vaccines that may affect the travellers. For example, travellers should be aware that unsafe drinking water is a classic source of infections such as diarrhea and parasitic diseases in developing countries (WHO, 2000). Precautions can be taken in many countries to prevent foodborne and waterborne infectious agents. Clinical manifestations may appear long after the traveller returns, so the link between travel and an infectious disease must be considered by the health care professional.

Diseases with Multiple Transmission Modes

CHNs often are challenged with the need to manage cases of disease that do not fit one specific mode of transmission and therefore make case and contact follow-up complex and multifaceted. For example, hepatitis A can be transmitted through contaminated food and water or through sexual contact. Therefore, the CHN must identify contacts and recommend post-exposure prophylaxis based on all possible modes of transmission, and prevent further transmission by providing comprehensive education and exclusion. Hepatitis A vaccine is used in most jurisdictions to prevent hepatitis A outbreaks by immunizing all contacts within 14 days of last exposure. Hepatitis A vaccine is also available in a form combined with hepatitis B vaccine for convenience and is often the preferred choice of travellers.

Nosocomial Infections

Nosocomial infections, such as health-care associated methicillin-resistant staphylococcus aureus (HA-MRSA), are acquired during a hospital stay and may involve patients, visitors, or staff; community-acquired staphylococcus aureus (CA-MRSA) emerges in community settings among children in daycare, soldiers, athletes, incarcerated people, persons involved in same sex practices, and Native populations (Allen, 2006). Effective surveillance systems and properly trained nurses in hospitals and other settings such as long-term care homes are essential in controlling the spread of infections to vulnerable clients. Infections of a bacterial nature may be treated with antibiotics; however, often the clients with nosocomial infections are the most prone to opportunistic infections, which may contribute to the development of antibiotic-resistant organisms. Hand hygiene is the most effective way of preventing the spread of nosocomial infections.

For instance, vancomycin-resistant enterococcus (VRE) is spread by direct contact with hands, surfaces, or objects that have been contaminated by the feces of an infected person. Enterococci bacteria are naturally present in our intestinal tract; healthy individuals usually are not at risk of this infection. However, some strains of enterococci can become resistant to vancomycin. Hospitalized patients with cancer, blood disorders, or immune deficiencies are particularly vulnerable, and the infections can be life-threatening to them. The significant rise in the incident rate for VRE patient admissions in Canada is alarming. It rose from 5.34/100 000 in 1999 to 15.52/100 000 in 2005 (PHAC, 2007b). Health care providers can help halt transmitting the nosocomial infections by practising infection-control precautions such as hand hygiene between patients.

REPORTABLE/NOTIFIABLE DISEASES

The terms *reportable* and *notifiable* diseases are commonly used interchangeably. A communicable disease is identified as a **notifiable disease** through the collaboration and consensus of experts in infectious disease. These experts from around the world study the impact of an identified disease by analyzing morbidity and mortality and then recommend the need for notification. The morbidity and mortality impact may be in a small defined area, or on a worldwide scale. As a result, reporting of some communicable diseases is required within provinces and territories, within Canada, and, in some instances, internationally to the WHO.

In Canada, the list of notifiable diseases at the federal level is agreed upon by consensus among provincial, territorial, and federal health authorities. This *National Notifiable Diseases* list helps to ensure uniformity among provincial/territorial efforts and conformity with international reporting requirements and to facilitate both tracking and required control efforts by public health personnel (PHAC, 2006d). Because the epidemiology of infectious diseases changes, this necessitates a periodic review of and modification to the National Notifiable Diseases list. (See Table 9.3.)

Non-reportable Diseases

Some communicable diseases are non-reportable. They commonly occur in the population and the burden of illness to the community is not considered great. Examples include the common cold, herpes, pediculosis, conjunctivitis, and scabies. The role of the CHN with regard to non-reportable diseases is usually an educational and supportive one. For example, in daycare outbreaks of non-reportable diseases, the CHN is often called upon to educate daycare staff and parents about transmission and management to prevent further occurrences.

Reporting of Communicable Diseases

In Canada, both provincial/territorial and national guidelines and legislation dictate which diseases must be reported, who is responsible for reporting, and what is the reporting format and the mechanism for reporting to the national surveillance system. Currently, some provinces and territories report within the integrated Public Health Information System (iPHIS) (B.C. Centre for Disease Control, 2006). If there is a requirement for international health reporting, the PHAC reports to WHO. The International Health Regulations (IHR) (WHO, 2006b) are the only legally binding instrument requiring the reporting of communicable diseases at the international level, currently limited to cholera, plague, and yellow fever (Heymann, 2004). The WHO updates and revises the IHR to address the threat of new and re-emerging infections and to accommodate new reporting sources. A number of diseases *under surveillance* by WHO (e.g., avian

TABLE 9.3
Notifiable Communicable Diseases, 2006

Acute Flaccid Paralysis	Hepatitis Non-A, Non-B	Salmonellosis
AIDS	Human Immunodeficiency Virus	Shigellosis
Amoebiasis	Influenza, Laboratory-Confirmed	Smallpox
Anthrax	Invasive *Haemophilus influenzae* Type b Disease	Syphilis, All
Botulism	Invasive Group A Streptococcal Disease	Syphilis, Congenital
Brucellosis	Invasive Meningococcal Disease	Syphilis, Early Latent
Campylobacteriosis	Invasive Pneumococcal Disease	Syphilis, Early Symptomatic
Chancroid	Legionellosis	(Primary and Secondary)
Chickenpox	Leprosy	Syphilis, Other
Chlamydia, Genital	Listeriosis (all types)	Tetanus
Cholera	Malaria	Tuberculosis
Creutzfeldt-Jakob Disease	Measles	Tularemia
Cryptosporidiosis	Meningitis, Pneumococcal	Trichinosis
Cyclosporiasis	Meningitis, Other Bacterial	Typhoid
Diphtheria	Meningitis, Viral	Verotoxigenic E. coli
Giardiasis	Mumps	Viral Hemorrhagic Fevers (Crimean Congo,
Gonorrhea	Paratyphoid	Ebola, Lassa, Margurg)
Gonococcal Ophthalmia Neonatorum	Pertussis	West Nile Virus Asymptomatic Infection
Group B Streptococcal Disease of the Newborn	Plague	West Nile Virus Fever
Hantavirus Pulmonary Syndrome	Poliomyelitis	West Nile Virus Neurological Syndromes
Hepatitis A	Rabies	West Nile Virus Unclassified/Unspecified
Hepatitis B	Rubella	Yellow Fever
Hepatitis C	Rubella, Congenital	

Sources: National notifiable diseases. *Retrieved December 9, 2006, from http://dsol-smed.phac-aspc.gc.ca/dsol-smed/ndis/list_e.html. Public Health Agency of Canada (2003). Reproduced with the permission of the Minister of Public Works and Government Services Canada, 2007.*

influenza and AIDS) are required to be reported at varied frequency depending on the disease and the geographic area in which it has occurred.

While some infectious diseases are common and mild (such as the common cold or pediculosis), others are serious enough to be defined as notifiable diseases (such as hepatitis C and HIV/AIDS) and must be reported to the local health authority. Local public health personnel are mandated by the provinces and territories to report all notifiable disease to their respective Ministry of Health, although some diseases are also required to be reported at the federal level. CHNs must know the principles of communicable disease transmission and be proactive and effective in protecting and improving the health of their communities through prevention, identification, control, surveillance, and management of these diseases.

CONTROL AND MANAGEMENT OF COMMUNICABLE DISEASES

The successful control and management of communicable diseases is integrally tied to using sound principles of epidemiology. (See Chapter 8.) **Surveillance** of a disease consists of "the process of systematic collection, orderly consolidation, analysis and evaluation of all pertinent data with prompt dis-

semination of the results to those who need to know, particularly those who are in a position to take action" (Heymann, 2004, p. 622). Through data analysis, the investigator may uncover the cause or source of the disease (e.g., investigation of a case of salmonella infection may identify a contaminated food item in a restaurant).

Active Surveillance

Monitoring of diseases, investigation of disease outbreaks, and observation of patterns of disease are responsibilities of the local health authorities. **Active surveillance** is the collection of data utilizing screening tools, interviews, and sentinel systems to identify disease occurrence in the community when individuals present with suggestive symptoms. Such surveillance depends on the creation of surveillance screening tools that heighten the awareness of health care practitioners in relation to a specific disease. It may occur in response to the identification of an outbreak or notification to the local health authority of a communicable disease or suspected communicable disease.

Active surveillance may be best illustrated by the screening created in response to the increasing risk across Canada of West Nile virus (WNV), first recognized as a threat in North America in 1999. When WNV was first reported, provincial and federal health authorities applied public health measures to identify the spread of this new communicable disease. WNV was detected for the first time in Canada in 2001, in birds and mosquitoes. In 2002, Canadian health authorities documented WNV activity in five provinces: Nova Scotia, Quebec, Ontario, Manitoba, and Saskatchewan. In 2005, 224 human cases were identified; 101 were from Ontario. In 2004, 29 human cases were identified in Canada, compared with more than 1300 in 2003 (PHAC, 2006e). The active surveillance activities during the early days of WNV infections in Canada were conducted partly through the development of a screening tool.

Similarly, a febrile respiratory illness (FRI) screening tool (see Figure 9.2) has been developed for active surveillance of influenza-like illnesses (ILI). The FRI screening tool is utilized in emergency rooms and other acute care settings to provide consistent and early identification of febrile respiratory illnesses such as influenza and SARS, in order to facilitate the necessary control activities to decrease transmission risks in hospitals and other settings. It is also utilized to quickly detect and contain clusters and outbreaks, and helps to identify any new or virulent microorganism-caused respiratory infections (Ontario Ministry of Health and Long-Term Care, 2006).

Passive Surveillance

Passive surveillance relies on the health care provider to notify the local health authority of clients with signs and symptoms associated with a reportable disease. It also relies on laboratory test results if the disease or infectious agent is on the reportable disease list for the respective province/territory. Completeness of the notification report depends on the health care workers' ability to recognize the signs and symptoms, their attention to the necessity for surveillance, and their interest in providing a detailed and comprehensive report. Communicable disease reports tend to differ in their completeness, which possibly is related to the perceived seriousness and burden of illness of the disease. A report must include all the necessary demographics of the person, the symptoms and date of onset of the presenting illness, and travel history, and may include social history, sexual history, diagnostic tests done to date, and prescribed treatment.

Surveillance, whether active, passive, or both, does not end with the notification of the disease case to the local health authority; rather, it initiates the next steps toward the control and management of the disease. Surveillance also plays a significant role in the management of reports of suspected cases of disease. CHNs provide guidelines to institutions, health care professionals, and others in relation to diagnostic tests and control measures to identify and manage a *suspected* case of disease in terms of transmission risk and potential community impact.

Contact Tracing

Contact tracing is a response to disease reporting. After a notifiable communicable disease is reported to the local health unit, the infected person is interviewed by a CHN regarding

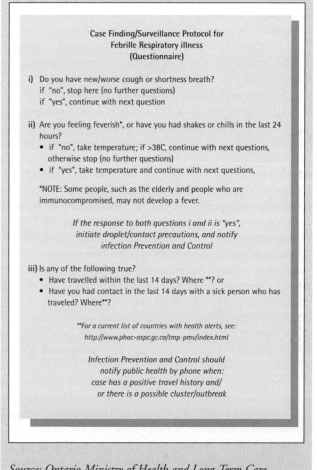

FIGURE 9.2 Sample Case Finding/Surveillance Protocol for Febrile Respiratory Illness (Questionnaire)

Case Finding/Surveillance Protocol for
Febrile Respiratory illness
(Questionnaire)

i)   Do you have new/worse cough or shortness breath?
     if "no", stop here (no further questions)
     if "yes", continue with next question

ii) Are you feeling feverish*, or have you had shakes or chills in the last 24 hours?
     • if "no", take temperature; if >38C, continue with next questions, otherwise stop (no further questions)
     • if "yes", take temperature and continue with next questions,

     *NOTE: Some people, such as the elderly and people who are immunocompromised, may not develop a fever.

     If the response to both questions i and ii is "yes", initiate droplet/contact precautions, and notify infection Prevention and Control

iii) Is any of the following true?
     • Have travelled within the last 14 days? Where **? or
     • Have you had contact in the last 14 days with a sick person who has traveled? Where**?

     ***For a current list of countries with health alerts, see: http://www.phac-aspc.gc.ca/tmp-pmv/index.html*

     Infection Prevention and Control should notify public health by phone when: case has a positive travel history and/ or there is a possible cluster/outbreak

Source: Ontario Ministry of Health and Long-Term Care. (2005). Preventing febrile respiratory illnesses: Protecting patients and staff: Appendix 1: Sample case findings/surveillance form. Provincial Infectious Diseases Advisory Committee. Retrieved September 11, 2006, from www.health.gov.on.ca/english/ providers/program/infectious/diseases/ic_fri.html.

contacts, people exposed to the client during the infectious period of the disease or who may already be ill with the disease. The CHN must know the mode of transmission, incubation period, and infective period of the particular disease in order to determine what constitutes a contact in each individual situation. The *initial case definition* must be formulated based on signs and symptoms and place and time of exposure. A list of contacts must be collected from the first identified case. With this list, the local health authority proceeds with further assessment and investigation and follows up with recommendations for treatment or post-exposure chemoprophylaxis as deemed necessary.

Contacts are identified based on the possibility of transmission, where the window of risk can be very short or quite long. For example, when investigating a case of measles the CHN would include in the contact list those people who were in contact with the infectious individual seven days prior to the onset of the rash; while investigating a case of tuberculosis the CHN may identify not just recent contacts but contacts as far back as three months ago. The **degree of exposure** (the time spent with the infected person) and where the exposure took place are included in the collected data. Not all reportable diseases warrant the same type of contact tracing, because of varying degrees of burden of illness (e.g., varicella), and/or because the nature of human to human communicability may be a low risk (e.g., rabies).

The ease with which public health professionals are provided with comprehensive and inclusive lists of contacts will depend on how the individual or community comprehends the scope of the issue, or an individual's or community's experience with the disease in the past. For example, obtaining contacts from those who have had an experience with an adolescent dying from meningococcal disease is easier than obtaining a comprehensive list of contacts from an infected food service worker whose perception is that hepatitis A infection is not a serious disease. The report is only as reliable and accurate as the person relaying the information and the parameters required for reporting. That is, if the health care provider is unsure of the signs and symptoms of the disease, the need for reporting will go unrecognized and the surveillance and contact tracing may be delayed.

Ongoing education of health care professionals helps to ensure detailed disease reporting. The **integrated Public Health Information System** (iPHIS) (PHAC, 2006f) is an electronic system of reporting that allows jurisdictions within a province to communicate disease patterns and contacts with one another. As well, the **Canadian Integrated Outbreak Surveillance Centre** (CIOSC) (2006), an outbreak-specific electronic system, has been developed for health care professionals to communicate outbreaks of respiratory or enteric illnesses interprovincially. It enables public health professionals to make links in person, place, and time for clients with similar presentation.

Contact tracing requires a confidential approach, since much of the information is disease- and client-specific. An exception to the confidential necessity and practice of contact tracing is occasionally required. During the SARS outbreak that occurred in Toronto during March through May of 2003, quarantine acts of the federal and Ontario Ministries of Health allowed health and safety authorities to conduct contact tracing in a public forum by naming those with SARS in the public media. Their purpose was to protect the public as well as to notify the contacts of those first infected persons in order to allow the contacts to self-identify and come forward for health assessment. Although contact tracing might be viewed as an infringement of a person's right to privacy, it is necessary to contain the spread of the virulent disease while providing ethically competent care. (See Chapter 4.)

Effective contact tracing requires comprehensive assessment of the infected individual and accurate disease reporting. While facilitating this process, the CHN is also assessing the individual as part of the community where they live, work, and play. For example, contact tracing conducted during a recent outbreak of TB in a homeless shelter required the local public health unit to become cognizant of the community defined by this unique population (Jamieson & Yang, 2004). This involved learning about the soup kitchens, drop-in centres, parks, and other areas where these individuals congregated. Local public health personnel could not achieve this task without the assistance of the ill individual (who provided information about the likely first case) and the community partners (who work closely with this population). These partners are not limited to health care providers but include all community agencies that provide services to the homeless. The result of the partnership was to develop a more focused and targeted screening of contacts.

Contact tracing can involve identification of individuals who have not had any proximal contact with the case. As our scientific knowledge and surveillance abilities have increased, donor organs and blood products that are transplanted/transfused have been identified as potential **indirect contact** modes of transmission in some diseases. For example, West Nile virus (WNV) was identified in four clients receiving organs from an asymptomatic donor in 2002 (Centers for Disease Control and Prevention, 2002). Changes to screening practices were subsequently made to organ and blood donor screening and testing practices as well as the clinical use of donated organs and blood. Canadian Blood Services (2006) now screens all blood products for known infectious diseases, such as HIV, syphilis, hepatitis B and C, and WNV. Other emerging diseases such as Creutzfeldt-Jakob disease (CJD) necessitate that the CHN thoroughly understand modes of transmission in order to perform thorough history taking in contact tracing. It would be important to know, for example, if instruments used in invasive procedures involving brain or neural tissue on a client diagnosed with CJD may have been contaminated.

Response to Outbreaks

An *outbreak* can be identified when expected symptoms in the population exist at an increased level. These symptoms may exist in the general population or in institutions such as hospitals, long term care homes, or daycares. An outbreak may not necessarily be a reportable disease, but may initially be of unknown etiology suggestive of a communicable disease. An outbreak can be identified when a group of persons present with similar signs and symptoms—such as fever, coughing, and malaise in the case of an outbreak of influenza-like illness. Generally, *outbreak reports* are communicated to public health authorities as soon as possible to allow investigation for a cause of illness. In addition, early notification facilitates early institution of appropriate control methods, such as cohorting (separation) of well and ill clients into separate areas.

The terms "case" and "index case" are used throughout any discussion of outbreaks. A **case** refers to a single ill individual. When an individual person is identified as the likely first case in an outbreak, this person is referred to as the **index** case. Often, the index case in an outbreak is identified after other persons become ill and surveillance data indicate that the outbreak began with the identified individual. The purpose in identifying a common source (contaminated food) or an index case (infectious person) is two-fold: (a) to interrupt further transmission of the disease by identifying the route of transmission, and (b) to understand the cause of the outbreak by identifying the origin of the pathogen. The information that a CHN gathers to understand and define an outbreak is often like pieces of a puzzle and requires the CHN to possess critical-thinking and analytic skills.

Steps in Managing an Outbreak The initial investigation of an outbreak includes review of the signs and symptoms the ill clients share in common, the onset and whether some clients are recovering, the usual course of the illness, and the source of the outbreak (e.g., source of outbreak can be a contaminated air conditioning unit in a legionella outbreak or an infected person in the case of a pertussis, measles, or mumps outbreak). Heymann (2004) outlines six general steps in the management of an outbreak:

1. *Verifying the diagnosis*—The investigator utilizes laboratory results and anticipates the diagnostic specimens required. Laboratories are involved in testing specimens. Autopsies may be required. At this point a surveillance case definition is determined in order to identify others with the same symptomatology.

2. *Confirming the existence of an outbreak*—The CHN commonly plots the existence of illness on a graph or an epidemiological curve. This graph represents the number of people presenting with symptoms as per the case definition, with incidence over time. An outbreak occurs when the incidence rises above what is normally expected.

3. *Identifying affected persons and characteristics*—The CHN records complete case histories to obtain a comprehensive understanding of the outbreak. Additional cases may be identified as enquiry or active surveillance reveals additional cases.

4. *Defining and investigating the population at risk*—This group of people is identified as those who may present with the illness and may require laboratory testing to ensure the remaining cases are identified. This provides the denominator when calculating specific attack rates. For example, out of the 100 people exposed only 10 were infected, which is a 10% attack rate.

5. *Generating a hypothesis*—This is the determination of the cause of the outbreak. A thorough investigation into the relevant conditions that existed before the outbreak occurred, the existence of a reservoir, the mode of exit from the source, the mode of transmission, the mode of entry, and the susceptibility of the host must be considered. In foodborne outbreaks, for example, a contaminated product may have been consumed by all those who were ill with similar symptoms. The food may be tested and the pathogen identified.

6. *Containing the outbreak*—Coordination of control measures early in an outbreak is key to ending the outbreak. Response may include working on a multidisciplinary team including CHNs, public health inspectors, physicians, microbiologists, epidemiologists, and communication specialists. Immediate and properly maintained isolation or quarantine of ill persons can prevent spread of the illness. Ongoing disease surveillance also continues. Periodic reports are provided in order to communicate to the public, and outbreak reporting to provincial/ territorial authorities is provided.

Generally, an outbreak report is generated after the outbreak is determined to be over, although in large outbreaks reporting may occur through the course of the outbreak. Scientific study and learning is generated after each outbreak as each outbreak presents differently. Debriefing sessions with all those involved in any aspect of the outbreak is an important and often missed learning opportunity. Efforts should be made to approach debriefing sessions with a structured format to avoid placing blame on individuals and to ensure behaviour change occurs to prevent similar outbreaks from happening again.

Case Study

In a pertussis outbreak the CHN initially gathered the following information: seven ill children, all in elementary schools, only two children in the same school, all children in the same city; there appeared to be no other common links—they did not know each other, no common social events or travel, and no shared activities. The CHN could not identify a common source. Then an adult was diagnosed with pertussis, and on investigation, the CHN found that the adult was a teacher's spouse who had been ill for several weeks with pertussis-like symptoms. The teacher was a special education teacher who travelled throughout the city to elementary schools. This teacher had been in every school that the ill children attended.

Discussion Questions

1. Who is the index case?

2. Would you do an active surveillance or passive surveillance? Why?

3. Outline the steps to control and manage the pertussis outbreak.

PREPAREDNESS FOR DELIBERATELY CAUSED OUTBREAKS OF INFECTIOUS DISEASE

The *natural occurrence of disease* in populations helps us identify when an unusual event may be occurring, if a disease occurrence is suspicious, and if it should be investigated. **Bioterrorism** can be defined as the deliberate act of using a microorganism such as bacteria or virus with the intent of causing infection and harm to achieve certain goals or gains (Shah, 2003). Agents considered to be a bioterrorism concern include anthrax, botulism, hemorrhagic fevers, plague, smallpox, and tularemia. For example, in 2001, anthrax spores were discovered in the United States postal system, causing 22 infections and 5 deaths (Centers for Disease Control and Prevention, 2006). More than 32 000 contacts of those who may have come into contact with anthrax-contaminated mail envelopes were provided antibiotics. Smallpox, although considered eradicated in 1977 (Heymann, 2004), is still considered a concern because of the belief that a stockpile exists somewhere in the world and that terrorists may access these sources.

It is expected that in deliberately caused outbreaks, the demand for acute care and public health services would be taxed to the limit. If an infectious agent is widely dispersed, then demand for active surveillance and contact tracing would greatly increase. Infections deliberately set may be a one-time occurrence or happen a number of times. The agent used will determine the risk of person to person transmission and communicability. Prevention of these activities requires training and current information about intelligence within our global community. There needs to be a strong public health infrastructure to deal with rapid and effective detection and response mechanisms through emergency preparedness and funding activities such as stockpiling of drugs, vaccines, and equipment. Strategies that have helped public health deal with infectious disease outbreaks such as SARS should be considered in preparation for a bioterrorist event. Special training may include basic emergency management, communicating within the Incident Management System, infection control, dealing safely with specimens, and decontamination procedures.

ROLE OF THE COMMUNITY HEALTH NURSE

History has shown that communicable diseases are controlled through changes in practice or environment. Typhoid and cholera are two communicable diseases that can be transmitted via contaminated water. The sanitation of water is one of the public health triumphs that occurred in the early 1900s. Improved sanitation and the development of vaccines for typhoid and cholera have virtually eliminated these diseases from the developed world. These diseases still continue to plague developing countries where water sanitation and vaccination programs are limited or not available (Heymann, 2004).

CHNs can break the chain of infection at the mode of transmission link by educating the public on personal hygiene and the importance of clean drinking water. Today, breaking the chain of infection is achieved through various methods, each one targeted at different links. For example, immunization programs (especially for children) modify the susceptible host into a resistant host, whereas prophylaxis can diminish or reduce the ability of the infectious agent to multiply after entry into the susceptible host. Sterilization of instruments, proper cooking of food in restaurants, and harm-reduction methods are strategies targeted at the reservoir, thereby altering the ability of the infectious agent to transmit from one host to another.

Immunization campaigns, screening, ensuring that quarantine requirements are met, instituting isolation, providing prophylaxis, and acting as consultants on communicable disease to community groups are some of CHNs' service delivery activities. CHNs working under the medical officer of health are responsible for monitoring and reporting communicable disease occurrence in the community as reported by other health care providers, schools, childcare agencies, laboratories, the general public, and health care institutions.

Levels of Preventive Measures

CHNs use the nursing process to implement primary, secondary, and tertiary prevention activities in controlling communicable diseases. *Primary prevention* attempts to prevent the disease from occurring. *Secondary prevention* detects a disease or condition in a certain population, usually by screening or testing for the disease. *Tertiary prevention* involves the reduction of the extent and severity of the health problem in order to minimize the disability.

The main **primary prevention measures** for controlling communicable disease include:

- promoting and implementing immunization programs, notifying the contacts, and making referrals for the needed follow-up diagnosis;
- providing chemoprophylaxis such as antimicrobial medications and antitoxin for prevention of diseases such as malaria and tuberculosis;
- working with public health authorities and community partners concerning protective and control measures for communicable diseases; and
- educating the public on safe sexual practices, optimal nutrition, healthy environments for better air quality and sanitation, and use of preventive measures such as universal precautions.

Secondary prevention measures include:

- screening, which includes case finding, referral, and mass screening for early detection;
- early diagnosis, which includes interpretation of diagnostic results;
- early treatment, which includes provision of antimicrobial medications for newly diagnosed contacts;

- teaching for medication and treatment compliance that includes provision of supportive care such as diet, rest, and exercise, and teaching for side effects of the medications; and
- advocacy for accessible diagnostic and treatment services for socially disadvantaged groups such as the poor, the underhoused, and people with language and cultural barriers.

Screening There are two reasons for testing or screening for a communicable disease. The first is in response to the disease being identified in the community. Epidemiological reports can reveal or identify a population that is at risk for disease. CHNs screen the population to validate these reports and to identify the at-risk individuals. The persons being tested have not been identified in the contact screening but are part of the population at risk. For example, a student is diagnosed with tuberculosis; all students in his/her school, and not just those with close contact to the index student, may be tested for tuberculosis. The list of exposures of the case must be analyzed to also identify the *index* or *first case*. As well, the history of the cases may help to determine the *index case*; that is, who first presented with the disease symptoms. The second and a more general strategy is testing and screening after broad immunization campaigns, which are done as a standard of practice (e.g., titres following a hepatitis B vaccination series). The **titres** check the efficacy of the immunization to ensure that those who received the vaccine now have antibodies to the disease. A random sample of those immunized is used as a strategy by pharmaceutical companies to demonstrate efficacy or *seroconversion rates*.

Isolation and Quarantine Isolation and quarantine are also secondary preventive measures. Treatment or management of some infectious agents includes isolation or quarantine to reduce the transmission and break the chain of infection. **Isolation** refers to separation of an *infectious person* for a period of time to prevent or limit the direct or indirect transmission of the infectious agent. Isolation period is calculated based on the infectious or communicability period, for example, the infectious period for mumps is 14 to 25 days, whereas the infectious period for influenza is 3 to 7 days, therefore the isolation period is much longer for mumps than influenza. **Quarantine** is the restriction of activities for a *well person* who has been exposed to a case of communicable disease during its period of communicability to prevent disease transmission. Generally, communicable diseases that are transmitted by direct or airborne routes require that the contacts be isolated from other people and possibly placed in quarantine. The length of time spent in quarantine is calculated as the time the disease or organism would be incubating. Thus, the length of the quarantine period is specific to each communicable disease. For example, the incubation period which determines the quarantine period for varicella is 14 to 21 days, whereas the incubation for influenza is 1 to 3 days. The communicable period is not always known for every disease, especially emerging diseases. SARS is considered to have an incubation period of up to 10 days (Heymann, 2004). During the SARS outbreak, it was uncertain when the infected person was most contagious or when the symptoms displayed by the patient equated to communicability. For this reason, contacts were placed in quarantine for a minimum of 10 days.

Prophylaxis Prophylaxis, a secondary preventive measure, is the utilization of chemoprophylaxic or immunoprophylaxic agents to prevent illness from a pathogen or an infectious agent following a known or possible exposure. Prophylaxic agents may be prescribed for exposed vulnerable hosts such as pregnant women, infants, people who have an immune disorder or transplant, or anyone who had contact with a disease that has high morbidity and mortality rates or a disease that has significant long-term effects.

Immunoprophylaxic agents are inclusive of both active and passive immunizing agents. **Active immunizing agents** are vaccines that stimulate the immune system to create antibodies. **Passive immunizing agents** include immune serum globulin, which is of human origin, and immune globulins that contain specific antibodies to a particular organism, such as hepatitis B immune globulin (HBIG) or rabies immune globulin (RIG), provide preformed antibodies.

Prophylaxis provides protection to vulnerable hosts in the general population. The role of the CHN is to identify vulnerable hosts, monitor the therapy if it is long term, and possibly administer or facilitate the administration of one-time prophylaxis. An example of the use of *chemoprophylaxis* includes the administration of Isoniazid (INH) to children younger than six years of age who are identified as contacts in a tuberculosis outbreak despite having a negative response to the tuberculin skin test. These children are given this medication daily for three months. It is recognized that young children may not have the ability to fight the TB organism as well as an older child or adult. The medication provides the child with the ability to fight the organism, reduces bacterial load, and reduces the possibility of disseminated disease. A tuberculin skin test is repeated after three months, and if the result continues to be negative and no other immune disorder appears to exist, the INH can be discontinued. *Immunoprophylaxis* can be an appropriate choice if, for example, during an outbreak of varicella in the community, contact tracing reveals that one of the contacts is a pregnant woman; she may be a candidate for varicella-zoster immune globulin (VZIG). The VZIG will either protect the woman from acquiring varicella or lessen the symptoms if the disease occurs, thereby protecting the fetus.

Tertiary prevention measures aim to reduce the extent and severity of the health problems in order to minimize the complications by:

- educating and monitoring treatment compliance to prevent complications, and
- monitoring effectiveness of treatment and identifying and referring for adverse effects.

Education of the public may be carried out at the individual, family, and community levels through community-based programs. Education is not directed at a single stage in the chain of infection; rather, it targets the whole chain and teaches measures that can be adopted into the individual's personal health habits. The goal is to help the client and the community return to baseline functioning, or a new state of health. Examples include the administration of **direct observed therapy (DOT)**, which is a mechanism utilized to ensure a tuberculosis client takes daily medications. The nurse observes the client taking the medications on a daily schedule. This is to prevent the risk of non-compliance and thereby reduce the possibility of drug-resistant tuberculosis, which could place communities of individuals at risk.

Through various levels of prevention activities, CHNs play major roles in education, health promotion, direct care, community development and mobilization, liaison, research, advocacy, program planning and evaluation, and policy formulation. All are essential skills in epidemiologic investigation for successful management and control of communicable diseases.

PRIORITIES IN CONTROLLING COMMUNICABLE DISEASES

Like other nations, Canada works in partnership with the WHO to reduce the incidence and impact of communicable diseases on its population. The role of the WHO in communicable disease control is to lead global efforts in surveillance, prevention, control, and research. What continues to be a challenge for all nations can be seen in the following priorities set by the WHO (2000):

- to reduce the negative consequences of malaria and tuberculosis
- to continue to strengthen surveillance, monitoring, and response to communicable disease
- to intensify routine prevention and control; and
- to generate new knowledge through research for development of tools and intervention methods.

Control of communicable disease must be an international effort. With increasing international cooperation in managing diseases and knowledge exchange, infrastructures for protecting public health become a priority for both developing and developed countries. An example can be seen in the 2005 conference in Ottawa, where the global community gathered to develop the first Canadian research agenda for best practices in pandemic influenza planning. Canadian Research Box 9.1 lists the ten research priorities that arose from the conference.

Canadian Research Box 9.1

Scheifele, D., & Tam, T. (2006). Addressing a public health priority: First Canadian research agenda on influenza prevention, control and management. *Canada Communicable Disease Report, 32*(22), 265–270. (Available from www.phac-aspc.gc.ca/publicat/ccdr-rmtc/06vol32/dr3222eb.html.)

More than 70 Canadian and international vaccine experts participated in a two-day Influenza Research Priorities Workshop in Ottawa in August 2005. The purpose of the workshop was to develop the first Canadian research agenda on the best practices to coordinate, control, and prevent influenza. Experts came from policy makers, academia, researchers, funding agencies, industry, public health, and international bodies such as the World Health Organization (WHO), the U.S. National Institute of Allergy and Infectious Disease, and the U.S. National Vaccine Program Office.

All participants attended plenary sessions on an overview of the current national and global knowledge from research of influenza such as communicability, pathogenesis, epidemiology, and the immune response to influenza infection in humans; new anti-influenza drugs; public health programs; and strategies, strengths, and opportunities. Then, in six break-out sessions held over two days, participants used a five-point Likert relevancy scale to identify three to five key research priorities in terms of urgency for public health, uniqueness to Canada, feasibility, impact on decreasing the burden of disease, and potential for rapid knowledge translation.

In the plenary session, research priorities were clustered into the following 10 priority areas: (1) influenza virus characterization and ecology; (2) influenza virus transmission; (3) public health preventive measures; (4) improving rapid diagnostic test availability; (5) clinical management of influenza patients; (6) development and optimal use of antiviral drugs; (7) surge capacity of the health care system; (8) more effective and acceptable influenza vaccines; (9) immunization programs; and (10) preparation for a pandemic vaccine. Based on the research agenda developed from this workshop, the federal government instilled $1 billion for pandemic and research activities in May 2006.

Discussion Questions:

1. Which possible disciplines/professionals would you most likely invite to participate in this multidisciplinary team to derive a research agenda on the prevention of influenza?

2. Review the 10 identified research priorities for control and management of influenza. Discuss what might be the role for CHNs in each of these initiatives.

Summary

This chapter has discussed the basic principles of communicable disease control including vaccine-preventable diseases and the role of the CHN in dealing with them. The topic of communicable disease control is broad, and each day the world faces a new disease that may or may not find its way into any community. CHNs must be prepared to respond to the unexpected. They must work in partnership with the local, national, and global communities to develop effective surveillance methods and screening tools, to enhance emergency response mechanisms, and to implement public health measures in primary, secondary, and tertiary prevention for communicable disease control. It is imperative that CHNs possess a strong relationship with their community partners, a solid knowledge base of epidemiology and current information on communicable diseases, knowledge of available resources, and strong decision-making and research skills. Integration of these skills will help the CHN to be successful in the role of protecting and promoting the health of Canadians.

KEY TERMS

communicable diseases
outbreak
endemic
epidemic
pandemic
foodborne infection
foodborne intoxication
foodborne outbreaks
outbreak of waterborne disease
vector-borne disease
zoonotic infections
nosocomial infections
notifiable diseases
surveillance
active surveillance
passive surveillance
contact tracing
contacts
degree of exposure
integrated Public Health Information System
Canadian Integrated Outbreak Surveillance Centre
indirect contact
case
index case
bioterrorism
primary prevention measures
secondary prevention measures
titres
isolation
quarantine
prophylaxis
active immunizing agents
passive immunizing agents
tertiary prevention measures
direct observed therapy

STUDY QUESTIONS

1. What is the link between epidemiology and control of communicable diseases?

2. What are the modes of transmission of communicable diseases?

3. A high school student is diagnosed with tuberculosis. How would you conduct contact tracing?

4. A daycare has just notified you, as a new CHN, that a child in its care has meningitis. The staff and parents of other children are very anxious. Describe your nursing interventions.

5. The local health authority has just hired you to work on hepatitis A management and control. Being new to the region, what would be your priority tasks?

6. What information would you need from the infectious individual and about the disease (e.g., HIV) to conduct comprehensive contact tracing?

INDIVIDUAL CRITICAL THINKING EXERCISES

1. You receive several laboratory reports for the same disease from the same geographical area. What steps are needed to differentiate between an increased incidence as opposed to a usual occurrence of the disease?

2. In question 1 above, what would be your sources of information for the investigation?

3. You are working in a downtown clinic that provides services to marginalized/vulnerable persons. A client presents to the clinic with non-specific ailments. You are collecting the history. The client reveals a history of addictions to crack cocaine and other substances and that he has multiple sexual partners. Your recommendation is to have a full work-up for sexually transmitted infections. The client refuses. Discuss your nursing responsibilities.

4. Refer to question 3 above; the client's HIV test shows a positive result. What should be your next steps?

GROUP CRITICAL THINKING EXERCISES

1. Large numbers of migrants come from regions where the prevalence of tuberculosis is high. This has resulted in the importation of a large burden of latent infection that can be expected to generate future active cases in aging migrants. Discuss the implications for caring for the future active cases. Healthy public policy should be included in the discussion as opposed to local health authority policy.

2. AIDS can manifest after years of HIV-positive status; a positive HIV test may not occur until three months after the contact. Similarly, in tuberculosis, the skin test can be negative up to 12 weeks post-exposure, and the manifestations of the disease may occur sometime in the person's lifetime. Discuss the implications of contact tracing for these two diseases.

3. Emerging diseases, changes in antibiotic resistance, and threats of terrorism with biological agents have heightened the awareness of surveillance needs worldwide. Since September 11, 2001, the threat of smallpox and anthrax has been in the media. Discuss the information needed to control the spread of smallpox.

REFERENCES

Allen, U. A. (2006). Public health implications of MRSA in Canada. *Can. Med. Assoc. J., 175* (2), 161–162.

B.C. Centre for Disease Control. (2006). *Integrated public health information system.* Retrieved December 6, 2006, from www.bccdc.org/content.php?item=10.

Canadian Blood Services (2006). *Testing.* Retrieved September 10, 2006, from www.bloodservices.ca/centreapps/internet/uw_v502_mainengine.nsf/page/testing?OpenDocument.

Canadian Food Inspection Agency. (2006). *Number of cases of hantavirus.* Retrieved September 5, 2006, from www.inspection.gc.ca/english/animal/heasan/disemala/hanta/hantafse.shtml.

Canadian Integrated Outbreak Surveillance Centre. (2006). *Enteric Alerts.* Retrieved September 10, 2006, from www.hc-sc.gc.ca/ed-ud/respond/food-aliment/fiorp-priti_11_e.html.

Centers for Disease Control and Prevention. (2002, September 6). Public health dispatch: West Nile virus infection in organ donor and transplant recipients—Georgia and Florida, 2002. *MMWR, 51*(35), 790. Retrieved December 26, 2006, from http://www.cdc.gov/mmwr/preview/mmwrhtml/mm5135a5.htm.

Centers for Disease Control and Prevention. (2006). *Questions and answers about Anthrax.* Retrieved September 10, 2006, from www.cdc.gov/ncidod/EID/index/htm.

Drebot, M. A., & Artsob, H. (2006). West Nile virus: A pathogen of concern for older adults. *Geriatrics and Aging, 9*(7), 465–471.

Health Canada. (2003). *Notifiable disease on line: Glossary.* Retrieved December 5, 2006, from http://dsol-smed.phac-aspc.gc.ca/dsol-smed/ndis/glossa_e.html

Heymann, D. L. (2004). *Control of communicable diseases manual: An official report of the American Public Health Association* (18th ed.). Washington, DC: American Public Health Association.

Jamieson, F. B., & Yang, J. (2004). Uncovering a TB outbreak: Using DNA fingerprinting. *Ontario Thoracic Review, 16*(4), 1, 4.

Kakkilaya, B. S. (2006, April 14). *Malaria site: What is Malaria?* Retrieved April 24, 2007, from http://www.malariasite.com/malaria/WhatIsMalaria.htm.

McKay, M. (2005). Community health nursing in Canada. In L. Stamler & L. Yiu (Eds.). *Community nursing: A Canadian perspective* (pp. 1–15). Toronto: Pearson Education Canada.

Ontario Ministry of Health and Long-Term Care. (2006). *Ontario's best practice manual: Preventing febrile respiratory illnesses,* 2006. Retrieved August 27, 2006, from www.health.gov.on.ca/english/providers/program/infectious/syndromes/fri.html.

Pan American Health Organization. (2004). *Number of cases of Hantavirus Pulmonary Syndrome* (Region of the Americas, *1993–2004).* Retrieved December 8, 2006, from www.paho.org/english/ad/dpc/cd/hantavirus2004.ppt#257,1,Slide1.

Pubic Health Agency of Canada. (2000). *Waterborne outbreak of gastroenteritis associated with a contaminated municipal water supply, Walkerton, Ontario.* Communicable Disease Report (CCDR). Retrieved from http://www.phac-aspc.gc.ca/publicat/ccdr-rmtc/00vol26/dr2620eb.html.

Public Health Agency of Canada. (PHAC). (2001). *Waterborne Cryptosporidiosis outbreak, North Battleford, Saskatchewan.* Communicable Disease Report (CCDR). Retrieved from http://www.phac-aspc.gc.ca/publicat/ccdr-rmtc/01vol27/dr2722ea.html.

Public Health Agency of Canada. (2006a). *Understanding influenza.* Retrieved December 6, 2006, from http://www.phac-aspc.gc.ca/influenza/influenza-undrstnd_e.html#3.

Public Health Agency of Canada. (2006b). *Canadian immigration guide* (7th ed.). Minister of Public Works and Government Services Canada: Author.

Public Health Agency of Canada. (2006c). *Number of cases of Lyme disease.* Retrieved September 5, 2006, from www.phac-aspc.gc/id-mi.lyme-fs_e.html.

Public Health Agency of Canada. (2006d). *Notifiable diseases on line.* Retrieved September 9, 2006, from http://dsol-smed.phac-aspc.gc.ca/dsol-smed/ndis/list_e.html

Public Health Agency of Canada. (2006e). *West Nile Virus MONITOR: Human surveillance (2003–2005).* Retrieved September 10, 2006, from www.phac-aspc.gc.ca/wnv-vwn/mon-humsurv-archive_e.html.

Public Health Agency of Canada. (2006f). *Canadian Integrated Public Health Surveillance.* Retrieved October 4, 2007, from http://www.phac-aspc.gc.ca/php-psp/ciphs_e.html.

Public Health Agency of Canada. (2007a). *Creutzfeldt-Jakob Disease (CJD).* Retrieved July 13, 2007, from http://www.phac-aspc.gc.ca/hcai-iamss/cjd-mcj/cjdss-ssmcj/stats_e.html#canada.

Public Health Agency of Canada. (2007b). *The Canadian nosocomial infection surveillance program.* Retrieved April 24, 2007, from http://www.phac-aspc.gc.ca/nois-sinp/projects/vre_e.html.

Riemann, C., & Cliver, D. (2005). *Foodborne infections and intoxications* (3rd ed.). Academic Press, Elsevier.

Shah, C. P. (2003). *Public health & preventative medicine in Canada* (5th ed.). Toronto: Elsevier Canada.

World Health Organization. (1998). Report of the director-general. *1998 world health report: Health in the 21st century: A vision for all.* Geneva, Switzerland: Author.

World Health Organization. (2000). *Communicable diseases 2000: Highlights of activities in 1999 and major challenges for the future.* Retrieved December 6, 2006, from www.who.int/infectious-disease-news/CDS2000/PDF/cd2000-e.pdf.

World Health Organization. (2003). *Communicable diseases cluster: Highlights of communicable disease activities, major recent achievements.* Retrieved September 9, 2006, from www.who.int/infectious-disease-news/IDdocs/highlights-2003/CDS-highlights-2003.pdf.

World Health Organization. (2006a). *Five keys to safer food.* Retrieved December 6, 2006, from http://www.who.int/fsf/Documents/5keys-ID-eng.pdf.

World Health Organization. (2006b). *International health regulations.* Retrieved December 6, 2006, from http://www.who.int/csr/ihr/en/.

ADDITIONAL RESOURCES

Websites

Centers for Disease Control and Prevention (CDC).
MMWR: Morbidity and Mortality Weekly Report
www.cdc.gov/mmwr/

Community and Hospital Infection Control Association
Canada (CHICA)
www.chica.org

Pan American Health Organization
www.paho.org/english/ad/dpc/cd/res-tdr-home.htm

Public Health Agency of Canada (PHAC)
www.phac-aspc.gc.ca/publicat/ccdr-rmtc/

World Health Organization: Integrated Disease Surveillance
Programme
www.who.int/csr/labepidemiology/projects/surveillance/en/print.html

Readings

Ellis, E., Gallant, V., Phypers, M., Scholten, D., & Miron, M. (2007). *Tuberculosis in Canada, 2003.* Ottawa: Public Health Agency of Canada. (Also available at http://www.phac-aspc.gc.ca/publicat/2007/tbcan03/index.html.)

About the Authors

Leeann Whitney, RN, BScN (Laurentian), MAEd (Central Michigan), is the Director of Infectious Diseases at the North Bay Parry Sound District Health Unit. Ms. Whitney's background includes teaching with Canadore College and Laurentian University, as well as working in acute care and community health. Her current focus is communicable disease control, and vaccine-preventable disease has become a passion during her work on a multi-disciplinary team at the health unit. She has lately become the lead pandemic influenza planner for the district.

Sheila Marchant-Short, RN, BScN (Western Ontario), MScN (British Columbia), has worked in Communicable Disease Control in Newfoundland and Labrador and at the Epidemiology and Disease Control Centre in Victoria, B.C., and with the B.C. Ministry of Health. She is now Manager of the Communicable Disease Control Program in North Bay, Ontario.

Lucia Yiu, RN, BScN, BA (Windsor), BSc (Toronto), MScN (Western Ontario), is an Associate Professor in the Faculty of Nursing, University of Windsor, and an Educational and Training Consultant in community nursing. Her practice and research include multicultural health, international health, experiential learning, community development, breast health, and program planning and evaluation.

Family Care

Linda J. Patrick and Kathryn Edmunds

OBJECTIVES

After studying this chapter, you should be able to:

1. Define family and its basic purposes.

2. Explain the difference between viewing the family as context and the family as client.

3. Describe the theoretical underpinnings of family health care nursing.

4. Discuss the components and basic characteristics of family assessment models.

5. Describe how family assessments shape nursing interventions.

6. Discuss the opportunities and challenges for community health nurses who provide care to families.

INTRODUCTION

Family health nursing has evolved considerably over the past 20 years to become a "specialty body of knowledge in nursing" (Harmon Hanson, 2005, p. 4). Community health nurses (CHNs) in Canada have a long history of caring for individuals as members of a family and/or entire families. MacDonald (2002) reinforces the importance of family nursing practice in the following statement: "Nursing practice with individuals and families is essential for providing the grounding for community or population-focused practice ... Nurses draw on their practical skills and situated knowledge of individuals and families to change policies, and develop programs for the benefit of the larger population, and to build responsive communities" (p. 17). In this chapter, you will study the family as context and the family as client and develop an understanding of family assessment and relevant theories applied in community nursing settings. You will also examine the skills needed for planning nursing interventions for families, including the case management approach to care.

WHY STUDY FAMILY NURSING?

Canadians are spending less time in acute care settings during illness or following surgery, resulting in an increasing amount of community-based and family-provided health care. Earlier discharges from hospital settings mean that family caregivers are continuing treatments previously done only in a hospital setting (e.g., medication administration, wound management, and intravenous therapy). This shift also means that nurses

who work in community health settings need to develop knowledge and skill in helping families cope with often very complex caregiving situations. In the mid 1990s, Green (1997) suggested that "nurses need an understanding and appreciation of the interactive complexity of family life, and they need to know how to 'think family'" (p. 230). Nearly a decade later, Hartrick Doane and Varcoe (2006) challenge CHNs to go beyond just thinking family, and begin to "understand family as a relational experience, understanding nursing and culture as relational processes and conceptualizing difference as a basis for connection" (p. 7). This approach is viewed as having the potential for more equitable and compassionate family nursing practice.

WHAT IS FAMILY?

A **family** is "society's most basic small group" (Hitchcock, Schubert, & Thomas, 2003, p. 590) and is central to society by providing core ingredients that determine the quality of life for its members at all ages (Bomar, 2004). The Vanier Institute of the Family (2006) defines family as "any combination of two or more persons who are bound together over time by ties of mutual consent, birth and/or adoption or placement."

Family forms in Canada include nuclear families, extended families, single-parent families, blended families, and homosexual families. (See Table 10.1.) Same-sex marriage has been legalized across Canada by the Civil Marriage Act enacted on July 20, 2005 (Department of Justice Canada, 2005). A pet may even be considered a family member for the person who lives alone (Lepage, Essiembre, & Coutu-Wakulczyk, 1996). Best practice guidelines published by the Registered Nurses' Association of Ontario (RNAO) (2006) reinforce that the CHN who works with families should respect each family as being unique and assess individuals in the context of the family as they define it.

Family Function

Denham (2003) describes **family function** as "the individual and cooperative processes used by developing persons as to dynamically engage one another and their diverse environments over the life course" (p. 277). The functions or responsibilities assumed by a family may include:

- physical maintenance and care of group members;
- addition of new members through procreation or adoption;

TABLE 10.1
Varieties of Family Forms

Statistics Canada (2006) describes family forms as comprised of:

1. couples (married or common-law, including same-sex couples*)
- living in the same home.
- with children or without children.

2. single parent or lone-parent families (male or female)
- living with one or more children.

3. persons who are not matched to a family
- living alone.
- living with a family (related to).
- living with a family (not related to).
- living with other non-family persons (non-family persons may live with their married children or with their children who have children of their own).

Notes:

Same-sex couples have been counted as couple families since 2001.

Families can be described in the following terms: nuclear (parents with one or more children); single-parent; extended (grandparents, aunts, and uncles); blended (remarried with children); adoptive; foster; and boomerang (adult children who return to live at home).

Though the majority of definitions refer to common living arrangements, the linkages between members of a family can be (1) biological, (2) psychological, or (3) social.

Source: Statistics Canada. (2006, July 3). Census family. Retrieved October 5, 2007, from http://www.statcan.ca/english/concepts/definitions/cen-family.htm.

- socialization of children;
- social control of members;
- production, consumption, distribution of goods and services; and
- affective nurturance-love (Vanier Institute of the Family, 2006).

CHNs can address a family's functional processes, as identified above, during health care visits. Families may benefit from intervention by CHNs during times of family transitions and health crisis. Interventions may include health teaching or counselling to promote family health and those that specifically target strengthening a family's social support system through referrals to other support services (Denham, 2005).

Societal Changes Affecting the Canadian Family

The "traditional" Canadian family was once defined as mother, father, and children. According to the 2006 Statistics Canada census data, the proportion of traditional families is declining with married couples being in the minority and the number of childless couples surpassing those with children (Alphonso, 2007). Other trends include growing numbers of young adults aged 20 to 29 staying at home with their parents instead of moving into separate dwellings, and seniors living with their children as part of a three generation household. Statistics Canada (2007a) cites the aging of the Canadian population along with increasing life expectancy as impacting on the composition of the family. Particularly, the large cohort of baby-boomers (born between 1946 and 1965) moving into their senior years. Younger adults sometimes referred to as "baby-busters" are fewer in number and have lower fertility rates leading to the increasing numbers of couples without children. Specifically, "since 1986, the proportion of married couples with children has declined from 49.4%, to 34.6%" (p.1).

Statistics Canada (2007b) reports that married couples are now in the minority in Canada with over half of Canadian adults falling into a cohort of never having married, living common-law, or being divorced, separated or widowed. A significant increase was reported for the number of same-sex couples with the first ever count of same-sex marriages. In July 2005, Canada became the fourth country in the world to legalize same-sex marriage. Broad changes in policy on same-sex couple rights and entitlements and greater social tolerance may have led to same-sex couples self-identifying in larger numbers (Fenlon & Agrell, 2007).

Other characteristics of Canadian families taken from the 2006 census also have implications for community health nursing practice. For instance, one in four Canadian families with children are lone-parent families (Fenlon & Agrell, 2007) with substantially lower incomes than two-parent families resulting in poverty being a common thread. According to Statistics Canada (2007b), there are 2.1 million children in 1.4 million lone-parent families. Lone-mother families are more likely to experience financial difficulties than other family structures. Canadian women are also delaying having children in lieu of pursuing education and employment opportunities with a resulting increase in the number of children aged 4 and under who had mothers in their forties (Statistics Canada, 2007c). This translates into a larger age gap between mothers and children and may change childhood and family experiences. Future studies will hopefully shed more light on the impact of this upward trend and the changes to the family experience when grandparents move in.

As the age of women having children rises and life expectancy increases, there is an overlap with the result being three generation households (Fuller-Thompson, 2007). This trend is also the result of increased immigration from countries where extended families are the norm. With this family form come both advantages and disadvantages. The crisis in daycare and rising house prices create financial and emotional burdens that can be lightened by sharing a home and a division of labour with an older generation. If the motivation for this family arrangement is purely financial necessity and not their choice, the consequences can increase the stress for all members of the family. The impact of multigenerational living arrangements on family stress, especially couple relationships, requires further investigation.

Many Canadians are born into families that have lived in this country for generations, but numerous families have also chosen to immigrate here. It is anticipated that Canada will continue to encourage immigration in the future as a means of building its population. This is in part due to an aging society, with people who are living longer lives and choosing to have smaller families. It is also due to ten years of decline in the fertility rate in Canada, which reached a record low of 1.49 in 2000. The fertility rate is an estimate of the average number of children each women aged 15 to 49 will have in her lifetime. Statistics Canada (2006) reported that the total fertility rate in 2004 was unchanged from the 2003 rate of 1.53 children per woman. The birth rate had declined from 10.6 live births per 1000 population in 2003 to a record low of 10.5 in 2004. Immigrants have impacted on Canada's birth rate; their fertility rates are higher compared with Canadian-born women, but their rates decline to national levels with the second-generation.

FAMILY HEALTH NURSING PRACTICE

Family health nursing is defined in the literature in different ways, and though there is no one overall theory, family nursing is based on theory guided by evidence-based knowledge (Rowe Kaakinen & Harmon Hanson, 2004). In a recent definition by Harmon Hanson (2005), **family health care nursing** was defined as "a process of providing for the health care needs of families that are within the scope of nursing practice. This nursing care can be aimed toward the family as context, the family as a whole, the family as a system, or the family as a component of society" (p. 9). Nurses in community settings who have the family as client must take a broader and more comprehensive approach to nursing care. Health promotion of the whole family, as well as individual members, is a primary goal of family nursing (Bomar, 2004). For the care to be most effective, the CHN works within the family's context. Five principles that guide and enhance family nursing practice (Allender & Spradley, 2005a) are:

- "work with the family collectively,
- start where the family is,
- adapt nursing intervention to the family's stage of development,
- recognize the validity of family structural variations, and
- emphasize family strengths." (p. 521)

Family as Context

The CHN focuses on either the individual within the context of his or her family or on the family with the individual as context. Viewing the family as context is the traditional focus of nursing, in which the individual is the foreground and the family is in the background (Friedman, Bowden, & Jones, 2003; Harmon Hanson, 2005). The nurse who interviews a newly married woman with cancer and her husband concerning the woman's experience with the life-threatening illness is an example of concentrating on the individual within the context of family. The nurse who focuses on the family with the individual as context would interview the adult children of a woman with Alzheimer's disease to discover how the family copes with caring for their mother at home.

There are five ways of viewing the family in family nursing (Friedman et al., 2003):

- The first level is to view the family as context to the client. The CHN focuses nursing care on the individual, with the family as a secondary focus.
- In the second level, the family is viewed as a sum of its individual family members or parts. Health care is provided to each individual family member and this is viewed as providing family health care. This is not the same as viewing the whole family as the focus of care.
- In the third level of family nursing practice, the focus is on family subsystems. Family dyads, triads, and other family subsystems are the focus of care, for example a CHN who focuses on the care of the new mother and her baby during a home visit. Other areas of focus could be caregiving issues and bonding attachment issues.
- Family as client is the fourth way of viewing the family. The unit of care is the entire family. The nurse does not focus on either the individual or the family, but concentrates on both the individual and the family simultaneously. The interaction that occurs among members of the family is emphasized. In the family-as-client approach to care, the family is in the foreground and individuals are in the background. (See Figure 10.1, Level IV.) The nurse would assess each person within the family and provide health care for all family members.
- A fifth level of family nursing conceptualizes family as a component of society. The family is seen as one of society's basic institutions. Nursing practice that focuses on the family as client is **family systems nursing**. Nurses who practise at this level will have extensive knowledge about family dynamics, family systems theory, and family assessment and intervention.

Health Promotion of the Family

"Family health promotion is the process of achieving family well-being in the biological, emotional, physical, and spiritual realms for individual members and the family unit" (Bomar, 2004, p. 11). This means that **family health promotion** can occur for an individual family member within the context of the family or for the family system as a unit. Areas that a CHN should assess when planning health promotion for the family as a whole include family functioning, family dynamics, communication patterns in the family, relationships between members, and the family's interaction with the community (Friedman et al., 2003).

FIGURE 10.1   Five Ways of Viewing the Family Practice

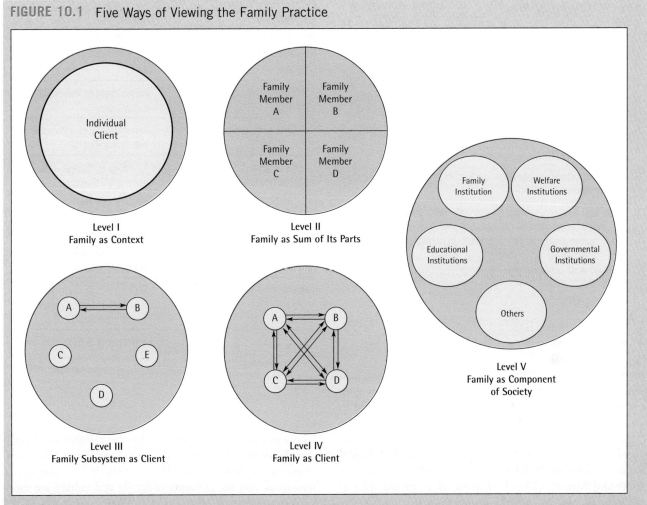

Source: Reproduced with permission from Friedman, M. M., Bowden, V. R., & Jones, E. G. (Eds.). (2003). Family nursing: Research, theory, & practice *(5th ed.). Upper Saddle River, NJ: Prentice Hall, p. 37 © Reprinted by permission of Pearson Education, Inc. Upper Saddle River, NJ.*

A role of the CHN caring for families is to assist the family to, "attain, maintain, and regain the highest level of family health possible" (Bomar, 2005, p. 244). A primary strategy may be to assist families to make informed choices about healthy lifestyle behaviours by increasing their knowledge and skills. Mandle (2002) describes the first step as creating awareness about actual or potential problems. The second step is to recognize families who are at a particular risk and to then offer them "the benefits of nursing knowledge about motivating and supporting behavioural change" (p. 195).

Canadian Research Box 10.1

Sword, W. A., Krueger, P. D., & Watt, M. S. (2006). Predictors of acceptance of a postpartum public health nurse home visit: Findings of an Ontario survey. *Canadian Journal of Public Health, 97*(3), 191–196.

The researchers in this study were interested in determining the predictors of acceptance of a home visit offered through Ontario's universal Hospital Stay and Postpartum Home Visiting Program, as well as the rates of offer and

the uptake of a home visit. The method used was a self-report questionnaire (in four languages) given to 1250 women recruited from across Ontario who met the inclusion criteria of a vaginal birth to a live singleton infant and who were also discharged home with the infant. Four weeks following discharge, 890 (or 71.2%) of the women participated in a structured telephone interview.

The results of this study are relevant for CHNs working in public health settings who have responsibility for developing and implementing home visiting programs for new mothers. The offer of a home visit by a public health nurse was high across sites, but there were statistically different rates of acceptance of a home visit by a new mother. Predictors of acceptance included "first live birth, lower social support, lower maternal rating of services in labour and delivery, poorer maternal self-reported health, probable postpartum depression, lower maternal rating of services on the postpartum unit, and breastfeeding initiation" (p. 193). The findings of this study lend support for the universal public health nurse postpartum visit initiated in the province. The authors concluded that future studies should explore the reasons for women accepting or declining a visit, the perceived value of the visits by the mothers, the characteristics of women who accept a selective visit vs. a universal home visit, and a comparison of effectiveness between telephone visits and home visits since telephone visits are less costly.

Discussion Questions:

1. How important a resource do you think the CHN is for a new mother?

2. How can nursing programs prepare future CHNs to gain the knowledge and skills required to participate in the development of evidence-based postpartum programs and policies that address the needs of postpartum women and their infants?

Theoretical Underpinnings of Family Health Nursing

Family social science theories, family therapy theories, and nursing models and theories all contribute to the emerging field of family nursing theories. Theories that are oriented to practice are relevant to nurses working with families (Friedman et al., 2003); for example, Neuman's System Model is frequently used by CHNs. The McGill Model (Feeley & Gottlieb, 2000) and the Developmental Model of Health and Nursing (Allen & Warner, 2002) are examples of family theories emerging within nursing.

Although every family is unique, all families share some universal characteristics. Allender and Spradley (2005b, p. 497) list five of the most important characteristics for CHNs to consider:

- Every family is a small social system.
- Every family has its own cultural values and rules.
- Every family has structure.
- Every family has certain basic functions.
- Every family moves through stages in its life cycle.

These universal characteristics reflect the importance of culture as well as structural-functional theory, systems theory, and theories of family development—all theories from the social sciences that have been applied to families. **Structural-functional theory** focuses on how the family structure contributes to and affects family functions. **Systems theory** focuses on the interaction between members of the family system and between the family system and other systems (Artinian, 1999). **Family developmental theory** refers to stages and tasks as presented in Table 10.2. This is a life-cycle approach, which suggests that families move through typical and shared developmental stages, experiencing growth and development in a similar manner to individuals (Hitchcock et al., 2003).

The theoretical concept of culture is discussed in Chapter 20. **Family culture** "is the acquired knowledge that

TABLE 10.2
Family Life Cycle Developmental Stages and Tasks (North American middle class)

Stage	Tasks
Forming partnerships and/or marriage	Commitment to and establishing a new family
Child bearing families	Adjustment to parenthood and new family members
Families with • Preschool children • School-age children • Teenagers	Adjusting to changes in the partner relationship Meeting age-appropriate developmental needs of children
Launching children	Adjustment to needs of young adults leaving and/or re-entering the family
Middle-aged parents	Maintenance of supportive relationships with children and across generations
Aging parents	Adjustments to retirement, end of life

family members use to interpret their experiences and to generate behaviours that influence family structure and function" (Allendar & Spradley, 2005b, p. 500). It is important to remember that the concepts of family and culture are intertwined and that the shared values, beliefs, and practices (i.e., culture) within families shape the meaning of life experiences and behaviours of family members. It is a limitation that "[a]lthough most family social science and nursing theories recognize culture as a significant variable in client health behaviours, these theories do not specifically focus on culture and cultural influence on family and family nursing care" (Ferguson-Marshalleck & Miller, 2005, p. 198).

Clarke (1998) adds another level to the discussion of family nursing theory by discussing two paradigms, community-based nursing and community-focused nursing. "*Community-based nursing* is focused on the individual within the family in the community . . . . *Community-focused nursing* is directed toward the health of the family and community as a whole" (p. 47). The theories discussed in this chapter centre on how the person and family are viewed within the community. Epidemiological models and social change theories are examples of how models and frameworks are applied when communities are viewed in their entirety.

Theories help us to "make sense" of our world and theories that are relevant to families inform and guide nursing practice. However, no one theory or conceptual model is sufficient for describing the multifaceted nature of family processes and relationships (Harmon Hanson & Rowe Kaakinen, 2005; Hartrick Doane & Varcoe, 2005; RNAO, 2006). In order to fully understand a variety of perspectives about families and thereby increase the potential for a variety of nursing interventions, CHNs will need to have the knowledge and skill to utilize and integrate multiple theories within the contexts of health promotion and determinants of health. The guiding question becomes: "How do these theories sensitize me to particular families and how will they enhance and/or constrain my ability to responsively attend to particular families at particular times?" (Hartrick Doane & Varcoe, 2005, p. 48).

FAMILY ASSESSMENT

"A *family assessment* is an exploration between the nurse and family to gain insight into the family's perspective of the event, their strengths and need for support" (RNAO, 2006). Regardless of the concepts, models, and tools utilized, a comprehensive **family assessment** uses open-ended questions and is detailed and inclusive. Nursing assessments are ongoing, which mean they change, are added to, and develop over time as data are shared with and observed by the nurse. An assessment is not "done to" the family, but is rather a process that the nurse facilitates. The act of facilitation starts to build a relationship between the nurse and the family. The assessment process is part of the nursing process, being the foundation upon which planning, interventions, and evaluation are based. However, conducting assessments may actually limit the CHN's discovery and potential for strengthening family health if the focus becomes completing a prescribed checklist and task rather than building relationships (Hartrick Doan & Varcoe, 2005). Another challenge in working with families is establishing relationships that connect across difference and diversity. Hartrick Doane and Varcoe (2006) state that nurses need to strive to understand complexity and difference as an opportunity to become more responsive in relationships, aware of the context in which family strengths are enacted, and open to possibilities and potential within clients and ourselves. CHNs need to always be aware that the family may have different meanings of what the promotion of their health means for them. Family health promotion is also influenced by local, provincial, and federal structures and policies that relate to the determinants of health, such as funding for health care, education, and social services.

Some aspects of nursing in community settings can help the nurse and family in the assessment process:

- The interviews will often take place in the family's home, where the family is likely to be more comfortable.
- Other family members are more likely to be present, which adds to the family assessment data.
- There will often be multiple visits, which promote trust and the development of a relationship between the nurse and the family over time.
- The nurse gathers data about the family in its own context.

Much of the care provided by CHNs takes place in clients' homes (although care may also be provided in community or hospital-based settings, for example, hospital liaison for discharge planning). Home visits have many advantages; however, it is a standard of practice for CHNs that a holistic assessment occurs in collaboration with the client (individual, family, or community) wherever the care is provided. It is also an expectation that the nurse can negotiate and provide care that is appropriate to the values of clients in a variety of settings (Community Health Nurses Association of Canada, 2003).

Leahey and Harper-Jaques (1996) describe five core assumptions relating to the family–nurse relationship. These assumptions underlie the family nursing models that are reviewed in this chapter.

- The family–nurse relationship is characterized by reciprocity.
- The family–nurse relationship is nonhierarchical.
- Nurses and families each have specialized expertise in maintaining health and in managing health problems.
- Nurses and families each bring strengths and resources to the family–nurse relationship.
- A feedback process can simultaneously occur at several different relationship levels.

Each family member and the nurse bring their own perceptions, values, and beliefs to the interactions. These assumptions are central to the forming of collaborative relationships between nurses and families. What is common to all assessments is that respect is demonstrated for the client's values and beliefs, so that practice is guided and improved through appropriate nursing interventions that are meaningful to the family. This also means that the family has the right to choose the level at which they wish to participate in the nurse–client relationship (RNAO, 2006).

An illustration of this is the field of genetics, with increasing knowledge, testing, and interventions resulting in complex implications for families. Genetic testing carries benefits, risks, and limitations. Risk of or actual disease may be caused by shared genetic factors (such as chromosomal abnormalities) within families. However, families that live together share multifaceted gene–environmental influences that can make risk difficult to establish (Williams & Skirton, 2005). Nevertheless, careful assessment of genetic factors will continue to be a greater focus in nursing care (Esplen, 2006). According to the Canadian Nurses Association (2005), nurses working with families across the lifespan will increasingly encounter people who are living with genetic information. CHNs may be involved in pre-conception counselling, and helping families cope with childhood and adult-onset diseases, including chronic diseases. Nursing interventions will focus on supporting individuals and families as they determine how genetic information will be utilized (Williams & Skirton, 2005).

The Friedman Family Assessment Model (Friedman et al., 2003), the Calgary Family Assessment Model (Wright & Leahey, 2005), the McGill Model (Feeley & Gottlieb, 2000; Gottlieb & Rowat, 1987), and the Developmental Model of Health and Nursing (Allen & Warner, 2002; Ford-Gilboe, 2002) are examples of family assessment models. The latter three were developed in Canada. Essential features of the models are presented in Table 10.3.

TABLE 10.3
Components of Family Assessment Models

Friedman Family Assessment	Calgary Family Assessment Model	McGill Model	Developmental Model of Health and Nursing
Identifying data	Developmental stage and history of family	The family as the subsystem	The family as the primary social system
Developmental stage and history of family	Structural	Health as the focus of work	Health work
Environmental data	Developmental	Learning as the process through which health behaviours are acquired	Health potential
Family structure	Functional		Competence in health behaviours
Family functions		Family collaborates with the nurse in the learning process	Health status
Family coping			

Source: Adapted from Supporting and strengthening families through expected and unexpected life events *(p. 42), by the Registered Nurses Association of Ontario, 2006, Toronto: Author.*

The Friedman Family Assessment Model has six broad categories (see Table 10.3) (Friedman et al., 2003). Identifying data include family composition, cultural background, religious identification, social class status, and recreational activities. The developmental stage is assessed along with the family's history and the history of both parents' family of origin. Environmental data include characteristics of the home, neighbourhood, and community; the family's geographic mobility; associations with the community and use of community resources; and the family's social support system. Family structure looks at communication patterns, power structure, role structure, and family values. Affective, socialization, and health care functions are assessed in the family functions category. The sixth category, family stress and coping, includes assessment of stressors and strengths along with coping strategies (Friedman et al., 2003). Each category has many subcategories. The nurse and the family decide which areas need in-depth exploration based on the focus for nursing intervention.

Wright and Leahey (2005) first developed the Calgary Family Assessment Model (CFAM) in 1983 at the University of Calgary. The CFAM has been conceptualized as a branching model with three major categories: structural, developmental, and functional. As in Friedman's model, it has many subcategories. Each nurse decides which subcategories should be explored and assesses each family accordingly. The nurse and the family move back and forth across the branches to build a story of the family and its interactions.

Interventions are conceptualized in the Calgary Family Intervention Model (CFIM), which complements the CFAM and provides a framework for family functions in three domains: cognitive, affective, and behavioural. Interventions focus on promoting, improving, and sustaining effective family functioning. The most effective interventions are congruent with the family's beliefs and values, the articulation of which is facilitated during the assessment (Wright & Leahy, 2005).

The McGill Model has been developed and refined over time by faculty and students at the McGill University School of Nursing (Gottlieb & Rowat, 1987). This model emphasizes family, health, collaboration, and learning. The family is an active participant, with the nurse, in its own health care. "One of the goals of nursing, based on the McGill Model, is to help families use the strengths of the individual family members and of the family as unit, as well as resources external to the family system, to cope, achieve their goals, and develop" (Feeley & Gottlieb, 2000, p. 10). Health consists of processes that are dynamic and multidimensional, especially the processes of coping and development.

The assessment phase of the McGill Model requires an exploratory approach by the nurse, with the nurse creating a supportive environment so that the family's perceptions and strengths can emerge. Learning needs are identified and the initiative for planning can be with the nurse or the family (Gottlieb & Rowat, 1987). It is during the implementation phase that the family becomes an active learner in collaboration with the nurse. Arising from the McGill Model, the Developmental Model of Health and Nursing emphasizes health as a process, the nurse as an empowering partner, and the potential for families to demonstrate strengths and positive growth (Ford-Gilboe, 2002).

A valuable tool for all assessments is the genogram (see Figure 10.2), which is used to build a picture of family structure, relationships, and boundaries. Another tool that is especially useful for CHNs is the ecomap (see Figure 10.3), which visually represents a family's connections and the nature of relationships with the larger community and can be used to assess resources and strengths (Tarko & Reed, 2004; Wright & Leahy, 2005). As derived from Wright and Leahy (1999), some general questions to guide the family-assessment interview are listed in the text box "Examples of Family Assessment and Interview Questions."

Examples of Family Assessment and Interview Questions

1. How can I be the most helpful to you and your family at this time? (clarifies expectations and builds partnership between the family and the nurse)

2. What has been most/least helpful to you and your family in the past? (identifies past difficulties, strengths, and achievements)

3. Who of your family and friends would you like to share information with and who not? (identifies alliances, resources, and conflicts)

4. What is the greatest challenge facing your family right now? (identifies actual/potential stress, roles, values, and beliefs)

5. What do you need to best prepare you/your family for _____? (identifies appropriate community resources)

6. What strengths does your family have right now? (identifies current positive resources and assists with planning)

7. What is the one question you would like to have answered right now? (identifies the most pressing issue or concern)

8. How have I been most helpful to you today? How could we improve? (demonstrates willingness to learn from the family and work collaboratively)

FIGURE 10.2 Sample Genogram: The B. Family

Another valuable tool during assessment is the genogram, which is used to build a picture of family structure, relationships, and boundaries. This genogram shows the family of Mr. and Mrs. B., who were married in 2000. Mrs. B. is 27 years old and has just given birth to her third child, a girl. She lives with her 28-year-old husband and their other two children, boys, who are six and two years old. The oldest son has asthma and attends Grade 1 at the local elementary school. Mrs. B.'s father died of cancer in 1998. Her mother and large extended family live close by. Mr. B. provides for the family financially by working as a high-school teacher. The B. family is used for the case study later in the chapter.

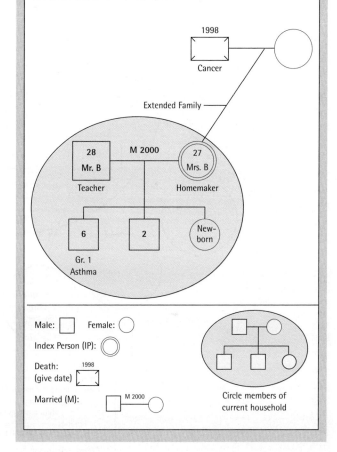

During the assessment process, the nurse facilitates the family in discovering and articulating the often unexamined assumptions, context, and expectations underlying its perception of reality. This means that:

- The assessment process takes time, sensitivity, and flexibility.
- The assessment process starts from the perspective of the family and/or the community.
- Assessments take place in an atmosphere of openness, awareness, mutual collaboration, and relationship-building.
- Assessments are holistic.
- Assessment tools can be adapted and adjusted to identified needs (identified by the client and the nurse), such as time and area of focus.

Many family assessment tools are available (Allender & Spradley, 2005a; Friedman et al., 2003; Rowe Kaakinen & Harmon Hanson, 2004; RNAO, 2006; Tarko & Reid, 2004). So how does the CHN decide on an assessment tool that will then guide interventions? It is not a case of "one size fits all" or of designing the "perfect" model. Rather, it is having the openness, knowledge, and skill to evaluate existing theories, models, and tools in light of what would be most appropriate and effective for the client, and integrating and adapting as necessary.

The theories, frameworks, and assessment models discussed in this chapter have in common that the CHN and the family are engaged in a social process of exploration, negotiation, and mutual goal setting, centred within the family–nurse relationship. Interventions are grounded in the contexts of family structure and function, family development, family support and environment, health work and potential, health promotion, education and advocacy, determinants of health, and the principles of primary health care. (See Figure 10.4.)

FIGURE 10.3 Sample Ecomap: The B. Family

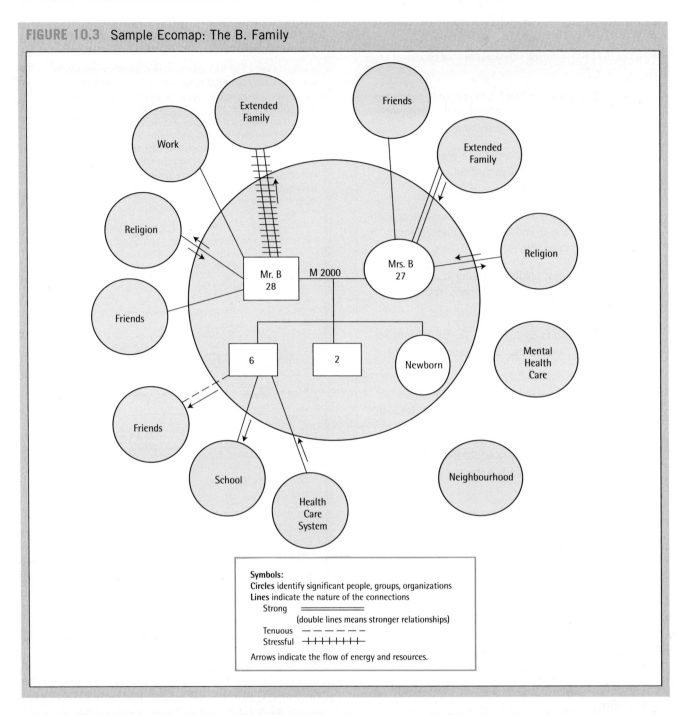

Symbols:
Circles identify significant people, groups, organizations
Lines indicate the nature of the connections
Strong ═══════
(double lines means stronger relationships)
Tenuous – – – – – –
Stressful +++++++
Arrows indicate the flow of energy and resources.

Canadian Research Box 10.2

Ford-Gilboe, M., Wuest, J., & Merritt-Gray, M. (2005). Strengthening capacity to limit intrusion: Theorizing family health promotion in the aftermath of woman abuse. *Qualitative Health Research, 15,* (4), 477–501.

The purpose of this feminist grounded theory research was to develop a substantive and explanatory theory illuminating the health promotion processes of diverse single-parent families (SPFs) headed by mothers who had experienced intimate partner violence (IPV). SPFs (usually headed by mothers) make up 25% of Canadian families. Defined as "a pattern of physical, sexual, and/or emotional violence by an intimate partner in the context of coercive control" (p. 478), IPV is often a significant factor when women decide to leave relationships. Women in 40 SPFs living with the aftereffects of IPV in Ontario and New Brunswick were recruited and interviewed twice. Eleven children older than age 12 also participated (with their consent and that of their mothers). The families represented a diversity of cultural, ethnic, socioeconomic, and urban/rural backgrounds.

Intrusion, a central concept in the theory, is the unwanted and "external control or interference that demands attention, diverts energy away from family priorities, and limits choices" (p. 482). After leaving an abusive partner/father, families engaged in the focal health promotion process of strengthening capacity in order to limit intrusion through four subprocesses: providing, regenerating family, renewing self, and rebuilding security. These subprocesses are intertwined, affected by the intensity and sources of intrusion, and are acted upon in an effort to achieve the goals of surviving and positioning for the future. Four conditions—family ideals; the quality of connections with family, friends, and community; developmental stages of the children; and accessibility and sustainability of needed services—are also of influence.

Promoting health through positioning for the future is accomplished by proactive and intentional efforts to develop the skills and strengths needed for long-term goals. Surviving is a reactive process focusing on gaining control of basic and daily demands in order to reduce intrusion. These are evolving and cyclical processes. Positioning for the future (such as leaving an abusive partner) entails risk and may have negative consequences that increase intrusion and result in intensified efforts toward surviving. Yet successful surviving builds control and confidence. Over time, and because of the work done by surviving, family capacity for health promotion to limit intrusion is strengthened.

Discussion Questions:

1. What are the implications of this research for family nursing that supports strengths and reduces intrusion?

2. Do you think a health promoting cyclical process of survival and positioning for the future occurs in families where IPV has not happened? How would you research this question?

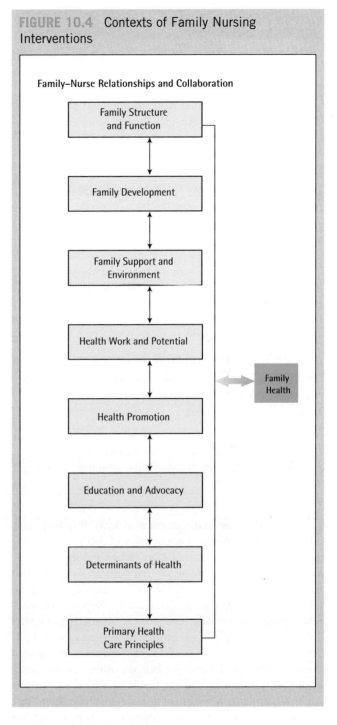

FIGURE 10.4 Contexts of Family Nursing Interventions

CASE MANAGEMENT AND FAMILY-CENTRED CARE

Case management is a collaborative approach used by CHNs to coordinate and deliver health care services. It is also referred to in the literature as service coordination and service facilitation. A community health nurse case manager works with individuals, families, and other health care providers to facilitate all necessary services for care provided in community settings during times of illness and other health care conditions requiring nursing intervention. The model was first introduced in 1985 as an outgrowth of primary care nursing and described by Cohen and Cesta (2001) as an opportunity

for the nursing profession to define its role in the changing health care industry (p. 3). Traditional nursing care delivery systems are not able to deal with "the many constraints, economic limitations, and continual changes in today's health care settings" (Cohen & Cesta, p. 9). The model also challenges the profession to define nurses' work in terms of its autonomous value to the client.

Case Study

Figures 10.2 and 10.3 show the genogram and ecomap of the B. family. The family lives in a comfortable three-bedroom home in an established neighbourhood. They value being active in their religious organization. Mrs. B feels supported by her extended family; however, she also feels she is not able to support them in return at this time. Mr. B has stressful and distant relations with his family. Their six-year-old son enjoys school but has had difficulty making friends. You are a CHN required to make follow-up telephone calls to new mothers following discharge from hospital. During your phone conversation, Mrs B. tells you that she is feeling "very overwhelmed and tearful" after having the new baby. She voices concern and fear that she is not bonding with the baby. She has never experienced anything like this before and has not shared her feelings with her husband or her family.

Discussion Questions

1. How soon should you make the home visit?

2. What should you do if you are unable to personally make a home visit within an appropriate length of time?

3. Discuss which assessment model you will use, and describe what beginning information you have about family strengths, challenges, and community supports.

The goal of case management is to arrive at quality, cost-effective client outcomes. The provision of client care by using a case manager is becoming a more recognized strategy. Case management is meant to ensure that patients receive needed care and services and that those services are delivered in an efficient manner (Cohen & Cesta, 2001). Nurses in community settings use the case management approach to identify and assess clients, plan care, provide or delegate care, and follow up with an evaluation of care. For nurses working with families, this would mean the best outcomes for individual clients within families and the family as a whole. Canadian nurses have a lengthy history of providing family-centred care to vulnerable individuals and connecting them to services with the purpose of promoting health and preventing disease (Jack, 2000; Rafael, 1999; Sword, Krueger, & Watt, 2006).

In Canada, restructuring during the 1990s resulted in two major mechanisms for managed care to save health care dollars. The first was decreasing the length of stay in hospitals (early discharge); the second was decreasing the time spent delivering home care services. The danger of these was that cost containment, not quality of life, became the main determining factor (Daiski, 2000). The result has been many complaints about deteriorating home care services and the detrimental impact of the changes on patients and their families. "Inadequate professional follow-up care often forces families to take over these responsibilities" (Daiski, 2000,

p. 75). Currently, there is a demographic shift toward an aging population occurring in Canada that is similar to other developed Western nations. As the population of seniors grows, more pressure will be put on informal caregivers with a simultaneous increase in the number of nurses necessary for providing care in community settings (O'Sullivan Burchard, 2005).

Once embraced as a model to increase nursing's influence in the system, case management has come under criticism for its focus on cost containment. Nurses as case managers are challenged to creatively "integrate financing mechanisms and appropriate utilization management, and ensure high-quality service delivery by prioritizing outcomes (Daiski, 2000, p. 75). This is a very challenging situation for nurses, who must determine the most appropriate services to meet the needs of the client while providing the most benefit at the least cost.

Summary

This chapter is an overview of family care in community settings. It is not all-encompassing, but rather provides a glimpse into a nursing specialty. Changing family composition and increasing cultural diversity of families are discussed, a key message being that it is important for nurses to remain open to the perceptions, values, and beliefs of families and to gather that information as part of a holistic assessment. The nurse does not only "conduct" an assessment but facilitates the optimal process for family functioning. In community health, this process often occurs in the client's home. Over time, strong relationships between the nurse and the family can develop. Planning, implementation, and evaluation interventions are also collaborative processes between the nurse and the family. Many assessment models are available, most based on multidisciplinary theories, but there is no perfect assessment model, tool, or plan of care. CHNs need to be aware of and utilize the theories and models consistent with the underlying concepts and assumptions that will "make sense" of the situation for the nurse and the family. As mutual priorities are set, appropriate tools can be focused and adapted.

> The future of family health nursing will be influenced by health policy, health promotion agendas, economics, changes in the nursing profession, family demands, health promotion lifestyle changes, and the growing emphasis by family and health care professionals on capacity building with families to transform their health. (Bomar, 2004, p. 34)

KEY TERMS

family
family form
family function
family health care nursing
family systems nursing
family health promotion
structural-functional theory
systems theory
family developmental theory

family culture
family assessment
case management

STUDY QUESTIONS

1. What are some of the key challenges facing families today?

2. What are some of the reasons that young people are moving back home or leaving home at a later age?

3. What are some of the terms used to describe nurses' work with families?

4. Describe attributes of a collaborative relationship with a family.

5. Develop your own definition of a Canadian family.

6. How does a CHN provide effective care while working with the family as client?

INDIVIDUAL CRITICAL THINKING EXERCISES

1. What are some examples of how determinants of health could affect families?

2. Discuss the responsibilities families need to meet for healthy functioning.

3. What are some of the shared assumptions for facilitating relationships with families?

4. Discuss the societal changes that have influenced family life in Canada.

5. How does the CHN assist families to strengthen their capacity to act on their own behalf for health promotion?

GROUP CRITICAL THINKING EXERCISES

1. Describe how approaches to family health nursing in the community differ from acute care settings.

2. Case management requires a balance between quality client care and cost-effectiveness.

3. How do family assessment models help you to meet this goal as a CHN?

4. Explain how the changing demographics of the Canadian family influence community health nursing care.

5. Differentiate between viewing the family as client and the family as context.

6. Elaborate on what it means to "think family."

REFERENCES

Allen, F. M., & Warner, M. (2002). A developmental model of health and nursing. *Journal of Family Nursing, 8*(2), 96–135.

Allendar, J., & Spradley, B. (2005a). Assessment of families. In J. Allendar & B. Spradley (Eds.), *Community health nursing: Promoting and protecting the public's health* (6th ed.) (pp. 516–538). Philadelphia: Lippincott, Williams & Wilkins.

Allendar, J., & Spradley, B. (2005b). Theoretical bases for promoting family health. In J. Allendar & B. Spradley (Eds.), *Community health nursing: Promoting and protecting the public's health* (6th ed.) (pp. 495–514). Philadelphia: Lippincott, Williams & Wilkins.

Alphonso, C. (2007, September 13). Canadians redefine the family. *The Globe and Mail*, p. 1.

Artinian, N. T. (1999). Selecting a model to guide family assessment. In G. D. Wegner & R. J. Alexander (Eds.), *Readings in family nursing* (2nd ed.) (pp. 447–459). Philadelphia: Lippincott.

Bomar, P. J. (2004). Introduction to family health nursing and promoting family health. In Bomar, P. J. (Ed.), *Promoting health in families: Applying family research and theory to nursing practice* (3rd ed.) (pp. 3–37). Philadelphia: Saunders.

Bomar, P. J. (2005). Family health promotion. In S. M. Harmon Hanson, V. Gedaly-Duff, & J. Rowe Kaakinen (Eds.), *Family health care nursing: Theory, practice & research* (3rd ed.) (pp. 243–264). Philadelphia: F. A. Davis.

Canadian Nurses Association. (2005). Nursing and genetics: Are you ready? *Nursing Now: Issues and Trends in Canadian Nursing, 20*, 1–5.

Clarke, P. N. (1998). Nursing theory as a guide for inquiry in family and community health nursing. *Nursing Science Quarterly, 11*(2), 47–48.

Cohen, E. L., & Cesta, T. G. (2001). *Nursing case management: From essentials to advanced practice application.* St. Louis: Mosby.

Community Health Nurses Association of Canada (CHNAC). (2003). *Canadian community health nursing standards of practice.* Ottawa: Author.

Daiski, I. (2000). The road to professionalism in nursing: Case management or practice based in nursing theory? *Nursing Science Quarterly, 13*(1), 74–79.

Denham, S. A. (2003). Relationships between family rituals, family routines, and health. *Journal of Family Nursing, 9*(3), 305–330.

Denham, S. A. (2005). Family structure, function, and process. In S. M. Harmon Hanson, V. Gedaly-Duff, & J. Rowe Kaakinen (Eds.), *Family health care nursing theory, practice and research* (3rd ed.)(pp. 119–156). Philadelphia: F.A. Davis.

Department of Justice Canada. (2005). *Civil Marriage Act.* Retrieved May 16, 2007, from http://canada.justice.gc.ca/en/news/nr/2005/doc_31378.html.

Esplen, M. J. (2006). Mapping the human genome: Psychosocial impacts and implications for nursing. *Canadian Journal of Nursing Research, 38*(2), 115–123.

Feeley, N., & Gottlieb, L. N. (2000). Nursing approaches for working with family strengths and resources. *Journal of Family Nursing, 6*(1), 9–24.

Fenlon, B., & Agrell, S. (2007, September 12). Canada's changing family. *Globe and Mail Update and Canadian Press*, pp. 1-4. Retrieved September 29, 2007, from http://www.theglobeandmail.com/servlet/story/RTGAM.20070912.wcensusrelease0912/BNStory/National/

Ferguson-Marshalleck, E., & Miller, J. K. (2005). Sociocultural influences on family health. In S. Harmon Hansen, V. Gedaly-Duff, & J. Rowe Kaakinen (Eds.).

Family health care nursing: Theory, practice & research (3rd ed.) (pp. 197–214), Philadelphia: F. A. Davis.

Ford-Gilboe, M. (2002). Developing knowledge about family health promotion by testing the developmental model of health and nursing. *Journal of Family Nursing, 8*(2), 140–156.

Friedman, M. M., Bowden, V. R., & Jones, E. G. (Eds.). (2003). *Family nursing: Research, theory, & practice* (5th ed.). Upper Saddle River, NJ: Prentice Hall.

Fuller-Thompson, E. (2007, September 13). Cited in "Then your in-laws move in." Article by Agrell, Siri . *The Globe and Mail*, p. 1 & 2.

Gottlieb, L., & Rowat, K. (1987). The McGill model of nursing: A practice-derived model. *Advances in Nursing Science, 9*(4), 51–61.

Green, C. P. (1997). Teaching students how to "think family." *Journal of Family Nursing, 3*(3), 230–246.

Harmon Hanson, S. M. (2005). Family health care nursing: An Introduction. In S. M. Harmon Hanson, V. Gedaly-Duff, & J. Rowe Kaakinen (Eds.), *Family health care nursing theory, practice and research* (3rd ed.) (pp. 3–37). Philadelphia: F. A. Davis.

Harmon Hanson, S., & Rowe Kaakinen, G. (2005). Theoretical foundations for nursing of families. In S. Harmon Hansen, V. Gedaly-Duff, & J. Rowe Kaakinen (Eds.), *Family health care nursing: Theory, practice & research* (3rd ed.) (pp. 69–95). Philadelphia: F. A. Davis.

Hartrick Doane, G., & Varcoe, C. (2005). *Family nursing as relational inquiry: Developing health-promoting practice.* Philadelphia: Lippincott Williams & Wilkins.

Hartrick Doane, G., & Varcoe, C. (2006). The 'hard spots' of family nursing: Connecting across difference and diversity. *Journal of Family Nursing, 12*(1), 7–21.

Hitchcock, J. E., Schubert, P. E., & Thomas, S. A. (Eds.). (2003). *Community health nursing: Caring inAction.* Albany: Delmar.

Jack, S. (2000). *Mandating public health nurses to become case managers. Is it necessary?* Unpublished manuscript, McMaster University, Hamilton, Ontario.

Leahy, M., & Harper-Jaques, S. (1996). Family–nurse relationships: Core assumptions and clinical implications. *Journal of Family Nursing, 2*(2), 133–151.

Lepage, M., Essiembre, L. G., & Coutu-Wakulczyk, G. (1996). Variations sur le theme de la Famille. *Canadian Nurse, 92*(7), 40–44.

MacDonald, M. (2002). Health promotion: Historical, philosophical and theoretical perspectives. In L. Young & V. Hayes (Eds.), *Transforming health promotion practice: Concepts, issues and applications* (pp. 22–45). Philadelphia: F. A. Davis.

Mandle, C. L. (2002). Health promotion and the family. In C. L. Edelman & C. L. Mandle (Eds.), *Health promotion throughout the lifespan* (5th ed.) (pp. 169–198). Toronto: Mosby.

O'Sullivan Burchard, D. J. H. (2005). Family nursing: Challenges and opportunities: What will the challenges for family nursing be over the next few years? *Journal of Family Nursing, 11*(4), 332–335.

Rafael, A. R. F. (1999). From rhetoric to reality: The changing face of public health nursing in Southern Ontario. *Public Health Nursing, 16*(1), 50–59.

Registered Nurses' Association of Ontario (Revised). (2006). *Supporting and strengthening families through expected and unexpected life events.* Toronto: Author.

Rowe Kaakinen, J., & Harmon Hanson, S. (2004). Theoretical foundations for family nursing practice. In Bomar, P. J. (Ed.), *Promoting health in families: Applying family research and theory to nursing practice* (3rd ed.) (pp. 93–116). Philadelphia: Saunders.

Statistics Canada. (2006). Birth rate. *The Daily, August 14, 2006.* Retrieved on October 9, 2007, from http://www42. statcan.ca/smr04/2006/08/smr04_22606_04_e.htm.

Statistics Canada. (2007a). Family portrait: Continuity and change in Canadian families and households in 2006: National portrait: Individuals. Retrieved September 30, 2007, from http://www12.statcan.ca/english/census06/ analysis/famhouse/ind5.cfm.

Statistics Canada. (2007b). 2006 Census: Families, marital status, households and dwelling characteristics. *The Daily*, p. 1-3. Retrieved September 23, 2007, from http://www. statcan.ca/Daily/English/070912/d070912a.htm.

Statistics Canada. (2007c). Study: Canada's immigrant labour market, p 1-4. Retrieved September 30, 2007, from http:// www.statcan.ca/Daily/English/070910/d070910a.htm.

Sword, W. A., Krueger, P. D., & Watt, M. S. (2006). Predictors of acceptance of a postpartum public health nurse home visit: Findings of an Ontario survey. *Canadian Journal of Public Health, 97*(3), 191–196.

Tarko, M., & Reed, K. (2004). Family assessment and intervention. In Bomar, P. J. (Ed.), *Promoting health in families: Applying family research and theory to nursing practice* (3rd ed.) (pp. 274–303). Philadelphia: Saunders.

Vanier Institute of the Family. (2006). *Profiling Canada's families II.* Ottawa: CNA.

Williams, J., & Skirton, H. (2005). Genomics, family nursing, and families across the life span. In S. Harmon Hansen, V. Gedaly-Duff, & J. Rowe Kaakinen (Eds.), *Family health care nursing: Theory, practice & research* (3rd ed.) (pp. 437–455), Philadelphia: F. A. Davis.

Wright, L. M., & Leahy, M. (1999). Maximizing time, minimizing suffering: The 15-minute (or less) family interview. *Journal of Family Nursing 5*(3), 259–274.

Wright, L. M., & Leahy, M. (2005). *Nurses and families: A guide to family assessment and intervention* (4th ed.). Philadelphia: F. A. Davis.

ADDITIONAL RESOURCES

Websites

Canadian Nurses Association
www.cna-nurses.ca

Child and Family Canada
www.cfc-efc.ca

Registered Nurses' Association of Ontario
   www.rnao.org
Statistics Canada
   www.statcan.ca
The Vanier Institute of the Family
   www.vifamily.ca

Readings

Kearney, M. H., York, R., & Deatrick, J. A. (2000). Effects of home visits to vulnerable young families. *Journal of Nursing Scholarship, 32,* 369–376.

McNaughton, D. B. (2004). Nurse home visits to maternal-child clients: A review of intervention research. *Public Health Nurse, 21,* 207–219.

Registered Nurses' Association of Ontario. (2002). *Supporting and strengthening families through expected and unexpected life events.* Toronto: Registered Nurses' Association of Ontario.

Registered Nurses' Association of Ontario. (2006). *Supporting and strengthening families through expected and unexpected life events* (rev. suppl.). Toronto: Registered Nurses' Association of Ontario.

Sword, W. A., Krueger, P. D., & Watt, M. S. (2006). Predictors of acceptance of a postpartum public health nurse home visit: Findings from an Ontario survey. *Canadian Journal of Public Health, 97*(3), 191–196.

About the Authors

Linda J. Patrick, RN, BScN (University of Windsor), MA (Central Michigan with a specialization in post secondary education), MSc (Nursing, University of Windsor), PhD (McMaster University), has been involved in nursing education since 1989 and has experience in both acute care settings and community health working as a nurse with the Victorian Order of Nurses and as a diabetes educator in a community health centre. Current theoretical and research interests include existential phenomenology, embodiment and chronic illness, and the prevention or delay of type 2 diabetes in women with previous GDM.

Kathryn Edmunds, RN, BN (University of Manitoba), MSN (Wayne State University with a specialization in transcultural nursing), is currently a Doctoral Student in the School of Nursing at the University of Western Ontario. She has been a faculty member in nursing at the University of Windsor and has extensive experience as a public health nurse with the Windsor-Essex County Health Unit working in rural southwestern Ontario. Current theoretical and research interests include the effects of uprootedness, displacement, and marginalization on culture and health.

Community Care

Lucia Yiu

OBJECTIVES

After studying this chapter, you should be able to:

1. Describe the concept of community and discuss its functions and dynamics.

2. Briefly describe the selected common models and frameworks used in community health nursing practice.

3. Explain the community health nursing process and its application in caring for community clients.

4. Discuss the purposes, methods, parameters, and participatory tools used in community assessment, planning, and intervention.

5. Explain the importance of population health promotion, risk assessment, community engagement, community governance, and community development.

6. Discuss the nurse's role in caring for a community.

INTRODUCTION

Community health nurses (CHNs) care for people where they live, learn, play, and work. Their goal is to improve the health of the community by promoting, preserving, and protecting the health of individuals, families, aggregates, and populations. Their practice includes promoting health, building individual/ community capacity, connecting and caring, facilitating access and equity, and demonstrating professional responsibility and accountability (Community Health Nurses Association of Canada, 2003). When entering the practice of community health nursing, novice nurses often ask, "What does caring for a community mean?" "Where and how do I begin?" and "What is a healthy community?" Unlike having clients in hospitals or acute care settings, who actively seek episodic care for their presenting problems, community health nurses must determine *who* and *where* their clients are—and *when, why, what,* and *how* best to promote their health in the community. They must understand the complexity and needs of their diverse populations and the relationship of environment and health, and must work autonomously to build community partnerships that are based on a philosophy of primary health care. This chapter provides an overview of the community health nursing process including community assessment, selected community health practice models, population health promotion, community development, and community participatory tools.

COMMUNITY DEFINED

Developing an understanding of a community, its functions and dynamics, and the relationships between these and the health of the people is fundamental to providing competent community care. A **community** may be defined as a group of people who live, learn, work, and play in an environment at a given time. They share common characteristics and interests and function in a social system that meets their needs within a larger social system such as an organization, a region, a province, or a nation.

The core of any community is its *people,* who are characterized by their age, sex, socioeconomic status, education level, occupation, ethnicity, and religion. A community may be defined by its *place* or geopolitical boundaries, which often are used to determine the location of service delivery (Vollman, Anderson, & McFarlane, 2004). **Geopolitical boundaries** refer to both *geographic boundaries* such as mountains, rivers, or lakes, and *political boundaries* such as program or agency service districts. **Aggregate communities** refer to groups of people with common interests, culture, beliefs, or goals. More recently, CHNs also have begun to examine **virtual communities**, where members meet in various internet communities—such as chat rooms, MySpace, and Facebook—to share their common interests.

Community Functions

Communities, though unique, carry out various functions to sustain the day-to-day livelihood of their residents. These **community functions** include provision of:

- space and infrastructure for housing, schools, recreation, government, and health and social service;

- employment and income, including productivity and distribution through consumption of goods, trading, and economic growth;

- security, protection, and law enforcement to protect the public from crime;

- participation, socialization, and networking for all community members; and

- linkages with other community systems for opportunities for growth and capacity building.

Community Dynamics

Community functions are supported by three interactive **community dynamics**: effective communication, leadership, and decision making (Clemen-Stone, Eigsti, & McGuire, 2002).

Communication Competent communities possess strong and cohesive vertical, horizontal, and diagonal patterns of communication among the community key partners. *Vertical communication* enables communities to link to larger communities or to those with higher decision-making power. *Horizontal communication* allows the community to connect to and work collaboratively with its own members, environment, and other service systems. *Diagonal communication* reinforces the cohesiveness and communication of all system components, both horizontally and vertically, and helps reduce the silo effects when communication is done only vertically and horizontally.

Leadership Formal and informal leaders lead their members by influencing the decision-making process, using their status and position in the community. *Formal leaders* are elected official politicians such as mayors, members of parliament, or the prime minister. *Informal leaders* are those with prominent positions in the community, such as religious leaders, executives or representatives of community organizations or professionals, elders of community groups, philanthropists, or local heroes.

Decision Making Formal leaders use government policies to guide their decision making for the community, while informal leaders use their status to influence community groups and to effect change. Based on community needs, these leaders collaborate and negotiate with community groups to advocate for optimal change.

Competent community dynamics foster public participation, mutual support, and community action to promote community growth and ultimately healthy communities. What, then, does a healthy community look like? See the box "Characteristics of Healthy Communities."

SELECTED MODELS AND FRAMEWORKS OF COMMUNITY HEALTH NURSING PRACTICE

CHNs use models and frameworks to systematically collect data and analyze the relationships of various data components. The selected model or framework for practice must be easy to use and reflect one's practice philosophy. A number of existing nursing models and frameworks focus only on individual and not community care. This section briefly describes those frameworks commonly used in community nursing practice.

Characteristics of Healthy Communities

- Clean and safe physical environment
- Conservation of natural environment and resources
- Affordable and adequate access to food, water, housing, recreation, and transportation
- Accessible and quality health and social services
- Opportunities for education and skill development
- Robust economy with high employment rate
- Peace and low crime rates
- Supportive family and work life
- Strong sense of community belonging
- Strong culture, heritage, and spiritual beliefs
- Equity, social justice, and diversity
- Citizen participation in decision-making
- Committed leadership
- Healthy public policy

Source: Adapted from Ontario Healthy Communities Coalition. (2003). What makes a community healthy? *Retrieved November 12, 2006, from http://www.healthycommunities.on.ca/about_us/healthy_community.htm.*

Community-as-Partner Model

Vollman et al. (2004) described community and nursing process as the two main attributes in their community-as-partner model. The *community attribute* is the **community assessment wheel**, which shows that a community comprises nine interacting subsystems: physical environment, education, safety, transportation, politics and government, health and social services, communication, economy, and culture and religion. At the core of this community assessment wheel are the community residents, who have their unique history, demographics, values, and beliefs.

The nursing attribute reflects Betty Neuman's stress adaptation model, which is derived from the general systems theory. Within the community are the *lines of resistance* or strengths that protect the community from harm or threats. Surrounding the community are the *normal lines of defence* that reflect the normal state of health attained by the community. *Flexible lines of defence* form the outer layer around the community. They serve as a buffer zone that represents the community's temporary health response to stressors. These stressors create tension-producing stimuli and may, in turn, penetrate the various lines of defence surrounding the community, affecting the system equilibrium. CHNs assess and analyze the degree of reaction to the stressors experienced by the community and implement purposeful primary, secondary, and tertiary interventions to promote client optimal health.

Epidemiologic Framework

CHNs may use the *epidemiologic triangle* (host–environment–agent) to examine the frequency and distribution of a disease or health condition in the population being studied. They determine *what* the community is, *who* is affected (host), *where* and *when* the condition occurred (environment), and *why* and *how* (agent) it occurred. They may also use the "web of causation" to study the chains of causation and their effects on a health problem. (See Chapter 8.)

Community Capacity Approach

Capacity building is a process that strengthens the ability of an individual, organization, community, or health system to develop and implement health promotion initiatives and sustain positive health outcomes over time (Joffres et al., 2004). It involves organizational development, human resource development, leadership, partnership, resource allocation, and policy formulation. Optimal capacity building is realized when the community is committed to change, has resources to draw from, and has a strong infrastructure to support its functions and dynamics (Sahay, 2004). According to McKnight and Kretzmann (1997), a capacity-building approach is about building community strengths and not community deficits. A *community assets map* may be used to outline the assets and capacity of the community and identify strengths and potential resources for interventions. Data for creating the community assets map include skills and experiences of individuals and organizations, services, and physical and financial resources within and outside the community.

Community Health Promotion Model

Over the past four decades, health promotion research has supported that approximately 25% of the health of the population is attributed to the health care system and the remaining 75% is determined by a multiplicity of factors that include social and economic environments (50%), biological and genetic endowment (15%), and physical environments (10%) (Kirby, 2002). The *community health promotion model* (Figure 11.1) therefore incorporates the four health fields (Lalonde, 1974) and determinants of health (Public Health Agency of Canada [PHAC], 2003) to assess the health of the community and uses Epp's (1986) health promotion strategies, the Ottawa Charter of Health Promotion (World Health Organization [WHO], Canadian Public Health Association, & Health and Welfare Canada, 1986), and primary health care principles (WHO, 1978) to guide community planning, intervention, and evaluation. (See Chapters 6, 7, and 13.) Nursing process is an integral part of the Community Health Promotion Model and is used to systematically assess, plan for, intervene in, and evaluate the health of the community.

The Community Health Promotion Model provides a holistic approach to promoting the health of the population so that a higher quality of community life and equity in health can

FIGURE 11.1 Community Health Promotion Model

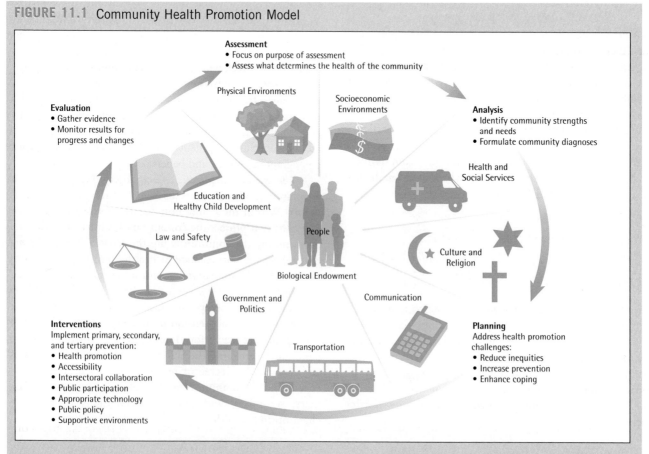

Credit: Camillia Matuk.

be attained. It recognizes that a community's health is impacted by more than just genetics, health care services, and lifestyle risk factors such as poor nutrition, lack of physical activity, and tobacco use. It emphasizes the importance of social determinants of health or social and economic factors in influencing the health of the community. These factors include employment, housing, food, education, childhood years, workplace safety, social inclusion, and access to health systems. They impact how people cope with their environment and thereby influence health inequities among people of various social positions within and between communities and countries (PHAC, 2004; Raphael, 2004; WHO, 2006). For example, a young single mother's decision to feed a high-carbohydrate diet to her children may not be her poor lifestyle choice, but rather her inability to meet her family's nutritional needs because of her low education and income and lack of family support and resources. Community health nursing process using the Community Health Promotion Model is described below.

COMMUNITY HEALTH NURSING PROCESS

As depicted in the Community Health Promotion Model, the *process of community health nursing* is continuous and cyclical; it consists of four phases: assessment, planning, implementation, and evaluation. CHNs may enter at any of these phases, but must first determine the purpose or goal of their nursing involvement. This goal-oriented activity enables CHNs to critically analyze the problem or issue, make inferences on the implications and consequences of the problems or issues, formulate community nursing diagnoses, plan and implement the interventions, and evaluate the outcomes. This chapter focuses on community assessment and related tools. Please refer to Chapter 13 for community planning, intervention, and evaluation.

Community Assessment

Community assessment is an ongoing quantitative and qualitative systematic appraisal of the community. It can be a comprehensive process because of the complexity of community functions and dynamics. Some key questions that guide the beginning steps of community assessment are:

- What is the purpose of my community assessment and why is it needed?
- Who and where is my target population?
- What are the characteristics of my community?
- What information about the community do I need to know and where can I obtain this information?
- What approaches or techniques should I use to get my community data?
- What are my resources or constraints to complete this community assessment (e.g., time, political environment, expertise, labour, and cost)?
- Whose community and whose needs are being assessed?
- Am I meeting the community *needs* or community *wants*?

Purpose of Community Assessment

Community assessment must be guided by the purpose of the assessment. The reason for community assessment may be one or a combination of environmental scan, needs assessment, problem investigation, and/or resource evaluation.

Environmental Scan The most preliminary and fundamental assessment of the community is an **environmental scan**, in which one scans the overall environment through a **windshield survey**. CHNs can drive around the neighbourhood or take a walking tour, and use their senses of sight, touch, hearing, and smell to collect information and form their preliminary assessment of their community. They can see the people, the housing conditions, the geography, and the physical layout of various services in the community. During a walking tour, CHNs can listen to what languages people speak to one another and what concerns them during their daily conversations in their neighbourhood cafés or markets. They can smell the air quality or taste the water, and they can feel the oppression or friendliness of the people. By scanning the environment, CHNs can familiarize themselves with their work environment and connect people to the resources and environment in which they live. Windshield surveys are best done at two different times of day and on different days of the week for data comparison purposes.

Needs Assessment Appropriate and cost-effective services that meet the health needs of the population are based on the community's needs, not on its unrealistic wants or desires. **Needs** are what the community perceives as the gap between its current situation and desired situation. To perform a needs assessment, CHNs must (a) investigate the nature of the needs, (b) determine whether the expressed needs represent the opinions of the community, and (c) determine whether the community is willing and has the resources to take action.

Problem Investigation Problem investigations are done specifically in response to a problem or concern. For example, with an outbreak of E. coli, tuberculosis, or sexually transmitted infections in a community, CHNs investigate the occurrence and distribution of the disease, explore the roots or causes of the problems and their effects, and develop plans to respond appropriately.

Resource Evaluation To be financially accountable, service providers are expected to plan for cost-effective, efficient, and seamless services through resource allocation and re-allocation. **Resource evaluation** involves the assessment and evaluation of existing community resources and services. This includes an examination of the adequacy of human, financial, and physical resources, community partnerships, service utilization, gaps and duplications, affordability, and accessibility to the target populations.

Components in Community Assessment

Various community health nursing practice models may view the community differently, but they all study the basic community components or subsystems as follows:

Community History and Perception Understanding the past allows the CHN to build on existing strengths and avoid repeating the same failures. Areas for examination include history of the issues of concern and community actions taken in the past. The perceptions of the residents on the community issues; the attitudes of officials and local politicians; and the community's attitudes, beliefs, and felt needs for health, education, and health care services should be specifically explored.

Population The very core of any community is people. A **population** is a diverse group of people or aggregates residing within the boundaries of a community. A group refers to two or more people, while an **aggregate** is a group of people based on shared common interests, demographics, cultural heritages, and socioeconomic and education levels. Population and aggregates are terms commonly used interchangeably. A **target population** refers to the population for whom nursing intervention is intended. **Population at risk** refers to a group of individuals who have a high probability of developing illness. People who are susceptible to inequity, injury, disease, or premature deaths are described as a **vulnerable or indigent population**. Personal characteristics and health behaviours of the aggregates or populations may have negative or positive impacts on their own health status and that of the community. For example, communities with a high number of smokers may not reject the anti-smoking by-law despite the rising rates of chronic respiratory diseases and cancer; and employ-

ees may encourage their peers to attain a healthy weight by joining a weight-loss or walk-fit program in their workplace.

In addition to *biology and genetic endowment,* an understanding of the *composition of the population* by age distribution, sex, marital status, social class, occupation, birth rate, employment, religion, education level, family size, and other factors enables CHNs to assess who their population is in terms of their developmental and situational needs. *Health status data* of the community, such as trends in mortality rates (especially maternal and infant death rates), morbidity rates (e.g., common infectious diseases and chronic conditions), and life expectancy give indications regarding the health of the population. Studying the *rate of population growth or decline* also allows the CHN to examine the population trends and anticipate needed services (e.g., chronic health conditions in the aging population put more demands on home care services). A scenario is to note the aging Canadian population in Figure 11.2 and the recent hospital admission statistics, where 59% (67 876) of the fall-related hospital admissions were for people over 65 years of age (Canadian Institute for Health Information [CIHI], 2004). Such community data should alert the CHN to consider fall prevention and strengthening community support services as priority interventions for elderly clients living alone in their homes.

People tend to reside in areas for a variety of reasons: proximity to their employment and extended family, accessibility to education, amenities, recreational facilities, crime

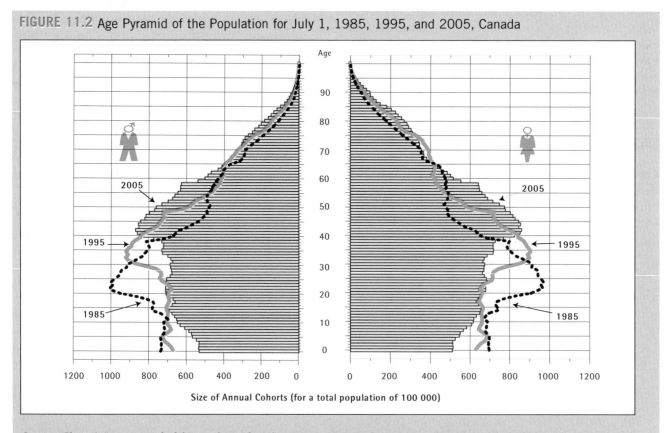

FIGURE 11.2 Age Pyramid of the Population for July 1, 1985, 1995, and 2005, Canada

Sources: Chart 4: "Age pyramid of the population for July 1, 1985, 1995, and 2005, Canada," adapted from the Statistics Canada publication "Annual Demographic Statistics," 2005, Catalogue 91-213, released April 4, 2006, page 6: http://www.statscan.ca/english/freepub/91-213-XIB/0000591-213-XIB.pdf.

rate, political reasons, and climate. The *density of the population* may shift with time and demographic makeup. For example, an influx of refugees or unemployed workers into a community may be driven by economic or political changes.

Communities are not static. The needs, characteristics, makeup, and health status of the population also change over time within its physical and social environments. For example, a surge in a community's unemployment rate may result in high family stress, a poor economy, and the relocation of many young people to other communities for work; strengthening community and social services for these communities would then become a health priority. Similarly, promoting healthy lifestyles and community support to combat social isolation and poverty is much needed in the remote northern communities because of their higher rates of smoking, obesity, suicide, and alcohol use compared with the nation's averages (Statistics Canada, 2002). CHNs must clearly identify the target population in relation to the scale of the problem experienced by the community as a whole; collect relevant population data; and examine, compare, and estimate the health outcomes and risk factors within the community or at the regional, provincial, and/or national conditions.

Boundaries The boundary of the community refers to where the target population lives, works, plays, and learns. Healthy communities do not exist in isolation. They are separated or connected to other communities by physical or artificial boundaries. **Physical boundaries** include geographic boundaries such as mountains, valleys, roads, lakes, rivers, or oceans. **Artificial boundaries** include (a) *political boundaries,* which depict governance of various townships, counties, cities, and provinces; and (b) *situational boundaries,* which are governed by specific circumstances such as zoning for school children, traffic patterns, or smoking areas. Health communities have permeable boundaries for the exchange of services between communities.

Physical Environments The health of the people in a community is affected by levels of exposure to contaminants in their immediate environment. For example, air and water pollution may cause respiratory problems, digestive problems, cancer, and birth defects; geographic isolation may lead to poor access to health services and subsequent inequity in health status (Federal, Provincial, Territorial Advisory Committee on Population Health [FPTACPH], 1999). Physical environmental factors that affect community health include:

- Biological and chemical characteristics: vegetation and forestry, animals and insects, bacteria and other microorganisms, food and water supply, chemicals, and toxic substances.
- Physical characteristics: geography, climate, and natural resources such as soil, mountains, valleys, rivers, lakes, oceans, water, air, oil, and designs of communities, buildings, and roads.

Socioeconomic Environments Despite strong economic growth and federal surpluses in 2000, the rate of child poverty in Canada rose from 14.9% in 1989 to 15.6% in 2002. One in

six children lives in poverty; only half of all Canadians have full-time employment. The income gap between the rich and the poor is wider than ever. Low-income families pay between 30% and 50% of their income toward rent. In 2004, 41% of food bank users were children. Income equality, employment, housing, and food security all affect people's health and their sense of well-being (Campaign 2000, 2005; Raven & Frank, 2004).

Income and Social Status Income and social status are positively associated with education level, good health, and quality of life (PHAC, 2003). People with low income tend to have low education and reside in geared-to-income housing. They are in poorer health than the well-educated professionals whose income level allows them to live in middle- to upper-class locales. However, upward or downward mobility can be seen in various social classes during economic turmoil. High employment rates, new housing, and business developments are common signs for communities with a healthy economy and/or industrial capacity.

Employment and Working Conditions Employment and working conditions significantly affect one's physical, mental, and social health and general well-being. People who are employed in a safe workplace experience less stress, live longer, and have fewer health problems.

Social Supports and Networks Early hospital discharge, an aging population, and rising chronic diseases have led to the need for strong formal and informal social supports and networks in communities. Research shows that there is a positive relationship between social support and health status and perceived health (Larni & Johnson, 2004; PHAC, 2003).

Diversity and Social Inclusion Healthy communities embrace harmony, safety, and diversity as the social norm. For example, schools instill cultural awareness and sensitivity in young children thereby reducing racism or bullying; service agencies provide classes to strengthen parenting skills and promote family relationships, which indirectly prevents family violence; and neighbourhood watches reduce crime rates. Social inclusion by gender, age, ability, sexual orientation, race, ethnicity, and religion will create a community where people feel they belong and so strive to reach their full potential as members (PHAC, 2003).

Recreation Recreation provides a form of socialization and a means for healthy physical and mental activity for people outside of their family, school, and work life. CHNs can assess where and how people spend their time together after school or work, whether local recreational facilities/activities are appropriate to people of all ages, and whether these activities are accessible and affordable to the public.

Education and Healthy Child Development Health status is directly associated with levels of education and socioeconomic status. Education provides people the life skills needed for their day-to-day living and the technical skills for their career advancement. Canadians with low literacy skills are more likely to be poor and unemployed and suffer from poor health than those with higher levels of education (FPTACPH, 1999).

Educational institutions are ideal settings in which children can learn to adopt societal norms and health behaviours in their early years. Youth with positive assets such as parental nurturing and monitoring, school engagement, volunteerism, and peer connections are more likely to report high self-worth and healthy lifestyles (CIHI, 2005).

Canadian Research Box 11.1

Yiu Matuk, L., & Ruggirello, T. (2007). Culture connection project: Promoting multiculturalism in elementary schools. *CJPH, 98*(1), 26–29.

This school-based community project aimed to promote multiculturalism among grade-school students through drama education in Windsor-Essex County, Ontario. Participants included a total of 665 Grade 3 to 6 students from 6 targeted schools, with 158 lead-class students representing each school. Using a non-experimental design approach, cultural themes from group discussions with each lead class were developed into an interactive drama performance and performed for all participants. A follow-up drama workshop was offered to each lead class one week after the drama performance. All students completed a questionnaire before and after the drama performance and after the drama workshop. With the enhanced awareness of multiculturalism, lead-class students then developed their own strategies to promote multiculturalism within their own school settings. Statistical analysis on the effects of drama education on students' attitudes toward multiculturalism revealed that drama education was an effective experiential tool for promoting multiculturalism in a school setting. Lead-class students used multi-strategies (murals, cultural trips, puppets, drama, etc.) to promote cultural awareness in their own schools. The key to promoting interracial harmony is to respect and accept individual differences and to broaden the social determinants of health by providing culture safety care.

Discussion Questions:

1. Discuss the benefits of using drama education to promote multiculturalism in schools.

2. Why is it important to promote multiculturalism in schools or communities?

3. Discuss the implications of social exclusion (such as racism or discrimination) on health.

Healthy physical, cognitive, and emotional development in children is determined by effects ranging from preconception health and prenatal care to the quality of parental nurturing and supervision. Disadvantaged children tend to not perform well in school. Low-income children are at greater risk for poor health. Poor early childhood developmental characteristics, such as low birth weight or poor nutrition, can delay language or brain development and compromise physical and mental health through to adulthood (CIHI, 2005; Graham, 2004).

With 65% to 85% of Canadian mothers working in dual-income families, limited childcare spaces, poverty, and wider income gaps (Friendly, 2002), CHNs must attend to more than just teaching parenting skills when caring for families in community settings; they must be responsive to the adequacy of social policy surrounding issues such as parental leaves, national childcare policy, unemployment benefits, and social assistance, and the impact of these factors on the health needs of families and children.

Culture and Religion   Canada is second to Australia in terms of vast numbers of people of different races or ethnic groups, colours, and religions, and one in every five Canadians belongs to a visible minority group (Badets, 2003). **Culture** is the way we think, live, act, and feel. Various ethnocultural groups in many Canadian communities strive to preserve their heritages through their own social events, language classes, and educational programs. Visible minority or new Canadians with language and cultural barriers are often alienated from the mainstream society and experience inequities in health from poverty, social isolation, bullying, and poor access to care (e.g., high unemployment rate in newcomers and high incidence of suicide and diabetes in Aboriginal people) (Craig, 2004; Hyman, 2001). Despite effort from the government to promote multiculturalism, many ethnic groups tend to live and work in their own ethnic communities to avoid marginalization. CHNs can address the diversity and health needs of the community population and how the various cultural practices may affect its health beliefs and practices. (See Chapter 20.)

Religion offers a form of spiritual support for many people, especially those in crisis. Some religions can affect the health care practices of various members of the population. For example, Jehovah's Witnesses refuse blood transfusions, and Muslims and Jews require adjustment of family, school, and work routines during their religious celebrations and prayers.

Health and Social Services   Most people, whether sick or healthy, seek health services at some time in their lives. Health services include primary, secondary, and tertiary care, ranging from promotion and protection of health to hospital, rehabilitative, and palliative care services. Social services including welfare, employment, mothers' allowance, and disability pensions are examples of assistance for those who are single parents, unemployed, or have physical and/or mental disabilities. An infrastructure of a wide range of health and social services can help people emerge from their crises, and service availability alone will not improve the health status of the community.

Territorialism and unwillingness to share information or resources among community agencies for fear of losing funding to support their own programs often result in fragmentation and/or duplication of services. CHNs assess what and how health and social services are used and delivered to their communities, and whether service gaps, unmet needs, duplications, and strengths exist. They work with the community to make these services better coordinated, accessible, affordable, and known to the people in need. Assessment of services needs can also be made by examining individual lifestyle choices such as physical activity, healthy eating, healthy weights, tobacco, alcohol, and drug use, workplace safety, gambling, safe sex, HIV testing, and multiple risk behaviours. Adoption of personal health practices and coping skills can prevent disease and promote personal health. How these skills are practised is influenced by individuals' culture, social relationships, sense of belonging, and the socioeconomic environments in which they live, work, learn, and play (FPTACPH, 1999; PHAC, 2003).

Transportation   An established and reliable transportation system is essential to ensure that community members have access to all the services they need. CHNs assess the transportation needs for rural clients, the poor, the frail elderly, and those with physical limitations, and seek ways to mobilize local resources to meet their needs (e.g., reduced taxi fare for seniors or volunteer drivers).

Communication   Effective and efficient communication is crucial for building supportive and collaborative relationships and thereby the delivery of quality care to community members. In addition to conveying clear messages, the methods, location, and timing of communication are also pivotal in the communication process. The common modes of formal and informal communication for community members are usually the local newspapers, newsletters, notice boards, radio, television, flyers, and community forums.

Governments and Politics   Governments provide an organized structure that sets policies to ensure all essential services are in place and will meet the basic needs and goals of the community. They provide formal leadership to work with communities and reinforce compliance to their policies (e.g., smoke-free regulations). While formal leaders hold authority in making decisions, informal leaders and community members often have the power to implement them. CHNs must examine the extent to which a community engages and empowers its community members in making decisions on issues that affect their health.

CHNs must be aware of the existing government policies, work with both formal and informal leaders, and be involved in the decision-making process. They can also assess evidence of community development, relationships between the community and other agencies, the degree of cooperation or conflict between agencies and decision-making bodies, and the effectiveness of the decisions made.

Law and Safety   Governments set rules and regulations as *law*. Such crimes as homicides, assaults, and thefts are symptoms of family and community response to stress (e.g., family violence, unemployment, and drug use). *Safety* is a prerequisite to quality of life. Communities grow and prosper economically in peaceful times, and wealth therefore is the most important determinant of health (Health Canada, Statistics Canada, & the Canadian Institute for Health Information, 1999; Lynch et al., 2004). Peace is achieved when society has law and order. CHNs can assess whether residents are feeling safe in their community by examining the occurrences of crimes (i.e., types, rates, and locations) and collaborating with the police in crime prevention to create a safe place for people to live in.

Sources of Community Data

Because communities have multi-system components, data concerning them can be abundant and complex. Therefore, the data collected for community assessment must be realistic,

and credible sources and appropriate data collection techniques must be used to ensure the validity of the assessment. There are two main types of community data:

- *quantitative data,* such as facts and figures that are commonly found in population statistics or health status reports, and
- *qualitative data,* such as statements or opinions gathered from windshield surveys, focus groups, open forums, key informants, or public meetings.

Generally, existing data should be examined before gathering new data. New data can be gathered from surveys and meetings with community residents and leaders. With today's sophisticated computerized information-management systems, much of the existing data is now easily accessible on the internet and in local libraries.

Common community data may be obtained from these sources:

- Statistics Canada (e.g., for census data and vital statistics);
- Local, provincial, and federal health departments and the Canadian Institute for Health Information (e.g., vital statistics related to determinants of health and diseases);
- Municipal planning departments (e.g., housing and business and industrial developments);
- Environment Canada (e.g., environmental indices);
- Police departments (e.g., crime statistics and trends);
- Local organizations, such as hospitals, school boards, and agencies (e.g., annual reports on service delivered);
- Municipal traffic departments and provincial transportation departments (e.g., traffic accidents and resulting injuries and deaths); and
- Workers' Compensation Board (e.g., work-related injuries and deaths).

Methods for Community Data Collection

Once the needed data are identified for the purpose of community assessment, CHNs decide how best to obtain the data within the resources available and the time constraints. In addition to *record review* and *observation methods* such as windshield surveys and walking tours mentioned earlier, they may observe the stakeholders and/or residents through community surveys, community forums, and focus groups.

Community Surveys   **Community surveys** are a series of questions addressing the issue(s) or population(s) being studied. They can produce a broad range of data from a representative sample population in a short period of time. They can be conducted via regular mail, email, telephone, or face-to-face interviews. The data collected provide a snapshot of the population being studied and may be generalized to describe the larger population. Major community surveys (e.g., the National Population Health Survey and the Canadian Community Health Survey) are usually repeated every five years to examine changes in behaviours over time.

Community Forums **Community forums** are public meetings in which community members discuss issues of concern with their community leaders or decision makers. They provide a two-way dialogue through which members can share their experiences and opinions. They are usually held in neighbourhood community centres, schools, or service clubs. This approach is an inexpensive way to collect community data. The people who attend these meetings are either directly involved in or affected by the topic being discussed. Community forum topics may include the impact of a school closure, service restructuring in a community, or crime reduction in a neighbourhood. Often, one person or a few people may dominate these forum discussions; their opinions may not represent the majority's view, and the purpose of the forum may be derailed. CHNs must use effective facilitation skills to elicit maximum public response for the priority issues or concerns being addressed in these community forums.

Focus Groups **Focus groups** are small group interviews with an average of 8 to 12 people that usually last 1 to 2 hours. There may be a series of focus groups on the same topic across the community, region, province, or nation. Though similar in format and low in cost compared with the community forums, focus groups are smaller in scale and the participants are more homogeneous in their characteristics or experience related to the topic being discussed. These participants may be aggregates such as women, school children, elderly, or caregivers, or community leaders such as key informants, politicians, or health care providers. Focus groups provide opportunities for *community dialogue* by allowing people to openly exchange experiences and express opinions.

No single source or method can provide all the assessment data on a community. CHNs must use multiple strategies to collect the needed data. Epidemiological and research skills are particularly important for analyzing and interpreting vital statistics and figures. (See Chapters 8 and 13.) Community data collection can be an overwhelming experience, but it need not be a time-consuming process. The key is to focus on the purpose of the assessment and to know what the health indictors are and where and how to collect the needed data. Table 11.1 lists selected population health indicators that describe the characteristics of the community or health system.

Population Health

The concept of population health reflects the WHO's definition of health and builds on the traditional practice of health promotion and public health in which the focus is on preventive activities and disease management. What makes people healthy? The health of a population is measured by health status indicators and is influenced by broad social, economic, and physical environments; personal health practices; individual capacity and coping skills; human biology; early childhood development; and health service. **Population health** aims to maintain and improve the health status of (1) the entire population (i.e., community-focused), (2) a specific target population (i.e., systems-focused), or (3) the individuals (i.e., individual-focused) within the community (Minnesota Department of Health, 2001). It strives to reduce inequities in health status between population groups by addressing what determines their health (PHAC, 2002a).

Healthy populations contribute to the overall productivity and quality of life in the community and to a sustainable and equitable health care system. Based on this belief, the Public Health Agency of Canada (2002b) developed a **population health template** with eight key elements and corresponding action steps for health practitioners, educators, and researchers. (See Appendix 11A and Chapter 5.) Implementing a population approach involves the process of analyzing the health issue, setting priorities, taking action, evaluating results, and gaining stronger evidence/developing knowledge.

Although providing care to the community or population is not new to CHNs (see Chapter 1), there are various personal and system barriers that challenge CHNs to conduct population health promotion. (See Canadian Research Box 11.2.) Until CHNs are able to overcome these barriers, the "noble goal of developing a health care system that emphasizes health promotion . . . will never be attainable, and PHNs [CHNs] will never have an opportunity to play the leadership role in health promotion that has been envisioned for them" (Cohen, 2006, p. 65).

Canadian Research Box 11.2

Cohen, B. (2006). Barriers to population-focused health promotion: The experience of public health nurses in the province of Manitoba. *CJNR, 38*(3), 52–67.

This descriptive study explored the perceptions of 24 public health nurse (PHNs) on the nature of their population-focused health promotion practice in three geographically and demographically diverse regions. Results from the standardized, open-ended interviews revealed remarkable similarities in PHNs' perceptions about their practice. Most barriers identified were related to individual PHNs' attitudes, professional education, organizational infrastructure and culture, and health system constraints. While PHNs have a leadership role to play in population-focused health promotion, many PHNs in this study revealed that they were more comfortable with providing individual and family-focused care than advocacy or population-focused care. Other identified barriers included lack of educational preparation for population-focused care, lack of human resources, high workload, and reluctance from the staff/managers to buy in to the importance of population-focused health promotion. The author called for a concerted effort to address these identified barriers in order to truly deliver population-focused health promotion.

Discussion Questions:

1. Discuss what might be the barriers in providing population-focused health promotion at the individual level, organizational level, and community level.

2. Discuss ways to overcome the barriers identified in the previous question.

3. Discuss how your nursing program can better prepare you to practise population-focused health promotion.

TABLE 11.1
Selected Population Health Indicators and Data Sources

Health Status

Well-being	Self-rated health, self-esteem
Health conditions	Body mass index, asthma, arthritis, rheumatism, pain, diabetes, hypertension, low birth weight, cancer incidence, injuries
Living and working conditions	Education, income, labour force, housing, crime
Personal resource	Life stress, social support
Human functions	Life expectancy, functional health status, participation and activity limitation
Death	Potential years of life lost, mortality by selected causes

Non-medical Determinants of Health

Health behaviours	Physical activity, breastfeeding practices, fruit and vegetable consumption, type and behaviour of smoker, frequency of heavy drinking
Environmental factors	Exposure to secondhand smoke

Health System Performance

Acceptability	Patient satisfaction
Accessibility	Pap smear, influenza vaccination
Appropriateness	C-section
Effectiveness	Readmissions
Efficiency	Expected compared to actual stay
Safety	In-hospital hip fracture

Community and Health System Characteristics

Community	Teen pregnancy, visible minority, population estimates, urban and rural population
Health system	Hip replacement, hysterectomy
Resources	Doctor rate

Source: Adapted from Health Indicators: Data tables and maps, *from the Statistics Canada publication "Health Indicators," Catalogue 82-221, 2006, no.1, released June 13, 2006: http://www.statcan.ca/english/freepub/82-221-XIE/2006001/tables.htm#hs.*

Case Study: What Does Health Mean to People in a Slum Area?

Study the community scene illustrated in Figure 11.3. List and rank what you think the people in this community would say was needed to improve their health. In a group of 4 to 6 students, compare the individual rankings and discuss the following questions.

Discussion Questions

1. Who are the experts in identifying the local needs of a community? By priority, rank the areas that you feel would improve the health of this community and relate them to the determinants of health.

2. If you were a resident of this community, how would you feel if someone made judgments about your living situation? Why? What do you see as the priority area to improve the health of your community?

3. What data sources and data collection methods would you use to establish a community profile as depicted in this figure?

FIGURE 11.3   A Slum Area

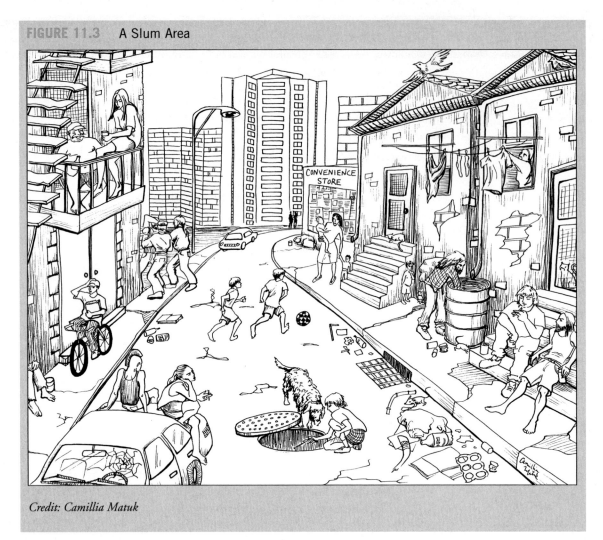

Credit: Camillia Matuk

Risk Assessment   CHNs do not necessarily work with every member in the community. Rather, they assess the conditions of risks and benefits that apply to the entire population or to its significant aggregates and deliver health services to those who are at risk. **Risk** refers to the probability or likelihood that healthy persons exposed to a specific factor will acquire a specific disease. These specific factors, called **risk factors**, can be environmental, lifestyle, and psychosocial factors (e.g., sources of exposure, cultural practices, patterns of behaviours, local concerns, direct impact from the service delivery system) or biological factors (e.g., age, sex, or genetic makeup). When doing **risk assessment,** CHNs identify and target clients who are most likely to contract the disease or develop unhealthy behaviours, and assess attributes that affect or potentially affect their health. For example, teens have a higher risk than adults of contracting STIs or getting pregnant as they tend to experiment more with their sexuality; similarly, older adults are more likely to have falls than are younger adults due to the aging process.

Community Analysis and Nursing Diagnoses

The purpose of data analysis is to identify actual and potential community strengths and needs that are relevant to the improvement of existing health services. Competent **community analysis** relies on a clear conceptual or philosophical understanding of health, community dynamics, and community health nursing. Community data are systematically summarized into categories and compared with other relative community systems for significance; inferences are then made to formulate **community nursing diagnoses**.

Community nursing diagnoses and nursing diagnoses are similar. They differ in that community nursing diagnoses are broad, addressing a community or aggregate, whereas nursing diagnoses address individuals or families. All communities have strengths as well as problems. Community health nursing diagnoses should therefore include both problem and wellness diagnoses, with statements consisting of the following components:

- The specific aggregate or target group;
- The actual or potential unhealthy or healthy response/situation that a nurse can change;
- The etiology or cause for the unhealthy or healthy response/situation; and
- The characteristics (i.e., signs and symptoms) or evidence that describe the response or situation.

There is no classification or taxonomy for community-oriented diagnoses to date, but this should not deter CHNs from developing their own community diagnoses. Their community analysis will help develop and organize nursing knowledge and further the continued development of nursing diagnoses. Table 11.2 illustrates examples of nursing diagnoses formulation.

Planning, Implementation, and Evaluation

Once the community needs are prioritized, nursing interventions will be devised to resolve those needs. The intervention plan must address the *challenges* to achieving health for all: reducing inequalities, increasing prevention, and enhancing community coping (Epp, 1986). (See Chapter 6.) The goals and objectives for intervention are derived from the community nursing diagnoses. Nursing interventions include pri-

mary, secondary, and tertiary preventive services that reflect the five principles of primary health care: accessibility, promotion and prevention, inter-sectoral cooperation, appropriate technology, and public participation (WHO, 1978). (See Chapter 7 and Figure 7.1.) To provide population-focused health promotion, strategies used may include but are not limited to advocacy for healthy public policy, strengthening of community action, and the creation of supportive environments (CHNAC, 2003; Epp, 1986; Raphael, 2004).

Though some CHNs, such as home health nurses, may focus on direct-care services to individuals and families, public health nurses apply a different set of skills for population-focused care. Specific public health interventions include consultation, counselling, health teaching, case management, referral and follow-up, screening, outreach, disease surveillance, policy development and enforcement, social marketing, advocacy, community organizing, coalition building, and collaboration (CHNAC, 2003; Minnesota Department of Health, 2001). (See Chapter 3.)

TABLE 11.2
Examples of Community Health Nursing Diagnosis

Components of Nursing Diagnosis	Focus Population	Problem or Wellness Diagnosis	Etiology	Characteristics
What do the components mean?	Who is your target group or community?	What is the potential/actual community issue, concern, situation or response you need to manage or intervene?	Why is there this community issue, concern, situation, or response? Identify the causation factors.	How did you make this etiologic inference? Give supporting community data/evidence or manifestations (signs or symptoms).
Example 1	For students in high school	Have a potential for healthy lifestyles	Related to their desire to learn about nutrition and physical activities	As evidenced by integrated school curriculum with an emphasis on healthy lifestyles components
Example 2	Residents in Kent community	Potential dysfunction in value–belief pattern: ethical conflicts between the public and government	Related to introducing users' fees to the health care system	As evidenced by debates and public demonstrations over the need for a two-tiered health care system
Example 3	In west-end community	Optimal waste disposal	Related to effective management of the community recycling system	As evidenced by 98% of utilization of the recycling programs, and 25% reduction of rodents in the city area
Example 4	Among newcomers	Aggregate energy deficit (inadequate income and resources and high family stress level)	Related to inadequate language and skill trades program to prepare newcomers to be employable	As evidenced by high unemployment rates at 25%, unable to find work because of lack of language skills and Canadian work experiences/requirements, high anxiety and stress expressed by family.

Nursing interventions will be successful when the community is fully engaged and empowered throughout the nursing process. At the same time, CHNs themselves must feel empowered to challenge the expectations of the top-down approaches to planning and management. To truly advocate for bottom-up planning, CHNs must possess competent knowledge, skills, critical judgment, and, most importantly, confidence in their practice.

Subjective and objective data collected during the community assessment help form the needed indicators for evaluation of any evidence of success. (See Chapter 13.) Community planning and interventions will be effective when public policy and supportive environments are addressed. Above all, there needs to be *commitment* from the community to work on the identified need or issue.

Community Participatory Tools for Community Planning

A **community participatory approach** is key to community planning. The community decides what makes a need into a priority; who is to take the action; what the action will be; when and how it is to be done; and who, when, and how to do what. Community participatory tools assist community dialogue among the residents, community leaders, government officials, and service providers to help quantify and qualify the health issues, needs, or concerns that they identify (Yiu, 2001). Active participation and sharing of their experiences can empower people to take responsibility and ownership in health and to effect change.

Community Needs Matrix Tool CHNs may use a community needs matrix tool to ask participants to discuss, name, rate, or explain what they perceive to be the most important health problems or the most feasible interventions in their community. The degree of concern about each issue is tallied on a blank chart similar to that in Table 11.3. Table 11.3 indicates that this community is more concerned about accidents than

about pneumonia. CHNs use good listening and facilitation skills to learn what the community has to say about their lived experiences. Through mutual planning, they can also validate the data collected, educate the community, and increase their awareness of their choices of action.

Community Mapping Community mapping is a schematic map of the community indicating the distribution and occurrence of illness, disease, and health; major resources; environmental conditions; and accessibility and barriers to various services. CHNs may ask the community members to look at their accessibility and the resources in their living environment as part of the intervention plan. The participants could use community mapping to express their perceptions and experiences. Figure 11.4 illustrates an example of community map on case distribution of spina bifida.

Present–Future Drawing A present–future drawing (Figure 11.5) can be drawn by the community clients to reflect upon their present situation and what resources and constraints contributed to it, and to visualize how the future might appear. The tool allows the nurse to see where the community wants to go and, hence, to formulate mutual intervention goals and objectives.

TABLE 11.3 Example of the Results of a Community Needs Matrix Tool				
Identified Health Need	Not a Concern	Somewhat Concerned	A Concern	Very Concerned
Accidents	*	***	***	****
Nutrition	*	**	**	****
Pneumonia	*	**	***	*
STIs	*	***	***	*

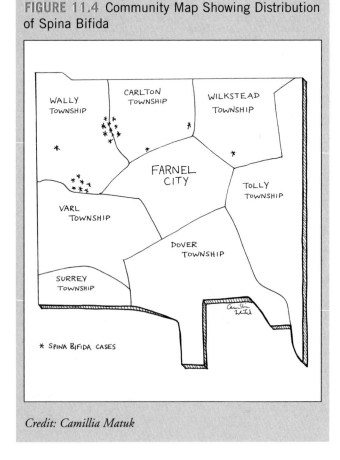

FIGURE 11.4 Community Map Showing Distribution of Spina Bifida

Credit: Camillia Matuk

FIGURE 11.5 Present–Future Drawing

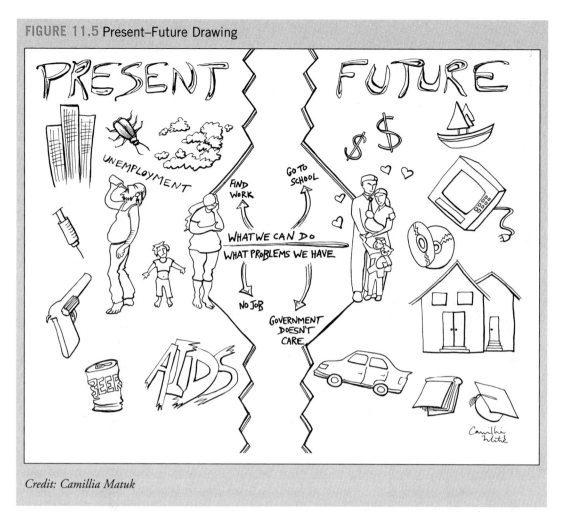

Credit: Camillia Matuk

Community Engagement and Community Governance

Community engagement and community governance are keys to achieving sustainable programs and program accountability, as well as to building community capacity and ownership (Ktpatzer Consulting, 2006). (See Figure 11.6.) **Community engagement** is "a process involving citizens at various levels of participation based on interpersonal communication and trust and a common understanding and purpose" (p. 4). Local community members or representative aggregates start by receiving the information from the health care providers or government, and through consultation, involvement, collaboration, and partnerships they eventually are empowered with the authority to make decisions on issues that affect the health of their own communities. **Community governance** is a "method of community engagement that ensures effective involvement and empowerment of local community representatives in the planning, direction setting and monitoring of health organizations to meet the health needs and priorities of the populations within local neighbourhood communities" (p. 4).

Community Development

Community development is the "process of involving a community in the identification and reinforcement of those aspects of everyday life, culture and political activity which are conducive to health. This might include support for political action to modify the total environment and strengthen resources for healthy living, as well as reinforcing social networks and social support within a community and developing the material resources and economic base available to the community" (Canadian Public Health Association, 1990, p. 19). The community begins with a need or a vision for change. CHNs work in partnership with their communities as they define their own goals, mobilize resources, and develop action plans for collectively identified issues or problems. All the stakeholders are engaged in this consensus building process. Community development involves a range of practices to *improve, strengthen,* and *sustain* community life and local conditions and to enable people, particularly those in disadvantaged situations, to engage in decision making and to achieve control over their circumstances. One example can be

FIGURE 11.6 Community Engagement and Community Governance

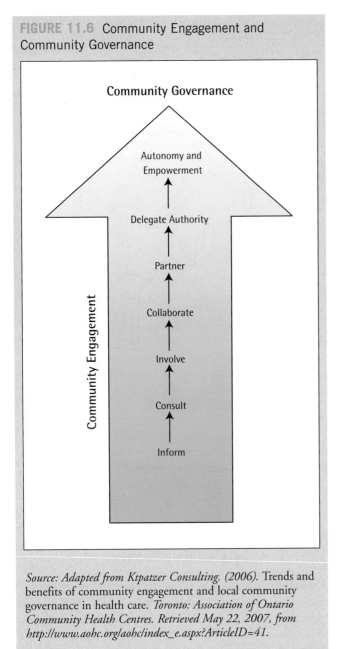

Source: Adapted from Ktpatzer Consulting. (2006). Trends and benefits of community engagement and local community governance in health care. *Toronto: Association of Ontario Community Health Centres. Retrieved May 22, 2007, from http://www.aohc.org/aohc/index_e.aspx?ArticleID=41.*

seen in groups in various urban communities working with governments on health and social issues to provide safe and affordable housing for those who are homeless. Another example is with rural residents, addressing suicide as a community problem and through consensus building and resource mobilization with their stakeholders finding solutions to strengthen community social support and improve mental health for the residents.

Community interventions must be evaluated to measure whether the expected results were achieved and where the successes and problems lie. The steps involved in **community evaluation** (van Marris & King, 2002) are (a) getting ready

to evaluate, (b) engaging stakeholders, (c) assessing resources for the evaluation, (d) designing the evaluation, (e) determining appropriate methods of measurement and procedures, (f) developing a work plan, budget, and timeline for evaluation, (g) collecting data by using agreed-upon methods and procedures, (h) processing and analyzing the data, (i) interpreting and disseminating the results, and (j) taking action.

Successes should be shared with the community so that the work can be sustained within the community and become a model to benefit other communities. Lessons learned from challenges or barriers can teach others to avoid making the same mistakes. Plans should be made for any future changes needed in the community. Interventions should be evaluated and documented to support evidence-based practice. Table 11.4 provides a summary guide that CHNs may use to assess the health of a community and develop a community intervention plan.

Summary

When promoting the health of communities, CHNs use a population approach to work with individuals, families, aggregates, populations, and the community. They are expected to demonstrate essential knowledge, skills, and attitude as expected in the *core competencies* for public health practice in Canada (PHAC, 2007). (See Appendix B for core competency statements and practice examples.) Problems identified at the individual and family levels (such as poverty and teen pregnancy) may call for further actions at the system or community level. CHNs must be able to conduct accurate community assessment before they can provide community health promotion.

An understanding of the community makeup and dynamics will guide the implementation of the community nursing process. Sound community assessment requires the CHNs to know the purpose of the assessment, the techniques to use, the data to collect, and where to collect them. The use of a population health approach to community health promotion allows the nurse to look beyond the traditional delivery of health services and to examine various determinants of health, including how social and political environments impact community health. Community analysis requires CHNs to work with the community to analyze the data and devise a mutual plan for community action and evaluation. Throughout this community health nursing process, CHNs may use various community participatory tools to interact with community stakeholders and population groups to address the community's health needs. They must understand the importance of community engagement, community governance, and community development to advocate positive change. If CHNs are to improve the health of the community and achieve social justice and health for all, they must display competent leadership in community health promotion.

TABLE 11.4
Guide to Community Health Nursing Process

QUESTIONS/AREAS FOR CONSIDERATION	DATA/OBSERVATIONS
A. ASSESSMENT	
1. Purpose of Community Assessment, Target Group, and Location • For environmental scan, needs assessment, problem investigation, or resource evaluation? • Rationale for the assessment in relation to the target group? • Who is the target group? What are their characteristics? • Boundaries where target group resides? • Supportive evidence for the health needs of the target group?	
2. Community Historical and Perception • Previous history of community actions by local groups or government? • Perceptions of the residents on the community issues, problems, attitudes, beliefs, felt needs?	

3. Population
• Total and composition of the population in the community: age group distribution, gender, marital status, birth rate, family size, etc.?
• Density and rate of population growth: increased or decreased?
• Health status
  – Mortality rates: Overall, age specific, and cause-specific
  – Morbidity rate for specific diseases, their incidence and prevalence
  – Comparison of mortality and morbidity rates with previous years, with regional, provincial and national rates
  – Life expectancy and trends
  – Biologic and genetic endowment
  – Health status: indicators and influencing factors related to purpose of assessment (e.g., nutrition, immunization, lifestyles, stress, sexually transmitted infections, unplanned pregnancy, prenatal care, emergency care, primary, secondary, and tertiary care, etc.)	

4. Physical Environments
• Location: boundaries, geography, climate, plants, and animals posing threats to health; percentage of urban or rural area?
• Housing: type, condition, slum areas, sanitation, adequacy, crowding?
• Shopping facilities: types, location, and accessibility?
• Safety
  – Crime rates, types, and where? Feeling of safety?
  – Police and relationships with the community?
• Water supply: quality and adequacy?
• Sanitation: sewage and waste disposal?	

5. Socioeconomic Environments
• Income levels: poverty rate, number receiving social assistance?
• Social status and mobility
  – Percentages for each social class?
  – Patterns and impact of mobility on health needs and health service planning?
• Employment and working conditions
  – Major industries and business establishments?
  – Employment rate, primary occupations?
  – Occupational hazards?
  – Safe and supportive worklife?
• Social supports and networks: support groups and community group involvement?
• Social inclusion: embrace diversity and share social experience by gender, sex, sexual orientation, race, ethnicity, and religion?
• Recreation: facilities, affordability, accessibility, and appropriate for all ages?	

→

TABLE 11.4
continued

QUESTIONS/AREAS FOR CONSIDERATION	DATA/OBSERVATIONS

6. Education and Healthy Child Development
• Education: literacy rates, attitudes, and facilities/programs for life skills and technical skills?
  – Peer connection and engagement in school?
  – Relationships to health status and employment?
• Healthy child development: preconception health, prenatal and parenting class, and daycare?	

7. Culture and Religion • Ethnic and racial group composition and subcultures, culture, and languages spoken? • Cultural diversity and tolerance, positive and negative influence on health practices? • Cultural adaptation, perceptions of health? • Religious affiliations and spiritual support and influence on health practices?	

8. Health and Social Services
• Services and community organizations
  – Location, ratios of health workers to rural and urban populations?
  – Number of beds availability and type, health service utilization? Health budgets priority, amount per capita and spending?
  – Provision of primary, secondary, and tertiary care? Service gaps and duplications?
  – Evidence of community engagement and community governance (e.g., inter-sectoral cooperation, health promotion, public participation and appropriate technology used in service delivery)?
  – Available and adequate social assistance to meet community needs?
• Personal health practices and coping skills
  – Healthy lifestyle practices?
  – Effective or maladaptive coping?	

9. Transportation • Type, availability, accessible, affordable, and usage?	

10. Government and Politics
• Communications
  – Methods, timing, and locations of verbal and non-verbal communication (e.g., newspapers, radio, television, flyers, and forums)?
  – Relationships with other organizations, degree of conflict and collaboration?
  – Evidence of interpersonal relationships, commitment, and partnerships?
• Leadership
  – Formal and informal leaders and visions for the community?
  – Power structure, delegations, politics?
• Decision making: effective and efficient process of decision making (e.g., policy formulation, human resources, etc.)?	

B. ANALYSIS **1. Wellness Nursing Diagnoses** • Potential and actual community strengths? **2. Problem Nursing Diagnoses** • Potential and actual community needs and gaps?	
C. PLANNED INTERVENTIONS • Implementation of primary, secondary, and tertiary preventive care focusing on health promotion challenges such as reducing inequities, increasing prevention, and enhancing coping? • Evidence of incorporation of primary health care principles, public policy, and supportive environments in nursing care planning? • Expected outcomes and target dates clearly defined?	
D. EVALUATION • Monitoring of progress and gathering of evidence of success based on outcomes objectives? Lessons learned and knowledge transfer?	

KEY TERMS

community
geopolitical boundaries
aggregate communities
virtual communities
community functions
community dynamics
community assessment wheel
capacity building
community assessment
environmental scan
windshield survey
needs
resource evaluation
population
aggregate
target population
population at risk
vulnerable or indigent population
physical boundaries
artificial boundaries
culture
religion
community surveys
community forums
focus groups
population health
population health template
risk
risk factors
risk assessment
community analysis
community nursing diagnoses
community participatory approach
community engagement
community governance
community development
community evaluation

STUDY QUESTIONS

1. Name four community settings where CHNs work, and describe their role and functions.

2. What are the characteristics of a healthy community?

3. What nursing process skills will you use to promote the health of the community?

4. What assessment components are used when assessing community health?

5. Define population health, community engagement, community governance, community development, and capacity building.

6. Discuss the benefits of community dialogue between community health nurses and Aboriginal communities or any other population groups.

INDIVIDUAL CRITICAL THINKING EXERCISES

1. Why is it important for the nurse to provide care to the community?

2. How does the community health nursing process differ from the individual nursing process?

3. How would you work with your community to identify their health needs and share their community experiences?

4. In developing a health profile for a community, what assessment questions would you ask for each category of the community components? Where and how would you collect the needed data?

5. Why is it important to use participatory tools for community planning?

GROUP CRITICAL THINKING EXERCISES

1. Based on the community needs matrix tool (Table 11.3), what are some of the questions you would want to ask the community about their ratings? What would be the next steps?

2. In a group of 2 to 4, spend about an hour visiting and talking to people in your local neighbourhood. Describe your community visit and explain your impression about the felt needs, real needs, and wants of the community. Formulate your nursing diagnoses and propose your actions.

3. Discuss possible ways to engage your community to meet the identified health needs in question 2.

REFERENCES

Badets, J. (2003). Update on cultural diversity. In Statistics Canada, *Canadian social trends.* Summer 2003, No. 70. Retrieved May 22, 2007, from http://www.statcan.ca/bsolc/english/bsolc?catno=11-008-X20030026623.

Campaign 2000. (2005). *Decision time for Canada: Let's make poverty history: 2005 report card on child poverty in Canada.* Retrieved May 22, 2007, from http://www.campaign2000.ca/rc/index.html.

Canadian Institute for Health Information (CIHI). (2004). *National trauma registry 2004 report: Major injury in Canada.* Ottawa: Author.

Canadian Institute for Health Information (CIHI). (2005). *Improving the health of young Canadians, 2005.* Retrieved May 21, 2007, from http://secure.cihi.ca/cihiweb/dispPage.jsp?cw_page=PG_380_E&cw_topic=380&cw_rel=AR_1217_E.

Canadian Public Health Association. (1990). *Community health-public health nursing in Canada: Preparation & practice.* Ottawa: Author.

Clemen-Stone, S., Eigsti, D., & McGuire, S. (2002). *Comprehensive community health nursing* (6th ed.). Toronto: Mosby.

Cohen, B. (2006). Barriers to population-focused health promotion: The experience of public health nurses in the province of Manitoba. *CJNR, 38*(3), 52–67.

Community Health Nurses Association of Canada. (2003). *Community health nursing standards of practice.* Retrieved May 22, 2007 from http://www. communityhealthnursescanada.org/Standards.htm.

Craig, W. (2004). Bullying and fighting. In Boyce, W. (Ed.). *Young people in Canada: Their health and well-being* (pp. 87–96). Ottawa: Health Canada.

Epp, J. (1986). *Health for all: A framework for health promotion.* Ottawa: Health and Welfare Canada.

Federal, Provincial, and Territorial Advisory Committee on Population Health [FPTACPH]. (1999). *Toward a healthy future: Second report on the health of Canadians.* Ottawa: Minister of Supply and Services.

Friendly, M. (2002, November). *Early childhood education and care.* Paper presented at The Social Determinants of Health Across the Lifespan Conference. Toronto.

Graham, H. (2004). Childhood disadvantage and health inequalities: A framework for policy based on life course research. *Child: Care, Health & Development, 30*(6), 671–678.

Health Canada, Statistics Canada, & the Canadian Institute for Health Information. (1999). *Toward a healthy future: Second report on the health of Canadians.* Ottawa: Author.

Hyman, H. (2001). *Immigration and health.* Cat. No. H13-5/ 01-5E. Ottawa: Minister of Public Works and Government Services Canada.

Joffres, C., Heath, S., Farquharson, J., Barkhouse, K., Hood, R., Latter, C., & MacLean, D. R. (2004). Defining and operationalizing capacity for heart health promotion in Nova Scotia, Canada. *Health Promotion International, 19*(1), 39–49.

Kirby, M. (2002). *The health of Canadians—The federal role final report, Vol. 6: Recommendations for reform. Part VI: Health promotion and disease prevention.* The Standing Senate Committee on Social Affairs, Science and Technology. Retrieved May 20, 2007, from http://www. parl.gc.ca/37/2/parlbus/commbus/senate/com-e/soci-e/rep-e/repoct02vol6part5-e.htm.

Ktpatzer Consulting. (2006, June). *Trends and benefits of community engagement and local community governance in health care.* Toronto: Association of Ontario Community Health Centres. Retrieved May 23, 2007, from http:// www.aohc.org/aohc/index_e.aspx?ArticleID=41.

Lalonde, M. (1974). *A new perspective on the health of Canadians.* Ottawa: Government of Canada.

Larni, K., & Johnson, M. (2004). An evaluation of a volunteer-support program for families at risk. *Public Health Nursing, 21*(4), 297–305.

Lynch, J., Smith, G. D., Harper, S., Hillemeier, M., Ross, N., Kaplan, G. A., & Wolfson, M. (2004). Is income inequality a determinant of population health? Part 1: A systematic review. *The Milbank Quarterly, 82*(1), 5–99.

McKnight, J. K., & Kretzmann, J. P. (1997). Mapping community capacity. In M. Minkler (Ed.), *Community organizing and community building for health* (pp. 157–172). New Brunswick, NJ: Rutgers University Press.

Minnesota Department of Health. (2001). *Public health interventions: Applications for public health nursing practice.*

Retrieved May 22, 2007, from http://www.health.state.mn. us/divs/cfh/ophp/resources/docs/wheel.pdf.

Public Health Agency of Canada (PHAC). (2002a). *Population health: What is population health approach?* Retrieved May 22, 2007, from http://www.phac-aspc.gc. ca/ph-sp/phdd/approach/index.html#What.

Public Health Agency of Canada (PHAC). (2002b). *Summary table of population health key elements.* Retrieved May 23, 2007, from http://www.phac-aspc.gc.ca/ph-sp/phdd/pdf/ summary_table.pdf.

Public Health Agency of Canada (PHAC). (2003, March). *What determines health?* Retrieved May 23, 2007 from http:// www.phac-aspc.gc.ca/ph-sp/phdd/determinants/index.html.

Public Health Agency of Canada (PHAC). (2004). *The social determinants of health: An overview of the implications for policy and the role of the health sector.* Retrieved May 20, 2007, from http://www.phac-aspc.gc.ca/ph-sp/phdd/ overview_implications/01_overview.html.

Public Health Agency of Canada (PHAC). (2007). *Core competencies for Public Health Practice, Release 1.0.* Retrieved October 1, 2007, from http://www.phac-aspc.gc.ca/ccph-cesp/pdfs/cc-manual-eng090407.pdf.

Raphael, D. (Ed.). (2004). *Social determinants of health: Canadian perspectives.* Toronto: Canadian Scholars' Press.

Raven, P., & Frank, L. (2004). *The Nova Scotia child poverty report card.* Canadian Centre for Policy Alternatives Nova Scotia. Retrieved May 20, 2007, from http://www. policyalternatives.ca/documents/Nova_Scotia_Pubs/ ns_child_poverty_2004.pdf.

Sahay, T. (2004). *A review of the literature on the links between health promotion capacity building and health outcomes.* Toronto: Ontario Health Promotion Resource System. Retrieved May 22, 2007, from http://www.ohprs.ca/ resources/tina_finalreport_27dec2004.pdf.

Statistics Canada. (2002). *How healthy are Canadians? Annual report 2005, Health Reports supplement.* Retrieved May 23, 2007, from http://www.statcan.ca/english/freepub/82-003-SIE/82-003-SIE2005000.htm.

Van Marris, B., & King, B. (2002). *Evaluating health promotion programs.* The University of Toronto: The Health Communication Unit.

Vollman, A., Anderson, E., & McFarlane, J. (2004). *Community as partner: Theory and practice in nursing* (Canadian ed.). Philadelphia, PA: Lippincott, Williams and Wilkins.

World Health Organization (WHO). (1978). *Primary health care: Report on the International Conference on Primary Health Care, Alma Ata, USSR, 6–12, September 1978.* Geneva, Switzerland: Author.

World Health Organization (WHO), Canadian Public Health Association, & Health and Welfare Canada. (1986). *Ottawa Charter of health promotion.* Ottawa: Health and Welfare Canada.

World Health Organization (WHO). (2006). *Commission on social determinants of health.* Retrieved May 22, 2007, from http://www.who.int/social_determinants/en/.

Yiu, L. (2001). *Monitoring and evaluation: A handbook for maternal and child health workers.* Ottawa: University of

Ottawa, Canada-China Yunnan Maternal and Child Health Project & the Yunnan Public Health Bureau.

Yiu Matuk, L., & Ruggirello, T. (2007). Culture connection project: Promoting multiculturalism in elementary schools. *CJPH, 98*(1), 26–29.

ADDITIONAL RESOURCES

Websites

Canadian Public Health Association
  www.cpha.ca
Canadian Institute for Health Information (CIHI)
  www.cihi.ca
Public Health Agency of Canada
  www.phac-aspc.gc.ca
Statistics Canada, *Canadian Community Health Survey (CCHS), 2000/01*
  www.statcan.ca/english/sdds/3226.htm

Readings

Diem, E., & Moyer, A. (2005). *Community health nursing projects: making a difference.* Toronto: Lippincott Williams & Wilkins.

Statistics Canada. (2006). *Research projects from the Canadian Community Health Survey (CCHS).* http://www.statcan.ca/english/rdc/rdcprojectscchs.htm.

About the Author

Lucia Yiu, RN, BScN, BA (Psychology, Windsor), BSc (Physiology, Toronto), MScN (Administration, Western Ontario), is an Associate Professor in the Faculty of Nursing, University of Windsor, and an Educational and Training Consultant in community nursing. She has worked overseas and served on various community and social services committees involving local and district health planning.

Appendix 11A

TABLE 11A — Summary Table of Population Health Key Elements	
Key Element	**Actions**
1. Focus on the health of populations	• Determine indicators for measuring health status. • Measure and analyze population health status and health status inequities to identify health issues. • Assess contextual conditions, characteristics, and trends.
2. Address the determinants of health and their interactions	• Determine indicators for measuring the determinants of health. • Measure and analyze the determinants of health and their interactions to link health issues to their determinants.
3. Base decisions on evidence	• Use best evidence available at all stages of policy and program development. • Explain criteria for including or excluding evidence. • Draw on a variety of data. • Generate data through mixed research methods. • Identify and assess effective interventions. • Disseminate research findings and facilitate policy uptake.
4. Increase upstream investments	• Apply criteria to select priorities for investment. • Balance short- and long-term investments. • Influence investments in other sectors.
5. Apply multiple strategies	• Identify scope of action for interventions. • Take action on the determinants of health and their interactions. • Implement strategies to reduce inequities in health status between population groups. • Apply a comprehensive mix of interventions and strategies. • Apply interventions that address health issues in an integrated way. • Apply methods to improve health over the life span. • Act in multiple settings. • Establish a coordinating mechanism to guide interventions.
6. Collaborate across sectors and levels	• Engage partners early on to establish shared values and alignment of purpose. • Establish concrete objectives and focus on visible results. • Identify and support a champion. • Invest in the alliance-building process. • Generate political support and build on positive factors in the policy environment. • Share leadership, accountability, and rewards among partners.
7. Employ mechanisms for public involvement	• Capture the public's interest. • Contribute to health literacy. • Apply public involvement strategies that link to overarching purpose.
8. Demonstrate accountability for health outcomes	• Construct a results-based accountability framework. • Ascertain baseline measures and set targets for health improvement. • Institutionalize effective evaluation systems. • Promote the use of health impact assessment tools. • Publicly report results.

The goals of a population health approach are to maintain and improve the health status of the entire population and to reduce the inequities in health status between population groups.

Source: The Population Health Template: Key Elements and Actions that Define a Population Health Approach, *Public Health Agency of Canada, (2002) © Reproduced with the permission of the Minister of Public Works and Government Services Canada, 2006.*

Occupational Health

Sharon L. Chadwick and Bernice Doyle

OBJECTIVES

After studying this chapter, you should be able to:

1. Discuss the components of an occupational health and safety program.
2. Identify the legislation and standards that apply to workplace health and safety.
3. Identify the different types of occupational hazards to which workers may be exposed.
4. Describe the occupational health team.
5. Outline the roles and competencies of occupational health nurses.
6. Identify linkages between occupational and community health.
7. Consider occupational health principles when working in the community health setting.
8. Recognize occupational hazards to which community health nurses may be exposed and identify controls.

INTRODUCTION

Workplace fatalities, injuries and illnesses remain at unacceptably high levels and involve an enormous and unnecessary health burden, suffering, and economic loss amounting to 4–5% of GDP. According to WHO and ILO estimates for the year 2000 there are 2.0 million work-related deaths per year. WHO estimates that there are only 10–15% of workers who have access to a basic standard of occupational health services." (World Health Organization, 2002)

These are significant numbers. Because work affects every part of our lives, injuries and illnesses can significantly affect individuals, families, and communities. It is important for all nursing professionals, regardless of work setting, to be aware of the basic principles of occupational health and safety.

The purpose of this chapter is to provide an overview of the specialty nursing practice of occupational health. General principles and the components of occupational health and safety programs are outlined and include the roles of various members of the occupational health and safety team. Occupational health nursing practice is explained in more detail. The role, competencies, and benefits (to both employees and employers) of occupational health nursing are described and related to the community health setting. Legislation and research are presented in the Canadian context. Health promotion is discussed as an integral part of all

components. Community health nurses (CHNs) can only benefit from this brief introduction to the world of occupational health and safety.

GENERAL PRINCIPLES OF OCCUPATIONAL HEALTH AND SAFETY

Health and safety programs support the development of the highest level of worker health by creating a safe and healthy work environment. Basic **occupational health theory** states that it is "aimed at prevention" and includes "health promotion and protection in the context of the work environment" (Doyle, 2006, p. 3-3). In other words, **occupational health and safety programs** prevent ill health from work-related injury or illness and protect workers from existing or potential health and safety hazards at work. This section describes the components of a comprehensive program to meet these objectives

Workplace health and safety programs are often developed because of specific legislated requirements in health and safety. As a minimum, an employer's health and safety program must contain the elements necessary to meet the legislated requirements for the jurisdiction in which a particular work site exists and operates. In addition, numerous standards are related to the field of health and safety at work. The legislation and other standards that may apply in a comprehensive health and safety program are outlined in this section.

Health and safety **hazards** at work are categorized into five basic types: physical, chemical, biological, ergonomic, and psychosocial. Categories of hazards are discussed later in the chapter.

The nurse is just one member of the team that delivers comprehensive occupational health and safety programs. In the next section we discuss the components of an occupational health and safety program, followed by a description of all the members of the team.

COMPONENTS OF AN OCCUPATIONAL HEALTH AND SAFETY PROGRAM

Management Commitment

A number of components make up an occupational health and safety program, and many factors determine the extent to which each component can be developed and implemented at a work site. The first and most important component necessary for an effective program is **management commitment**.

Management is responsible for the overall operation of the workplace, including the development and enforcement of any policies and procedures. Without management commitment to health and safety, an effective program is simply not possible. Evidence of this commitment in any workplace can be seen by policies, procedures, and programs that focus on pertinent issues and are well-known throughout the workforce. In other words, the program not only must address the health and safety hazards, but also must be communicated to the workers.

Having appropriate and adequate resources is also evidence of the extent of management commitment to health and safety. Worker commitment, support, and cooperation are more likely to follow when management commitment, focus, and communication are evident. To be effective, policies and procedures must be followed by the workers, and systems must be in place so that workers have support in addressing health and safety issues that arise. A workplace culture in which everyone knows the health and safety rules, takes ownership, and is held accountable at all times for preventing injuries or ill health goes a long way in maintaining worker health and safety at all levels.

Worker Involvement

An effective program promotes health and safety at work in a variety of ways. Training, job analyses, health assessments, and health and safety committees are important components that directly involve workers and impact workplace health and safety.

Training Workers Training begins when workers are hired or transferred into any new job, whether on a permanent, temporary, part-time, or full-time basis. Training is also appropriate if new procedures, new equipment, or different tasks are introduced to existing jobs or processes. Worker training should encompass all aspects of health and safety that apply to the job, including:

- hazards;
- company policies;
- legislative responsibilities;
- duty to refuse unsafe work;
- safe operating procedures for performing work and using equipment;
- requirements, care, and use of personal protective equipment;
- first-aid services, equipment, and supplies;
- emergency procedures for alarms or evacuations; and
- reporting requirements for injuries, illnesses, hazards, incidents, and near misses.

Assessing the Jobs of Workers Ensuring that jobs are analyzed as part of the health and safety program helps to identify potential inherent hazards as well as determine the skills or physical

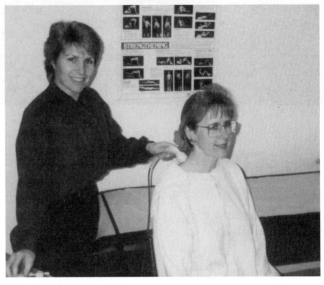

Photo 12.1

Occupational health and safety nurse on job site with workers.

Credit: Provided by the Canadian Nurses Foundation from the Canadian Nursing History Collection

requirements of a job. Often called a **job demands analysis**, this is also known as job task analysis or critical task analysis. Regardless of the name, this component can prevent work-related injury or illness. To assess a job's demands, the job is divided into specific tasks and each task is analyzed to determine the physical or mental requirements. In addition, the hazards posed to a worker while performing the work are specified. Information from the analysis is useful in other areas of health and safety. A job demands analysis is essential when conducting a worker health assessment, which determines whether the worker is physically and mentally able to perform a job. This is used for screening workers either on initial hiring or when returning to work after illness or injury. When job accommodation is necessary, the results of a job demands analysis can help identify the job changes that are required so that a worker can perform tasks without risking health and safety.

Formally Involving the Workers The most common mechanism for involving workers in health and safety at work is through a joint health and safety committee. This committee usually consists of both worker and management representatives and is a forum to address workplace health and safety issues. While many jurisdictions in Canada have legislation that requires employers to establish joint health and safety committees, there is no reason for employers to wait for legislation or official orders to establish such a committee. The committee can:

- participate in development and implementation of programs to protect the employees' safety and health;
- deal with employee complaints and suggestions concerning safety and health;
- ensure the maintenance and monitoring of injury and work hazard records;
- monitor and follow up hazard reports and recommend action;

- set up and promote programs to improve employee training and education;
- participate in all safety and health inquiries and investigations;
- consult with professional and technical experts;
- participate in resolving workplace refusals and work stoppages;
- make recommendations to management for accident prevention and safety program activities; and
- monitor effectiveness of safety programs and procedures. (Canadian Centre for Occupational Health and Safety [CCOHS], 2007)

Committees can go a long way in motivating workers in health and safety and therefore protecting worker health so that injuries and illnesses are prevented.

The Work Environment

An assessment of the work environment, an essential component of a health and safety program, should be done in order to recognize and control hazards. Recognition is the first step in protecting workers from workplace hazards. Hazard identification can be done by trained members of the health and safety committee, other workers who are trained in hazard recognition, or by health and safety specialists who have training in measuring hazards. These people must consider all aspects of the work-site operations, including all processes, all materials used (i.e., from raw materials to end products), and all the actual and potential points of worker contact or exposure. Hazard identification can involve walk-throughs of the work site, either on a regular basis or in response to specific concerns. Review of work-injury statistics can also point to areas on a work site that need to be surveyed and assessed to identify hazards. Another method for identifying hazards is to complete a *job hazard analysis*. This involves identifying each component of a particular job and then examining it to ascertain any actual or potential hazards. This can be done by using a form such as the one found in Figure 12.1. Once the hazards have been identified for each job task, the actual risk must be assessed.

The type of assessment or expertise required depends on the type of hazard. For example, noise is a common hazard in workplaces. Taking a simple noise measurement requires a sound level meter. A more complex measurement of noise exposure involves dosimetry, which requires workers to wear a measuring device throughout a workday. Exposure time and noise levels are then calculated to determine a worker's actual exposure to noise as well as the risk of hearing being affected and occupationally induced hearing loss caused.

Hazard evaluation can help to determine the risk to workers' health from any type of workplace hazard. In addition, hazard evaluation points to those hazards that require controls so that worker exposure and consequent health effects are eliminated or minimized as much as is practicable.

Hazard control can be divided into three general categories: engineering controls, administrative controls, and personal protective equipment. The controls identified or implemented should be entered as part of the job hazard analysis (Figure 12.1).

Engineering controls are the first choice, because hazards are removed at the source, preventing exposure and therefore eliminating the risk of harmful health effects. A simple example of an engineering control is a muffler on a car, which reduces the noise of a vehicle. Isolation of either a hazard source (e.g., enclosing noisy machinery) or the workers (e.g., by placing them in a control room) is a common engineering control in many industries.

Administrative controls include such strategies as job rotation to minimize the time a worker is exposed to a hazard in a particular process and the instituting of safe work procedures. When safe work procedures are followed, they can significantly reduce the risks to health posed by hazards.

The use of **personal protective equipment** is very common in industry to prevent exposure to health hazards. Examples of such equipment include respiratory protective equipment (RPE), gloves, protective eye goggles, hard hats, or fall protection equipment. Personal protective equipment is used as a last resort when a hazard cannot be eliminated or controlled by any other means. Rogers (2003, p. 201) gives five things to consider when using personal protective equipment:

- selecting the proper type of equipment;
- ensuring proper fit;
- instructing workers in the proper use of equipment;
- enforcing of standards for using the equipment, whether legislated or workplace based; and
- conducting effective equipment sanitation and maintenance.

FIGURE 12.1 Sample Job Hazard Analysis Worksheet

Occupation/Job Classification: _____

Location/Site: _____

Department: _____

Specific Job: _____

_____

Prepared by: _____

_____

_____

Date: _____

Job Tasks by Sequence of Events	Potential Hazards	Preventive Actions or Controls

It's important to remember that using personal protective equipment does not eliminate a hazard, but it can minimize exposure if it is properly fitted, used, and maintained.

Addressing Injuries, Illnesses, and Incidents

Despite the best intentions and the preventive focus of occupational health and safety programs, injuries and illnesses still occur in the workplace. Because of this, such elements as first aid, health surveillance for hazard exposures, rehabilitation of workers, incident investigations, and emergency preparedness for major incidents need to be addressed in a program. As a minimum, most jurisdictions require employers to provide first-aid services—the most basic form of worker health assessment, as work-related injuries and illnesses must be reported, assessed, treated, and documented by a first-aider. In more comprehensive health and safety programs, more extensive health assessments are done, including health surveillance and rehabilitation. This will be discussed in more detail in the "Occupational Health Nursing" section.

Conducting workplace investigations is another part of a health and safety program. Some investigations are mandated by legislation, such as those done because of a serious injury or a major incident that could cause serious injury or significant property damage. Workplace investigations are done to determine causes and prevent recurrence; they are not intended to find fault. Often, a number of factors or events, not just a single one, lead to injuries, property damage, or near misses. Thorough investigations are necessary so that all factors can be addressed when recommendations are made to prevent future incidents.

Preparing for emergencies is critical for any work site, regardless of the size or type. Being prepared minimizes not only injuries to workers but also damage to property. "Emergency management is a dynamic process. Planning, though critical, is not the only component. Training, conducting drills, testing equipment, and coordinating activities with the community are other important functions" (Federal Emergency Management Agency, 2007). Although emergency preparedness does not prevent an emergency, it ensures that both human and economic losses are minimized.

Program Administration

Comprehensive records are a necessary component of an effective health and safety program. A variety of records must be kept for the purposes of:

- meeting legislated requirements (e.g., first-aid records or material safety data sheets);
- informing and communicating;
- maintaining baseline measurements (e.g., worker baseline tests);
- determining hazards (e.g., if a number of workers from one department report the same types of health problems, a hazard investigation may be warranted);

- preventing injuries or illnesses (a review of injury or illness records can identify problem areas and preventive steps can be taken to reduce additional problems);
- proving or disproving exposures to hazards (e.g., for insurance or compensation claims);
- program tracking (program objectives should be measurable and tracking helps determine whether objectives are being met); and
- evaluating and planning a program.

Each company will have preferences for different types of records and reports, including policies, procedures, tracking, and evaluation. In addition, members of the health and safety team may have specific professional requirements for record keeping. It is important to constantly assess the records to ensure they are well maintained and kept up to date.

LEGISLATION AND STANDARDS

Health and Safety

Each province and territory in Canada has legislated standards for health and safety in the workplace. In general, the legislation outlines the rights, responsibilities, and fundamental principles for achieving and maintaining workplace health and safety. Most importantly, health and safety legislation sets standards so that health problems or safety risks at work are minimized. Consequences of not meeting the minimum requirements are also outlined in the legislation.

Both employers and employees have obligations under health and safety legislation. Employers have overall responsibility for ensuring health and safety at their work sites. In turn, workers are responsible for working safely and cooperating with the employer by following health and safety policies and procedures. Standard-setting agencies, such as the government, have legislated duties of inspection and enforcement.

Legislation can set overall general objectives, or it can be very specific and include detailed procedures for preserving health and safety at work, such as fall protection or confined space entry. First-aid requirements or the need for joint health and safety committees may also be addressed. The laws also deal with specific hazards such as noise, chemicals in the workplace, or biological hazards. Legislation may require that workers have a specific level of competence to perform work safely and can require training in certain areas. Some laws apply to all industries in a given jurisdiction while some are industry specific. Both employers and workers are well advised to find out the legislated requirements for health and safety for their specific workplace.

While provincial or territorial legislation applies to employers and workers within its boundaries, not all work sites fall under provincial or territorial jurisdiction. Industries that cross provincial or territorial boundaries, such as banks and some communications and transportation businesses, fall under federal jurisdiction.

The legislation that pertains to hazardous products is slightly different from other health and safety legislation because both federal and provincial/territorial legislation apply. The federal Hazardous Products Act governs all jurisdictions. In addition, each jurisdiction has its own laws in this area, commonly known as the **Workplace Hazardous Materials Information System (WHMIS)**. From a practical point of view, there are three major components of WHMIS legislation:

- workers must be informed of the nature of the hazards posed by any hazardous products at work;
- hazardous products must be labelled; and
- hazardous products must have a material safety data sheet that outlines components, physical properties, health hazards, first aid, toxicity, and any other aspects that pertain to health and safety.

Workers' Compensation Legislation

Workers' compensation legislation goes hand in hand with occupational health and safety legislation. It was introduced to protect both workers and employers when work-related injuries or illnesses occur. Workers' compensation is a form of no-fault insurance that protects employers from being sued by workers who become injured or ill due to work. In turn, workers receive compensation for work-related injuries or illnesses and do not have to take legal action against an employer to obtain it.

Compensation legislation is in every Canadian jurisdiction. The laws of each dictate reporting requirements, compensation allowances, and procedures for obtaining and providing compensation. Different commissions or boards throughout Canada administer their respective legislation.

Human Rights Legislation

Canada has a Charter of Rights and Freedoms that protects basic human rights. In addition, each jurisdiction has legislation that protects human rights, and this legislation applies at the workplace as well as any other setting. From a health and safety point of view, human rights legislation protects individuals from discrimination at the workplace due to any of the listed protected areas, which include disability, sex, family status, or religion. It requires employers to consider individual differences and outlines a duty to accommodate those differences. For example, if a worker is returning to work after suffering an injury and is unable to perform the job held prior to the injury, the employer must accommodate the worker's new disability. An employer who claims that such accommodation is not possible must prove that it would cause undue hardship.

Other Legislation

Many other pieces of legislation can apply at a workplace and affect health and safety programs. Though a complete list would be too lengthy, some examples include:

- employment standards;
- cross-jurisdictional legislation (e.g., drug-testing requirements in the transportation industry in the United States);
- public health legislation, including communicable disease reporting or immunization;
- privacy legislation;
- building standards and codes;
- fire codes;
- disaster services;
- Good Samaritan legislation; and
- legislation pertaining to health and safety professionals.

Other Standards

In addition to the laws of the land, many other standards can apply at a workplace and impact a health and safety program. Manufacturers of equipment and supplies, regardless of the type of industry, often have safety standards that apply to their products. Workers and employers must know and follow these standards to maintain health and safety.

Many industries have what are commonly known as industry-based standards, best practices, or industry safety codes for health and safety at work. An industry association often writes these and recommends that they be used by employers. These types of standards help employers to comply with legislation, and many go further than the minimum legislated standards. Professional associations often develop minimum practice standards for their members. As well, safety associations are a common source for guidelines and recommended practices in health and safety.

Still other standards are set by organizations for equipment, policies, or procedures. The Canadian Standards Association (CSA) is a prominent standards-setting organization. Examples of CSA standards that apply to health and safety programs include those for personal protective equipment such as eye protection, face protection, and respiratory protection. Some, but not all, standards are referenced in legislation and made mandatory. Regardless of whether the standards are a requirement, they are a useful resource for health and safety programs and can provide guidance on a variety of issues. Some standards or guidelines are distributed by governments. While these may not be requirements, they are a valuable resource for anyone developing an effective health and safety program or implementing the requirements of the legislation.

TYPES OF HEALTH AND SAFETY HAZARDS

Safety Hazards

Safety or mechanical hazards are a significant source of injury in the workplace. These types of hazards are generally fairly obvious and include unguarded belts, unprotected gears, shafts without railings, ladders that do not provide proper support, poor housekeeping, or unsecured items that can fall on workers' heads or toes to cause injury. The list is endless.

Physical Hazards

The Canadian Centre for Occupational Health and Safety defines **physical hazards** as "sources of energy that may cause injury or disease" (CCOHS, n.d., c). Types of physical hazards and some examples include:

- noise: chain saw,
- vibration: jackhammer,
- ionizing radiation: checking welds on pipelines,
- ultraviolet radiation: welding,
- excessive heat: foundry, and
- excessive cold: winter outdoors.

Noise in the workplace is as ubiquitous at work as it is in our homes and other environments. Our ears can tolerate certain levels without long-term effects, but hearing loss can occur after exposure to high noise levels over a period of time. Once the inner ear is damaged from excessive noise, there is no cure. This makes prevention of hearing loss due to exposure to excessive noise extremely important.

Vibration sources in the workplace including tools such as jackhammers, sanders, stamping machines, and drills can cause long-term effects to fingers and hands. Workers who operate excavating equipment can experience effects to their whole body if they sit in a seat that vibrates. "The risk of injury from exposure to either type of vibration depends on the intensity and frequency of the vibration, the duration of exposure (usually measured in years), and the part(s) of the body affected" (Alberta Employment, Immigration and Industry, Workplace Health and Safety [WHS], 2004, p. 1). Local effects of using vibrating tools can include Raynaud's syndrome, while whole-body vibration can produce a wide range of effects, including back and neck problems.

The uses of ionizing radiation, such as X-rays and radiation for cancer treatment, are well known in the health care industry; however, ionizing radiation is also used in other industries. One example is the use of a radioactive source for checking welds on pipes. The health effects of ionizing radiation can range from mild skin erythema to cancer. Non-ionizing radiation includes various types along the electromagnetic spectrum. The ultraviolet rays of sunlight are probably the best known of the non-ionizing radiation hazards. Ultraviolet radiation, a common hazard in welding, can cause a painful injury known as welder's flash, in which the cornea is burned.

A wide variety of industries can expose workers to excessive heat or excessive cold. Factors that determine whether workers suffer heat stress, and the extent of the health effects, include air temperature, humidity, amount of radiant heat, air speed, clothing, physical activity, and individual factors (Alberta Employment, Immigration and Industry, WHS, 2007). Health effects can include heat cramps, heat exhaustion, heat stroke, and death. Working outside during a hot summer day in a foundry near molten metal, or in many other work situations, can cause heat stress in workers. Exposure to the other temperature extreme, cold, can occur either outside (e.g., in the construction industry) or inside (e.g., working in refrigeration units, immersing hands in cold water, or using cold equipment or tools). As with heat, a number of factors determine the health effects, which vary from reduced dexterity to hypothermia and death.

Chemical Hazards

Found in almost any work setting, chemicals are a significant hazard in the workplace. **Chemical hazards** can be in liquid, solid, or gaseous form, in mists, vapours, or fumes. Chemicals enter the body in many ways, including ingestion, injection, and skin absorption. Probably the most common route of entry is via inhalation (CCOHS, 1997–2006). The most prudent way to prevent chemical exposures is to become informed about the chemicals used and to minimize exposure as much as possible by using the controls available, including personal protective equipment. Material safety data sheets, required under health and safety legislation, include information about the toxicity of different chemicals, their potential health effects, first-aid measures, and protection from exposure.

Biological Hazards

Biological hazards, such as bacteria, viruses, insects, plants, birds, animals, and even other humans, can cause a variety of health effects, such as skin irritation, allergies, infections, and cancer (CCOHS, n.d., a). Workers who may be exposed to biological hazards include health care workers (to bacterial or viral diseases from their patients), forestry workers (to insects, plants, birds, and animals), and maintenance workers (who may clean an area where there are mouse droppings and therefore may be exposed to hantavirus).

Ergonomic Hazards

Ergonomic hazards are workplace conditions that can cause injury to the musculoskeletal system of the worker (CCOHS, n.d., b). Examples of ergonomic hazards in the workplace include repetitive work, static postures, improper lighting, and poor tool design.

Psychosocial Hazards

Psychosocial hazards can be defined as "factors and situations encountered or associated with one's job or work environment that create or potentiate stress, emotional strain, and/or interpersonal problems" (Rogers, 2003, p. 148). Examples of psychosocial hazards include anything that may cause a worker to experience stress, such as high workloads, harassment, inflexible work arrangements, uncertainty, shift work, or conflict in the workplace.

THE OCCUPATIONAL HEALTH AND SAFETY TEAM

Occupational health nurses are members of occupational health and safety teams. Their roles on these teams will be discussed in the next section. Other team members include occupational physicians, occupational hygienists, safety professionals, ergonomists, and other specialists who address either work environment issues or workers themselves.

Occupational Health Physicians

Occupational health physicians are medical doctors who have specialized in the field of occupational medicine. They deal specifically with worker health to diagnose and treat injuries, illnesses, and diseases that may stem from workplace exposures. Companies hire these medical specialists on a full-time, part-time, or consultant basis, depending on the needs of the company, its commitment to health and safety, and its

economic situation. Occupational health nurses and occupational physicians work closely together to prevent illness and to promote the highest level of health in workers.

Occupational Hygienists

Occupational hygienists focus primarily on recognizing, measuring, evaluating, and controlling health hazards in the workplace. Usually, their educational background emphasizes the sciences, plus special training in the principles and concepts of work environment assessment. They use special equipment to quantitatively measure hazards such as noise or chemicals. Occupational hygienists also understand the health effects of different hazards on the human body.

In Canada, there are two recognized professionals: registered occupational hygienists (ROH) and registered occupational hygiene technologists (ROHT). To qualify as an ROH, the Canadian Registration Board of Occupational Hygienists (CRBOH) requires a university degree plus experience. An ROHT must have experience in occupational hygiene, the amount of which varies according to the level of education achieved. Professionals must maintain competency in their respective areas to register with the CRBOH.

Ergonomists

An **ergonomist** is a professional who "applies theory, principles, data, and methods to . . . optimize human well-being and overall system performance" (Association of Canadian Ergonomists, 2007, p. 1). Though these professionals have diverse educational backgrounds, all have an interest in and work to improve work situations by addressing the "physical, cognitive, social, organizational, environmental, and other relevant factors" in the workplace (p. 1). In other words, ergonomists look at both worker characteristics and work environment characteristics (such as equipment) to prevent injuries and illnesses. For example, ergonomists examine the potential for musculoskeletal problems from repetitive work or inappropriate tools, eyestrain caused by computer screens or improper lighting, or physical or psychological problems caused by shift work.

Safety Professionals

Safety professionals, or safety officers, are also integral members of health and safety teams. In Canada, safety professionals can register and receive professional designation as a Canadian Registered Safety Professional (CRSP) from the Board of Canadian Registered Safety Professionals (BCRSP). A safety professional promotes workplace health and safety in a variety of ways. A safety professional with a CRSP designation is an individual (BCRSP, 2007, p. 1):

- who has met the academic, experience and examination requirements of a national registration authority.

- with in-depth knowledge of health and safety principles and practices who uses this knowledge to develop systems in the workplace in order to achieve optimum control over hazards detrimental to people, equipment, material, and the environment.

■ committed to the principles of loss control, accident prevention, and environmental protection.

■ whose knowledge and skills are continually upgraded through a certification maintenance program to ensure the organization always has a qualified, up-to-date professional managing health and safety interests.

■ committed to managing the organization's health and safety issues and concerns according to a code of ethics.

Others

Other specialists or professionals may be part of the health and safety team at one time or another. These include counsellors, psychologists, physiotherapists, massage therapists, case managers, and rehabilitation specialists. The extent to which these individuals work in health and safety is based on need, economics, and management commitment.

OCCUPATIONAL HEALTH NURSING

Occupational health nursing is a recognized specialty practice under the Canadian Nurses Association (CNA). It is defined by the American Association of Occupational Health Nurses (AAOHN) as "the specialty practice that provides for and delivers health and safety programs and services to workers, worker populations, and community groups. The practice focuses on promotion and restoration of health, prevention of illness and injury, and the protection from work related and environmental hazards" (AAOHN, 2007, p. 1).

Conceptual Framework

An occupational health nursing conceptual framework presents values and beliefs about four aspects: the individual, health, occupational health nursing, and the environment. (See the box "Conceptual Framework of Occupational Health Nursing.") The interrelationship of these four components reflects the assumptions and philosophy of occupational health nursing practice (Canadian Occupational Health Nurses Association [COHNA], 2002).

Role of the Occupational Health Nurse

Nurses have been working in occupational health since the late 1800s, when they were employed by industries to care for ailing workers and their families (Levy, Wegman, Baron, & Sokas, 2006; Rogers, 2003). Since then, the role of the occupational health nurse (OHN) has expanded to include the areas of epidemiology, industrial hygiene, environmental health, toxicology, safety, management, health education, early disease detection, disease prevention, health promotion, and health and environmental surveillance (Levy & Wegman, 2006).

Rogers (2003) identifies major roles in occupational health nursing practice: clinician/practitioner, case manager, health promotion specialist, manager, educator, researcher, and consultant. Many OHNs function in several or all of these roles. The **clinician/practitioner** applies the nursing process to direct care for occupational, and often non-occupational, injuries and illnesses at the workplace. The OHN also collaborates with other members of the occupational health team to maintain a safe and healthy work environment.

The **case manager** role has emerged and become increasingly more prominent over the past decade as employers demand cost-effective health management for their injured and ill workers. The goal of the OHN's case management role is timely coordination of health services so that worker needs are met in a manner that protects health in a cost-effective manner for the employer (Rogers, 2003, p. 87). Case management includes managing occupational as well as non-occupational injuries and illnesses of workers.

Conceptual Framework of Occupational Health Nursing

The individual is unique in biological, psychological, social, spiritual, and cultural characteristics. The individual has rights to confidentiality of health records, advocacy, and information about health status and potential hazards. The individual also has the right to work in a safe and healthy environment, choose or refuse participation in occupational health programs, and refuse unsafe/unhealthy work. In addition, the individual has responsibilities to maintain his/her own health, know the hazards of the workplace, assume responsibility for the consequences of his/her actions, respect the rights and needs of others, and maintain safe work practices for self and others.

Health is the extent to which an individual or group is able to realize aspirations to satisfy needs and to change or cope with the environment. Health is, therefore, seen as a resource for everyday life, not the objective of living. Health is a positive concept emphasizing social and personal resources as well as physical capacities.

Occupational health nursing is that specialty area of nursing practice that focuses on the worker group by promoting health, preventing illness/injury, protecting workers from risks associated with exposure to occupational health hazards, recommending placement of workers in jobs suited to their physiological and psychological health status, and restoring workers' health in a safe and healthy work environment.

Environment consists of dynamic forces that interact with each other and the individual. The environment can be social, economic, political, physical, and cultural as well as the internal psychological status of the individual. A major focus of occupational health nursing is the work environment because of its unique health hazards.

Source: Canadian Occupational Health Nurses Association. (2002). Occupational health nursing practice guidelines. Retrieved April 25, 2007, from www.cohna-aciist.ca. Reproduced with permission.

The OHN can play a key role in developing and implementing health promotion programs. Although not a legislated part of occupational health and safety, health promotion programs encompass best practice in occupational health nursing. Health promotion programs can prevent illness and injury by increasing awareness of lifestyle risks to health, encouraging behaviour modification, and promoting lifestyle changes.

A manager serves an important function in the operation of the occupational health service by providing the structure and direction for the development, implementation, and evaluation of the program. The **administrator** is also responsible for communicating and interpreting the occupational health program to management and other members of the occupational health team.

The OHN **educator** teaches and prepares nursing students in the occupational health nursing specialty. The educator must have the appropriate education to teach, as well as experience and knowledge in the concepts of occupational health. The educator must be able to integrate theory with actual practice in the workplace.

The role of the OHN as a **researcher** is growing, and there is increasing focus on this area. The researcher develops researchable questions, conducts research, and communicates the research findings to other occupational health nurses, other researchers, and the public.

The OHN **consultant** serves as a resource to other occupational health professionals, management, and organizations; assists in the development and evaluation of occupational programs and services; and recommends strategies and options for improvement. The consultant generally does not have direct responsibility for implementing or enforcing the recommendations. Consultants must be aware of the "business" of occupational health, as well as having excellent communication skills (both oral and written). OHN consultants may function either internally or externally to the organization.

Occupational Health Nursing as a Specialty Practice

Occupational health nursing is a specialty in which registered nurses generally work outside the traditional health care system. Most OHNs work independently and may be the only health care professional in the workplace setting. Consequently, OHNs must ensure that they have the appropriate education, training, and expertise to practise competently in order to provide a variety of services such as:

- health promotion and injury/illness prevention;
- health surveillance for those workers who may be exposed to health hazards (e.g., audiometric testing for noise-exposed workers; blood-lead levels for lead-exposed workers);
- health monitoring for workers who have health conditions that may impact on their ability to do their jobs safely, or where workplace exposures may have a detrimental effect on their health;
- pre-placement health assessments to match fitness for work with bona fide occupational requirements such as job demands;
- primary care and case management for ill or injured workers;
- counselling;
- referral to employee assistance programs;
- management and administration;
- research;
- worker education;
- job hazard analysis; and
- ergonomic assessments.

CNA Certification OHN Competencies

The Canadian Nurses Association outlines key competencies for occupational health nurses to complete the certification exam. The high-level competencies are listed below. For more detail refer to the CNA website.

1. Provision of Occupational Health, Safety, and Environmental Nursing

The occupational health nurse:

- practises in accordance with occupational health, safety, and environmental nursing standards of practice, code of ethics, and applicable professional legislation,
- practises in compliance with legislation, codes, regulations, and standards, and
- complies with legislative requirement for due diligence regarding record keeping.

2. Recognition, Evaluation, and Control of Workplace, Environmental Health, and Safety Hazards

The occupational health nurse:

- identifies potential and existing workplace/environmental health and safety hazards,
- assesses the level of risk and severity of hazards based on probability that harm may occur in a specific situation,
- applies principles of hazard control, and
- makes recommendations for control measures based on risk assessment findings.

3. Health Assessment, Planning, Implementation, Monitoring, and Evaluation

The occupational health nurse:

- assesses, plans, implements, recommends, and monitors interventions to promote employee health and wellness,
- develops, implements, and evaluates programs and procedures for health surveillance, and
- collects, analyzes, uses, and communicates aggregate date for prevention, identification of trends, statistical or research purposes.

4. Assessment, Care, and Case Management of Injuries and Illnesses

The occupational health nurse:

- applies the nursing process to implement appropriate interventions to minimize the effects of illness and injury,
- uses a combination of ongoing data gathering activities to evaluate ill or injured employees,
- identifies the implications for fitness to work for identified health disorders,
- identifies occupational or non-occupational injuries and illness, assesses limitations, and recommends workplace accommodation as required,
- provides and coordinates ability/case management, and
- counsels employees in the prevention and management of both occupational and non-occupational illnesses and injuries.

5. Environment, Health, Safety, Wellness Promotion, and Prevention

The occupational health nurse:

- provides leadership to empower employees and management to adopt strategies directed toward both organizational and individual health, safety, and wellness.

6. Environment, Health, Safety, and Wellness Management

The occupational health nurse:

- manages environment, health, safety, and wellness services.

Source: Adapted from Canadian Nurses Association (2006). Occupational health nursing certification: The occupational health nursing examination list of competencies. Retrieved September 27, 2007, from www.cna-nurses.ca/cna/documents/pdf/publications/CERT_Occup_e.pdf.

Education In Canada, OHNs are registered nurses who hold a diploma or degree in nursing and have a variety of additional qualifications and experience. OHNs may also have a certificate, diploma, or degree in occupational health and safety from a community college or university. Courses may include such topics as hazard identification and control, toxicology, ergonomics, occupational environments, health surveillance, program development, audiometric testing, spirometry, and disability case management. To ensure their competency, registered nurses who choose to work in this field should take this specific education.

Certification OHNs in Canada may obtain national certification in their specialty by writing the Canadian Nurses Association certification exam. The first to develop a specialty certification exam, OHNs did this through their own association, the Canadian Council for Occupational Health Nurses Incorporated (CCOHN), in 1984. This certification earned international recognition, and many specialty nursing groups followed. In 1992, the CCOHN certification process was transferred to the jurisdiction of the Canadian Nurses Association.

OHNs who are certified in occupational health nursing have met specific eligibility requirements and passed a written exam to show that they have met a national standard of competency in Occupational Health Nursing. In Canada, expertise unique to this specialty is recognized with the initials COHN(C), granted by the Canadian Nurses Association. The initials COHN or COHN-S recognize U.S. certification. These are marks of distinction for occupational health nursing excellence.

The six major competencies for occupational health nursing required for the Canadian Nurses Association (CNA) certification exam are headlined in the text box "CNA Certification OHN Competencies." Each major competency is followed by a list of standards.

Specialty Associations and Networking OHNs from across Canada have been meeting informally since 1980. The formal association was founded in 1984 and incorporated in its current form in 1994. The Canadian Occupational Health Nurses Association/Association Canadienne des Infirmières et Infirmiers en Santé du Travail (COHNA/ACIIST) continues to evolve and is the voice of OHNs in Canada.

COHNA/ACIIST has more than 2000 members. Members of the provincial occupational health nursing associations are automatically members of COHNA/ACIIST. The Board of Directors is composed of representatives from each provincial association. Nine provinces are represented. Information on the association is available on the COHNA/ACIIST website.

The objectives of COHNA/ACIIST are:

- to improve health and safety of workers by speaking with a national voice to influence health and safety regulations legislation;
- to enhance the profile of OHNs at provincial, territorial, national, and international levels;
- to advance the profession by providing a national forum for the exchange of ideas and concerns;
- to contribute to the health of the community by providing quality health services to workers;
- to promote national standards for OHNs; and
- to encourage continuing education and ensure the certification process meets COHNA/ACIIST (COHNA, 2000a) standards.

Benefits of Occupational Health Nursing

OHNs are a valuable part of an organization's team. Benefits of having an OHN on staff have been outlined by the Alberta Occupational Health Nurses Association (AOHNA) and by COHNA/ACIIST.

Benefits to Employees Having an OHN at the work site benefits employees (AOHNA [n.d.]) by:

- decreasing the risk of workplace illness and injury;
- educating them on health and safety issues that may affect them both on and off the job;
- increasing job satisfaction and morale;
- placing them in jobs that they can perform safely;
- training them in healthy and safe work practices; and
- facilitating a safe return to work following illness or injury by helping such employees maintain a sense of self-worth and connection with the workplace, perform modified work, and minimize loss of income from time away from work.

Benefits to the Employer OHNs in the workplace are a valuable asset to the organization and assist the employer (AOHNA, [n.d.]; COHNA, 2000b) by:

- increasing compliance with federal and provincial occupational health and safety legislation;
- allowing managers to spend less time dealing with unfamiliar health and safety issues;
- reducing costs of premiums and penalties on WCB and other insurance and benefit plans;
- lowering the risk of workplace illness and injury;
- reducing lost time/downtime related to both on-the-job and off-the-job illness and injury;
- improving employee morale and productivity;
- decreasing absenteeism;
- assisting in placement of employees in jobs that are suitable to their physical and mental abilities;
- enhancing corporate image; and
- decreasing employee turnover, which reduces costs of recruiting and retraining staff.

Cost–Benefit and Cost-Effectiveness Analyses OHNs must be able to demonstrate their contributions, value, business relevance, and return on investment for employers (Morris & Smith, 2001). In today's corporate climate, this must be done by using business principles like cost–benefit and cost-effectiveness analyses. Programs that cannot demonstrate that they are financially beneficial will not be maintained.

Cost–benefit analysis is a technique that represents both costs and benefits of the outcomes of a program in monetary terms, permitting a comparison between unlike elements and yielding a benefit-to-cost ratio (American Association of Occupational Health Nurses [AAOHN], 2004). It asks what is the benefit of the program (e.g., reduced WCB costs, increased productivity) compared with what it costs to run the program.

Cost-effectiveness analysis is used to determine which activities or interventions achieve the program's goals and objectives with the most value or greatest impact on cost (AAOHN, 2004). It involves comparing alternative options for the same services. An example of this would be comparing the costs for in-house versus contracted occupational health services.

AAOHN (2004) outlines the following steps for cost–benefit and cost-effectiveness analyses for OHNs.

1. Determine the program/service for financial analysis.
2. Formulate the objectives and goals of the program/service.
3. List alternative ways objectives and goals can be achieved.
4. Determine costs/benefits for all alternatives. Include appropriate cost categories such as personnel costs, supplies, capital expenditures, facility costs, and lost productive time.
5. Determine monetary value for costs/benefits, or determine outcome measures such as absenteeism rates, health services utilization, claims utilization, risk behaviours (such as smoking, obesity, seat belt use, and alcohol use), workers' compensation claims, lost-time incidents, and productivity rates.
6. Calculate discounting. Discounting reduces future costs to their present worth. It answers the question, "What is the cost of providing this service now compared with what it will cost in the future?"
7. Calculate the cost–benefit ratio or cost-effectiveness of the program/service (Ossler, 1984).

ORGANIZATIONAL CULTURE AND OCCUPATIONAL HEALTH

Organizational culture can be defined as the values, perceptions, beliefs, and behaviours that create a social system within a workplace. The impact of organizational culture on employee health behaviours is well documented (Allen, Allen, Kraft, & Certner, 1987; Bachmann, 2000; O'Donnell, 2000; Pratt, 2001; Rogers, 2003). The literature indicates that employees are more likely to be guided by the cultural "norms" of the organization than by their own values (Allen et al., 1987; Allen & Leutzinger, 1999). These norms may be positive or negative. An organization that values a "safe and healthy" workplace must have organizational goals that reflect this through the implementation of occupational health and safety programs and through role modelling of organizational behaviours that support, promote, and protect health (Rogers, 2003). Successful occupational health and safety programs must focus on the development of initiatives that go beyond the traditional physical component, addressing the areas of physical, emotional, social, intellectual, spiritual, and environmental well-being. The key to the success of all comprehensive occupational health and safety programs is to create a culture that supports safe and healthy activities and behaviours and moves toward both personal and organizational health, safety, and well-being. To be successful, this must involve participation from all levels within the organization.

OCCUPATIONAL HEALTH NURSING: LINKAGES WITH COMMUNITY HEALTH

Occupational health nursing is closely linked to community health nursing in both theory and practice (Rogers, 2003). Both nursing types emphasize prevention and health promotion as strategies for improving health and reducing the risks of illness (Rogers, 2003). Community health nurses focus on the public, while OHNs focus on the worker population.

Occupational health nursing functions may be categorized into the three levels of prevention: primary, secondary, and tertiary. Primary prevention by OHNs includes health promotion (such as nutrition, physical activity, coping) and disease prevention (such as incident and injury prevention, health risk appraisals, health education, smoking cessation, weight control, and stress management). Secondary prevention activities may include pre-placement assessments, health surveillance, incident reporting, and injury treatment. Tertiary prevention in occupational health includes return-to-work programs, work hardening, and monitoring employees for chronic health conditions (Rogers, 2003).

Occupational Health and Safety in the Community Health Setting

Community health nurses, as workers themselves, have a responsibility to maintain the health and safety of their workplace and to protect themselves and their co-workers from work-related illness or injury. Whether working on-site at a health facility, in the client's home, or on the road, the community health nurse must be aware of the occupational health and safety hazards and their appropriate controls, as outlined in the beginning of this chapter. Hazards for CHNs may include such things as workplace violence, working alone, driving, exposure to blood and body fluids, repetitive strain injuries, lifting and transferring of materials and clients, and exposure to chemicals. Identified hazards, near misses, and incidents must be reported promptly and investigated to prevent future incidents resulting in illness or injury. Working in a safe and healthy manner should become the "norm" of the community health workplace and part of everyday work performance.

CANADIAN RESEARCH

How does one measure the extent to which occupational health nursing care helps the clients? This is challenging for the occupational health and safety profession because it is difficult to quantify the promotion and maintenance of physical, mental, emotional, and spiritual health as well as the prevention of ill health. In the field of occupational health nursing, as with all other areas of nursing, quantifying effectiveness is particularly important because significant costs are associated

with health care. Determining the effectiveness of our nursing practice is a challenge (Graziani, 1996), and any tools for this purpose are valuable.

Canadian nursing research in occupational health is limited and therefore provides opportunities for nurses in the future. Although only a handful of academic research studies have been done by OHNs, research is being done by industry and by other occupational health professionals. Canadian Research Box 12.2 illustrates one example of Canadian nursing research in occupational health nursing.

Case Study

Marie is a 47-year-old community health nurse who has worked in a rural community health setting in northern Saskatchewan for 15 years. Marie works primarily at the local community health centre and frequently travels to visit new mothers and babies in the surrounding area.

Discussion Questions

1. What hazards might Marie encounter when she visits her clients?

2. How might these hazards differ from those of a community health nurse working in an urban setting?

3. What controls should be in place?

4. Identify the responsibilities of the employer for ensuring Marie's health and safety.

Canadian Research Box 12.2

Skillen, D. L., Anderson, M. C., Seglie, J., & Gilbert, J. (2002). Toward a model for effectiveness: What Alberta occupational health nurses think. *AAOHN Journal, 50*(2), 75–82.

Four Alberta nurses conducted a study and proposed a model for determining the effectiveness of occupational health nursing practice. The model (see Figure 12.2) identifies five occupational health nursing goals:

■ balance,
■ communication,
■ leadership,
■ continuing competence, and
■ trust.

To achieve these five goals, ten occupational health nursing functions as well as nine relationships were suggested and discussed. The model states that the base or foundation for occupational health nursing practice is education and experience as a registered nurse as well as baseline competence in occupational health nursing, which includes education and experience in occupational health nursing along with knowledge of a number of related disciplines.

The model brings together a number of elements of occupational health nursing in a comprehensive format and provides a basis for further research, discussion, and development. The researchers acknowledge that further work and discussion is needed so that the effectiveness of occupational health nursing practice can be measured using their model.

Discussion Questions:

1. Of what practical use is a model such as this for the practice of nursing?

2. How would you suggest the model be used when effectiveness measures are developed?

Source: Skillen, D.L., Anderson, M.C., Deglie, J. and Gilbert J. (2002). Toward a model for effectiveness: what Alberta occupational health nurses think. AAOHN Journal, 50(2), 75–82.

FIGURE 12.2 Model for Determining the Effectiveness of Occupational Health Nursing Practice

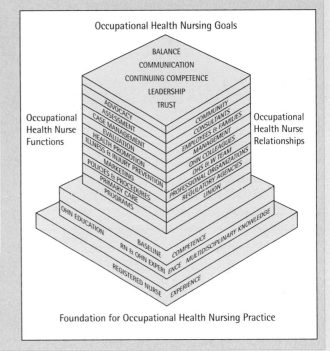

Foundation for Occupational Health Nursing Practice

Summary

Occupational health nursing is a specialized area of nursing requiring specific education and competence. As well, occupational health and safety issues affect *all* nurses in their everyday work experience. It is important that registered nurses in the community health setting be aware of occupational health and safety issues, which may impact the health of their clients as well as themselves.

This chapter has looked at the components of an occupational health and safety program. Management commitment, worker involvement, legislation and standards, and program administration have all been discussed. The different categories of health and safety hazards were introduced. Occupational health nursing was portrayed both as an integral part of the occupational health and safety team and as a specialty of nursing. A conceptual framework for occupational health nursing and the roles and competencies of OHNs were presented. Finally, the necessity of considering occupational health and safety in all aspects of nursing, particularly community health, was considered.

As you continue your studies and your work in nursing, think about how a patient's work setting can affect health, what nursing care may be required, and what referrals may be indicated. If your patient is young and hasn't yet been introduced to the work world, think about how a family

member's work could be a factor in the presenting problem or the family's health. If you're working with a senior, think about how previous work exposures may be a factor in current health issues that senior may be facing. Finally, and most importantly, think about your own health and safety as you work and the steps you can take to protect yourself as a worker and to promote your own health and safety.

KEY TERMS

occupational health theory
occupational health and safety programs
hazards
management commitment
job demands analysis
engineering controls
administrative controls
personal protective equipment
Workplace Hazardous Materials Information System (WHMIS)
safety or mechanical hazards
physical hazards
chemical hazards
biological hazards
ergonomic hazards

psychosocial hazards
occupational health physicians
occupational hygienists
ergonomist
safety professionals
occupational health nursing
clinician/practitioner
case manager
administrator
educator
researcher
consultant
cost–benefit analysis
cost-effectiveness analysis
organizational culture

STUDY QUESTIONS

1. List the components of an effective occupational health and safety program.

2. Who are the members of the occupational health and safety team?

3. Outline the roles of the occupational health physician, occupational hygienist, and the safety professional.

4. Name the categories into which hazards are divided, and give one example of each type of hazard.

5. Pick any one member of the occupational health and safety team and describe the similarities and differences between the focus of that member's role and an OHN's role.

6. What are the benefits of having an occupational nurse at the workplace for employees? for employers?

7. Name five hazards to which CHNs may be exposed in their work setting. In addition, state the category of hazard for each.

INDIVIDUAL CRITICAL THINKING EXERCISES

1. What is your role and responsibility as a CHN for occupational health and safety at work?

2. Who is responsible for identifying hazards in the workplace?

3. As a CHN, how can you provide input into a joint health and safety committee?

4. Consider the linkages, similarities, and differences between community health nursing and occupational health nursing.

GROUP CRITICAL THINKING EXERCISES

1. How would you set up a joint health and safety committee in the community health unit? Why would you want to?

2. Identify the legislation pertinent to health and safety in your jurisdiction.

3. Using the job hazard analysis form (Figure 12.1), identify five hazards in a community health nursing workplace. Specify the controls that could be used to eliminate or minimize exposure to these hazards.

REFERENCES

Alberta Employment, Immigration and Industry, Workplace Health and Safety. (2004). *All shook up—Understanding vibration.* Edmonton, AB: Author. Retrieved April 26, 2007, from http://employment.alberta.ca/documents/WHS/WHS-PUB_erg026.pdf

Alberta Employment, Immigration and Industry, Workplace Health and Safety. (2007). *Working in the heat.* Edmonton, AB: Author. Retrieved April 26, 2007, from http://employment.alberta.ca/documents/WHS/WHS-PUB_mg022.pdf

Alberta Occupational Health Nurses Association. (n.d.). *What is occupational health nursing?* Retrieved July 25, 2007, from http://www.aohna.ab.ca/.

Allen, R., Allen, J., Kraft, C., & Certner, B. (1987). *The organizational unconscious: How to create the corporate culture that you want and need.* Morristown, NJ: Human Resources Institute.

Allen, J., & Leutzinger, J. (1999). The role of culture change in health promotion. *The Art of Health Promotion, 3*(1), 1–10.

American Association of Occupational Health Nurses. (2004). *Advisory: Cost benefit and cost effectiveness analysis.* Retrieved April 25, 2007, from http://www.aaohn.org/practice/advisories/upload/advisory_costbenefit.PDF.

American Association of Occupational Health Nurses. (2007). *Occupational and Environmental Health Nursing Profession Fact Sheet.* Retrieved April 25, 2007, from http://www.aaohn.org/press_room/fact_sheets/aaohn.cfm.

Association of Canadian Ergonomists. (2007). *About ergonomics.* Retrieved July 25, 2007, from http:/// http://www.ace-ergocanada.ca/index.php?contentid=142.

Bachmann, K. (2000). *More than just hard hats and safety boots: Creating healthier work environments.* Ottawa: Conference Board of Canada.

Board of Canadian Registered Safety Professionals. (2007). *Home page.* Retrieved April 25, 2007, from www.bcrsp.ca/.

Canadian Centre for Occupational Health and Safety. (1997–2006). *How workplace chemicals enter the body.* Retrieved April 25, 2007, from www.ccohs.ca/oshanswers/chemicals/how_chem.html.

Canadian Centre for Occupational Health and Safety. (2007). *What is a joint health and safety committee?* Retrieved April 26, 2007, from www.ccohs.ca/oshanswers/hsprograms/hscommittees/whatisa.html.

Canadian Centre for Occupational Health and Safety. (n.d., a). *Biological hazards.* Retrieved April 25, 2007, from www.ccohs.ca/oshanswers/biol_hazards/.

Canadian Centre for Occupational Health and Safety. (n.d., b). *Ergonomics.* Retrieved April 25, 2007, from www.ccohs.ca/oshanswers/ergonomics.

Canadian Centre for Occupational Health and Safety. (n.d., c). *Physical agents.* Retrieved April 15, 2007, from www.ccohs.ca/oshanswers/phys_agents/.

Canadian Nurses Association. (2006). *Occupational health nursing certification: The occupational nursing examination list of competencies.* Retrieved September 27, 2007, from www.cna-nurses.ca/cna/documents/pdf/publications/CERT_Occup_e.pdf.

Canadian Occupational Health Nurses Association (COHNA-ACIIST). (2000a). *About us.* Retrieved April 25, 2007, from http://www.cohna-aciist.ca.

Canadian Occupational Health Nurses Association (COHNA-ACIIST). (2000b). *Canadian occupational health nurses information booklet.* Author.

Canadian Occupational Health Nurses Association (COHNA-ACIIST). (2002). *Occupational health nursing practice guidelines.* Retrieved April 25, 2007, from http://www.cohna-aciist.ca.

Doyle, B. (2006). *Introduction to occupational health nursing.* Edmonton, AB: Grant MacEwan College.

Federal Emergency Management Agency. (2007). *Emergency management guide for business and industry.* Retrieved April 26, 2007, from http://www.fema.gov/business/guide/index.shtm.

Graziani, C. (1996). Defining "effectiveness" in health development. *Synergy: Canadian Initiatives for International Health, 8*(3), 1, 5.

Levy, B., Wegman, D., Baron, S., & Sokas, R. (2006). *Occupational and environmental health: Recognizing and preventing disease and injury* (5th ed.). Philadelphia, PA: Lippincott, Williams & Wilkins.

Morris, J., & Smith, P. (2001). Demonstrating the cost effectiveness of an expert occupational and environmental nurse. *AAOHN Journal, 49*(12), 547–556.

O'Donnell, M. P. (2000). *How to design workplace health promotion programs* (5th ed.). West Bloomfield, MI: American Journal of Health Promotion.

Pratt, D. (2001). *The healthy scorecard: Delivering breakthrough results that employees and investors will love.* Victoria, BC: Trafford.

Rogers, B. (2003). *Occupational and environmental health nursing: Concepts and practice* (2nd ed.). Philadelphia, PA: Saunders.

World Health Organization. (2002). *Good practice in occupational health services: A contribution to workplace health.* Accessed April 25, 2007, from http://www.euro.who.int/document/e77650.pdf.

ADDITIONAL RESOURCES

Websites

Canadian Nurses Association
  www.cna-aiic.ca
Canadian Occupational Health Nurses Association
  www.cohna-aciist.ca

About the Authors

Sharon L. Chadwick, RN, BScN, MSc, COHN(C), COHN-S, has been working in the field of Occupational Health and Safety for more than 16 years. Her varied experience in this specialty includes consulting, transportation, health care, and government. Sharon has also taught in the Occupational Health Nursing Certificate Program at Grant MacEwan College for more than 10 years and has experience writing and developing courses for distance delivery. Currently, Sharon is Senior Manager, WHS Program Planning, Research and Audit in the Workplace Innovation and Continuous Improvement Branch of the Alberta Government. Sharon has served as President of the Canadian Occupational Health Nurses Association/Association Canadienne des Infirmières et Infirmiers en Santé du Travail (COHNA/ACIIST) and is a currently a member of the American Board for Occupational Health Nurses (ABOHN).

Bernice Doyle, RN, COHN(C), has been working in the Occupational Health Nursing specialty for more than 20 years. Her experience includes working in a variety of industries including government. She also has experience writing and developing occupational health nursing courses for distance delivery and teaching occupational health nursing students. Currently, Ms. Doyle is a manager in the Workplace Health and Safety Policy and Standards Branch for the Alberta Government, Edmonton, Alberta.

Community Health Planning, Monitoring, and Evaluation

Nancy C. Edwards, Josephine Etowa, and Margaret Ann Kennedy

OBJECTIVES

After studying this chapter, you should be able to:

1. Describe the importance of program planning, monitoring, and evaluation in the practice of community health nursing.

2. Develop a planning-implementation-evaluation plan by using a logic model.

3. Describe how the socio-ecological determinants of health can be reflected in our approach to planning, monitoring, and evaluation.

4. Describe components of the assessment-planning-evaluation cycle and the involvement of community stakeholders in this process.

5. Describe elements of the multiple interventions framework and its application to a complex community health issue.

6. Explain how commonly used evaluation models and the choice of indicators may be structured to address program accountability.

INTRODUCTION

Planning, monitoring, and evaluating community health programs are fundamental processes used by community health nurses (CHNs) as they work in partnership with the community. With more scrutiny of how public funds are being expended and increased demands for evidence-based programs, these processes have become even more critical. Nurses are in a position to plan new programs, redesign existing services, monitor the implementation of programs, and evaluate their impact. Nurses often make important contributions to these processes with the substantial involvement of community representatives, key stakeholders from a variety of service sectors, and colleagues from multiple disciplines.

There are many tools available to assist community health nurses in program planning, but their utility will be diminished if underlying determinants of health are ignored and programs are developed without considering social justice issues. Bringing evidence and theory to bear on complex community health problems is a necessary yet insufficient approach to planning. The authentic engagement of the community in planning, monitoring, and evaluating community health programs is essential if underlying social determinants are to be addressed.

PROGRAM PLANNING AND EVALUATION

The planning–evaluation cycle involves several key components. Although there are many versions of planning models in common use, all contain similar elements. A classic **planning–implementation–evaluation cycle** (Figure 13.1) involves the following steps:

- conducting a situational analysis or community assessment;
- identifying the problems or issues of concern;
- considering possible solutions or actions to address the problem;
- selecting the best alternative(s);
- designing and implementing the program;
- monitoring and evaluating the program;
- analyzing and interpreting results of the monitoring and evaluation process; and
- using results to make modifications to the program or to inform decisions about other programs.

The steps in this cycle may need to be repeated as one develops a better understanding of an issue and obtains additional input from partners. It may be necessary to cycle back to other steps in the process to try to develop a more complete picture of the factors affecting the problem and the potential solutions that need to be considered.

FIGURE 13.1 Planning–Implementation–Evaluation Cycle

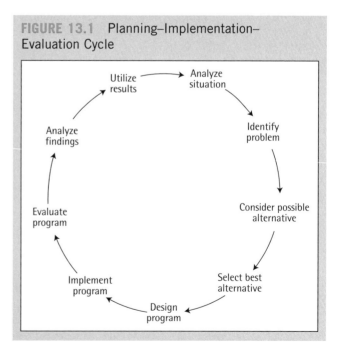

SELECTING A PROGRAM PLANNING AND EVALUATION FRAMEWORK

Many program planning and evaluation frameworks are available. **Frameworks** provide a guide for the types of information that need to be assembled and the organization of this information into a coherent plan. Several factors should be considered in selecting a framework for use. First, most community health agencies will have a standard planning framework that is used across departments. Use of a common framework allows for a coherent and consistent approach to planning within an organization. Second, the use of a particular framework may be a requirement of those who fund programs as this allows them to compare results across funded programs. Third, a framework may be chosen because it helps detail a particular aspect of the planning process that is vexing or challenging. For instance, a framework may be chosen because it is particularly useful in defining the underlying *socio-ecological determinants* of a problem, it guides the choice of theory that will help define program elements, or it is more appropriate for addressing the needs of marginalized populations. Finally, the selection of a framework may be influenced by a set of underlying values or principles such as an intention to use participatory approaches throughout the planning and evaluation process, or consistency with a social justice approach.

The **program logic model** is used extensively in many public health agencies in Canada, at both regional and municipal levels (Porteous, Sheldrick, & Stewart, 2002). It is also used by provincial and federal government agencies. A program evaluation tool kit provides a detailed description of its application (Porteous, Sheldrick, & Stewart, 1997). Logic models provide a coherent structure for complex health programs, help to expose gaps, and yield an overview of programs with appealing visual clarity.

As a support to planning, analysis, and program evaluation preparation, the logic model provides a diagram of "what the program is supposed to do, with whom, and why" (Porteous et al., 2002, p. 116). Cooksy, Gill, & Kelly (2001) note that the logic model is unique among tools for its simplicity in demonstrating program interrelationships and linkages. Logic models should be developed in collaboration with community and academic partners. In this way, both experiential learning and research findings can inform model development. Joint preparation of a logic model will help build consensus about program priorities among the planning team. In using a logic model, one should avoid positioning it as a rigid guideline that prevents iterative evolution or lateral exploration of the program under review.

Development of a logic model consists of two planning stages, referred to as **CAT** (components, activities, and target groups) and **SOLO** (short-term outcomes and long-term outcomes). For the CAT stage, activities are first clustered thematically into components for the program under review. For example, a suicide prevention program for youth might include the components of risk assessment, crisis intervention, and peer support. Activities are the specific intervention strategies to be used for each component. Using the suicide prevention example, the crisis intervention component may include training youth workers in crisis management, developing community supports for youth in crisis, and establishing better communication among social and health services organizations about youth in crisis. Target groups are the intended recipients of a program. In this example, this might be homeless youth and youth having difficulty in school, and the frontline workers for youth in schools, homeless shelters, and other health and social service organizations.

The purpose of the SOLO stage is to identify program outcomes. *Short-term outcomes* are the immediate and direct results of the program, while *long-term outcomes* reflect the ultimate goals of the program. Building the knowledge and skills of youth workers to identify and support youth in crisis would be a short-term outcome, while reducing youth suicide rates would be longer term. Many extraneous factors may influence the achievement of long-term outcomes. Thus, they are more difficult to directly and exclusively attribute to the program.

The program evaluation tool kit identifies how evaluation processes may be used to inform decision making during program planning and implementation. **Evaluation** is an ongoing, dynamic process that supports further refinement of program activities and helps to identify gaps or flaws in the original program design. It is critical to involve community partners in the evaluation process. They can play key roles in helping with data interpretation and identifying recommendations emerging from program evaluation.

TOOLS AND PROCESSES TO SUPPORT PLANNING AND EVALUATION PROCESSES

Many tools and processes may be used in combination with an organizing framework. Environmental scans, assessing strengths, weaknesses, opportunities, and threats; key informant interviews; focus groups; and round tables engage partners in a planning process. The efficient involvement of community partners is important because those working in service-delivery sectors have many demands on their time. Involving them in the planning process helps build commitment to the program and aids the design of a program that reflects the dynamic realities and strengths of the community.

Gathering Information about Community Needs and Priorities

There are practical tools available to help with gathering information about community needs and priorities. However, these must be used in conjunction with approaches that build relationships and create opportunities to hear the voices of disadvantaged groups. Additional examples of tools used to assess needs are provided in Chapter 11.

Assessment of Strengths, Weaknesses, Opportunities, and Threats (SWOT) A **SWOT analysis** identifies internal strengths and weaknesses of the organization or program,

FIGURE 13.2 PHAC Tool Kit Decision-Oriented Model for Program Evaluation

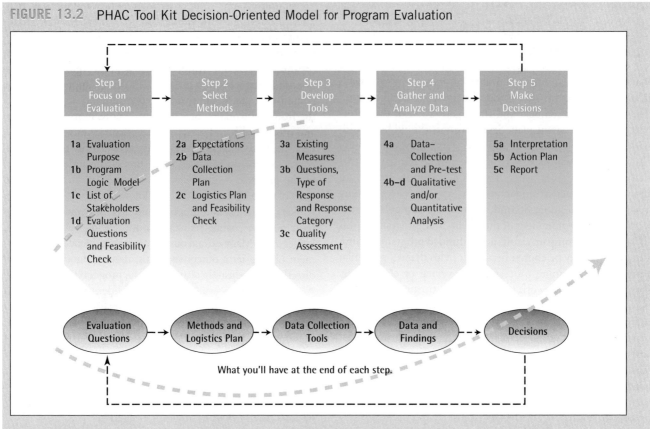

Source: Public Health Agency of Canada. (2006). Program evaluation tool kit. Retrieved October 1, 2007, from http://www.phac-aspc. gc. ca/php-psp/toolkit.html.

along with external opportunities and threats. A SWOT analysis may involve document and policy reviews, community meetings, key informant interviews, and focus groups. It helps those planning a program to customize the fit between the organization (or in this case the program) and its environment (Fraser & Stupak, 2002). A SWOT analysis may also assist in determining the feasibility of initiating or continuing a program and may help identify service gaps. SWOT analyses are frequently used as part of a strategic planning process when managers are developing long-term plans for the organization.

Assessing Needs through Qualitative Interviews and Focus Groups The use of qualitative research strategies such as individual interviews and focus groups elaborates those issues and experiences that are not readily understood through quantitative and statistical tools (Pope & Mays, 1995). For example, although quantitative evaluation tools may demonstrate that a particular subpopulation is less likely than another to use community health services, they may not be able to explain *why and how*. Similarly, quantitative data may not shed light on the perceived appropriateness of community health services and programs (Dana, 2002). Qualitative research tools not only address these gaps but also can be used to assess the meanings of health and care (Sofaer, 1999). Qualitative data can increase the relevance and interpretability of quantitative data generated during a needs assessment.

Individual interviews allow for exploration of first-person experiences and prompt interactive discussions that centre on the perspectives of participants (Patton, 2002). In-depth interviews may yield pertinent examples and rich descriptions of experiences (Rubin & Rubin, 2005). Focus groups are used "to elicit and validate collective testimonies" (Kamberelis & Dimitriadis, 2005, p. 897). The composition of focus groups must be carefully planned. Although some diversity of viewpoints is important, one should try to assemble a group in which there is not an underlying power structure among its members that may discourage some participants from openly sharing their viewpoints. For example, it may not be appropriate to have a focus group consisting of both frontline workers and their managers because front-line workers may hesitate to discuss issues concerning organizational leadership or working conditions when their managers are present. Focus groups provide opportunities for members to share and validate their individual experiences. The discussion may stimulate participant ownership of the program under development and may prompt participants toward action.

Organizing Information and Setting Priorities

The second set of tools helps with organizing and understanding data and information, and guides priority setting. See Chapters 11 and 14 for additional examples.

Analyzing and Representing Qualitative Data Analyzing qualitative data involves describing, classifying, and connecting the data. *Content analysis* is frequently used for planning purposes. It is a systematic, replicable technique for compressing large volumes of text data into fewer content categories based on explicit rules of coding (Stemler, 2001). This involves assigning codes or labels to the text data. Data are then grouped into categories to reflect emerging patterns of responses. Systematic counting and recording techniques may also be used to help identify patterns of responses such as the predominant use of certain kinds of phrases by some respondents but not others (Silverman, 2000).

Analyzed qualitative data can be packaged in text, matrix, or figure formats. A text format involves the use of illustrative quotes. Matrices are used to compare major categories of data and highlight differences and similarities among subgroups. For example, a matrix of needs assessment information may be used to compare responses from homeless men and shelter staff regarding the fairness of the shelter rules; or the perspectives of teachers, parents, and students regarding the acceptability and need for school sexual health clinics. Figures may be a useful visual tool to reflect emerging relationships among categories of coded data.

Using Quantitative Data Many sources of quantitative data may be accessed as you plan a program. These include local and provincial data documenting the magnitude of the problem and contributing factors. These data often are obtained through sources such as special surveys (e.g., school surveys to document patterns of smoking among youth), routinely collected information (e.g., police and ambulance reports), and surveillance data (e.g., reports of communicable diseases). There are many excellent examples of reporting formats that have been developed to display quantitative data. A useful starting point is to examine existing reports (e.g., health status reports) and to enlist the assistance of someone with epidemiological training.

A second use of quantitative data is to help with estimating program costs and the potential return on investments. Various methods and tools may be of relevance here, including the use of the balanced scorecard (Kaplan & Norton, 1996) and the application of health economics methods (Drummond & McGuire, 2001). The work of Dr. Gina Browne and her team (2005) provides a particularly useful illustration of how important it is to consider the costs and cost savings that may be incurred from implementing a program.

Interpreting systematic reviews is a third use of quantitative data. *Systematic reviews* assemble findings from studies with a common research objective (e.g., to examine the effectiveness of exercise and balance programs to reduce the risk of falls among seniors). Those undertaking systematic reviews use a thorough and rigorous set of methods to both identify all potentially relevant studies and to review the methodological quality of these studies. Studies deemed to be relevant and of adequate quality are included in the review. Outcome data are extracted using standard procedures. When possible, the quantitative findings from two or more studies are collapsed into a single estimate of effect. This is done by using statistical techniques, and the review process is then called a **meta-analysis**.

The illustration in Figure 13.3 is from a Cochrane review on the effectiveness of fall prevention interventions. It summarizes results from several studies. There are three important things to understand in looking at this diagram. First, the relative risk is used to indicate whether the study group that received the intervention has a lower rate of falls than the study group that did not receive the intervention. If there is no difference between the groups, the relative risk is one. If the intervention group has a lower rate of falls than the control group, the relative risk will be less than one (indicating a protective effect). Each of the four studies had a relative risk less than 1 (range 0.60 to 0.75). Second, if this intervention effect is statistically significant (indicating that if we repeated the experiment, we are 95% certain that we would again find a difference between groups), then the confidence interval around the relative risk will also be less than one. In Figure 13.3, the confidence interval is shown as a horizontal line on the diagram and listed in the right-hand column. We can see from the diagram that only Wagner's study (1994) found a statistically significant protective effect of the intervention. Third, results are then pooled across the four studies (the meta-analysis part of the exercise). A weighting factor is used in making this calculation so that studies with small sample sizes will contribute less weight to the pooled estimate than studies with large sample sizes. In this example, the pooled relative risk is 0.73 and the result is statistically significant—test for overall effect yields a p value < 0.00006. Thus, it follows that the recommendation in the abstract for this review concludes that "multidisciplinary, multifactorial, health/environmental risk factor screening/intervention programmes in the community for an unselected population of older people (4 trials, 1 651 participants, pooled relative risk (RR) 0.73, 95% confidence interval (CI) 0.63 to 0.85) is likely to be beneficial" (Gillespie et al., 2003, p. 1).

Priority Setting

Setting priorities is a vital step in the planning process. An in-depth examination of a problem in the community may leave one overwhelmed at the thought of narrowing down the possibilities for action. Several guiding principles for priority setting need to be kept in mind. These are *buy-in, transparency*, and *communication*. Setting priorities inevitably means that one can neither address all of the identified needs nor operationalize all of the proposed interventions. Engaging community members and key stakeholders in discussing the problem may initially help with *buy-in* but runs the risk of backfiring if the selection of priorities suggests that their input and ideas were not considered. Thus, it is also important to look at ways to engage the community in the process of setting priorities as one begins to more clearly define program components and activities. While it may not be realistic to involve a large community in a priority-setting exercise, one can invite input on

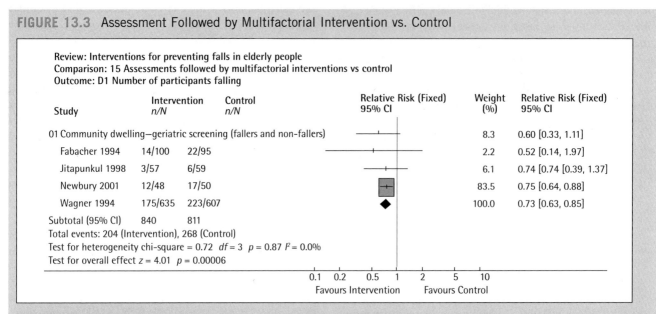

FIGURE 13.3 Assessment Followed by Multifactorial Intervention vs. Control

Source: Gillespie, L.D., Gillespie, W.J., Robertson, M.C., Lamb, S.E., Cumming, R.G. & Rowe, B.H. *Interventions for preventing falls in elderly people*. Cochrane Database of Systematic Reviews 2003, *Issue 4. Art. No.: CD000340. DOI: 10.1002/14651858.CD000340.*

the selection of criteria to inform priority setting. Agreement among senior managers on a common priority-setting process for an organization will help ensure managerial support for the priorities identified.

The second principle is *transparency*—whereby the process for selecting priorities is made apparent to those who were not directly involved in the process. In other words, key stakeholders are able to understand how you got from point A (understanding problem and considering possible intervention strategies) to point B (priority definition of the problem and strategies). Various criteria have been applied to identify priority interventions. Both objective and subjective criteria are important. Objective criteria are measurable facets of a problem and its solutions. For example, what is the magnitude (prevalence or incidence) of a problem? What are the short- and long-term consequences of the problem (e.g., mortality or morbidity)? Are there effective strategies to address the problem? And how cost-effective are the strategies relative to other approaches? Subjective criteria require judgment calls that are based on underlying values about the issue and the implementing organization. For instance, will working on the problem lead to new and stronger partnerships with other community agencies? Is tackling the problem within the mandate of our organization? Is there community readiness and political will to address this problem in both the short and the long term?

The third principle is *communication*. A clear communication strategy needs to accompany efforts to set priorities. Both internal and external communication processes are vital. Internally, the identification of priorities should be directly linked to the approval mechanisms for program funding. Externally, one needs to communicate priorities to partners who have provided input on the program. This will help to ensure more buy-in for program implementation.

THE SHIFT TO MULTIPLE INTERVENTIONS

Increasingly, community health programs are targeting the complexity and root causes of problems. This requires a socio-ecological examination of the issue of interest, and a planning–intervention–evaluation cycle that addresses these underlying determinants. Raphael (2004) defines *social determinants of health* as "the economic and social conditions that influence the health of individuals, communities and jurisdictions as a whole" (p. 1). Several key features of these social determinants are shaping contemporary community health programs. The determinants do not reside in isolation from each other. Rather, determinants are nested; that is, they are interrelated and as one determinant changes, another may also shift. Some determinants are deeply embedded, following from historical inequities such as the oppression that Aboriginal populations have experienced (Smith, Varcoe, & Edwards, 2005) and stigma faced by marginalized groups (Carr & Gramling, 2004).

The **Multiple Intervention Program (MIP) framework** arises from earlier work by Edwards and Moyer (1999). In Ontario in the late 1980s, there was a shift away from public health programs that predominantly involved home visits and clinically oriented services in schools and workplaces. As evidence on socio-ecological determinants increased, and as considerations of how best to distribute scarce resources in public health were debated, programs increasingly began to focus on interventions targeting multiple layers of the system. Nurses were being asked to expand their repertoire of interventions, to include not only those appropriate for individuals and families (such as home visits and primary care clinics) but also those targeted at community, organizational, and policy levels (such as community action, environment change, and policy strengthening and enforcement). With the input of frontline public health nurses and managers in Ottawa, a program framework was developed to reflect the integration of self-care capacity and action, collective care capacity and action, and environmental supports (Edwards & Moyer, 1999).

The next generation of this framework was developed 10 years later (Edwards, Mill, & Kothari, 2004). Its evolution arose from the observations and reflections of practitioners and from research. Managers identified the challenges of trying to plan and evaluate multiple intervention programs. Research findings were shedding light on a related set of issues. Through the 1990s, results from some well-designed experimental studies of multiple intervention programs were yielding unexpected and disappointing findings (Bauman, Suchindran, & Murray, 1999; Merzel & D'Afflitti, 2003; Sorenson, Emmons, Hunt, & Johnston, 1998). For instance, the COMMIT trial (COMMIT Research Group, 1995a) was a four-year, multiple intervention study that targeted tobacco cessation and compared 11 matched pairs of communities in the United States and Canada. Eleven communities were in the control group and received no intervention. Eleven communities received a very well developed and theory-based intervention that aimed to increase cessation rates among heavy smokers. The intervention program that was designed was considered "state of the art and science." It included more than 50 strategies that were aimed at various levels of the system including individual behaviour change strategies, community mobilization, and organizational and policy change. However, the goal of reducing smoking rates among heavy smokers was not reached (COMMIT Research Group, 1995b). Authors (Zanna et al., 1994) have attempted to describe reasons for the failures of the COMMIT trial and other multiple interventions to achieve their expected outcomes. Common reasons include the failure to involve the community in the planning process, the short duration of programs that does not allow enough time for policy change, failure to plan for long-term sustainability, and inadequate funding (Edwards, MacLean, Estable, & Meyer, 2006; Merzel & D'Afflitti, 2003).

Yet, in apparent contradiction to some of the research on multiple intervention programs, there have been compelling examples of significant multiple intervention program successes in such fields as tobacco control and injury prevention. Prolonged efforts (often over more than a decade) have yielded substantial improvements in health outcomes from multi-strategy and multi-level interventions. These efforts have required coordinating strategies in many sectors. In the case of injury prevention, for example, multiple intervention programs have included a combination of strategies aimed at raising awareness (e.g., public media campaigns); supporting behaviour change (e.g., infant car seat clinics); changing social norms (e.g., a generation of children now think that wearing a seat belt is the norm, it is no longer socially acceptable to drink and drive); and developing regulations or passing legislation and setting up enforcement approaches (e.g., using traffic calming strategies, police checkpoints for seat belt use and drunk driving).

THE MULTIPLE INTERVENTION PROGRAM FRAMEWORK

The MIP framework consists of five main elements. (See Figure 13.4.) Use of the framework involves an iterative cycle whereby emerging lessons from program implementation and

FIGURE 13.4 Multiple Interventions Framework

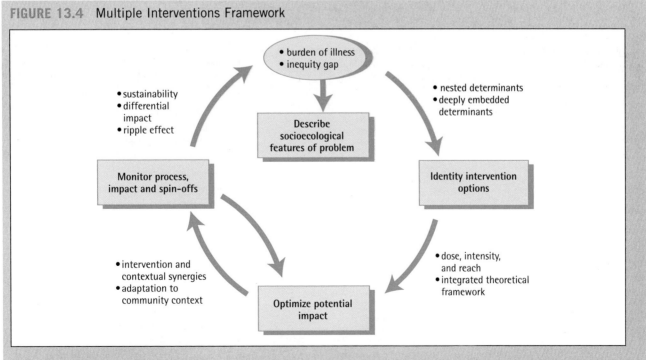

Source: Edwards, N., Mill, J., & Kothari, A. (2004). Multiple intervention framework, 36(1), 44. Reprinted by permission of CJNR.

new research findings continuously inform program adjustments. Optimal application of the framework should be based on in-depth knowledge of the local community (tacit knowledge), expertise with relevant theories, and up-to-date familiarity with good-quality research evidence (both primary studies and systematic and integrative reviews). We describe each element of the framework, using illustrative examples for the problem of preventing falls among seniors. Table 13.1 provides a summary of the types of research studies that are relevant to each element of the model. These are described in more detail below.

Identification of Community Health Issue

The first element is the identification of a community health issue that is the program focus. When an issue is identified, it is important to identify population subgroups that may be disadvantaged because they bear an unequal or inequitable burden of the health problem.

Description of Socio-ecological Determinants

The second element involves describing the socio-ecological determinants of the problem. Here, a socio-ecological perspective helps to expose the factors that may be contributing to and/or causing the problem. Similarly, strengths and capacities at different levels of the system may reveal potential solutions to the problem.

Several types of research inform this element of the framework. Etiological research examines putative causes of health problems. Both qualitative and quantitative studies may reveal

TABLE 13.1
Assembling the Research Evidence

Element of Framework	Description of Relevant Research Studies and Data	Examples from Research on Preventing Falls
Burden of illness and inequities	Prevalence and incidence of disease burden Age- and gender-specific rates of disease Policy coverage for sub-populations	*Burden of Illness:* One in three seniors falls each year. Approximately 25% of all falls result in injuries. Falls are the 6th leading cause of death among seniors in Canada. *Inequities:* Although seniors living in publicly subsidized apartment buildings have worse health status than seniors living in privately owned apartment buildings, they are significantly more likely to have universal access to grab bars (Edwards, Birkett, Nair et al., 2006).
Socioecological determinants of problem	Etiological studies, laboratory studies, integrative reviews, qualitative and quantitative studies of determinants	Findings from individual studies and reviews (Gill, Williams, & Tinetti, 2000; O'Loughlin, Robitaille, Boivin, & Suissa, 1993; Rawski, 1998) indicate that major risk factors for falls among community-dwelling seniors are: • Use of benzodiazepine sedative hyponotics • Polypharmacy (using 4 or more drugs) • Problems with balance and peripheral neuromuscular dysfunction • Environmental hazards Qualitative and quantitative studies identify the perspectives of seniors on risk factors for falls and identify the outcomes that are most important to them (e.g., loss of independence) (Aminzadeh and Edwards, 1998). Laboratory studies identify specific features of the built environment (e.g., configuration of grab bars, height of stairs, dimensions of handrails) that may interact with personal variables (e.g., chronic illness, balance, hand grip strength, cognition) to increase the risk of falls. (Maki, Perry, Scovil, Mihailidis, & Fernie, 2006; Sveistrup, Lockett, Edwards, & Aminzadeh, 2006). Policy studies examine policy gaps and the influence of the policy environment on the risk of falls (Perdue, Stone, & Gostin, 2003).

TABLE 13.1
continued

Element of Framework	Description of Relevant Research Studies and Data	Examples from Research on Preventing Falls
Intervention options	Efficacy and effectiveness studies, cost-effectiveness or cost–benefit studies, program evaluation, systematic reviews, best practice guideline documents, theories	Cochrane reviews and primary studies provide evidence of effectiveness on strategies to prevent falls and fall-related injuries (Gillespie et al., 2003; McClure et al., 2005; Parker, Gillespie, & Gillespie, 2006). Best practice guidelines for preventing falls (Scott, Dukeshire, Gallagher, & Scanlan, 2001) are informed by effectiveness studies. Community health evaluation studies yield promising strategies from fall prevention programs (Gallagher & Scott, 1997).
Optimal blend of strategies	Effectiveness studies of multi-strategy and multi-level interventions Studies informed by integrated theories Studies that examine contextual influences on intervention strategies	Evidence that exercise programs are effective when used in combination with modifications to the built environment (Gillespie et al., 2003). Evidence that multifactor approaches are more effective in reducing falls than single strategies (Tinetti et al., 1994). Socio-behavioural factors explain underutilization of efficacious interventions (Edwards, Lockett, Aminzadeh, & Nair, 2003; Fisher, Li, Michael, & Cleveland, 2004; George, Binns, Clayden, & Mulley, 1988; Naik & Gill, 2005). Studies examining the application of theory to fall prevention (Sampson & Morenoff, 2000)
Monitoring and evaluating process, impact, spin-offs, and sustainability	Identification of potential indicators, ways of assembling data to support decision making	Mandatory Core Program Guidelines for Public Health in Ontario (Ontario Ministry of Health and Long-term Care, 1997) Identify indicators to monitor fall prevention programs.

the complex relationships among determinants. Laboratory studies may yield insights into biological or environmental factors that are at play; while organizational and policy studies may reveal determinants that operate at a macro level. While individual primary studies may be useful, systematic or integrative reviews that identify causal factors from a synthesis of the best available evidence are more informative. Integrative reviews use findings from both qualitative and quantitative studies (Mays, Pope, & Popay, 2005). The phases of an integrative review process include: (1) problem formulation, (2) data collection or literature search, (3) evaluation of data from diverse research designs, (4) data analysis, and (5) interpretation and presentation of results (Whittemore & Knafl, 2005). Integrative reviews may also contribute to the identification of theoretical insights to guide program strategies.

Evidence on socio-ecological determinants is lined up with relevant levels of the socio-ecological model (Table 13.2). In consultation with the community, priority levels for action are then selected based on community characteristics and knowledge of the policy context.

The nature or scope of different health issues may render various levels of the model more relevant than others. For instance, in the case of injury prevention, features of the built environment are likely to be a central concern, whereas with tobacco control, addiction and social norms are particularly

influential determinants. Furthermore, the level(s) of government (municipal, provincial, federal) to target is determined by who has budgetary and policy jurisdiction over the problem. Community partners will provide much-needed input on the joint action of determinants in their setting and the opportunities for influencing these determinants during the program period.

Intervention Options

The third element of the framework specifies intervention options. Here, one considers strategies that have demonstrated effectiveness and are theoretically sound. This knowledge must be coupled with community input on the feasibility of implementing interventions in their setting and the need to adapt interventions to ensure cultural and geographic relevance. For instance, while there is strong evidence of efficacy from laboratory studies and some evidence of effectiveness from studies with nursing home residents that hip protectors will reduce the risk of a hip fracture when a fall occurs, problems with compliance in using hip protectors have been reported (Parker et al., 2006). Reasons for non-compliance include inconvenience when busy nursing staff in long-term care settings have to help residents with dressing,

TABLE 13.2
Socio-ecological Determinants of Falls among the Elderly

Level of Socio-ecological Model	Example and Reference to Supporting Empirical Literature
Individual	Patterns and type of exercise (Benjamin, Edwards, & Bharti, 2005) Seniors' perceptions of barriers to physical activity (Lockett, Willis, & Edwards, 2005)
Interpersonal	Buddy systems in apartment buildings where neighbours check on each other to see if anyone has had an injurious fall
Community	Coalitions or other organized collectives taking action on preventing falls by raising awareness and addressing policy change (Edwards, 1999)
Built/physical environment	Presence of grab bars in bathrooms (Aminzadeh, Edwards, Lockett, & Nair, 2001) Features of safe stairs (Maki et al., 2006)
Social environment	Accessibility of esthetically pleasing and safe walking areas near seniors' housing (Giles-Corti & Donovan, 2003)
Organizational policy (e.g., workplace, places of worship, housing)	Skilled volunteers organized in the community to make home modifications such as installing handrails on indoor and outdoor stairs (Edwards, Benjamin, & Lockett, 2006)
Municipal policy	Policies regarding the marking of cracks in public sidewalks and length of time to fix these cracks (Gallagher & Scott, 1997)
Provincial policy	Provincial building codes for private and public housing (Edwards, Birkett et al., 2006)
National policy	Recommendations for building codes provided by National Research Council and uptake of empirical evidence in modifications to building codes (Pauls, 1991)

seniors try hip protectors but find them to be bulky under regular clothing, and seniors accidentally soil their hip protector garments due to urge incontinence. These factors reduce the effectiveness of hip protectors as an injury-prevention strategy.

A mix of studies is required to inform intervention choices. For example, etiological studies indicate that the use of benzodiazepine sedative hypnotics is consistently a risk factor for falls. This suggests that minimizing use of these medications would be a useful fall prevention strategy. For those planning a program, however, the question that arises is who is the most effective target—the seniors or those physicians who prescribe the medication? Studies from the field of addictions indicate that it is difficult to wean an individual off this class of drugs following long-term use. However, studies that have targeted changes in prescribing practice suggest that academic detailers (e.g., representatives from pharmaceutical companies who directly market new drugs to physicians) and audit and feedback strategies are effective in modifying physician prescribing behaviour (Foy et al., 2002). This combination of evidence indicates that a public health strategy targeting individual counselling for those who are taking benzodiazepines is less likely to have a population impact than a public health strategy that targets prescribing patterns among family physicians.

When selecting intervention options, planning teams also need to pay close attention to the *reach, dose,* and *intensity* of strategies that are required (Glasgow, Vogt, & Boles, 1999) to have their intended effect. The **reach** of an inter-

vention concerns what proportion and which particular segments of an intended target population receive the interventions. For example, a public service advertisement intended for all seniors will reach only those who are watching television or listening to the radio when the advertisement is run. The **dose** is the amount of intervention required to have an effect. Multiple exposures to a public service announcement are required to change awareness. The **intensity** of the intervention refers to its quality and whether it is tailored to the population subgroup receiving the intervention. For instance, a media campaign about the importance of walking regularly may have adequate intensity for seniors who have good functional status but is unlikely to be a suitable message for very frail seniors who are not independently mobile. A note of caution is important here. If strategies that appear promising are watered down due to funding constraints or other limitations on program delivery capacity, the dose and intensity required for the intervention to make a difference may be diluted and the expected outcome is unlikely to be achieved.

Choosing strategies requires in-depth knowledge of the community characteristics that may influence uptake and effectiveness of the intervention strategies. The readiness and capacity of the community for the intended change is an important consideration that can best be gauged by community partners. The identification of *policy windows* and *policy levers* is also important. **Policy windows** are periods of opportunity to get an issue on the policy agenda. Policy windows may open because of a community crisis; mounting concern about a growing problem among the public and substantial press coverage on this issue; or a period of planned change such as the amalgamation of municipalities. These policy windows can create the momentum and public support required for policy change. Identifying **policy levers** requires an understanding of the ways in which different kinds of policies (e.g., community health nursing standards, National Research Council building code recommendations, legislation) can be introduced or changed. Involving those with expertise in policy change processes—such as individuals with political science, public administration, or legal backgrounds—in content-specific areas will help your planning team.

In addition to evidence on what works and knowledge of the community, theoretical considerations should also drive the planning process. We are often inclined to apply those theories most familiar to us, rather than those theories most pertinent for the problem at hand. Since a multiple intervention program approach tackles more than one level of the socio-ecological determinants (Stokols, 1996), a mix of theories is required to guide the program. This involves integrating theories from various disciplines and is likely to require the expertise of individuals from different disciplines who know the theories well. Identifying a range of relevant theories may expand the intervention options to be considered.

Optimization of Intervention Strategies

The fourth framework element focuses on optimizing intervention strategies. That is, how can we increase the likelihood that the combination of interventions works in a well-orchestrated fashion and how can we adapt our interventions to a dynamic context? Sorting this out requires that we attend to the sequence and combination of strategies, and to the ways in which the political, social, organizational, and policy environments (contexts) are changing. The integrated theory that guides our program should inform decisions on how to optimize intervention strategies. Since intervention strategies may work together either positively or negatively, questions to consider when discussing how to optimize them include:

■ What is a particular program trying to achieve, and how can we combine intervention strategies to potentiate this?

■ Are there ways in which a particular combination of interventions might nullify each others' effects?

■ What is going on in the community that might enhance or reduce the impact of the intervention?

Two examples of how selected interventions might be optimized are provided in Table 13.3. The first example,

TABLE 13.3
Optimizing Interventions

Examples of Intervention Strategies and Intended Effect	Underlying Theory and Research to Support Plan for Optimizing Intervention Strategies	Optimizing the Intervention
Media campaign to raise awareness about the risk of hazardous stairs, and volunteer program to encourage seniors to take action to improve safety of home stairs.	Social marketing theory, media communication studies and stages of change theory (Prochaska et al., 1994) indicate that a media campaign can shift a segment of the population from precontemplation to contemplation for a short interval (days or weeks).	Media campaign should be timed to coincide with accessible options for action such as a help line for seniors to call to obtain volunteer assistance to make modifications to stairs (e.g., installation of handrails).
Collective action by a fall prevention coalition to increase community awareness of the importance of bathroom grab bars in combination with providing input to technical review committee for 5-year review process of building codes.	Kingdon's (1995) theory indicates that public opinion is a critical influence in the policy change process, both with respect to creating a demand for the change and the support necessary for introducing a new policy or modifying one that already exists. Kingdon's theory also identifies the importance of policy windows, periods of time when a particular policy change is more likely to happen.	Because the process of changing the National Research Council's building codes recommendations and, subsequently, provincial building code legislation involves an extended period, coalitions must be ready to mobilize public support for changes to the building codes at several time points. Effective and strategic application of Kingdon's (1995) theory by a coalition requires an understanding of how the building code revision process works and how public input on proposed changes is obtained, and knowledge of whether other key stakeholders such as the home building industry are supporting or opposing proposed changes to the building codes. The action by fall prevention coalitions through this process will require timely interventions to (a) mobilize public awareness and support, (b) work with key stakeholders to mobilize action by them, and (c) network with other coalitions.

which involves using the media and a risk counselling approach, illustrates how intervention strategies can be combined to potentiate their effect. The second example shows how a planned intervention strategy can be successfully combined with a *contextual influence*. Although programs have no direct control over contextual influences, anticipating those that may arise and making program adjustments to reflect contextual influences that do emerge may either optimize the planned intervention strategies or mitigate the negative influences of contextual changes.

Canadian Research Box 13.1

Etowa, J., Bernard, W. T., Oyinsan, B., & Clow, B. (In Press). Participatory Action Research (PAR): An approach to improving Black women's health in rural and remote communities. *International Journal of Transcultural Nursing*.

Based on the principles of participatory action research (PAR), this three-year, community–academic collaborative research not only engaged community members in the exploration of their health issues but also facilitated the process of innovative social actions to address these issues. The project involved 237 Black women living in the towns and villages along the southern and western shores of Nova Scotia. Evaluation indicators included the project process, impact, and outcomes. Process evaluation measures examined community participation in the planning, implementation, and dissemination phases of the project. Activities of the project included focus groups, community workshops, individual interviews, and personalized training programs on a number of topics such as research skills, use of computer software, conflict resolution, public speaking, professionalism, and trouble-shooting in Microsoft. As a result of their involvement in the project, community facilitators have become community health advocates, serving on community health boards, presenting at public events, organizing health forums, and using research findings to develop a play and travelling quilt titled "From Research to Action: Breaking the Silence." Community facilitators indicated that the project was instrumental in building their health knowledge, research skills, and confidence, especially in the area of community activism. The PAR approach fostered a two-way capacity-building process and "mutual-mentoring" as knowledge was exchanged between community and academic participants.

Discussion Questions:

1. What components of the research process would be transferable to other communities?

2. What strategies would you employ to implement this kind of participatory process in other communities?

3. Read two other articles on community development programs that have used a participatory process and compare their evaluation measures with those used in this study.

Monitoring and Evaluating Impacts, Spin-offs, and Sustainability

In the final element, monitoring and evaluating program processes, impacts, spin-offs, and sustainability are the central concern. **Processes** are intermediate outputs indicating that a program is doing what was intended. Assessing processes involves looking at the critical steps that are required for the program. For instance, developing solid partnerships with other community organizations, engaging community members on a coalition, and getting a health issue on a political agenda may all be necessary to ultimately achieve policy change. **Impacts** are the longer-term results of a program, often taking some years to achieve. As with processes, impacts may be assessed at various levels of the socio-ecological model. Thus, one might expect to see *impact indicators* of individual behaviour change, increased community awareness of falls and their prevention, changes to the built environment or policy change, all depending on the original intent of the program.

The selection of impact indicators should be guided by what we know about effective interventions and the "dose" of intervention expected to achieve a particular effect. Programs that are overly ambitious may appear ineffective because their resources are spread too thinly. When program managers cannot demonstrate an improvement in program outputs or outcomes, ongoing funding for the program may be threatened.

Spin-offs are unintended effects of a program. They may be positive or negative. One rarely sees formalized plans to assess spinoffs as they are largely unintended. They may, however, be identified through reflective approaches such as the maintenance of field notes during program implementation or team meeting discussions regarding observed spin-offs, and via mid- or end-of-program interviews with key informants and others who have participated in the program.

Sustainability concerns the longer-term viability of the program interventions. Evidence of sustainability at an organizational level may occur when an intervention becomes part of the routine. For instance, the introduction of a new assessment form during a program may become routinized when this form becomes part of standard data collection within the agency. Sustainability at a policy level may occur when the policy is established and enforcement strategies are routinely put in place. Sustainability does not necessarily refer to the ongoing funding of a program or imply that a program will be organized the way it started out or run by the same organization. Rather, the intent of sustainability is to continue addressing the problem and to evolve strategies to match how the problem is changing.

Summary

Community health nurses are key players in health program delivery and must also be integral to the dynamic process of program planning and evaluation. Familiarity with the tools and processes described in this chapter will help you contribute fully as a member of a program planning and evaluation team. As our examples have illustrated, community health programs are often aimed at community issues with a complex set of underlying determinants. It is not surprising that the planning process needs to be informed by a diverse set of data and evidence. Planning and evaluation should not occur in isolation. Rather, one must pull together an inter-disciplinary team with a wide range of experience to help with different facets of this process. By working together, community health workers with program planning experi-ence, academic researchers who are familiar with the theo-retical and empirical literature, and community partners who bring important insights and essential experiential learning can substantially strengthen the design and evalua-tion of multiple intervention programs in community health. This in turn will help us meet the complex needs of populations while demonstrating better accountability for the public funds used when programs are delivered.

KEY TERMS

planning–implementation–evaluation cycle
frameworks
program logic model
CAT
SOLO
evaluation
SWOT analysis
meta-analysis
Multiple Intervention Program (MIP) framework
reach
dose
intensity
policy windows
policy levers
processes
impacts
spin-offs

STUDY QUESTIONS

1. Are the steps in the planning–evaluation cycle always fol-lowed in a linear fashion?

2. List four factors that influence the choice of a program planning and evaluation framework.

3. Identify some tools commonly used in planning programs.

4. List three uses of quantitative data in planning and evalu-ating a program.

5. Identify the three principles of priority setting.

6. List the five main elements of the Multiple Intervention Program framework.

INDIVIDUAL CRITICAL THINKING EXERCISES

1. Your health care agency is collaborating with a community advocacy group to address escalating substance use among youth (ages 12 to 17). What are some of the underlying socio-ecological determinants of substance abuse in this age group?

2. Using the substance abuse problem above, what types of evidence would you assemble to support the development of the program plan and why?

3. What are the strengths and weaknesses of each type of evi-dence you have selected for the substance abuse problem?

4. What are some examples of indicators you can use to assess the impact of the substance abuse program at individual, organizational, community, and policy levels?

5. Identify a community health issue of interest. What are some examples of synergies that might be expected to occur between program strategies and community context?

GROUP CRITICAL THINKING EXERCISES

1. You are part of a team evaluating a childhood obesity pro-gram delivered through the local schools. What informa-tion would you need to develop a logic model for this initiative? Describe to the members of your team why it is important to spend time developing the logic model.

2. Locate a good example of a community health program plan that illustrates the integration of several different the-ories. Do these theories reflect different levels of socio-ecological determinants?

3. You have been asked to develop a multiple intervention program and evaluation plan to address homelessness among older adults. What community partners would you involve in this process and why? How would you get com-munity partners involved?

REFERENCES

Aminzadeh, F., & Edwards, N. (1998). Exploring seniors' views on the use of assistive devices in fall prevention. *Public Health Nursing, 15*(4), 297–304.

Aminzadeh, F., Edwards, N., Lockett, D., & Nair, R. C. (2000). Utilization of bathroom safety devices, patterns of bathing and toileting, and bathroom falls in a sample of community living older adults. *Technology and Disability, 13*(1), 95–103.

Bauman, K. E., Suchindran, C. M., & Murray, D. M. (1999). The paucity of effects in community trials: Is secular trend the culprit? *Preventive Medicine, 28*(4), 426–429.

Benjamin, K., Edwards, N., & Bharti, V. (2005). Attitudinal, perceptual, and normative beliefs influencing the exercise decisions of community-dwelling physically frail seniors: An application of the theory of planned behaviour. *Journal of Aging and Physical Activity, 13*(3), 276–293.

Browne, G. (2005). System Linked Research Unit. Hamilton, Ontario: McMaster University. Retrieved November 24, 2006, from http://www.fhs.mcmaster.ca/slru/interview.htm

Carr, R. L., & Gramling, L. F. (2004). Stigma: A health bar-rier for women with HIV/AIDS. *Journal of the Association of Nurses in AIDS Care, 15*(5), 30–39.

COMMIT Research Group. (1995a). Community Intervention Trial for Smoking Cessation. (COMMIT). I: Cohort results from a four-year community intervention. *American Journal of Public Health, 85*(2), 183–192.

COMMIT Research Group. (1995b). Community Intervention Trial for Smoking Cessation. (COMMIT). II: Changes in adult cigarette smoking prevalence. *American Journal of Public Health, 85*(2), 193–200.

Cooksy, L. J., Gill, P., & Kelly, P. A. (2001). The program logic model as an integrative framework for a multimethod evaluation. *Evaluation and Program Planning, 24(2),* 119–128.

Dana, R. H. (2002). Mental Health Services for African Americans: A Cultural/Racial Perspective. *Cultural Diversity and Ethnic Minority Psychology, 8*(1), 3–18.

Drummond, M., & McGuire, A. (2001). *Economic evaluation in health care: Merging theory with practice.* Oxford: University Press.

Edwards, N. (1999). Prevention of falls among seniors in the community. In M. Stewart (Ed.), *Community Nursing: Promoting Canadians' Health* (2nd ed.; pp. 296–316). Toronto: W.B. Saunders.

Edwards, N., Benjamin, K., & Lockett, D. (2006, September 25–27). *Environmental hazards and falls prevention: Defining a new research agenda.* Poster presented at the 2006 Australian Public Health Association conference, Sydney, Australia.

Edwards, N., Lockett, D., Aminzadeh, F., & Nair, R. (2003). Predictors of bath grab-bar use among community-living older adults. *Canadian Journal on Aging, 22*(2), 217–227.

Edwards, N., MacLean, L., Estable, A., & Meyer, M. (2006). *Multiple intervention program recommendations for Mandatory Health Program and Services Guidelines Technical Review Committees.* Ottawa: Community Health Research Unit, University of Ottawa.

Edwards, N., & Moyer, A. (1999). Community needs and capacity assessment: Critical component of program planning. In M. Stewart (Ed.), *Community Nursing: Promoting Canadians' Health* (2nd ed.; pp. 420–442). Toronto: W. B. Saunders.

Edwards, N., Mill, J., & Kothari, A. (2004). Multiple intervention research programs in community health. *Canadian Journal of Nursing Research, 36*(1), 40–54.

Edwards, N., Birkett, N., Nair, R., Murphy, M., Roberge, G., & Lockett, D. (2006). Access to bathtub grab bars: Evidence of a policy gap. *Canadian Journal on Aging, 25*(3), 295–304.

Etowa, J., Thomas-Bernard, W., Clow, B. & Oyinsan, B. (2007). Improving Black Women's health in Rural and Remote Communities through Participatory Action Research (PAR). *International Journal of Transcultural Nursing, 18*(4), 349–357.

Fisher, K. J., Li, F., Michael, Y., & Cleveland M. (2004). Neighborhood-level influences on physical activity among older adults: A multilevel analysis. *Journal of Aging and Physical Activity, 12*(1), 45–63.

Foy, R., Penney, G. C., Maclennan, G., Grimshaw, J., Campbell, M., & Grol, R. (2002). Attribute of clinical recommendations that influence change in practice following audit and feedback. *Journal of Clinical Epidemiology, 55*(7), 717–722.

Fraser, D. L., & Stupak, R. J. (2002). A synthesis of the strategic planning process with the principles of andragogy: Learning, leading and linking. *International Journal of Public Administration, 25*(9), 1199–1220.

Gallagher, E. M., & Scott, V. J. (1997). The Steps Project: Participatory action research to reduce falls in public places among seniors and persons with disabilities. *Canadian Journal of Public Health, 88*(2), 129–133.

George, J., Binns, V., Clayden, A., & Mulley, G. (1988). Aids and adaptations for the elderly at home: Underprovided, underused, and undermaintained. *British Medical Journal, 296,* 1365–1366.

Giles-Corti, B., & Donovan, R. J. (2003). Relative influences of individual, social environmental, and physical environmental correlates of walking. *American Journal of Public Health, 93*(9), 1583–1589.

Gill, T., Williams, C., & Tinetti, M. (2000). Environmental hazards and the risk of nonsyncopal falls in the homes of community-living older persons. *Medical Care, 38*(12), 1174–1183.

Gillespie, L. D., Gillespie, W. J., Robertson, M. C., Lamb, S. E., Cumming, R. G., & Rowe, B. H. (2003). Interventions for preventing falls in elderly people. *Cochrane Database of Systematic Reviews,* Issue 4. Art. No.: CD000340. DOI: 10. 1002/14651858. CD000340.

Glasgow, R. E., Vogt, T. M., & Boles, S. M. (1999). Evaluating the public health impact of health promotion interventions: The RE-AIM framework. *American Journal of Public Health, 89*(9), 1322–1327.

Kamberelis, G., & Dimitriadis, G. (2005). Focus groups: Strategic articulations of pedagogy, politics and inquiry. In N. K. Denzin & Y. S. Lincoln (Eds.), *The Sage handbook of qualitative research* (3rd ed.; pp.887–907). Thousand Oaks, CA: Sage.

Kaplan, R. S., & Norton, D. P. (1996). *The balanced scorecard.* Boston: Harvard Business School Press.

Kingdon, J. W. (1995). *Agendas, alternatives, and public policies.* (2nd ed.), New York, NY: Addison-Wesley.

Lockett, D., Willis, A., & Edwards, N. (2005). Through seniors' eyes: An exploratory qualitative study to identify environmental barriers to and facilitators of walking. *Canadian Journal of Nursing Research, 37*(3), 48–65.

Maki, B. E., Perry, S. D., Scovil, C. Y., Mihailidis, A., & Fernie, G. R. (2006). Getting a grip on stairs: Research to optimize effectiveness of handrails. In R. N. Pikaar, E. A. P. Koningsveld, & P. J. M. Settels (Eds.), *Proceedings IEA 2006 Congress* (pp. 4669–4674). Amsterdam: Elsevier.

Mays, N., Pope, C., & Popay, J. (2005). Systematically reviewing qualitative and quantitative evidence to inform management and policy-making in the health field. *Journal of Health Services Research & Policy, 10*(S1), 6–20.

McClure, R., Turner, C., Peel, N., Spinks, A., Eakin, E., & Hughes K. (2005). Population-based interventions for the prevention of fall-related injuries in older people. *Cochrane Database of Systematic Reviews,* 1, Art. No.: CD004441. DOI: 10. 1002/14651858. CD004441. pub2.

Merzel, D., & D'Afflitti, J. (2003). Reconsidering community-based health promotion: Promise, performance, and potential. *American Journal of Public Health, 93*(4), 557–574.

Naik, A. D., & Gill, T. M. (2005). Underutilization of environmental adaptations for bathing in community-living older persons. *Journal of the American Geriatrics Society, 53*(9), 1497–1503.

O'Loughlin, J., Robitaille, Y., Boivin, J. F., & Suissa, S. (1993). Incidence of and risk factors for falls and injurious falls among the community-dwelling elderly. *American Journal of Epidemiology, 137,* 342–354.

Ontario Ministry of Health and Long-term Care. (1997). Review of the Mandatory Health Programs and Service Guidelines. Ontario: Ontario Ministry of Health and Long-term care. Retrieved December 7, 2006 from http://www.health.gov.on.ca/english/providers/program/pubhealth/manprog/mhpsg_mn.html

Parker, M. J., Gillespie, W. J., & Gillespie, L. D. (2006). Effectiveness of hip protectors for preventing hip fractures in elderly people: Systematic review. *British Medical Journal, 332,* 571–574.

Patton, M. Q. (2002). The nature of qualitative inquiry. In *Qualitative research & evaluation methods* (3rd ed.; pp. 3–29). Thousand Oaks: Sage.

Pauls, J. L. (1991). Safety standards, requirements, and litigation in relation to building use and safety, especially safety from falls involving stairs. *Safety Science, 14,* 125–154.

Perdue, W. C., Stone, L. A., & Gostin, L. O. (2003). The built environment and its relation to the public's health: The legal framework. *American Journal of Public Health, 93*(9), 1390–1394.

Pope, C., & Mays, N. (1995). Qualitative research: reaching the parts other methods cannot reach: An introduction to qualitative methods in health and health services. *British Medical Journal, 311,* 42–45.

Porteous, N. L., Sheldrick, B. J., & Stewart, P. J. (1997). *Program evaluation tool kit: A blueprint for public health management.* Ottawa: Ottawa-Carleton Health Department.

Porteous, N., Sheldrick, B., & Stewart, P. (2002). Introducing program teams to logic models: Facilitating the learning process. *The Canadian Journal of Program Evaluation, 17*(3), 113–141.

Prochaska, J. O., Velicer, W. F., Rossi, J. S., Goldstein, M. G., Marcus, B. H., Rakowski, W., Fiore, C., Harlow, L. L., Redding, C. A., Rosenbloom, D., & Rossi, S. R. (1994). Stages of Change and Decisional Balance for Twelve Problem Behaviours. *Health Psychology, 13*(1), 39–46.

Raphael, D. (Ed.). (2004). *Social determinants of health: Canadian perspectives.* Toronto: Canadian Scholars' Press Inc.

Rawski, E. (1998). Review of the literature on falls among the elderly. *Image: Journal of Nursing Scholarship, 30*(1), 47–52.

Rubin, J. H., & Rubin, I. S. (2005). Listening, hearing and sharing social experiences. In *Qualitative interviewing: The art of hearing data* (2nd ed.) (pp. 1–18). Toronto: Sage Publications.

Sampson, R. J., & Morenoff, J. (2000). Public health and safety in context: Lessons from community-level theory on social capital. In B. Smedley & L. Syme, (Eds.), *Promoting Health: Intervention Strategies from Social and Behavioral Research.* Washington: National Academy Press.

Scott, V., Dukeshire, S., Gallagher, E., & Scanlan, A. (2001). *A best practices guide for the prevention of falls among seniors living in the community.* Prepared for the Federal/Provincial/Territorial Ministers of Health and Ministers Responsible for Seniors.

Silverman, D. (2000). Beginning data analysis. In *Doing qualitative research: A practical handbook* (Chap. 10, pp. 119–137). Thousand Oaks: Sage Publications.

Smith, D., Varcoe, C., & Edwards, N. (2005). Turning around the intergenerational impact of residential schools on aboriginal people: Implications for health policy and practice. *Canadian Journal of Nursing Research, 37*(4), 38–60.

Sofaer, S. (1999). Qualitative methods: What are they and why use them? *Health Services Research, 34*(5), 1101–18.

Sorenson, G., Emmons, K., Hunt, M. K., & Johnston, D. (1998). Implications of the results of community intervention trials. *Annual Review of Public Health, 19,* 379–416.

Stemler, S. (2001). An overview of content analysis. *Practical Assessment, Research & Evaluation, 7*(17). Retrieved November 13, 2006, from http://PAREonline.net/getvn.asp?v=7&n=17.

Stokols, D. (1996). Translating social ecological theory into guidelines for community health promotion. *American Journal of Health Promotion, 10*(4), 282–298.

Sveistrup, H., Lockett, D., Edwards, N., & Aminzadeh, F. (2006). Evaluation of bath grab bar placement for older adults. *Technology and Disability, 18,* 45–55.

Tinetti, M. E., Baker, D. I., McAvay, G., Claus, E. B., Garrett, P., Gottschalk, M., Koch, M. L., Trainor, K., & Horwitz, R. I. (1994). A Multifactorial Intervention to Reduce the Risk of Falling among Elderly People Living in the Community. *The New England Journal of Medicine, 331*(13), 821–827.

Whittemore, R., & Knafl, K. (2005). The integrative review: Updated methodology. *Journal of Advanced Nursing, 52*(5), 546–553.

Zanna, M., Cameron, R., Goldsmith, C. H., Poland, B., Lindsay, E., & Walker, R. (1994). Critique of the COMMIT study based on the Brantford experience. *Health and Canadian Society, 2*(2), 319–336.

ADDITIONAL RESOURCES

Websites

Multiple Intervention Toolkit
www.miptoolkit.com

Public Health Agency of Canada: Program Evaluation Toolkit
www.phac-aspc.gc.ca/php-psp/toolkit.html

Readings

Heymann, J., Hertaman, C., Barer, M. L., & Evans, R. G. (Eds). (2006). *Healthier societies: From analysis to action.* New York, NY: Oxford University Press.

Green, L. W., & Kreuter, M. W. (2005). *Health program planning: An educational and ecological approach.* (4th ed.). New York: McGraw Hill.

Sallis, J. F., Cervero, R. B., Ascher, W., Henderson, K. A., Kraft, M. K., & Kerr, J. (2006). An ecological approach to creating active living communities. *Annual Review of Public Health, 27,* 297–322.

About the Authors

Nancy Edwards, RN, is a Full Professor at the University of Ottawa, School of Nursing and Department of Epidemiology and Community Medicine. Nancy is Director of the Community Health Research Unit. She holds a Nursing Chair in multiple interventions for community health nursing, funded by the Canadian Health Services Research Foundation, the Canadian Institutes of Health Research, and the Government of Ontario.

Josephine Etowa, RN, is an Associate Professor at Dalhousie University, School of Nursing. She is a community health researcher and past chair of the Health Association of African Canadians. Josephine holds a post-doctoral fellowship, funded by the Canadian Health Services Research Foundation.

Margaret Ann Kennedy, RN, is Principal, Kennedy Health Informatics Associates. She is a nursing educator, consultant, and health care practitioner with expertise in nursing information management, nursing classification systems, and outcomes measurement. Margie is a member of the Clinical Standards Committee at Canada Health Infoway, and co-chairs the national Event Programme Task Force for Infoway's Partnership conferences.

Our thanks to Sabrina Farmer, Alex Budgell, and Diana Ehlers, who provided assistance with this manuscript.

Research

Donna Ciliska and Helen Thomas

OBJECTIVES

After studying this chapter, you should be able to:

1. Describe evidence-based practice as it relates to community health nursing.

2. Critically appraise research articles reporting on the effectiveness of treatment or prevention or qualitative research to judge whether they should be utilized in practice, management, or policy decisions.

3. Understand the barriers to utilizing research to change practice, management, and policy making.

4. Define how one might be involved in future community health research.

INTRODUCTION

Community health nurses (CHNs) continuously participate in research and have opportunities, frequently unrecognized, for improving their care by utilizing high-quality research. For example:

- One CHN role is to support breastfeeding, but you are not always sure that you are successful. Are there any interventions that have been shown to increase the duration and exclusivity of breastfeeding? If so, can breastfeeding interventions have any impact on infant eczema and gastrointestinal (GI) tract infections (Kramer, Chalmers, & Hodnett, 2001)?

- The local school board is concerned that there is too little time to teach the required curriculum, so they are considering reducing the time spent in physical activity. At the same time, the region is concerned about the increasing numbers of overweight children. Are school-based physical activity programs effective in improving fitness in children (Dobbins, Lockett, Michel, Beyers, Abate, & Feldman, 2001)?

- The rate of delayed development among school-age children is higher in your area than in the rest of the province. Can parenting programs led by CHNs reduce developmental delay in children (Thomas, Camiletti, Cava, Feldman, Underwood, & Wade, 1999)?

- As part of the mental health team, you visit families in which one member has a mental illness. How do family members experience the situation, and do they ever reach acceptance (Karp & Tanarugsachock, 2000)?

Every day, questions like these face CHNs. After graduation, how can nurses continue to be educated critical thinkers whose practice is based on high-quality research evidence?

How can busy nurses keep current with the research findings? This chapter highlights strategies that CHNs can use to develop and sustain evidence-based nursing practice.

WHAT IS EVIDENCE-BASED NURSING?

The term **evidence-based nursing (EBN)** has evolved from the initial work done in evidence-based medicine and is defined as the conscientious, explicit, and judicious use of current best evidence in making decisions about the care of individual patients. The practice of evidence-based medicine means integrating individual clinical expertise with the best available external clinical evidence from systematic research (Sackett, Rosenberg, Gray, & Haynes, 1996). We have conceptualized "evidence-based nursing" as broader in context than research utilization. The practice of EBN involves the following steps:

- formulation of an answerable question to address a specific patient problem or situation (Flemming, 1998);

- systematic searching for the research evidence that could be used to answer the question (McKibbon & Marks, 1998a, 1998b);

- appraisal of the validity, relevance, and applicability of the research evidence;

- decision making regarding the change in practice;

- implementation of the evidence-based practice decision; and

- evaluation of the outcome of the decision.

In evidence-based practice, research utilization is integrated with other information that might influence the management of health issues and problems, such as clinical expertise, client preference for alternative forms of care, and available resources (DiCenso, Cullum, & Ciliska, 1998). In Figure 14.1, elements in evidence-based decision making are presented. In the figure they all have equal weight; however, this is unlikely in reality. For example, CHNs have the skills to teach and support breastfeeding, know from the research evidence that breastfeeding intervention is effective (Kramer et al., 2001), and have employers who encourage them to utilize work time doing the intervention. However, some new mothers may see the home visit as intrusive and be unwilling to allow it to occur. Similarly, you tell your clients with osteoarthritis that glucosamine can be effective (Towheed, Anastassiades, Shea, Houpt, Welch, & Hochberg, 1999), but some of your patients do not have the money to purchase it. Historically, some people have misunderstood evidence-based practice to mean the application of research findings to a decision, regardless of the context or patient preferences. In an effort to overcome some of that connotation, some authors now call the process "evidence-informed practice," particularly in relation to the use of evidence in policy making (Canadian Health Services Research Foundation [CHSRF], 2004). What difference does the use of research make? Heater, Becker, & Olson (1988) conducted a meta-analysis to determine the contribution of research-based practice to client outcomes. They found 84 nurse-conducted studies involving 4146 patients and reported that clients who received research-based nursing care made "sizeable gains" in behavioural knowledge and physiological and psychosocial outcomes compared with those receiving routine nursing care.

So, why don't all nurses base their practice on evidence? Luker and Kenrick (1992) used qualitative techniques in an exploratory study of CHN decision making in the United Kingdom and determined that the nurses had an awareness of research but did not perceive it as informing their practice. Bostrom and Suter (1993) found that only 21% of 1200 practising nurses had implemented a new research finding in the previous six months. Nurses have reported difficulty in accessing and appraising published research, either because they do not have access to journals and libraries or because they have not been taught how to find and appraise research (Blythe & Royle, 1993; Pearcey, 1995).

Estabrooks (1998) surveyed staff nurses about their use of various sources of knowledge. Those most frequently used were found to be experiential, nursing school (even though the average length of time since completing their basic nursing education program was 18 years), workplace sources, physician sources, intuition, and past usual practice.

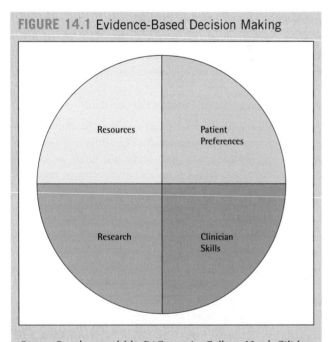

FIGURE 14.1 Evidence-Based Decision Making

Source: Based on model by DiCenso, A., Cullum, N., & Ciliska, D. (1998). Implementing evidence-based nursing: Some misconceptions. *Evidence-Based Nursing 1, 38–40, with permission from the BMJ Publishing Group.*

Literature (whether in textbook or journal form) was rated in the bottom five sources of information for frequency of use. The nurses were also asked to identify the one most common source from which they learned about research findings. Though 39% identified nursing journals, additional analyses revealed that the primary journals the nurses were reading were not research journals, but rather trade magazines published by nursing professional organizations.

The sheer volume of research is more than any nurse can manage. Nurses working individually cannot hope to find and read even the highest-quality research published each year. This is compounded by the fact that much of the research relevant to community health nursing is published in non-nursing journals.

There is a substantial time lag of 8 to 15 years between the time technical information is generated and the time it is used in actual practice (Lomas, 1991; Utterback, 1974). In addition to barriers faced by individual nurses, multiple political, cultural, economic, and other environmental barriers must be overcome in order to practise in an evidence-based way. However, this chapter will focus more on the abilities and strategies of individual nurses and teams of nurses to implement evidence-based practice.

THE PROCESS OF EVIDENCE-BASED NURSING

Asking Clinical Questions

Nurses need to maintain inquiring minds in order to evaluate interventions and consider options for other interventions. In order to find relevant research, **clinical questions** (also called **structured questions**) need to be structured, usually consisting of the situation, the intervention, and the outcomes (Flemming, 1998). The **situation** is the patient, client, population, or problem being addressed; the **intervention** is the action that is under consideration for some health promotion, disease prevention, or treatment effect; and the **outcome** is the result of interest from the client or clinical perspective. To return to some of the questions in the introduction, the phrasing of the questions might be:

- For new mothers (situation), does a structured breast-feeding support program delivered by a CHN (intervention), affect duration, exclusivity, GI infections, or eczema in the infants (outcomes)?
- Is glucosamine (intervention) effective in reducing pain and increasing functional ability (outcomes) in people with osteoarthritis (situation)?

Conducting an Efficient Search of the Literature

Structuring the question allows one to consider all the possible synonymous search terms for the conduct of an efficient search. The most efficient search is done with the help of a health sciences librarian, taking the original question, the list of synonyms for each component of the question, and any articles already found on the subject. The latter will allow the librarian to see how this type of article is indexed in the relevant databases. It is also important to be clear about the purpose in finding this literature. Is a systematic review needed (which would give direction regarding management or policy and procedure decisions; see the section "What Is a Systematic Review" on p. 233), or are the details of the interventions and their effectiveness needed (in which case the review would give the references for the studies, but one would probably want the individual primary studies as well)?

But what if you don't have access to a librarian? The most time-efficient sources of good data are the websites that critically appraise, rate, and summarize systematic reviews, such as www.health-evidence.ca, and journals of pre-appraised research, including *Evidence-Based Nursing, ACP Journal Club, Evidence-Based Medicine, Evidence-Based Cardiovascular Medicine, Evidence-Based Health Policy and Management,* and *Evidence-Based Mental Health.* These journals are similar in format in that they select high-quality research from published journals by using explicit quality criteria. Articles that report studies and reviews that warrant immediate attention by nurses attempting to keep pace with important advances are summarized in structured abstracts and commented on by clinical experts. The evidence-based journals are valuable resources that overcome the barriers of time (for example, the time to read all the issues of the more than 150 journals that are read for *Evidence-Based Nursing*), search skills, physical access to the original journals, and critical appraisal skills. While each issue of an evidence-based journal may contain only a few articles relevant to community health nursing, searchable online databases of abstracts and web-based updates for a specific user profile of clinical interests are available. Generally, *Evidence-Based Health Policy and Management* and *Evidence-Based Nursing* contain the most articles relevant to community health nursing.

Abstracts and commentaries from several abstraction journals (not *Evidence-Based Nursing*) are pooled on the *Best Evidence* CD-ROM (American College of Physicians, 2001). In addition, *Clinical Evidence* (in book format or online version; see Additional Resources) is an evidence-based tool organized around common primary care or hospital-based problems. It provides concise accounts of the current state of knowledge, ignorance, and uncertainty about the prevention and treatment of a wide range of clinical conditions based on thorough searches of the literature. *Clinical Evidence* uses information from the Cochrane Library (see below) and the abstraction journals. However, it starts not with the journals, but with clinical questions such as prevention and treatment of pressure sores or management of acute stroke or acute myocardial infarction.

The Cochrane Collaboration is an international organization that aims to help people make informed decisions about health by preparing, maintaining, and ensuring the accessibility of rigorous, systematic, and up-to-date reviews (including meta-analyses where appropriate) of the benefits and risks of health care interventions (Jadad & Haynes,

1998). Examples of the Cochrane Collaboration's relevance to community health include smoking cessation in the workplace, parent training for improving maternal psychosocial health, and prevention of falls in the elderly. The Cochrane Library is the product of the Collaboration's work and includes reports and protocols from more than 1000 systematic reviews produced within the Collaboration; abstracts of more than 1800 reviews summarized and critically appraised by the Centre for Reviews and Dissemination at the University of York, UK; and citations for more than 200 000 randomized controlled trials. One can search the Cochrane Library, without charge, for abstracts of reviews and, through subscription, for online access or the CD-ROM version, which is updated quarterly. Much smaller than Cochrane, the Effective Public Health Practice Project (Hamilton Public Health & Community Services, 2003) is an online site for high-quality systematic reviews relevant to public health practice in Canada. Public health practitioners, managers, policy people, and academics from around Ontario are involved in defining important practice and policy questions, setting priorities, conducting systematic reviews, and disseminating and utilizing the information.

If no answer is found to the structured question within the pre-appraised literature, it is necessary to go to other databases. Free online access is available for Pub-Med, which can be searched with key words, setting limits for type of publication, year of publication, language, a nursing subset of journals, and so on. Another useful place to search is Cumulative Index of Nursing and Allied Health Literature (CINAHL), but it is not free unless there is access through an academic centre. Similar to Pub-Med, it allows for limits to be set and to search by author or keyword.

Critically Appraising Retrieved Articles

Once the articles are found and retrieved, one must decide if their quality is sufficient that one can be confident in using them. Some health care research is too poor in quality to be used in decision making regarding clinical practice. As stated above, this is less critical with some of the pre-appraised sources of research. Several checklists for quality (validity), also known as "Users' Guides," have been developed to help people develop **critical appraisal skills**; that is, the ability to decide if an article is of sufficient methodological quality that it warrants attention for decision making. With a little practice, these skills become easier and quicker to apply.

Outcomes research or evaluative research answers questions about effectiveness or harm and has a quantitative design. As stated in Chapter 8 on epidemiology, different research designs are best for answering particular types of questions. For example, questions about effectiveness or harms of certain interventions and prevention are best answered by **randomized controlled trials** in which the investigators have no control over who is placed in the intervention group versus the control group. The most efficient article of this type is a systematic review of randomized trials. However, randomized trials may be unethical, such as randomizing mothers to breastfeed or not to see if breastfeeding is associated with eczema, or randomizing preteens to smoke to see if it causes lung cancer. Also, trials are very expensive. If a trial cannot be done (ethically or financially), the next best design to answer the question is a cohort design, where at least two groups are compared before and after one group receives an intervention. (See Chapter 8 or a basic nursing research text for more information on study designs.)

Questions exploring feelings and experiences are best answered through a qualitative design such as phenomenology or grounded theory. Questions and interventions that evolve through partnerships between researchers and participants are best dealt with through participatory action research. **Participatory action research** is action-oriented research in which the researchers and participants are partners in developing the question, intervention, and evaluation. It may be quantitative or qualitative and may involve triangulation of data (Burns & Groves, 2001). One principle when critically appraising articles is to ensure that the appropriate design was used to answer the question.

The Canadian Research Boxes in this chapter discuss criteria for critical appraisal of systematic reviews, single intervention studies, and qualitative research and demonstrate the application of the criteria to actual research studies.

Critical Appraisal of Studies of Interventions

The decision to use a study of intervention (usually a treatment or prevention) depends on the findings and the quality of the study design. The quality determines the level of confidence in the findings of the study. The major questions used to evaluate primary studies of interventions or prevention are:

- Are the results valid?
- What are the results?
- Will the results help me in improving the health of clients? (Ciliska, Cullum, & Marks, 2001; Sackett, Strauss, Richardson, Rosenberg, & Haynes, 2000)

The critical appraisal criteria shown in the box "How to Critically Appraise Studies of Treatment or Prevention" will be explained and applied in relation to the article by Ratner et al. (2004).

Are the Results Valid? This question considers whether the reported results are likely to reflect the true size and direction of the treatment effect. Was the research designed to minimize bias and lead to accurate findings?

Was the assignment of participants to treatment groups randomized, and was the randomization concealed? The purpose of randomization is to remove any control over who is assigned to an intervention or control group. As well, groups should be similar in all respects except for exposure to the intervention. Known and unknown factors (age, sex, socioeconomic status, disease severity) that could influence the outcome of the study

are evenly distributed among the groups. Different methods, such as a table of random numbers or computer-generated random numbers, ensure that all participants have an equal chance of being in each of the study groups. The methods section of the article should tell if and how participants were randomized.

The person recruiting the participants into the study should not know to which group each person is allocated. This is called *allocation concealment.* Concealment could happen through a process of calling a central office to get the allocation of the participant or through the use of numbered, opaque, sealed envelopes. In this way, the recruiter does not know until after participants are registered to which group they will be assigned, and the participant does not know at all. This prevents the recruiter from exercising bias in recruitment.

Was follow-up sufficiently long and complete? The first of these two criteria has to be judged by the clinician reading the paper. The definition of appropriate length of follow-up varies with different clinical questions. For example, success in weight loss measured at six months after a year-long intervention does not give a true picture of how many people are able to maintain the weight loss. A minimum expectation would be a one-year follow-up. Similarly, with early childhood interventions, follow-up for only two years may mean that some important outcomes that occur later in life for the child or family are missed.

The second part of these criteria relates to completeness of follow-up. Seldom are studies able to retain all participants until the end of the follow-up. If large numbers are lost, it reduces the confidence one can have in the results. To continue with the weight-loss example, large dropouts are usual during treatment and follow-up. If the author reports on only those who remained in the study, those participants are more likely to be doing well in terms of their weight loss. Participants who were unsuccessful with the intervention are more likely to drop out, making the intervention look far more effective than it is in reality. A retention rate of 80% is considered good; however, this is somewhat topic dependent, as one would expect the dropout rates of a transient population to be much higher.

Canadian Research Box 14.1

Ratner, P. A., Johnson, J. L., Richardson, C. G., Bottorff, J. L., Moffat, B., Mackay, M., Fofonoff, D., Kingsbury, K., Miller, C., & Budz, B. (2004). Efficacy of a smoking-cessation intervention for elective-surgical patients. *Research in Nursing and Health, 27*(3), 148–61.

Scenario: Your local hospital has contacted your community health agency to see if there could be any assistance for setting up a smoking cessation program for people scheduled to undergo elective surgery. Your agency is happy to partner on this initiative, and you volunteer to help the hospital team consider the program options. At your first meeting, you ask if there is any research on the topic. Since no one remembers seeing any such literature, they ask you to do a search and report back at the next meeting. You decide to try the search skills you learned at a recent seminar, which should allow you to find high-quality primary studies in a short time. You go to PubMed (www.pubmed.gov), and click "Clinical Queries" on the left side, under "PubMed Services." A screen comes up that allows you to search by "Clinical Study Category," "Systematic Reviews," or "Medical Genetics." You first try Find Systematic Reviews and enter the words "smoking cessation presurgical." There are no hits, so you repeat under Clinical Study Category using the category of "therapy." One hit comes up—a trial by Ratner and colleagues on the efficacy of smoking cessation for elective surgical patients (2004). You retrieve the full document.

Will you present this study to your committee next meeting?

In the article you retrieved by Ratner et al., the procedure section reports that the participants were randomized to receive either usual care or the smoking cessation intervention. After recruitment, the study personnel opened a sealed envelope containing a computer generated, randomly determined group allocation. Thus, participants were randomized, but we are not sure that allocation was concealed (by opaque envelopes) from personnel prior to recruitment. The intervention consisted of specially trained nurses who did three aspects of the intervention. The first was a 15-minute face-to-face counselling session in the pre-assessment clinic (1–3 weeks before surgery), followed by a review of progress in hospital within 24 hours after surgery, then telephone counselling starting about one week after the in-hospital session, which continued weekly for one month then biweekly for the second and third months. All encounters built on advice to stop smoking at least 24 hours before surgery, skill building and strategies to quit smoking, and a telephone hotline number.

The control group received "usual care" in which participants were managed by the usual pre and postoperative teaching, which may have included discussion about smoking cessation although there was no formal protocol to do so. Of the 418 people who met eligibility criteria, 57% agreed to participate. Though this is not as high as you would normally like for most interventions, you realize that it is probably a good participation rate for smokers. Follow-up lasted for one year, probably a reasonable length of time to assess an intervention like this for smoking cessation. Follow-up at one year was 71.3%; again this is less than you would hope to see, yet higher than follow-up for many smoking cessation studies. Intention-to-treat analysis was done. Outcome assessors were blinded; participants and clinicians were not, and could not be in an intervention like this. There were no differences between the two groups in demographic or smoking-related characteristics at baseline.

Smoking abstinence for at least 24 hours before surgery and 6- and 12-month abstinence rates were the primary outcomes. For presurgery, 73% of those in the intervention group abstained before surgery compared with 53% in the control group. This was statistically significant ($p < 0.003$).

In fact, the control group was more likely to increase the amount smoked before surgery (25.4% versus 9.9% in the control group, $p < 0.004$). At 6 months and 12 months, the authors used intention-to-treat analysis, attributing positive smoking status to participants lost to follow-up. In that analysis, there were no significant differences in smoking status at either measurement time. For example, the odds ratio for abstinence in the intervention group at 12 months was 0.92 (95% CIs 0.47 to 1.78). The odds ratio is close to 1, indicating little difference in rates between the two groups, and also the confidence interval crosses 1, indicating no statistical significance.

If the effect had been significant over time, the last area of the critique is to see if the article described the participants in enough detail to see if they might be similar to the population of interest. In this case, Ratner et al. gave details about the type of surgery and demographics. You could probably make a judgment about applicability to your population based on their description. You take this critique to the next committee meeting, and together you decide to explore other smoking-cessation programs, as presurgical abstinence is probably not enough to justify the expense of the program. You go back to the search phase!

Discussion Questions:

1. Let's say on your next search, you found several other interventions that had statistically significant findings at one-year follow-up. How would you use the research to argue for resources to be reallocated from the hospital pre-op programs and directed to a smoking cessation intervention described? Role play that you are the nurse and your classmates are the committee to whom you are reporting.

2. When it is difficult or impossible to randomize people (e.g., when a media or city/community-wide intervention is to be done), what is the next most rigorous design after a randomized controlled trial?

How to Critically Appraise Studies of Treatment or Prevention

1. Are the results of this study valid?
   a) Was the assignment of participants to treatment groups randomized, and was the randomization concealed?
   b) Was follow-up sufficiently long and complete?
   c) Were participants analyzed in the groups to which they were assigned?
   d) Were participants, clinicians, outcome assessors, and data analysts unaware of (blinded to or masked from) participant allocation?

e) Were participants in each group treated equally except for the intervention being evaluated?

f) Were the groups similar at the start of the trial?

2. What were the results?

a) How large is the effect? Is it clinically important?

b) How precise is the treatment effect?

3. Will the results help me in caring for my clients?

a) Are my clients so different from those in the study that the results do not apply?

b) Is the treatment feasible in our setting?

c) Were all the clinically important outcomes (harms as well as benefits) considered?

d) What are my clients' values and preferences for both the outcomes we are trying to prevent and the side effects that may arise?

Source: Adapted from Cullum (2000, 2001)

Were participants analyzed in groups to which they were assigned? This criterion relates to the fact that participants should be analyzed in the group to which they were randomized, regardless of whether or not they actually received the treatment or completed treatment as assigned. This is called **intention-to-treat analysis**. If the participants who discontinued treatment, for example, due to unpleasant side effects, were omitted from analysis, we would be left only with participants who had better outcomes, making the treatment look more effective than it actually is.

Were participants, clinicians, outcome assessors, and data analysts unaware of (blinded to or masked from) participant allocation? Several of the groups involved in a trial have the potential to bias the outcomes if they know whether a participant is in the intervention or control group. **Bias** means any systematic tendency to produce an outcome that differs from the truth. It includes the tendency to look more carefully for particular outcomes or to probe more deeply for outcomes in one group and not the other, as well as for participants to more likely recall an event or exposure that could have an impact if they have an adverse outcome than if they do not have an adverse outcome (Oxman, Guyatt, Cook, & Montori, 2002). Studies can be labelled single, double, or triple blinded depending on how many of the groups were unaware of the allocation of the participants. Authors should clearly state which groups were blinded or masked. For example, if participants know they are in the intervention group, they may have a sensitivity to the good or bad effects of the treatment. Participant blinding is easier to do in drug trials where placebos can be made to look identical to the active drug. However, it is far more difficult in community nursing to blind participants to a nurse coming to their home, or delivering a physical versus a primarily psychosocial intervention. It is often possible to minimize the potential bias by ensuring that the participant does not know the specific outcome. Similarly, clinicians who care for the participants and know the allocation may unconsciously alter the way they give care and may have a heightened awareness of good outcomes or adverse outcomes in a way that biases the evaluation.

The most important group to be blinded is the one that measures the outcomes. Ideally, they are not the clinicians providing care. The measurement of key outcomes can be unconsciously distorted by the clinicians' beliefs about the intervention and its side effects. Objective outcome measures, such as glycated hemoglobin, are less subject to outcome assessor bias. Similarly, data analyses should be done with coded data that does not allow for identification of treatment groups.

Consequently, readers of randomized trials should look for reports of which groups were and were not blinded to the participant allocation. If blinding is not possible, the authors should report on steps taken to minimize possible biases.

Were participants in each group treated equally except for the intervention being evaluated? Randomization should ensure that the only difference between study groups is the treatment being evaluated. An important principle is that additional treatments, or extra care, not be given. Readers of randomized trials should look carefully at the descriptions of interventions received by all groups, especially if the clinicians are not blinded to allocation.

Were the groups similar at the start of the trial? Randomization should ensure that the groups of study participants were similar at the beginning. Usually a table of baseline characteristics is prepared and some analysis is done to check that randomization actually "worked." If the groups show statistically significant differences at the beginning, the impact of the intervention may be altered, which can affect the validity of the result. If imbalances do exist at baseline, adjustment in the analysis can be done with statistical techniques.

What Were the Results? Once one has determined that the results are valid, it important to understand what the results really mean.

How large is the effect? Is it clinically important? How precise is the treatment effect? The effects of treatment are measured using one or more outcome measures. They can be dichotomous (yes/no; alive/dead; pregnant/not pregnant) or continuous (weight, adjustment score, blood pressure, self-esteem). Different statistical tests are used for different types of data. Often statistical test are reported as **p values.** The convention is that any p value less than 0.05 is considered statistically significant and means that the intervention has an effect on the outcome. More information may be gained about the extent of that difference by the use of other statistical tests such as relative risk reduction (RRR) and absolute risk reduction (ARR).

The **relative risk reduction** is the proportional reduction in rates of poor outcomes (e.g., death or readmission) between the experimental (better outcomes) and control (greater poor outcomes) participants. It is calculated as:

$$\text{Relative risk reduction} = \frac{\text{Event rate in control group} - \text{Event rate in experimental group}}{\text{Event rate in the control group}}$$

For example, an RRR of 50% means that there were 50% fewer deaths in the experimental group compared with the control group.

Relative risk (RR) is the proportion of participants experiencing an outcome in the intervention group divided by the proportion experiencing the outcome in the control group. However, RR does not take into account the number of people in the study who would have died anyway without the intervention.

This is called the **absolute risk reduction** and is calculated as:

$$\text{Absolute risk reduction} =$$
$$\text{Event rate in control group} - \text{Event rate in experimental group}$$

For example, an ARR of 2% means that there were 2% fewer deaths in the experimental group than the control group.

Yet another approach is to report the **number needed to treat (NNT)**. This describes the number of people who must be treated with the intervention in order to prevent one additional negative outcome (e.g., death) or promote one additional positive outcome (e.g., smoking cessation). The NNT is calculated as:

$$\text{NNT} = \frac{1}{\text{Absolute risk reduction}}$$

When researchers report statistical significance, it is imperative to ask if this is clinically important or meaningful. It is quite possible for results to be statistically significant but clinically unimportant. In a hypothetical example studying weight-loss interventions for obese women, the group with a more intensive intervention lost a mean of 5 kg more than the group in the less intensive intervention. Though the researchers found this statistically significant ($p = 0.03$), it did not meet the preset goal of a 10% weight loss in order to be a meaningful difference; that is, to be associated with health risk reduction. It also was not personally meaningful to the morbidly obese women.

Precision of the results can never be absolute but is estimated by calculating **confidence intervals** around the RRR or ARR. Confidence intervals (CI) are a range of values with a specified probability (usually 95%) of including the true effect, which can never be known absolutely. Wide confidence intervals indicate less precision in the estimated effect of the intervention. Precision increases with larger sample sizes.

Will the Results Help Me in Caring for My Clients?

- Are my clients so different from those in the study that the results do not apply?
- Is the treatment feasible in our setting?
- Were all the clinically important outcomes (harms as well as benefits) considered?
- What are my clients' values and preferences for both the outcome we are trying to prevent and the side effects that may arise?

In order to use the findings of a study, one needs to consider these questions and make judgments in relation to one's own client population. Consider how similar the characteristics of the study participants are to your own clients. Think about reasons why you should *not* apply the study results to your clients, rather than the looking for evidence that the clients are exactly the same as yours. Feasibility in your setting depends on such factors as cost, organizational resources, nursing skills, availability of special equipment, and acceptability to clients. Harms and benefits should be included in the reports by various obvious outcomes such as health but also other outcomes like quality of life and economics. In particular, negative effects or side effects should be included.

Critical Appraisal of Systematic Reviews

What Is a Systematic Review?   A **systematic review** is a summary of research evidence that relates to a specific question. It could involve causation, diagnosis, or prognosis, but more frequently involves **effectiveness** of an intervention. Basing a clinical decision on a single study may be a mistake, as the study may have an inadequate sample size to detect clinically important differences between treatments, leading to a false negative conclusion. Discrepant findings across studies of the same question may occur due to chance or subtle differences in study design or participants. Therefore, it is useful to look at a summary of all the research related to a single clinical question.

In a narrative review, authors may selectively pick articles that support their viewpoint and ignore those that do not, so that the conclusion is set before the articles are selected. Systematic reviews differ from an unsystematic narrative review in that they attempt to overcome possible biases by following a rigorous methodology of search, retrieval, relevance and validity (quality) rating, data extraction, synthesis, and report writing. Explicit pre-set criteria are used for relevance and validity. Two people conduct each stage independently, then compare results and discuss discrepancies before moving on to the next stage. Details of the methods used at every stage are recorded. A **meta-analysis** is the quantitative combination of results of several studies to get an overall summary statistic that represents the combined effect of the intervention across different study populations.

The terms "systematic review" and "overview" are often used interchangeably. The reviewers must decide whether the statistical combination (meta-analysis) is appropriate by using both clinical judgment and a statistical test for heterogeneity. The clinical judgment requires the reviewers to examine the methodologies and statistical tests completed in the studies under review and ascertain if it is reasonable to combine them in a meta-analysis. The statistical tests determine the extent to which the differences between results of individual studies are greater than one would expect if all studies were measuring the same underlying effect and the observed differences were due only to chance. The more significant the test of heterogeneity, the less likely that the observed differences are from chance alone and that some other factor, such as design, participants, intervention, or outcome, is responsible for the differences in the treatment effect across studies (Sackett et al., 2000). Readers must use their own expertise to decide whether the statistical combination is reasonable in terms of clinical and methodological sense.

Systematic reviews help to answer clinical questions without having to access large numbers of research reports; they overcome the obstacles of lack of time and, sometimes, lack of skills necessary to conduct the critical appraisal. But can one be confident in using all reviews? The search in the scenario of Canadian Research Box 14.2 yielded 195 reviews—are they all of equal value? What does one do if they give conflicting results?

Common misconceptions of systematic reviews are that many readers think they include *only* randomized trials, that they must adopt a biomedical model, and that they have to have some statistical synthesis (Petticrew, 2001). If these were true, there would be few reviews of interest in community health, as many community health questions have not been or cannot be addressed by randomized trials. Fortunately, review methods are improving to include non-randomized studies such as cohort studies, to use a population health model, and to synthesize without necessarily including meta-analysis. The Cochrane Collaboration Health Promotion/Public Health Field has been a leader in promoting the methods, conduct, and use of systematic reviews and meta-analyses in community health care. Many websites contain high-quality systematic reviews relevant to community health and resources for skill building in critical appraisal of reviews. (See Additional Resources.)

Appraising Systematic Reviews   In this section, we look at how to critically appraise systematic reviews to decide if the methods have sufficient rigour that the results may be applied to client or management decisions. The same major questions used for evaluation of intervention studies can be used to evaluate systematic reviews. (See the box "How to Critically Appraise Review Articles.")

Are the Results Valid?   *Is this a systematic review of randomized trials?* Questions about the effectiveness of treatment or prevention are best answered by randomized controlled trials if it is ethically possible to do so, whereas questions about harm or prognosis are best answered by cohort studies (Roberts & DiCenso, 1999). The reader of systematic reviews should look to see if the authors used randomized trials (if ethically possible) or the next most rigorous design that included a comparison group (quasi-randomized or cohort analytic designs).

Does the systematic review include a description of the strategies used to find all relevant studies? A thorough search for both published and unpublished studies should be done for a systematic review. The publication of research in a journal is more likely to occur in studies that have statistically significant results. Studies in which a new intervention is not found to be effective are frequently not published, a phenomenon known as publication bias (Dickersin, 1990). Systematic reviews that do not include unpublished studies may overestimate the effect of an intervention; that is, it will appear that the intervention is more effective than it really is. Therefore, in addition to searching through relevant databases such as CINAHL, MEDLINE, PsycINFO, ERIC, or Cochrane

Library, researchers should hand-search relevant journals, review reference lists from retrieved articles, contact authors and relevant manufacturing companies, and review abstracts presented at relevant scientific meetings. Unless the authors of the reviews tell us what they did to locate relevant studies, it is difficult to know if any were missed.

Every systematic review grows from a focused question, through the development of the search strategies and search terms for each database, to retrieval of studies. Explicit inclusion/exclusion criteria are predetermined, and two people independently review each article for inclusion.

Does the systematic review include a description of how the validity of individual studies was assessed? A narrative review often reports on study findings without considering the methodological strengths of the studies. Differences in study quality often explain differences in results across studies, with those of poorer quality tending to overestimate the effectiveness of the interventions (Kunz & Oxman, 1998). Quality ratings are sometimes used in the analysis to compare outcomes across studies by study strength. Or, if there are many studies to consider, the authors may choose to apply a quality rating threshold for inclusion or give greater attention and weight to the stronger studies.

Canadian Research Box 14.2

DiCenso, A., Guyatt, G., Willan, A., & Griffith, L. (2002). Interventions to reduce unintended pregnancies among adolescents: Systematic review of randomized controlled trials. *BMJ, 324*(7351), 1426–1434.

Scenario: You are the manager of the sexual health program at your health department. A local high school has asked you to offer a sexual health program in their school. They are concerned about the rates of both pregnancy and STIs. You guess that what they really want is an "abstinence" program. You decide to search the literature to find any evidence of effectiveness of sexual health generally or abstinence programs specifically. In PubMed you search "sexual health," limiting the search to "humans," "English," "adolescents," and the publication dates of "January 1995 to July 2002." You get 2071 hits. When you try adding "abstinence" you get the same number of hits. When you limit the primary search further by methods terms, the addition of "review" reduces the hits to 195; with "randomized trials," you still get 69 hits. Over lunch, you explain your discouragement to your colleagues. So many articles! So little time! How can you possibly be reasonably well prepared for the meeting at the school? One colleague suggests you try to further limit your search by choosing "meta-analysis" under publication type. You are elated because there are only four, and you can easily access the review cited above, which is available full-text and online. You don't have to retrieve and critically appraise 2071 articles!

The review included only randomized controlled trials, of which there were 22. The review question was narrowed from a starting-point scenario of sexual health. The authors wanted to know if primary prevention programs were effective in "delaying sexual intercourse, improving birth control use, and reducing incidence of pregnancy" in adolescents; this was a clear and focused question. The search strategy was extensive, involving the search of 12 electronic databases back to 1970, a hand search of ten key journals, and contact with experts to discover any unpublished studies. Criteria for study selection included:

- a target population of adolescents 18 years of age or less;
- the intervention being any primary prevention strategy (e.g., sex education classes, school-based clinics, community-based programs);
- the outcome measure being behavioural (e.g., initiation of sexual intercourse, birth control use, pregnancy);
- the study design being a randomized controlled trial; and
- the language being English or any language for which a translator was available.

Studies were excluded that were targeted to pregnant teens, high-risk populations, or the outcome of AIDS prevention, or that were conducted in a developing country. These criteria are quite explicit and help to ensure that the appropriate studies were included.

The appraisal tools used for validity (quality) rating included ratings of the appropriateness of the method of randomization, bias of the data collection, and number of withdrawals and dropouts. In the unplanned adolescent pregnancy review, there is consistency across the studies, with the test for heterogeneity showing no significant heterogeneity ($p = 0.99$).

The review found that interventions did not delay initiation of sexual intercourse for young women (OR: 1.12; 95% CI: 0.96–1.30) or young men (OR: 0.99; 95% CI: 0.84–1.16). Four abstinence programs and one school-based sexual education program were associated with an increase in number of pregnancies among partners of young male participants (OR: 1.54; 95% CI: 1.03–2.29). One study found significantly fewer pregnancies in young women who received a multifaceted program (OR: 0.41; 95% CI: 0.20–0.83).

These results are directly applicable to the introductory scenario. Potential negative effects of the abstinence programs were documented; costs were not reported. The review was done systematically; focused on a clearly delineated question; did quite an extensive literature search; focused on randomized trials; applied pre-defined inclusion, exclusion, and quality criteria; did a meta-analysis with pooled odds ratios; and considered both positive and negative outcomes. It is a high-quality review that found that primary preventions strategies do not delay initiation of sexual intercourse, improve use of birth control among young men or women, or reduce the number of pregnancies in young women. Four abstinence programs and one school-based sex education program were associated with an increase in number of pregnancies. There were significantly fewer pregnancies in young women who received a multifaceted program. Returning to the opening scenario, you can certainly present to the high school the evidence to not conduct the abstinence program and to consider a multifaceted intervention for the students.

Discussion Questions:

1. The media attend the meeting at the high school. They ask, "If abstinence does not work, and some of the other interventions do not work, then why should we spend any time or resources on sexual health education for adolescents?" How would you respond?

2. What components would you argue to be included in a multifaceted sexual health program for adolescents?

How to Critically Appraise Review Articles

1. Are the results of this systematic review valid?
   a) Is this a systematic review of randomized trials?
   b) Does the systematic review include a description of the strategies used to find all the relevant trials?
   c) Does the systematic review include a description of how the validity of individual studies was assessed?
   d) Were the results consistent from study to study?

2. What were the results?
   a) How large was the treatment effect?
   b) How precise was the estimate of treatment effect?

3. Will the results help me in caring for my clients?
   a) Are my clients so different from those in the study that the results do not apply?
   b) Is the treatment feasible in our setting?
   c) Were all the clinically important outcomes (harms as well as benefits) considered?
   d) What are my clients' values and preferences for both the outcomes we are trying to prevent and the side effects that may arise?

Source: Adapted from Ciliska, Cullum, & Marks, 2001 and Sackett et al., 2000.

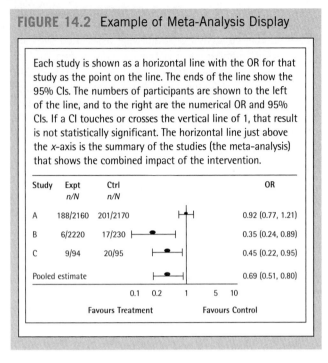

FIGURE 14.2 Example of Meta-Analysis Display

Each study is shown as a horizontal line with the OR for that study as the point on the line. The ends of the line show the 95% CIs. The numbers of participants are shown to the left of the line, and to the right are the numerical OR and 95% CIs. If a CI touches or crosses the vertical line of 1, that result is not statistically significant. The horizontal line just above the x-axis is the summary of the studies (the meta-analysis) that shows the combined impact of the intervention.

Study	Expt n/N	Ctrl n/N	OR
A	188/2160	201/2170	0.92 (0.77, 1.21)
B	6/2220	17/230	0.35 (0.24, 0.89)
C	9/94	20/95	0.45 (0.22, 0.95)
Pooled estimate			0.69 (0.51, 0.80)

0.1   0.2   1   5   10

Favours Treatment   Favours Control

across studies entered into a meta-analysis. Both OR and RR are used for dichotomous data (dead/alive, pregnant/not pregnant), while weighted mean difference is used for continuous data (blood pressure, blood glucose, stress measurement scale). (For more information on OR and RR, see Chapter 8.)

The precision of the results is estimated by calculating confidence intervals (CI, defined earlier) around the summary statistic. The CI is useful for decision making because we can look at both extremes of the effect. If the lower extreme is 1 or close to it, the effect of the intervention is quite small and probably not worthwhile. A hypothetical display is shown in Figure 14.2 to demonstrate how output tables are read. The summary odds ratio of the three studies in Figure 14.2 is 0.69 (95% CI: 0.51–0.90), which indicates that the treatment was effective in producing the desired outcome.

Will the Results Help Me in Caring for My Clients?

- Are my clients so different from those in the study that the study results do not apply?
- Is the treatment feasible in our setting?
- Were all the clinically important outcomes (harms as well as benefits) considered?
- What are my clients' values and preferences for both the outcome we are trying to prevent and the side effects that may arise?

These questions have to be answered by the readers in the context of their own work and client-encounter situations. For example, feasibility in the example in Canadian Research Box 14.2 would relate not only to the skills of the nurses and resources of the health department to do a multifaceted sexual health program, but also to the ability of the school board to withstand the parental pressures for abstinence programs.

Researchers try to look for all outcomes of interventions, both positive and negative, that might affect the participants and the health care system. Outcomes might include mortality, morbidity, costs, quality of life, and participant satisfaction. Participant and family values must be considered. If, in Canadian Research Box 14.2, families are unwilling to have their children exposed to multifaceted sexual health education programs, the students must be given an alternative during that school time.

Critical Appraisal of Qualitative Research

Qualitative research is important for the development of nursing knowledge. **Qualitative research** describes, explores, and explains phenomena and is concerned with the process or experience rather than outcomes. Done for the purpose of obtaining rich data, sampling is purposive as opposed to random or the probability sampling in quantitative research. Data collection is done in many ways, but the most common are observation and group or individual interviews. Data analysis is by codes, themes, and patterns, not by statistical techniques, and it produces rich, deep descriptions rather than numbers. Qualitative research does not allow inference

The predefined quality checklist minimizes reviewer bias by helping to ensure that reviewers appraise each study consistently and thoroughly. Having two or more raters helps to reduce mistakes and bias and increases the reader's confidence in the systematic review. The quality rating tools usually include criteria such as those presented for evaluating interventions. (Refer to Canadian Research Box 14.1 on p. 230.)

Were the results consistent from study to study? The reader would be most confident in using the results of a review if the results were similar in all included studies, that is, showing the same direction of effect, all being positive, all negative, or all showing no effect. But what if the direction of effect differs across studies? Differences may be due to types of clients included; the timing, duration, and intensity of the intervention; the outcomes measured; and/or the ways in which the outcomes were measured.

What Were the Results? *How large was the treatment effect? How precise is the estimate of treatment effect?* Comparing a simple count of studies that helped, harmed, or showed no difference in treatments would assume that all studies had equal validity, power of the sample size to detect a difference, and duration and intensity of interventions and follow-up. Meta-analysis, when appropriate, can assign different weight to individual studies so that those with greater precision or higher quality make a greater contribution to the summary statistic. Summary statistics usually used include odds ratio, relative risk (RR, defined earlier), and weighted mean difference. The **odds ratio (OR)** describes the odds of a participant in the experimental group having an event (e.g., pregnancy) divided by the odds of a participant in the control group having the event. In such a study as prevention of pregnancy, one would consider that an RR or OR of < 1 represents a beneficial treatment. **Weighted mean difference** is the mean of the difference found between control and intervention groups to a population as a whole, but allows the researcher to generalize to a theoretical understanding of the phenomena being studied (Ploeg, 1999).

Major types of qualitative research used in nursing include phenomenology, grounded theory, and ethnography. **Phenomenology** seeks to describe the lived experiences of people, such as the experience of people returning home after a stroke. **Grounded theory** generates theories or models of the phenomena being studied, such as the development of a model of coping used by family caregivers of people who have HIV. **Ethnography** describes a culture and answers questions such as what it is like to be a pregnant teen trying to continue with school. Reading qualitative research deepens our understanding of the potential and actual experiences of people we work with and has the potential to enrich our interactions and care.

Once again, the same major questions used to evaluate primary treatment studies or systematic reviews can be used to evaluate qualitative research. (See the box "How to Critically Appraise Qualitative Research Reports.")

Are the Findings Valid?   *Is the research question clear and adequately substantiated?* This question will determine whether the qualitative study will be read or not. The article should clearly establish the question and what is already known about the topic.

Is the design appropriate for the research question? On a grand level, it is important to determine that the authors used the appropriate method that fits the purpose of the study (e.g., that phenomenology is used to explore experience and meaning for clients following colostomy, rather than using an ethnographic approach). A more sophisticated appraisal considers the fit of the philosophical background of a particular perspective with the purpose of the study.

Was the method of sampling appropriate for the research question? The study should report on how participants were selected. Many different types of sampling are used in qualitative research, including sampling for maximum variation, typical cases, extreme cases, or critical cases.

Were data collected and managed systematically? The study should try to define the breadth (variation, multiple perspectives) and depth (numbers and types of data collected). Also, has each investigator kept track of the process, hunches, data collection, and data collection procedures through the use of journaling and memos?

Were the data analyzed appropriately? The researcher should report on how the data were organized and reduced in order to identify patterns. Often the analysis identifies further areas for data collection and analysis. Usually the researcher uses other team members to assist in the analysis, providing various interpretations of the data. Member checking (taking the results back to the participants or people associated with the issue under study) is sometimes done to gather alternative interpretations of the analysis.

What Are the Findings?   *Is the description of findings thorough?* Qualitative research is difficult to write for the word limit of

---

How to Critically Appraise Qualitative Research Reports

1. Are the findings valid?
   a) Is the research question clear and adequately substantiated?
   b) Is the design appropriate for the research question?
   c) Was the method of sampling appropriate for the research question?
   d) Were data collected and managed systematically?
   e) Were the data analyzed appropriately?
2. What are the findings?
   a) Is the description of findings thorough?
3. How can I apply the findings to patient care?
   a) What meaning and relevance does the study have for my practice?
   b) Does the study help me understand the context of my practice?
   c) Does the study enhance my knowledge about my practice?

Source: Russell, C. K., & Gregory, D. M. (2003). Evaluation of qualitative research reports. Evidence-Based Nursing, 6 , *36–40. Reproduced with permission of the BMJ Publishing Group.*

---

standard journals. It is difficult to fit the rich description and analysis into one publication. It is expected that authors have used direct quotations of the participants to illustrate the descriptions and conceptualizations.

How Can I Apply the Findings to Patient Care?

- What meaning and relevance does the study have for my practice?
- Does the study help me understand the context of my practice?
- Does the study enhance my knowledge about my practice?

The authors should establish the need and relevance of the research while both arguing why they conducted the research as well as discussing the results. Readers must use their critique of the study as well as the information presented in the report to decide if any parts of the research findings are potentially transferable to their own practice.

Making the Decision about Implementation

Each Canadian Research Box in this chapter shows high-quality evidence around the clinical scenario and clinical question. In community health nursing, many decisions to implement a change in practice are probably beyond the individual; they are decided by a team. In every case, the decision

Canadian Research Box 14.3

Wuest, J., & Merritt-Gray, M. (2001). Beyond survival: Reclaiming self after leaving an abusive male partner. *Canadian Journal of Nursing Research, 32,* 79–94.

Scenario: You work as a CHN. For several months you have been providing physical and supportive care for clients of a local women's shelter. You do not see them after they leave the shelter, and you would like to understand how these women further adjust after leaving an abusive partner. You decide to search on the Evidence-Based Nursing website to see if there are any pre-appraised studies. When you search "leaving" and "abusive partner," you get one hit, which is an abstract that describes a four-stage process of reclaiming self after leaving an abusive relationship (Wuest & Merritt-Gray, 2001). You decide to retrieve the full article (cited above) for critical appraisal.

You use the criteria from Russell & Gregory (2003) to critique the article. You find that the purpose was clear: to describe the experiences of women who have left abusive relationships and have not gone back. Feminist grounded theory was the design and was appropriate to the purpose. Theoretical sampling method was used; lay and professional helpers were asked to help identify women who had left abusive relationships. Fifteen women of diverse age, educational background, and socioeconomic status participated. Interviews were transcribed and analyzed, and at repeat interviews emerging themes were shared with participants for discussion and refinement.

The results are clearly described: *reclaiming self* was a central social psychological process that emerged in which women journeyed through four phases—*counteracting abuse, breaking free, not going back,* and *moving on.* Each of these themes is elaborated with quotations from the participants.

The thorough description of results, plus other literature findings (in the introduction and the discussion), provide meaning for women's shelter staff as well as for the CHNs, helping both understand the processes involved in leaving an abusive male partner. You decide that the methods used in this grounded theory study are more than adequate and that the findings are meaningful for your practice. The study raises several areas for possible assessment and confirmation with your client to see if they are issues and to discuss possible interventions, thus enhancing your knowledge about this area of practice. Qualitative research provides information for the development of interventions that may be tested in a quantitative evaluation.

Discussion Questions:

1. Qualitative research, such as grounded theory or phenomenology, does not tell us which interventions are effective, so how can qualitative research enrich our practice?

2. How could you use this research in an anticipatory way?

client values and choices. Furthermore, if the decision goes beyond individual clients or small groups, political and organizational elements become involved. This is particularly evident in the final decision of Canadian Research Box 14.2 to implement a comprehensive sexual health program. The students, parents, and high school would all have to be involved in the decision if there is any chance for a school-based intervention for sexual health to be successful.

What does one do if no research evidence is found during the database search? Or if the research that comes up is of consistently poor quality? In those cases, expert opinion or usual practice is the standard for decision making. One may be able to find practice guidelines on the topic. These depend on a thorough literature review, then consensus meetings with expert panels in order to make practice decisions, particularly where research evidence does not exist (Registered Nurses' Association of Ontario, 2002; U.S. Department of Health and Human Services, Agency for Healthcare Research and Quality, 2002). Similarly, "best practice" documents describe programs or interventions that seem to be effective but that may not yet have been rigorously evaluated.

Caution must be exercised when implementing interventions for which there is no good evaluation. CHNs must be particularly vigilant in observing for effects, both positive and negative, then charting them. Unfortunately, many effects are not evident until years after the intervention when no one is observing any longer! Areas of clinical interest where evaluation does not exist are prime research questions that should receive priority attention from funding agencies.

Planning for Dissemination and Implementation

Once a decision is made to change practice and organizational support is achieved, a comprehensive plan has to address how the others who work within the organization will be informed of the proposed change. Changing the practice of health professionals has been studied extensively with mixed, unclear results. The "Effective Practice and Organization of Care" review group within the Cochrane Collaboration conducted a systematic review of 44 existing reviews on the topic. They found that **passive dissemination** (as in sending out a report or directive) does not work. A range of interventions work in some circumstances but not consistently; multifaceted interventions targeting different barriers are likely to be more effective than single strategies. A diagnostic analysis should be done to identify factors likely to help and hinder the proposed change (University of York, NHS Centre for Reviews and Dissemination, 1999). For example, opinion leaders have been shown to be effective in some studies with physicians, but not others (University of York, NHS Centre for Reviews and Dissemination, 1999), and they were not successful as an intervention with nurses (Hodnett, Kaufman, O'Brien-Pallas, Chipman, Watson-MacDonell, & Hunsburger, 1996). Thus, evidence of the use of opinion leaders as a strategy of change has been inconclusive.

The diagnostic analysis (environmental scan) must consider barriers and supports in relation to the characteristics of the innovation (the change being introduced), individual clients and

involves all of the four aspects of Figure 14.1: the research evidence, available resources, skills of the practitioners, and the practitioners, the organization, and the environment so that barriers can be reduced and supports strengthened. It is important to consider characteristics of the innovation such as the resources it will require (will it cost more or actually be time/resource saving?) and how different it is from current practice. Relevant characteristics of individual practitioners include such issues as level of education, years of experience, and general acceptance or resistance to change. Organizational characteristics include affiliation with an academic setting, size, level of care, funding sources, organizational structure, research participation, research orientation, and usual valuing of research findings. The environment includes factors such as rural/urban, economic status of the community, and health issues valued by the community (Dobbins, Ciliska, Cockerill, Barnsley, & DiCenso, 2002).

Important stakeholders must be identified. They may include the nurses, medical staff, clients, and accounting staff. Each group should attend a different meeting to hear a tailored message about the proposed change, rationale, and timelines. The goal of each meeting is to get support for the practice change from each stakeholder group. A champion may be needed with the enthusiasm and energy to push for this practice change. Identifying opinion leaders and influencing their understanding and attitudes about the proposed practice change is another strategy worth pursuing, despite the inconclusiveness (mentioned above) that this strategy is effective. Interventions to promote dissemination, uptake, and utilization of research results is an area that requires further focused research in order to complete the cycle of evidence-based practice from question identification to implementation and evaluation.

Evaluation

After implementing a practice or policy change, an evaluation period is needed to see if it is working in the organization with the new population and staff. This does not mean replicating the original study that was used as a basis for the practice change. It does, however, mean a period of data collection or chart review to ensure that the desired outcomes are similar to the rates of those in the original study and that the client acceptability and negative outcomes are also similar.

Canadian Research Box 14.4

Arthur, H. M., Wright, D. M., & Smith, K. M. (2001a). Women and heart disease: The treatment may end but the suffering continues. *Canadian Journal of Nursing Research, 33,* 17–29.

Participatory action research scenario: You are a CHN working as part of a team delivering a cardiac rehabilitation program. You know that heart disease is the leading cause of death for both men and women, yet women have lower attendance and higher dropout rates in your program. The team has discussed this observation, trying to understand what the barriers are for women to attend the program or how the program is not meeting their needs

when they do attend. You suggest that some research literature might help address the problem. You are to report back at the next meeting. You again decide to do an initial search in the pre-appraised literature and go to the Evidence-Based Nursing website. You search "women" and "cardiac rehabilitation" and get eight hits. You have a brief look at the abstracts online, and one article is about women, their adjustment to heart disease, and their participation in a support group (Arthur et al., 2001b). You order the full-text article from the librarian (cited above).

The authors establish in the Background section that women have below-average attendance and higher dropout rates. They suggest, from their literature review, that women's primary need in cardiac rehab is support, particularly from women with the same experience. The purpose of this study was to develop and implement a community-based communication and psycho-educational support group for women with heart disease. Participatory action research, the methodology used, involves bringing representatives from stakeholders (those who will be affected by the intervention) as collaborators in defining the question, the intervention, and the evaluation. This strategy is used more frequently in broad-based community health interventions as it facilitates broad support for the new intervention. When used with disadvantaged groups, participatory action empowers them to have a voice in the program and in how the results will be disseminated (Burns & Groves, 2001). Participatory research strategies were originally developed by Friere, a Brazilian scholar who used these methods to promote social change, and methods of critical social theory to address power imbalances between the target community and the researchers (Friere, 1972). Participatory action involves a large commitment from participants and a variety of skills among the researchers, including group process, qualitative and quantitative design, and data collection and analysis.

Two groups of women met monthly for five months to develop the program. Sessions were facilitated jointly by a nurse clinician and a nurse researcher. Between sessions, participants kept diaries of their experiences. This particular participatory action research study used qualitative data. Sessions were videotaped and transcribed and used along with field notes and the women's diaries for data collection and final evaluation. Analysis revealed that the group helped the women cope with their emotional reactions, offered social support, and helped them manage their health problem. Further iterative analysis revealed that the overall benefit of the group was the acknowledgement and sharing of suffering.

For participatory action studies, use the critical appraisal criteria for qualitative research. To summarize the critical appraisal of this study: it included a clear and focused question; participatory action research was an appropriate method; there was adequate description of context; and data were collected and managed systematically

→

and analyzed appropriately. The report includes a thorough description of results, although few actual quotations from the participants are used to substantiate the analysis. The study makes a useful contribution to our knowledge of how women suffer from cardiac disease and how the group offered them social support and helped them manage.

You conclude that the study has been well done, and you will take it to your committee meeting as a possible model to use for program re-development to meet the needs of the women with established heart disease in your community.

Discussion Questions:

1. From your community experience, consider other identified problems or issues that you might approach from a participatory action research framework.

2. For each example in question 1, identify all the stakeholders who would need to be involved in order for the participatory action research to succeed.

USING RESEARCH FOR MANAGEMENT DECISIONS AND POLICY DEVELOPMENT

While research evidence is useful for individual practitioners working with individual clients, it is also important that management decisions be evidence based. Decisions regarding the implementation of a new intensive intervention in a community, such as the cardiac rehabilitation example, are usually made where there is no additional funding coming to an agency for the new program. Therefore, if the organization wishes to begin such a program, it needs to find the resources within what currently exists. This may mean taking staff away from some other programs or activities. Reviewing the research evidence for both the proposed activity and any existing programs helps managers to make those decisions. For example, following a string of four adolescent suicides, one school requested that the health department offer suicide prevention interventions at the school the following fall. During the summer, the health department conducted a systematic review of the effectiveness of school-based suicide prevention programs for teens. They found that the available research was of poor quality and no evidence supported the decision to implement the suicide prevention programs; furthermore, some studies indicated that there was harm to adolescent males who experienced such a program in that they were more likely to engage in negative coping behaviours and to commit suicide (Ploeg, 1999). The management decided to present this information to the school and to offer instead a comprehensive "healthy school" initiative, which would also be evaluated.

Similarly, people working at institutional or government policy levels are increasingly aware of and value the need for research evidence, yet they face other competing factors (public opinion and pressures, fiscal restraints) when making policy decisions.

The actual conduct (as opposed to the search and discovery) of systematic reviews has contributed to their use by clinicians and policy-level decision makers. Of the many examples, two are chosen from the chapter authors' experiences with the Effective Public Health Practice Project (Hamilton Public Health & Community Services, 2003). Potential review questions are sought from the policy, management, and frontline clinician perspectives. The review groups included the methodological experts along with the community practitioners who were chosen for their content expertise and their understanding of the context and relevance to community health. They assisted in identifying and refining the priority questions, rating articles for relevance to the question, reviewing drafts, and helping to write clinical, management, and policy implications. This process has also been used in Alberta by the Alberta Heritage Foundation for Medical Research.

In a second example, identification, prevention, or treatment of spousal abuse had not been included in minimum policy recommendations (Ontario Ministry of Health, Public Health Branch, 1997). This omission was identified as a weakness by community health clinicians in Ontario. A work group was set up and members carried out a systematic review (Mueller & Thomas, 2001) from which clear guidelines for clinicians, managers, and policy makers were developed. Later, these guidelines were included in new policy recommendations.

Participating in Community Health Research

CHNs are involved in many different types of research, the most common being program evaluation using process outcomes such as numbers of clients, numbers of groups, hours spent, and reasons for home visits. These types of data are important for tracking uses and users of services and how resources are spent within the agency. Client outcome measurement is the next most likely information collected, such as client mortality, morbidity, immunization status or coverage, communicable disease outbreak, goals met, or adolescent pregnancies after a school program. Nurses are usually asked to log these data, at least in formal records. They also may be required to report it in other formats, or the agency may conduct periodic chart reviews or database summaries. These local data often feed into provincial and national databases and registries of statistics. Some of these databases are available to regions within the provinces so that local rates can be followed.

Especially if associated with an academic setting, CHNs are also likely to be involved in effectiveness research; that is, testing an alternative intervention against usual or no intervention. They might deliver interventions such as a falls prevention program for the elderly or a child abuse prevention intervention for families already identified as abusers or at high risk for abuse. CHNs might also collect the data for an effectiveness study, such as assessing functional status in people who have suffered a stroke and who have received the specialist nurse home intervention. Initiation and maintenance of relationships with academic settings is beneficial from the perspective of agencies and the universities. The agency can gain consultation on research utilization and program evaluation, and the nursing faculty can be kept current on clinical issues in the community and priority research needs.

CHNs may also decide that stakeholders need to be consulted about a particular health problem such as inactivity in children, heart disease in women, or mental health needs of immigrant adolescents. In this case, one might do as Arthur et al. (2001a) did and develop a participatory action research program.

Summary

In this chapter, we reviewed evidence-based practice as it relates to community health nursing. While evidence can be observations made by the nurse, expert "gut hunches," or advice of colleagues, we too often ignore the evidence from research (Estabrooks, 1998). Therefore, this chapter focused on research evidence—finding, critiquing, and using it. Particular detail was presented in relation to critical appraisal of research articles on effectiveness questions (primary studies or systematic reviews) or qualitative research to judge whether they should be utilized in practice, management, or policy decisions.

The process of using quality research evidence does not end with the critical appraisal and individual decisions to implement with clients. In community nursing, it more often involves getting organizational "buy-in" and changing policies and procedures or care maps. Thus, we presented information about understanding the barriers to utilizing research to change practice, management, and policy making.

Research, in the form of process evaluation, currently takes place daily in every community organization in Canada. Therefore, CHNs can never avoid involvement in research. Further, as the valuing of research evidence increases in community health nursing, the critical attitude to practice will increase so that clinicians will more frequently ask relevant clinical questions. Since there is not a research-based answer for every clinical question within community health, the need to conduct research in community health will continue. CHNs will find they are asked to participate in research by collecting data, providing interventions, or developing research proposals.

KEY TERMS

evidence-based nursing (EBN)
clinical questions
structured questions
situation
intervention
outcome
critical appraisal skills
randomized controlled trials
participatory action research
intention-to-treat analysis
bias
p values
relative risk reduction
relative risk (RR)
absolute risk reduction
number needed to treat (NNT)
confidence intervals
systematic review
effectiveness
meta-analysis
odds ratio (OR)
weighted mean difference
qualitative research
phenomenology
grounded theory
ethnography
passive dissemination

STUDY QUESTIONS

1. Identify four factors to consider for evidence-based decision making.

2. What is the most critical attitude for a nurse in order to practise in an evidence-based way?

3. In what ways might you conduct research as part of your daily role in community health nursing?

4. Why would you seek out systematic reviews to answer clinical questions?

5. Name the four major categories of factors to consider when planning to implement a clinical practice or policy change. Give a few examples under each category.

INDIVIDUAL CRITICAL THINKING QUESTIONS

1. Pick an intervention that has been shown to be effective and discuss how you would plan to implement that practice change in a nursing agency. What factors would you assess? What processes would you use?

2. Answer the following by using Figure 14.3.

   a) How many studies were involved in this meta-analysis?

   b) Which of those studies had statistically significant findings?

   c) How would you interpret the result? Is the intervention effective? Is it statistically significant? Is it precise?

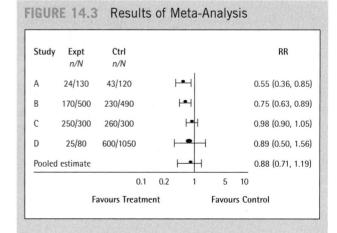

FIGURE 14.3 Results of Meta-Analysis

GROUP CRITICAL THINKING QUESTIONS

1. Select an article that evaluates an intervention relevant to community health nursing. Use the criteria in the first text box to critically appraise the article and come to a decision about using the intervention in your own practice.

2. As in question 1, critically appraise a systematic review article using the criteria in the second text box.

3. As in question 1, critically appraise an article on qualitative research using the criteria in the third text box. If it is a valid study, discuss what the study findings contribute to your understanding of the issue that was explored.

REFERENCES

American College of Physicians. (2001). *Best evidence.* (CD-ROM). Philadelphia, PA: Author.

Arthur, H. M., Wright, D. M., & Smith, K. M. (2001a). Women and heart disease: The treatment may end but the suffering continues. *Canadian Journal of Nursing Research, 33,* 17–29.

Arthur, H. M., Wright, D. M., & Smith, K. M. (2001b). Women and heart disease: The treatment may end but the suffering continues. *Canadian Journal of Nursing Research, 33,* 17–29. Abstract obtained from *Evidence-Based Nursing, 2002, 5,* 126. A support group created a caring environment where women with heart disease felt understood, supported, and strengthened by peers and nurse facilitators.

Blythe, J., & Royle, J. A. (1993). Assessing nurses' information needs in the work environment. *Bulletin of the Medical Librarians Association, 81,* 433–435.

Bostrom, J., & Suter, W. N. (1993). Research utilisation: Making the link to practice. *Journal of Nursing Staff Development, 9,* 28–34.

Burns, N., & Groves, S. K. (2001). *The practice of nursing research: Conduct, critique and utilization.* Philadelphia, PA: W.B. Saunders.

Canadian Health Services Research Foundation (CHSRF). (2004). *What counts? Interpreting evidence-based decision-making for management and policy.* Report of the 6th CHSRF Annual Invitational Workshop. Retrieved September 2006 from http://www.chsrf.ca/knowledge_transfer/pdf/2004_workshop_report_e.pdf.

Ciliska, D., Cullum, N., & Marks, S. (2001). Evaluation of systematic reviews of treatment or prevention interventions. *Evidence-Based Nursing, 4*(4), 100–104.

Cullum, N. (2000). Evaluation of studies of treatment or prevention interventions. *Evidence-Based Nursing, 3*(4), 100–102.

Cullum, N. (2001). Evaluation of studies of treatment or prevention interventions, part 2: Applying the results of studies to your patients. *Evidence-Based Nursing, 4*(1), 7–8.

DiCenso, A., Cullum, N., & Ciliska, D. (1998). Implementing evidence-based nursing: Some misconceptions. *Evidence-Based Nursing, 1,* 38–40.

Dickersin, K. (1990). The existence of publication bias and risk factors for its occurrence. *JAMA: The Journal of the American Medical Association, 263,* 1385–1389.

Dobbins, M., Ciliska, D., Cockerill, R., Barnsley, J., & DiCenso, A. (2002). A framework for the dissemination and utilization of research for health care policy and practice. *Online Journal of Knowledge Synthesis in Nursing, 9*(7). Retrieved December 3, 2003, from http://www.stti.iupui.edu/VirginiaHendersonLibrary/articles/090007.pdf.

Dobbins, M., Lockett, D., Michel, I., Beyers, J., Abate, N., & Feldman, L. (2001). *The effectiveness of school-based interventions in promoting physical activity and fitness among children and youth: A systematic review.* Hamilton: Public Health Research Education and Development Program. Effective Public Health Practice Project.

Estabrooks, C. A. (1998). Will evidence-based nursing practice make practice perfect? *Canadian Journal of Nursing Research, 30,* 15–36.

Flemming, K. (1998). Asking answerable questions. *Evidence-Based Nursing, 1,* 36–37.

Friere, P. (1972). *Pedagogy of the oppressed.* New York: Herder & Herder.

Hamilton Public Health & Community Services. (2003). *Effective public health practice project.* Retrieved June 9, 2003, from www.hamilton.ca/PHCS/EPHPP/EPHPP Research.asp.

Heater, B. S., Becker, A. M., & Olson, R. (1988). Nursing interventions and patient outcomes. A meta-analysis of studies. *Nursing Research, 37,* 303–307.

Hodnett, E. D., Kaufman, K., O'Brien-Pallas, L., Chipman, M., Watson-MacDonell, J., & Hunsburger, W. (1996). A strategy to promote research-based nursing care: Effects on childbirth outcomes. *Research in Nursing and Health, 19*(1), 13–20.

Jadad, A. R., & Haynes, R. B. (1998). The Cochrane collaboration: Advances and challenges in improving evidence-based decision making. *Medical Decision Making, 18,* 2–9.

Karp, D. A., & Tanarugsachock, V. (2000). Mental illness, caregiving, and emotion management. *Qualitative Health Research, 10,* 6–25.

Kramer, M. S., Chalmers, B., & Hodnett, E. (for the PROBIT Study Group). (2001). Promotion of breastfeeding intervention trial (PROBIT): A randomized trial in the Republic of Belarus. *JAMA: The Journal of the American Medical Association, 285,* 413–420.

Kunz, R., & Oxman, A. (1998). The unpredictability paradox: Review of empirical comparisons of randomized and non-randomized clinical trials. *BMJ, 317,* 1185–1190.

Lomas, J. (1991). Words without action? The production, dissemination, and impact of consensus recommendations. *Annual Review of Public Health, 12,* 41–65.

Luker, K. A., & Kenrick, M. (1992). An exploratory study of the sources of influence on the clinical decisions of community nurses. *Journal of Advanced Nursing, 17,* 457–466.

McKibbon, A., & Marks, S. (1998a). Searching for the best evidence, part 1: Where to look. *Evidence-Based Nursing, 1,* 68–70.

McKibbon, A., &; Marks, S. (1998b). Searching for the best evidence, part 2: Searching CINAHL and Medline. *Evidence-Based Nursing, 1,* 105–107.

Mueller, D., &; Thomas, H. (2001). *The effectiveness of public health interventions to reduce or prevent spousal abuse toward women: A systematic review.* Hamilton: Effective Public Health Practice Project. Retrieved November 30, 2003, from http://www.health.gov.on.ca/english/providers/pub/phero/pdf/phero_043003.pdf.

Ontario Ministry of Health, Public Health Branch. (1997). *Mandatory health program and services guidelines.* Toronto: Queen's Printer for Ontario.

Oxman, A., Guyatt, G., Cook, D., & Montori, V. (2002). Summarising the evidence. In G. Guyatt & D. Rennie (Eds.), *Users' guides to the medical literature: A manual for evidence-based clinical practice* (pp. 155–173). Chicago: AMA Press.

Pearcey, P. A. (1995). Achieving research-based nursing practice. *Journal of Advanced Nursing, 22,* 33–39.

Petticrew, M. (2001). Systematic reviews from astronomy to zoology: Myths and misconceptions. *BMJ, 322,* 98–101.

Ploeg, J. (1999). Identifying the best research design to fit the questions, part 2: Qualitative designs. *Evidence-Based Nursing, 2,* 36–37.

Ratner, P. A., Johnson, J. L., Richardson, C. G., Bottorff, J. L., Moffat, B., Mackay, M., Fofonoff, D., Kingsbury, K., Miller, C., Budz, B. (2004). Efficacy of a smoking-cessation intervention for elective-surgical patients. *Research in Nursing and Health, 27*(3), 148–61.

Registered Nurses' Association of Ontario. (2002). *Best practice guidelines.* Retrieved July 30, 2002, from www.rnao.org/bestpractices/

Roberts, J., & DiCenso, A. (1999). Identifying the best research design to fit the question, part 1: Quantitative designs. *Evidence-Based Nursing, 2,* 4–6.

Russell, C. K., & Gregory, D. M. (2003). Evaluation of qualitative research reports. *Evidence-Based Nursing, 6,* 36–40.

Sackett, D. L., Rosenberg, W., Gray, J. A. M., & Haynes, R. B. (1996). Evidence-based medicine: What it is and what it isn't. *BMJ, 312,* 71–72.

Sackett, D. L., Strauss, S. E., Richardson, W. S., Rosenberg, W., & Haynes, R. B. (2000). *Evidence based medicine: How to practice and teach EBM.* London: Churchill Livingstone.

Thomas, H., Camiletti, Y., Cava, M., Feldman, L., Underwood, J., & Wade, K. (1999). *The effectiveness of parenting groups with professional involvement in improving parent and child health outcomes.* Hamilton: Public Health Research Education and Development Program. Effective Public Health Practice Project.

Towheed, T. E., Anastassiades, T. P., Shea, B., Houpt, J., Welch, V., & Hochberg, M. C. (1999). Glucosamine therapy for treating osteoarthritis. *Cochrane Database of Systematic Reviews.* (Available to subscribers from The Cochrane Library, Chichester, UK, www.cochrane.org)

U.S. Department of Health and Human Services, Agency for Healthcare Research and Quality. (2002). *National guideline clearinghouse.* Retrieved July 30, 2002, from http://www.guideline.gov.

University of York, NHS Centre for Reviews and Dissemination. (1999). Getting evidence into practice. *Effective Health Care, 5*(1). Retrieved December 3, 2003, from http://www.york.ac.uk/inst/crd/ehc51.pdf.

Utterback, J. M. (1974). Innovation in industry and the diffusion of technology. *Science, 183,* 620–626.

ADDITIONAL RESOURCES

Websites

BMJ Journals Online
   www.bmjjournals.com

BMJ *Clinical Evidence*
   www.clinicalevidence.org

Cochrane Collaboration Health Promotion/
Public Health Field
   www.vichealth.vic.gov.au/cochrane

Cochrane Library
   www.thecochranelibrary.com

Evidence-Based Nursing
   www.evidencebasednursing.com

Health-evidence.ca
   www.health-evidence.ca

Teaching/Learning Evidence-based Practice
   www.mdx.ac.uk/www/rctsh/ebp/main.htm

Users' Guides Interactive
   www.usersguides.org

Books

McKibbon, A. (with Eady, A., & Marks, S.). (1999). *PDQ: Evidence-based principles and practice.* Hamilton: B. C. Decker.

Sackett, D. L., Strauss, S. E., Richardson, W. S., Rosenberg, W., & Haynes, R. B. (2000). *Evidence based medicine: How to practice and teach EBM.* London: Churchill Livingstone.

Articles

Greenhalgh, T. (1997). How to read a paper: Papers that summarise other papers (systematic reviews and meta-analyses). *BMJ, 315,* 672–675. Retrieved December 10, 2003, from http://www.bmj.com/cgi/content/full/315/7109/672.

Havelock, P. (1998). Teaching and learning evidence-based practice. In L. Ridsdale (Ed.), *Evidence-based practice in primary care* (pp. 173–190). New York: Churchill Livingstone.

U.S. Department of Health and Human Services, Agency for Healthcare Research and Quality (AHRQ). (2003). *National guideline clearinghouse.* Retrieved December 10, 2003, from http://www.guideline.gov.

Journals of Pre-appraised Research

Evidence-Based Nursing
   www.ebn.bmj.com

Evidence-Based Mental Health
   www.ebmh.bmj.com

Evidence-Based Medicine
   www.ebm.bmj.com

Evidence-Based Healthcare
   www.harcourt-international.com/journals/ebhc

About the Authors

Donna Ciliska, RN, PhD, is a Professor at the School of Nursing, McMaster University, and has an appointment as Nursing Consultant with Hamilton Public Health and Community Services. Dr. Ciliska is an editor of the journal *Evidence-Based Nursing.* Her research interests include community health, obesity, eating disorders, and research dissemination and utilization.

Helen Thomas, RN, MSc, is an Associate Professor in the School of Nursing at McMaster University and a Clinical Consultant with Hamilton Public Health and Social Services, Public Health Research Education and Development (PHRED) program. She is also the Director of the Effective Public Health Practice Project. Helen's research interests include adolescent health, homelessness, child abuse, and research dissemination, uptake, and utilization.

Information and Communication Technology

Ruta Valaitis and Linda Ferguson

OBJECTIVES

After studying this chapter, you should be able to:

1. Identify basic informatics competencies for community health nurses.

2. Describe the use of the internet to access health information by various Canadian population groups.

3. Evaluate the quality of a health website.

4. Describe a variety of internet technology applications with potential to support health promotion, disease prevention and chronic disease management.

5. Identify ways to increase accessibility to health information on the internet for the public.

6. List emerging technology tools that can support community health nursing practice, professional development, and knowledge exchange in community health nursing.

INTRODUCTION

Exponential growth has occurred in the use of internet-based **information and communication technologies (ICTs)** by health professionals and the public. The term ICT represents a variety of computer-based technology systems that support gathering, analyzing, archiving, retrieving, processing, and transmitting information and communication. ICTs can support people to increase control over their health through access to health information; provide social support; facilitate behaviour change; and support community mobilization. Primary health care nursing service delivery can be improved through the use of innovative, interactive **e-health** interventions that are tailored to individual needs. Eysenbach (2001) defined e-health as:

> an emerging field in the intersection of medical informatics, public health and business, referring to health services and information delivered or enhanced through the Internet and related technologies. In a broader sense, the term characterizes not only a technical development, but also a state-of-mind, a way of thinking, an attitude, and a commitment for networked, global thinking, to improve health care locally, regionally, and worldwide by using information and communication technology. (n.p.)

Community health nurses (CHNs) can support the effective use of ICTs to promote health, prevent illness, and manage chronic disease using e-health interventions.

CHNs are expected to meet the Canadian Community Health Nursing Standards of Practice (CHNAC, 2003), which include specific standards related to nursing informatics. (See Appendix A at the back of this book.) Nursing informatics (Staggers & Bagley Thompson, 2002) has been defined as:

> a specialty that integrates nursing science, computer science, and information science to manage and communicate data, information, and knowledge in nursing practice. Nursing informatics facilitates the integration of data, information, and knowledge to support patients, nurses, and other providers in their decision making in all roles and settings. This support is accomplished through the use of information structures, information processes, and information technology. (p. 262)

In this chapter, you will learn about CHN competencies as they relate to **nursing informatics** and gain an overview of current research on accessing and using the internet for health information and communication. You will explore innovations in technology that have shown potential to support health promotion, disease prevention, and chronic disease management. Finally, you will be introduced to ICTs that support professional development and knowledge exchange in community health nursing.

NURSING INFORMATICS COMPETENCIES

Public health informatics is defined as "the systematic application of information and computer sciences and technology to public health practice, research and learning" (Yasnoff, O'Carroll, Koo, Linkins, & Kilbourne, 2000). The Canadian Community Health Nursing Standards of Practice are based on the principles of primary health care that include the appropriate use of technology and resources. Specifically, the Standards state that CHNs are expected to "utilize nursing informatics (information and communication technology) to generate, manage and process relevant data to support nursing practice" (CHNAC, 2003).

Complementary to these standards is a set of public health informatics competencies developed in the United States for front-line staff, senior-level technical staff, and supervisory and management staff (O'Carroll & Public Health Informatics Competencies Working Group, 2002). These competencies were separated into three classes: (1) use of information for public health practice, (2) use of information technology to increase effectiveness as a public health professional, and

(3) management of IT projects to improve the effectiveness of the public health enterprise. The Canadian Nursing Informatics Association (CNIA) has also made recommendations concerning basic internet and computer competencies of nursing graduates (CNIA, 2003). CNIA identified a need to build strong links between nursing informatics and evidence-based practice; increase informatics skills of educators, clinicians, and students; identify how informatics is covered in curricula; build stronger human, material, and financial infrastructure for ICT in clinical and academic settings; and strengthen partnerships with the private sector.

USE OF THE INTERNET TO ACCESS HEALTH INFORMATION

Rapid growth has occurred in Canadians' use of the internet to access health information. Results from the General Social Survey and the Household Internet Use Survey showed that 46% of internet users over the age of 15 years searched for health or medical information (Stevenson, 2002). In 2002, almost 4 million households looked for health information on the internet, representing an increase of more than 262% from 1998 (Earl, 2004). The Household Internet Survey (Figure 15.1) illustrates the rapid growth of medical and health information searching by households between 1999 and 2003 (Statistics Canada, 2006). By 2006, 67.9% of Canadians over 18 years of age were reported to use the internet, with 35.6% of them accessing medical or health information (Statistics Canada, 2006).

This trend has been reported in other nations. The use of the internet for health information in the United States continues to grow. In 2004, 79% of internet users searched for health information (Rice, 2006). In the United States, the National Cancer Institute reported that 63% of adults used the internet and, of those, 63.7% searched for health information at least once within the last 12 months (Hesse et al., 2005).

Women were more likely to seek health information on the internet compared with men and young males (15–24 years of age), who were least likely to use it (Stevenson, 2002).

Other population groups more likely to search health information on the internet were families with children and health care workers. Thirty-eight percent of older Canadians who searched the internet for health information were specifically looking for information about specific diseases (65%), drugs (27%), and lifestyle issues such as diet, exercise, and health promotion (27%) (Silver, 2001).

Although participants viewed physicians as the most credible source of health information, 48.6% of respondents reported using the internet first, while 10.9% reported going to their physicians first (Hesse et al., 2005). They also found that internet usage was highest for younger, female, more educated, and more affluent users. Kivits (2006) noted similar trends in the United Kingdom, with internet users indicating the need for internet health resources to prepare for consultations with physicians or for follow-up on limited information provided to them. Accessibility of the internet makes it a source of choice for health information for the public.

Kivits (2006) conducted qualitative online interviews with 31 adults (most of whom were female) and found that internet use was a characteristic of healthy users, who may be seeking health promotion information for themselves or for others suffering from an illness or condition. In contrast, a random survey of 2038 adults in the Pew Internet Project found that although sick or disabled adults were less likely to go online, they searched for online health information more than their healthier counterparts (Goldner, 2006). Differences in findings may be explained by the samples and method of recruitment used. Kivits advertised the study through websites devoted to nutrition, fitness, and general health, which likely drew more health conscious and therefore healthier visitors. This finding should, therefore, be viewed with caution. Another trend noted by Hesse et al. (2005) was increasing internet use for personal health maintenance, with a corresponding increase in internet users (approximately 9%) who purchased pharmaceuticals online. Approximately 7% communicated with physicians via email—a phenomenon that will have significant management issues for physicians—and 4% participated in online support groups.

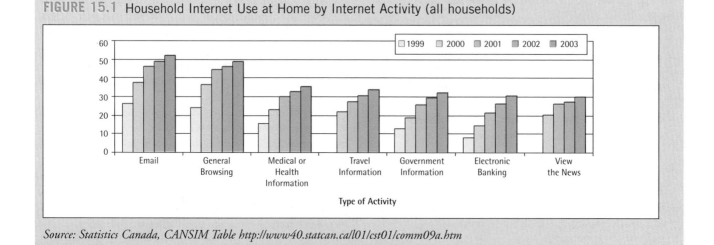

FIGURE 15.1 Household Internet Use at Home by Internet Activity (all households)

Source: Statistics Canada, CANSIM Table http://www40.statcan.ca/l01/cst01/comm09a.htm

Canadian Research Box 15.1

Skinner, H., Biscope, S., & Goldberg, E. (2003). How adolescents use technology for health information: Implications for health professionals from focus group studies. *Journal of Medical Internet Research, 5,* 32.

An Ontario study by Skinner et al. (2003) explored adolescents' use of technology for health information. Twenty-seven focus groups were conducted with 210 youth between the ages of 10 and 28 years, representing a variety of cultural, geographic, and socioeconomic backgrounds such as street youth and Aboriginal youth. Results indicated that the most common health topics searched were specific medical conditions (67%), body image and nutrition (63%), violence and personal safety (59%), and sexual health (56%). Mental health was another important, yet less often reported theme (22%). Two major challenges emerged in accessing health information. Youth found it difficult to find personally relevant, high-quality information and privacy when accessing the internet. Health professionals are encouraged to provide an interface between e-health applications and the health care setting, teach strategies to find and evaluate quality health information on the web, and use technology to build better interactions and connections with youth.

Discussion Questions:

1. CyberIsle (www.cyberisle.org) is a largely unmoderated Canadian health promotion website for youth. What are the potential implications with respect to the use of unmoderated versus moderated health promotion sites?

2. How can health information on the web be made more relevant for youth?

Despite the heavy use of the internet for health information, it is worrying that nurses and doctors are rarely asked for advice regarding where to search for health information online (Rice, 2006). This finding highlights an important health education role for CHNs, especially when working with internet users. Nurses are cautioned that online health information is only one approach to delivering health messages within myriad other communications media (Kivits, 2006).

Internet Access Issues

Although many populations use the internet for health information, do not assume that everyone has access. When designing health promotion programs for internet delivery, it is important to consider populations without access and non-users. Tapscott (1998) first identified the **digital divide** as information "haves" and "have-nots," which divided society into knowers and know-nots, doers and do-nots. The digital divide refers to the division of population groups who have and do not have access to—and/or the capability to use—information technology. A new digital divide was proposed differentiating three classes of access, including people with no access (22%), modest connections (such as dial-up) (40%), and the broadband elite (33%) (Fox, 2005). Further, Lenhart,

Horrigan, Rainie, Boyce, Madden, & O'Grady, (2003) described four main types of internet non-users. "Net-evaders" constitute 20% of non-users, who live in connected households and use family members as proxies to send and receive email and search the web. "Net dropouts" make up 17% of non-users (overlapping with "net-evaders"), who used the internet in the past but stopped because of technical problems or because they did not like it. Many of them think they may return to the internet someday. "Intermittent users" are made up of 27% to 44% of internet users who dropped out and have now returned to the internet. The last group is made up of 69% of non-users who are "truly disconnected." They have never used the internet and do not live with or know many internet users. Goldner (2006) warned health professionals to provide education to the sick about the quality of online health information despite their low internet use, because they will likely search the internet for health information.

Non-users in a New Zealand community were provided free internet access near their residence, but many were not interested in using it (Crump & McIlroy, 2003). The authors concluded that this population did not feel technology positively impacted their quality of life as they struggled to meet basic needs; technology was not a priority. Professionals should not assume, therefore, that all clients can or will access the internet for health information. Conversely, low-income communities in the United States have long been shown to use and benefit from community-based internet access to empower and build healthier neighbourhoods (Milio, 1996; Schon, Sanyal, & Mitchell, 1999).

Youth are early adopters in using technology, which has significant potential to enhance youth's health decision making. Their access issues differ from others. Skinner, Biscope, & Poland, (2003) studied 210 Ontario youth to explore their perceptions of the internet for health information and resources. The quality of internet access was significantly impacted by four factors. *Privacy* referred to youths' ability to search for information on sensitive topics without being observed by others; *gate-keeping* referred to blocks put on certain websites or limits to types of use; *timeliness* was related to the ability to have access to information for as long as needed (e.g., access limited during school hours or limitations from parents on internet time); *functionality* referred to technical issues such as speed of access and functions such as ICQ ("I Seek You"—an instant messaging program). The latter was strongly related to socioeconomic status and geographic location. Health and education professionals should support interventions to address the "access quality divide" for more vulnerable populations (Skinner et al. 2003).

Access for Disabled Populations

CHNs often work with disabled populations. The Canadian Council on Social Development (2005) reported that more than half a million adult Canadians have some form of vision loss, more than a million have some form of hearing loss, and a fair number have both. People with disabilities can benefit from using ICTs, since they can reduce isolation by helping them reach people with similar experiences (Seymour & Lupton, 2004), become better informed, increase communication, and enhance access to health information. The next

FIGURE 15.2 Screen Capture of Health Canada's Photo Gallery Website

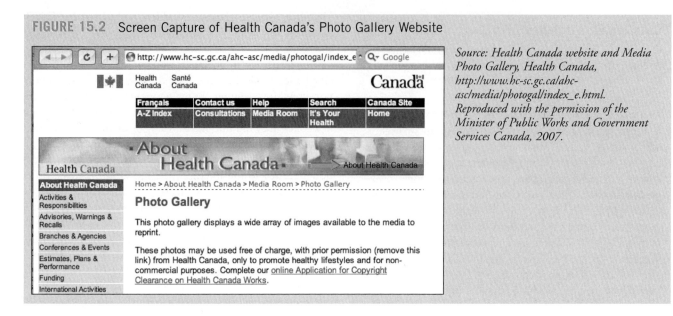

Source: Health Canada website and Media Photo Gallery, Health Canada, http://www.hc-sc.gc.ca/ahc-asc/media/photogal/index_e.html. Reproduced with the permission of the Minister of Public Works and Government Services Canada, 2007.

section will review accessibility standards that guide the design of health information websites, and provide a basic overview of technology tools to enhance disabled clients' internet access.

The World Wide Web Consortium (W3C) (www.w3.org) is an international organization that oversees the standardization and operation of the Web. In 1997, to ensure equitable and universal access to information for all populations including people with disabilities, W3C launched the **Web Accessibility Initiative (WAI)** (W3C, 2006). Under this initiative, accessibility standards for web content designers and developers were created. By 1999, the **Web Content Accessibility Guidelines (WCAG)** document was developed (Chisholm, Vanderheiden, & Jacobs, 1999) and has since been updated (Caldwell, Slatin, & Vanderheiden, 2006). These guidelines define **accessible** as "usable to a wide range of people with disabilities, including blindness and low vision, deafness and hearing loss, learning difficulties, cognitive limitations, limited movement, speech difficulties, photosensitivity and combinations of these." Standards were grouped into different priority levels. Disability advocates recommend that websites at a minimum meet the Priority Level One standard.

Priority Level One includes design standards that are relatively simple to meet. For example, web page images need clear text descriptions included in the html code. The code should include alt tags (alternative text tags) so that when a user rolls over the image, a text description appears. When browser preferences are set for "text only," the option for viewing images is turned off. This option is useful for the visually impaired. Screen readers turn screen text to speech and can read text programmed in the alt tag codes, thereby informing visitors what images are on the page (Figure 15.2 shows an example). Another simple Priority One standard includes the use of contrasting background and text colours. Such standards help to ensure that web documents are navigable. The Treasury Board of Canada has also identified a set of guidelines for all federal government department websites called the "Common Look and Feel for the Internet" (2004). These guidelines incorporate Priority One and Priority Two W3C checkpoints. These standards should be used when designing health information websites to ensure accessibility.

A cross-sectional evaluation conducted by Zeng and Parmanto (2004) of 108 consumer health information websites showed that none were completely accessible to the disabled. Every site had at least one violation of web accessibility rules. Educational and government health information sites fared significantly better than e-commerce, community, and corporate sites or portals. Accessible sites were more popular than less accessible sites, likely because accessible sites are easier to index. Thereby, they have a greater chance of being picked up by web crawlers that store page indexes for easier retrieval (Zeng & Parmanto). Second, more accessible sites are likely visited more often and may even be preferred by the non-disabled consumer. An evaluation of U.S. State Health Department websites indicated that public agencies "fall short of fair and equitable e-health accessibility and confidentiality" (West & Miller, 2006). There was also limited access to translations to meet the public's needs.

Case Study: Testing Website Accessibility

Identify your favourite health information website or your current clinical placement agency website. Once you have located the website, highlight and copy the URL (Universal Resource Locator—a unique identifier that provides an address for an internet site). Then proceed to an accessibility checker website. Three popular web accessibility checker sites are http://webxact.watchfire.com, www.cynthiasays.com, and http://checker.atrc.utoronto.ca (a Canadian site recently developed at the University of Toronto). Paste in the URL at the checker site. It will analyze your site and report how well it complied with W3C Web Content Accessibility Guidelines (Caldwell et al., 2006).

Discussion Questions

1. How accessible was your site?
2. Which standards did it fail?

Numerous software and hardware devices are available to assist disabled populations. Some commonly used devices for the visually impaired include screen readers, screen magnifiers, Braille displays, voice recognition technologies, data extraction tools that filter content from overly busy web pages, and optical character recognition software to turn a printed page into electronic text for screen reading (Fichten, Barile, & Asuncion, 2003). Portable note-taking devices can help people with speech communication disorders, and ergonomic adapters, dictation programs, and voice controlled software can assist the mobility impaired (Fichten et al.). Simple adjustments can be made with most Windows operating systems to enhance accessibility. Explore the "Accessibility Options" folder in the Control Panel to adjust settings for hearing, vision, and mobility. The Canadian Adaptech Network Project website (Adaptech Research Network, 2006) includes numerous useful resource links listing free or inexpensive products to assist the disabled.

QUALITY OF HEALTH INFORMATION ON THE INTERNET

Increased public access to health information on the internet has introduced both risks and opportunities. The public has a challenge in determining whether health information acquired on the internet can be trusted. At the same time, access to good-quality health information can empower clients to address their health issues. Health information on the internet includes health promotion information, screening tests, personal accounts of illness, patient testimonials about treatment effectiveness, patient opinions or perspectives on their illness experiences, product advertisers, treatment providers, patient/client discussion and support groups, peer-reviewed articles, and decision-making aids. Determining the quality of this information is challenging for clients, which may lead to their skepticism about the value of the information. A goal for CHNs includes assisting clients to become knowledgeable consumers of information available to them in this media (Jones, 2003). Recommendations for nurses are listed in Table 15.1.

Many internet users have indicated their concerns about the credibility of the health information on the internet and their willingness to judge it. They have also indicated interest in accessing both scientific and medical information along with patient testimonials about the illness experience (Kivits, 2006). Unfortunately, even though internet users may indicate they use criteria such as source credibility, language, and transparency to determine the value of online health information, they tended to disregard these criteria when actually conducting a search. In addition, internet users tended to rely on common sense or personal experience to judge the usefulness of the information (Eysenbach & Kohler, 2002; Silence, Briggs, & Herxheimer, 2004) and used correspondence with the content of other websites to judge its accuracy (Kivits). Users tended to develop a practical knowledge based on their experience to determine what information and sources of knowledge to select (Kivits).

TABLE 15.1
Recommended Nursing Actions with Respect to Health Information on the Internet

Develop skills in online health information retrieval and evaluation to identify and recommend the best online sites for health information.

Assess clients' internet access, computer competencies, health literacy, online activity, desired role in decision making, and need for assistive devices to access the Internet.

Identify local community resources for internet access.

Invite clients to discuss the health information they have found online.

Consider client–provider online communication options (email, bulletin boards, instant messaging), and develop guidelines for email triage in practice settings similar to telephone triage protocols.

When using internet-based communications with clients, learn about the security of the site and ramifications for client privacy.

Consider gender and culture preferences when developing Web-based health promotion interventions.

Teach clients how to evaluate quality and appropriateness of health information on the Web.

Sources: Adapted from Dickerson (2006) with permission. Sally Byers Blackwell Publishing.

In their usability study, Eysenbach and Kohler (2002) found that very few users noticed or remembered the websites from which they had acquired health information, and none of them used the "about us" links to find information about sponsoring organizations. These participants' search strategies tended to be broadcast rather than specific, using general search engines rather than medical portals or health websites as starting points. Participants may not know the differences among websites with domain names of .edu, .gov, .com, or .net (Changrani & Gany, 2005). Participants used links from the first screen of results displayed by the search engine and rarely refined their search terms or repeated the search. Most searches were concluded within five minutes. If participants repeated a search, they stated it was because they did not trust the source or understand the information. Though these findings were reported in 2002 (Eysenbach & Kohler), Kivits reported very similar findings in 2006. The lay public does not seem to be changing in terms of their critical appraisal of online information.

The quality of health information on the internet is highly variable. When the quality of condition-specific information on the internet was assessed for accuracy, some condition sites were identified as poor, including osteoarthritis (Maloney, Ilic, & Green, 2006), industry-sponsored tobacco-prevention information (Lin & Hullman, 2005), hypertension (Silence et al., 2004), lumbar disc herniation (Greene, Appel, Reinert, & Palumbo, 2005), scoliosis (Mathur et al., 2005), and postpartum depression (Summers & Logsdon, 2005). Other conditions or health issues were addressed more accurately, including living with HIV/AIDS (Kalichman et al., 2006), breastfeeding (Dornan & Oermann, 2006), and diabetes (Pearce, 2004). Essentially, consumers are left with having to determine the quality of online health information.

Tools Available for Rating Health Information on the Internet

Myriad tools are available to consumers and health care providers for evaluating the quality of health information on the internet. Unfortunately, as Gagliardi and Jadad (2002) demonstrated, most of the rating tools available have not been validated. Of the 47 rating tools that Jadad and Gagliardi identified in 1998, none provided information on reliability and validity. Five years later, they identified an additional 51 tools, with only 5 of the 98 providing information on validity and reliability. Consumers attempting to evaluate the quality may have difficulties determining the valuing of ratings provided on various websites. In addition, different consumers may have different purposes for the information, thus needing different criteria by which they will judge the quality of information. Various dimensions of internet resources can be evaluated, including content, journalistic value, targeted audience, website design, readability/usability, and ethical issues of privacy. These dimensions will change over time as technology evolves (Purcell, Wilson, & Delamothe, 2002). Because regulation of quality of internet health information is an ongoing yet unresolved issue (Purcell et al.), educating clients to be knowledgeable consumers of internet health information seems to be the most reasonable approach.

Providing clients with clear criteria of credible online information is the best means of enabling them to assess its quality. More and more often, clients are bringing printouts of online information to their health care providers, assuming the information to be reliable. Using the **HON code** (Health on the Net Foundation, 1997) to examine the information with clients is an effective way of teaching the criteria while simultaneously critiquing the online information. In Table 15.2, eight principles are listed and described.

Although health care professionals may be adept at applying HON criteria, most laypersons will not be. Table 15.3 illustrates questions that clients may use in assessing the health information they have accessed on the internet. Assisting clients to interpret and apply these criteria will empower them to use internet health information with greater confidence. HON (Health on the Net Foundation, 1997) also supports a service where health information consumers may submit a URL to the "WRAPIN" service (www.wrapin.org) to determine if the site is accredited or trustworthy (WRAPIN, 2001).

Assessment of Health Information Websites

The usability of health information websites may relate to more than the accuracy of the information provided. The Health Information Technology Institute provided another set of criteria that evaluate health information websites on their usability for consumers (Health Summit Working Group, 2007). These criteria include credibility, content, disclosures, links, design, interactivity, and caveats (Table 15.4) and relate to the presentation of information and ease of use.

TABLE 15.2
HON Code of Conduct for Medical and Health Websites

1. Authority	Any medical or health advice provided and hosted on this site will only be given by medically trained and qualified health professionals unless a clear statement is made that a piece of advice offered is from a non-medically qualified individual or organisation.
2. Complementarity	The information provided on this site is designed to support, not replace, the relationship that exists between a patient/site visitor and his/her existing physician.
3. Confidentiality	Confidentiality of data relating to individual patients and visitors to a medical/health website, including their identity, is respected by this website. The website owners undertake to honour or exceed the legal requirements of medical/health information privacy that apply in the country or state where the website and mirror sites are located.
4. Attribution	Where appropriate, information contained on this site will be supported by clear references to source data and, where possible, have specific HTML links to that data. The date when a clinical page was last modified will be clearly displayed (e.g. at the bottom of the page).
5. Justifiability	Any claims relating to the benefits/performance of a specific treatment, commercial product, or service will be supported by appropriate balanced evidence in the manner outlined above in Principle 4.
6. Transparency of authorship	The designers of this website will seek to provide information in the clearest possible manner and provide contact addresses for visitors that seek further information or support. The webmaster will display his/her email address clearly throughout the website.
7. Transparency of sponsorship	Support for this website will be clearly identified, including the identities of commercial and non-commercial organizations that have contributed funding, services or material for the site.
8. Honesty in advertising & editorial policy	If advertising is a source of funding, it will be clearly stated. A brief description of the advertising policy adopted by the website owners will be displayed on the site. Advertising another promotional material will be presented to viewers in a manner and context that facilitates differentiation between it and the original material created by the institution operating the site.

Source: Health on the Net (HON) Foundation, http://www.HealthOnNet.org.

TABLE 15.3
Questions for Clients to Use in Assessing Internet Health Information

1. Is the health information provided by a qualified medical practitioner or an organization that is committed to the public's health?
2. Does the website encourage you to discuss the health information with your physician or another health care professional?
3. Is your identity protected on this website?
4. Does the website indicate sources or references for the information provided? Are these sources credible?
5. Are claims of effectiveness of treatments supported by credible evidence?
6. Is the authorship of this website clear to you? Can you contact the webmaster for more information?
7. Is the sponsorship of the website clearly apparent to you?
8. Are the commercial advertisements clearly separated from the health information presented on the website? Is the advertising policy stated on the website?
9. Is there a link to the homepage of the sponsoring organization from the health information webpages?
10. Does the homepage explain the mission, purpose and objectives, sources of funding, and governance of the organization?

Readability of text is an important design aspect of every web page. Readability is a measure of how easily and comfortably text can be read. People with lower reading skills also use the internet. For websites intended for laypersons, reading levels should be focused approximately at a Grade 9 level. Reading experts suggest that the majority of the population prefers written materials three grades below the last grade attended at school (Gottlieb & Rogers, 2004). Although this level seems low, it may still be higher than the reading comprehension level of the general population, which is on average Grade 5–6 level (Boulos, 2005; Gottlieb & Rogers). Within the Canadian population, 7% of anglophones and 18% of francophones have not completed Grade 9 (Statistics Canada, 2006), and a large number of Canadians are not functional in prose, document, or numeracy literacy (Statistics Canada, 1997). Unfortunately, websites have much higher reading levels. Boulos found only one-third of internet diabetes mellitus websites were at a Grade 8 level or lower (using the Flesch Reading Ease Test and Flesch-Kincaid Readability Formula). The rest were significantly higher. Berland et al. (2001) identified that all internet materials on four common health conditions were written at high school or higher reading levels and exceeded recommended levels. This finding was supported by others (Boulos; D'Alessandro, Kingsley, & Johnston-West, 2001; Gottlieb & Rogers, 2004; Kaphingst, Zanfini, & Emmons, 2006).

TABLE 15.4
HITI Criteria for Assessing Health Information Websites

1. Credibility	Source: Sponsoring agency logo and information are displayed, along with relevant personal or financial associations. Disclosure of sponsorship is clear. Currency: Including date of posting and the date of the document on which information is based. Relevance: Content corresponds to intended purpose of website. Site evaluation: Editorial/content review process.
2. Content	Accuracy and completeness of content, with source identified Disclaimer: Statement that content is general health information and not medical advice.
3. Disclosures	Clear statement of the purpose of the site. Collection of user information: Indicating any user information collected from site and its intended purpose.
4. Links	Selection: Appropriate links are selected. Architecture: Ease of navigation to sites and back to original page. Content of links: Relevant to original website, accurate, external sites clearly identified.
5. Design	Accessibility: For lowest-level browser technology, use by hearing or visually impaired. Logical organization: Including design and layout, readability, language, balance of text and graphics. Navigability: Simple, internally consistent, and easy to use. Internal search capability: Highly desirable.
6. Interactivity	Feedback mechanisms: Feedback mechanisms and exchange of information among users.
7. Caveats	Clarification of the site's function to market products or services.

Source: Adapted from The Health Summit Working Group. (1999). Information Quality Tool. Retrieved April 12, 2007, from Mitretek Systems website: http://hitiweb.mitretek.org./docs/policy.html.

TABLE 15.5
SMOG Readability Assessment Tool: Document Assessment for Approximate Grade Level of Reading Skills

Step 1 Sample selection	Select 30 sentences from the text material: 10 consecutive sentences from the start, the middle, and the end of the material. A sentence is a complete idea with a period, question mark, or exclamation mark, a bulleted point, or both parts of a sentence with a colon included.
Step 2 Word count	Count the number of words with more than three syllables (polysyllabic) in the 30-sentence sample. Include all repetitions of a word, proper nouns, the full text of abbreviations, and hyphenated words as one word.
Step 3 Short text conversion	For documents of fewer than 30 sentences, multiply the number of polysyllabic words by a factor to simulate a sample of 30 sentences. For example, if the document contained 15 sentences, the factor would be 30 divided by 15 to equal a factor of 2. For documents of 24 sentences, the factor would be 30 divided by 24 to equal 1.25.
Step 4 Calculate	Determine the nearest square root of the number of words in the sample. A square root is a number multiplied by itself to equal a perfect square. For example, 8 multiplied by 8 (square root) equals 64 (perfect square). The number that is a square root is usually between 3 and 15.
Add the constant "3" to the square root obtained in step 4.	Example: A sample is assessed as having 86 polysyllabic words in 30 sentences. The nearest square root is 9 (9 times 9 equals 81).The constant of 3 is added to give an approximate reading level of 12, or more appropriately described as a reading level requiring the reading skills approximately at the Grade 12 reading level.

The result is the approximate grade level of reading skills required to read the document. The resultant grade level is correct within 1.5 grades in 68% of cases.

Source: Adapted from an article by McLaughlin (1969).

Health professionals who are recommending or creating websites for clients can assess the readability of written or internet text by using a relatively simple tool, the **SMOG (Simple Measure of Gobbledygook) Readability Test** (McLaughlin, 1969) (Table 15.5). SMOG reading levels correlate well with grade levels identified by other tests of readability (Gottlieb & Rogers, 2004). Because these tests are based on two variables of reading comprehension, word length and sentence length, the reading level of text materials can be reduced by using simple words and shorter sentences (Table 15.6). The Canadian Public Health Association (1999), in its National Literacy and Health Program, published the Directory of Plain Language Health Information to assist health educators in publishing clear and easily understood written materials. Key points are summarized in Table 15.7.

Health care professionals may refer clients to well-developed websites that are specific to their needs. Factors to be considered when judging the utility of online health information include ease of navigation and ease of accessing web pages within the site (Bensley, Brusk, Rivas, & Anderson, 2006). Internal links for ease of access are beneficial to users. External links should be assessed for their relatedness and ease of return to the original website. Use of graphics to illustrate concepts enhances usability; however, advertising on the website and irritating pop-ups may interfere with usability. Users also find a pleasing appearance and the opportunity for interactivity, such as calculations of body mass index (BMI), daily calorie counters, or self-report progress charts, to be beneficial (Ferney & Marshall, 2006). Ease of usage enhances the user's ability to read and use the information contained on a website. Clients can also be referred to government-sponsored health information websites, such as provincial governments (www.HealthyOntario.com), the Public Health Agency of Canada (www.phac-aspc.gc.ca), and the Canadian Health Network (www.canadian-health-network.ca).

Targeting Specific Users of Online Health Information

Online health information should also be designed for specific users. College students, most of whom are comfortable with internet use and have high reading levels, expressed interest in participating in online health courses or programs and accessing online health information (Escoffery, Milner, Adame, Butler, McCormick, & Mendell, 2005). Adolescents are major users and early adopters of the internet (Gray & Klein, 2006), with virtually all having access through home or school. Adolescents valued the internet for its accessibility, interactivity, availability of information, and ease of use, primarily through search engines such as Google, Yahoo, and Ask Jeeves (Parlove, Cowdery, & Hoerauf, 2004). Adolescents used the internet to access health information related to self-care, sexuality, and lifestyle issues. Preferred websites for adolescents included visual appeal, including music, modern look, and colourful and flashy design, and content appeal, including interactivity such as quizzes, games, advice sections, question and answer sections, and chat rooms. Aspects of health information websites that deterred these committed internet users included excessive advertising or intents to sell products or services and complicated internal navigation (Parlove et al.). Taking these findings into account permits better **targeting**. Targeting is "the development of a single intervention approach for a defined population sub-group that takes into account characteristics shared by sub-group's members" (Kreuter & Skinner, 2000). The concept comes from advertising principles that are related to market segmentation.

Individuals with stigmatized illnesses preferred online health education as a means of maintaining anonymity (Berger, Wagner, & Baker, 2005). They may also have a greater need for online support groups and other forums for

TABLE 15.6
Examples of Different Reading Levels

Grade 13 reading level*	Include exercise such as walking, biking, swimming, jogging, and active sports, according to your individual preferences. Consider other means of transportation or use stairs instead of elevators. Incorporate physical activities into your interactions with your children.
	The recommended amount of activity per week is 20 minutes of activity daily, on at least 5 separate occasions per week. Monitor your pulse rate, keeping it within the recommended target level during your activity. To stay physically fit, keep active and have fun.
Grade 9 reading level*	Include exercise such as walking, biking, swimming, jogging, and active sports, as you prefer. Consider walking to the store or using the stairs instead of elevators. Be active with your children.
	We recommend 20 minutes of activity daily, at least 5 times per week. Monitor your pulse rate, keeping it within the target level during your activity. To stay physically fit, keep active and have fun.
Grade 6 reading level*	Include walking, biking, swimming, jogging, and active sports in your daily life. Choose other ways of being active. Take the stairs. Walk to the store. Play with your kids.
	We suggest at least 20 minutes of exercise per day, 5 times per week. Include more time as you wish. Learn how to take your own pulse rate. Keep your pulse rate within the target level. Stay fit. Keep active. Have fun.

Approximate reading levels based on SMOG assessment

TABLE 15.7
Plain Language Strategies

- Use active voice by stating the subject of the action first, e.g., "You should eat 5 to 10 fruits and vegetables per day," instead of "5 to 10 fruits and vegetables should be eaten every day."
- Write directly to the reader, using "you" or implying "you" as the subject of the sentence, e.g., "Take this medication once per day," instead of "This medication should be taken once per day."
- Maintain a positive tone, stating actions as positive behaviours rather than avoidance behaviours, e.g., "Contact your doctor as soon as you feel sick," instead of "Avoid waiting too long to contact your doctor."
- Use common simple terms rather than technical jargon, e.g., "Medicine will relieve your child's pain," instead of "An analgesic will relieve your child's pain."
- Use short words and short sentences.
- Replace more difficult words with simpler words:
  — *drug* or *medicine* in place of *medication*
  — *heart* in place of *cardiac*
  — *doctor* in place of *physician*
  — *take part in* rather than *participate*
  — *problems* in place of *difficulties*
- When in doubt, ask your learners what words are most meaningful.
- Don't change verbs into nouns. The action word is a stronger depiction; e.g., "Decide when to involve your children in meal planning," instead of "Make decisions about your children's involvement in meal planning."
- List important points separate from the text.
  — Use bullets to highlight important points.
  — Keep bullets short.
  — Use boxes to highlight important information.
- Write instructions in the order that you want them to be carried out.
- List items in parallel form such as nouns or actions.
- Keep your writing in a conversational form.
- Test whatever you write with learners before you formalize it.

Source: Adapted from the Plain Language Service of the Canadian Public Health Association (1999), www.pls.cpha.ca/english/english.pdf.

online interactivity. Although immigrant women use the internet at the same rate as the general population, only 6% used the internet for health information, compared with 63% of the general population of internet users (Changrani & Gany, 2005). Many of these immigrant women indicated a preference for simple navigation sites, simple language, and simple URLs. They preferred soft soothing colours, images congruent with their culture, "not too much information," and interactive tools such as question-and-answer forums and video and slide show illustrations. They also valued information tailored to their health beliefs and specific needs.

Seniors over 65 years of age were the most underrepresented portion of the general population online. Approximately half of those using the internet (48.2%) sought health information for themselves (36.9%) or for others (31.3%) (Hesse et al., 2005). Only 18% of seniors with a high school diploma have gone online, compared to 65% of those with a college degree (Voelker, 2005). The National Institute on Aging (2002) identified challenges for seniors using online health information. Because scrolling through a website presents challenges for some seniors, designing websites or recommending those that present one paragraph per web page is a better alternative (Roush, 2006). The U.S. National Institute on Aging maintains a website with common health concerns (www.nihseniorhealth.gov) where text can be enlarged and a "talking function" can be activated as needed. The site provides links to other credible websites to assist seniors in making decisions about the value of the information they have accessed. Websites with these characteristics will be more useful to seniors.

Case Study: Helping Clients Assess Quality of Health Information on the Web

You are a nurse in a drop-in clinic. A breastfeeding mother with a three-month-old baby states that she wants to start feeding rice cereal to her baby to help him sleep through the night. Your experience tells you that parents often have questions about starting solids. The mother has found information on the internet that suggests starting solids when the baby can hold his head up and seems hungry after 8 feedings per day. The site stated, "When your baby is ready, baby cereals like rice make a perfect introduction to solid foods. They are fortified with additional iron that your growing baby may need." The mother regularly uses Google to search health information about her own care postpartum and caring for her baby. You asked her how she determines the quality of health information; she tells you that she uses sites that have professional images and refer to doctors or hospitals. The site she used was from a baby food manufacturer.

Discussion Questions

1. What advice would you provide the mother about searching for health information on the internet regarding infant care?

2. How would you teach her to assess the quality of a health website?

3. Which Canadian websites would you recommend for reliable health information about postpartum care and/or being a new parent?

TECHNOLOGY TO SUPPORT HEALTH PROMOTION, DISEASE PREVENTION, AND CHRONIC DISEASE MANAGEMENT

The use of ICTs to support e-health promotion interventions has grown. Evers (2006) attributed this growth to the increased internet use by the public, the low cost of delivery, and public willingness to actively manage their own health. It has been argued that e-health promotion interventions can be effective (Evers, 2006). Despite these claims, a review by Bessell, McDonald, Silagy, Anderson, Hiller, & Sansom (2002) showed that research methods used in studies to evaluate health promotion websites have lacked rigour, and thus firm conclusions can not be drawn. The authors did identify, however, that studies reporting on programs related to smoking cessation, education regarding eating habits, body image, and physical activity, as well as weight loss resulted in positive outcomes. A systematic review of e-health interventions cited in three journals between 1990 and 2003 addressed interventions of interest for CHNs such as support for rural women with chronic illness, diabetes, obesity, caregiver support, smoking cessation, and HIV/AIDS (Griffiths, Lindenmeyer, Powell, Lowe, & Thorogood, 2006). Table 15.8 lists their rationale and drawbacks to delivering health interventions using the internet.

TABLE 15.8
Summary of Findings from Systematic Review of Rationale and Drawbacks for Delivering Health Interventions by Using the Internet

Reasons for internet delivery	• reducing cost and increasing convenience for users • reduction of health services costs • reduction of isolation of users • the need for timely information • reduction of stigma • increased user and supplier control of the intervention
Possible drawbacks of internet interventions	• potential for reinforcing the problems the intervention was designed to help • may overcome isolation of time, mobility, and geography, but may be no substitute for face-to-face contact
Elements of future evaluations	• incorporate the cost; not just the cost to the health service, but also to users and their social networks • be alert to unintended effects of internet delivery of health interventions, and include a comparison with more traditional modes of delivery

It is not possible to describe all types of e-health applications in this chapter. Three main interventions with particular relevance to CHNs' practice with respect to health promotion and prevention relate to changing individual behaviour and providing support. These include tailored messaging systems, online support groups, and e-counselling interventions.

Tailoring E-Health Messages

The integration of features that enhance **interactivity** is thought to enhance learning (Stout, Villegas, & Kim, 2001). Interactivity refers to a process where a user is an active participant in using technology and information exchange occurs (i.e., chat rooms, calorie calculators, links). For example, computer programs that integrate social cognitive theory to promote behaviour change for management of weight and physical activity have shown positive results (Winett, Tate, Anderson, Wojcik, & Winett, 2005). Features in programs that generate personalized responses can increase positive attitudes and learning about health issues (Stout et al.), and have shown to result in positive health outcomes (Kypri & McAnally, 2005; Winett et al.). For example, generation of clear and understandable tailored messages that include the user's name and provide specific information addressing the user's individual health needs is important when designing computer-based health promotion interventions (Eakin, Brady, & Lusk, 2001). Compared with the concept of targeting, which focuses on interventions for groups, **tailoring** has been referred to as a "process of creating individualized intervention materials or strategies" (Kreuter & Skinner, 2000). Tailored messages are typically "pushed" to the user, as opposed to sites where users "pull" or search for information from fact sheets, booklets, videos, and images. Tailored messages are typically presented with self-comparison and recommendations based on authoritative research (Figure 15.3). The potential of technologies that provide assessment and feedback to support disease self-management is strong (Glasgow & Bull, 2001).

Tailored messages are particularly appropriate for online screening, which is an important prevention strategy. Various online screening interventions have been implemented with varying degrees of success, including screening for mental health (Farvolden, McBride, Bagby, & Ravitz, 2003; Houston, Cooper, Vu, Kahn, Toser, & Ford, 2001), chlamydia (Gaydos et al., 2006), fruit and vegetable consumption, fitness levels (Kypri & McAnally, 2005), and alcohol intake (Cunningham, Humphreys, Kypri, & van Mierlo, 2006). Although screening for alcohol is highly recommended in primary care, research shows that it is seldom done (Beich, Thorsen, & Rollnick, 2003). U.S. researchers (Saitz, Helmuth, Aromaa, Guard, Belanger, & Rosenbloom, 2004) found that screening and management of alcohol problems was a successful internet health promotion intervention. Many users were women reporting hazardous amounts of alcohol intake who might not have otherwise looked for help. Houston's et al. (2001) depression screening website was also very popular and reached younger individuals with depression more than previous public screening programs, indicating that it can be a useful addition to other mental health screening approaches. Gaydos et al. (2006) promoted women in Maryland to obtain home chlamydia screening kits through a website. Of the women who used the site, 97.2% requested the kit by email rather than a phone. Infection rates were 10.3%, indicating that the service was valuable, and users reported high satisfaction.

FIGURE 15.3 Portion of Tailored Final Report for a Fictitious Website User Created from Check Your Drinking (CYD)

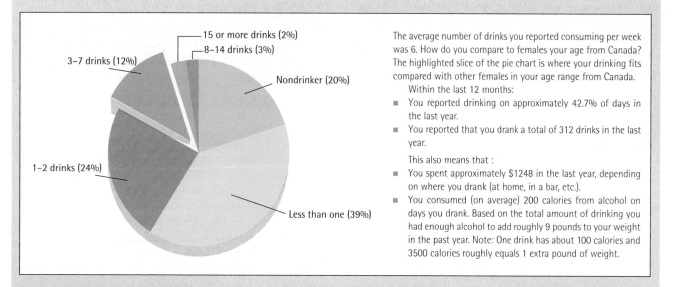

The average number of drinks you reported consuming per week was 6. How do you compare to females your age from Canada? The highlighted slice of the pie chart is where your drinking fits compared with other females in your age range from Canada.
Within the last 12 months:

- You reported drinking on approximately 42.7% of days in the last year.
- You reported that you drank a total of 312 drinks in the last year.

This also means that :

- You spent approximately $1248 in the last year, depending on where you drank (at home, in a bar, etc.).
- You consumed (on average) 200 calories from alcohol on days you drank. Based on the total amount of drinking you had enough alcohol to add roughly 9 pounds to your weight in the past year. Note: One drink has about 100 calories and 3500 calories roughly equals 1 extra pound of weight.

Average drinks per week for females age 35–44 from Canada

Source: AlcoholHelpCentre.net, http://www.alcoholhelpcentre.net/cyd, with permission.

Online Social Support Groups

Research from the United States shows that 9% of people who used the internet for health information have used an online social support group (Rice, 2006). In April 2007, Yahoo! listed 129 812 online support groups under the health and wellness topic. A systematic review (Eysenbach, Powell, Englesakis, Rizo, & Stern, 2004) of online support groups found 35 relevant studies. In addition to peer-to-peer support, most studies provided multiple interventions such as online communication with a professional and psychoeducation programs. Because of this, conclusions about the impact of peer-to-peer social support online as a single intervention can not be drawn. Studies tended to measure outcomes related to social support and depression, and often reported no effects. Despite this, the use of such groups appears to be growing, and no reported cases of harm were found.

The growth of online groups for new parents has been rapid. Parents use the internet to supplement information they receive from health professionals and books. The internet can also provide social support to parents who feel psychologically or geographically isolated and can meet the needs of parents with unique interests (i.e., adoption, bereavement, multiple births). In an Ontario study, pregnant and parenting teens in a large urban centre benefited from anonymous online discussions to obtain support and information as well as share experiences (Valaitis & Sword, 2005). However, time and access were major barriers to use. Key considerations for similar future interventions included involving teens in planning, ensuring a password-protected site, using pseudonyms to enhance anonymity, engaging and training teens to be moderators, and providing opportunities for synchronous (real time) as well as asynchronous (threaded) discussions. A parenting website in the U.K. called "Babyworld" was evaluated for its impact on the everyday lives of new mothers (Madge & O'Connor, 2006). This site was chosen for its high profile and heavy use. Semi-structured virtual group interviews and an online survey were conducted. Users visited the site to gain knowledge, for convenience, and to reach a broad audience. They valued that "the experience and knowledge of both experts and mothers can be shared, serving as a total support network and caring community" (Madge & O'Connor, 2006).

Online Counselling and Therapy

Online counselling and therapy interventions have been used for weight loss with type 2 diabetics (Tate, Jackvony, & Wing, 2003), mental health interventions (Ybarra & Eaton, 2005), and smoking-cessation programs (Etter, 2006). Online counselling interventions can be helpful for people who live in remote areas, value anonymity, or have access problems (transportation, scheduling). Online counselling has been delivered through email as an adjunct to traditional services, or as the main source of help to manage mental health issues (Ybarra & Eaton). Benefits of counselling through email include potentially more disclosure and better integration of therapy into day-to-day life. However, benefits may be offset by loss of nonverbal communication and potential miscommunication that can occur online.

Canadian Research Box 15.2

Cunningham, J. A., Humphreys, K., Kypri, K., & van Mierlo, T. (2006). Formative evaluation and three-month follow-up of an online personalized assessment feedback intervention for problem drinkers. *Journal of Medical Internet Research, 8,* 2–5.

Canadian researchers at the Centre for Addiction and Mental Health (2006) recruited 388 volunteers to complete the Check Your Drinking (CYD) screener (www.alcoholhelpcentre.net/cyd/Default.aspx). The tool uses the Alcohol Use Disorders Identification Test—the AUDIT alcohol screening tool (Saunders, Aasland, Babor, de la Fuente, & Grant, 1993). Registered users of the free web-based Stop Smoking Centre were recruited to participate via email. Users received an individualized tailored response (Figure 15.3) upon completing the tool. Responses were geared to each individual and presented a comparison of the participant's responses against similar population groups. Users were hot-linked to a feedback survey. Follow-ups were also conducted at three months following the initial screening. Participation rates were 40% (n = 138) and completion rates in follow-up were 70% (n = 97). Results showed that more women used the service. Problem drinkers found the tailored responses to be more useful and accurate than did moderate drinkers. There was also a reduction in drinking reported after use of the screener. This study did not use a control group; therefore, it can not be concluded that the screening tool caused a reduction in drinking. However, the study showed that online screening has potential to attract people who are less prone to seeking help from usual health care services.

Discussion Questions:

1. What do you think are the key features of online screening that make it attractive to this population?
2. How do you think this screening intervention would be received by university students? Why?
3. What other screening applications do you think could transfer well to an online environment?

Online smoking-cessation programs have been popular and incorporated the use of features such as self-help course materials, tools for self-monitoring, and regular email reminders (Etter, 2005; Lenert et al., 2003; Lenert, Munoz, Perez, & Bansod, 2004). Other programs included online counselling interventions (Woodruff, Edwards, Conway, & Elliott, 2001). Although there are claims of effectiveness of such programs, many have not been supported by published research (Etter, 2006). Computer programs that include interactive components are thought to be more effective. Examples of interactive components are calculators that estimate the cost of smoking, online social support groups where participants communicate with ex-smokers, features that permit posting of personal stories, and email follow-ups before and after quit dates for added support. Such programs can supplement face-to-face programs.

Ybarra & Eaton (2005) offered suggestions before providing online counselling services. Health professionals need to be comfortable with email or the internet or obtain education in it; they must be aware of security and confidentiality issues, as well as the potential consequences of the lack of nonverbal cues. They also need to set parameters with clients about response time and privacy and to protect the counsellor's privacy (i.e., not forwarding therapist emails to others) (Ybarra & Eaton).

POPULATION HEALTH AND TECHNOLOGY

Many internet technologies can support population health interventions. Computer and internet technologies have long been used to support community empowerment and capacity building (Korp, 2006; Mehra, Merkel, & Bishop, 2004; Milio, 1996; Schon et al., 1999). Youth in a large urban centre in Ontario have used ICTs to support a school-based community development project (Valaitis, 2005). Using technology reduced youths' anxiety in communicating with adults, increased their control, increased community participation, provided youth with better access to resources, and increased perception of their social status. An evaluation of the use of an interactive website to involve local citizens in driving policy related to a smoking bylaw in Calgary was very successful (Grierson, van Dijk, Dozois, & Mascher, 2006). The website sparked public debate about the issue, provided citizens with information about smoking, suggested messages to communicate to city councillors, and updated citizens on how council voted on the issue. Public response was very positive. The website was an effective community capacity-building tool and mobilization strategy that increased citizen participation in building local policy for a healthier community.

Numerous population-based **surveillance** systems exist within the public health system, which provide valuable data for program planning and evaluation. The Integrated Public Health Information System (iPHIS), which is being adopted across Canada, is a client health reporting surveillance system that supports tracking, follow-up, reporting, and management of cases related to immunization, communicable disease, and population health surveillance. Another national system has been implemented for tracking maternal and child health—the Integrated Services for Children Information System (iSCIS). It supports the national Healthy Babies, Healthy Children Program, where public health nurses track contacts and follow up with mothers of all newborns. CANSIM (Canadian Socio-economic Information Management System) tables report social trends impacting the lives of Canadians that can be accessed through E-STAT, which also provides access to Canadian census data and is available at no cost to students and educators through educational institutions (www.statcan.ca/english/Estat/intro.htm). These data are essential for program planners.

ELECTRONIC DOCUMENTATION FOR COMMUNITY HEALTH NURSING

The use of technology to support electronic documentation systems has been growing across Canada, including community health organizations. Three types of electronic documentation systems that have been developed are the *electronic medical record (EMR),* the *electronic patient record (EPR),* and the *electronic health record (EHR).* Nagle (2007) differentiated these terms with respect to access to information, scope of the information included in the documentation, and custodianship of the record. Typically, EMRs are found in primary health care settings and clinics, whereas EPRs are maintained by health care organizations. Access to both of these records is limited to authorized caregivers, and the content typically reflects information that used to be recorded in paper-based systems. The EHR is a more comprehensive record that includes contents from the EPR and EMR. It typically includes most information gathered from encounters with the health care system, such as primary care, pharmacies, laboratories, and diagnostic imaging units. The client controls access to his or her record, which is "owned" by the client but is hosted by a jurisdiction (Nagle, 2007). The EHR, which provides a longitudinal record of an individual's health history and care, is currently being tested in numerous provinces by Canada Health Infoway. Some organizations have incorporated handheld technologies to facilitate electronic recording to support highly mobile CHNs (Valaitis & O'Mara, 2005).

TECHNOLOGIES THAT SUPPORT KNOWLEDGE EXCHANGE AND PROFESSIONAL DEVELOPMENT

ICTs can greatly benefit CHNs through the provision of access to supports for professional development and evidence-based decision making. These technologies include online **communities of practice**, portals and repositories of evidence-based community health literature. A community of practice refers to groups of people who share common interests, values, and problems about a topic and interact together to deepen their knowledge (Wenger, McDermott, & Snyder, 2002). Canadian nursing researchers investigated the networking needs of community health nursing researchers and decision makers (Edwards & Kothari, 2004; Kothari et al., 2005). They identified a need for a formal community health network to assist decision makers, researchers, and practitioners to debate the management of complex community health problems supported by relevant research. Although face-to-face networks were preferred, there was willingness to try online networks. Findings resulted in the launch of an online networking project, CHNET-Works! All nurses are encouraged to join the web-enhanced teleconferences on current community health topics (www.chnet-works.ca).

The Canadian Nurses Association (CAN) recently launched the **NurseONE portal.** "NurseONE serves as a gateway to resources for health-care professionals in all domains of practice—direct care, education, administration and research—to support and enhance their clinical and professional careers" (CNA, 2006). NurseONE provides access to learning resources, news, bulletins, alerts, statistics, and plans to provide discussion boards to support nursing communities. The Public Health Agency of Canada (PHAC) (2006) has developed a portal for knowledge exchange: the Canadian Best Practices Portal for Health Promotion and Chronic Disease Prevention (http://cbpp-pcpe.phac-aspc.gc.ca). It aims to enhance knowledge exchange in best practices and provides a central access point for best practices approaches. PHAC also provides practitioners with online learning modules to enhance skills in public health practice (www.phac-aspc.gc.ca/csc-ccs/sehs-acss/index_e.html). Practitioners in public health can register to take the skills enhancement online modules in topics such as epidemiology, chronic disease, public health surveillance, and measurement of health status. A reliable source of evidence-based materials relevant to CHNs includes the fully searchable online service Health-Evidence.ca (http://health-evidence.ca). The Effective Public Health Practice Program also provides links to numerous valuable systematic literature reviews and summaries (www.hamilton.ca/ephpp).

Summary

ICTs have the potential to provide information, communication, and other supports to empower individuals, groups, and communities. The rapid growth of internet use by the public to access health information can not be ignored. CHNs need to incorporate this into their plan of care and take a leadership role in enabling the public to use this health information resource in a safe and effective manner. CHNs can also help ensure accessibility to quality health information for the populations that they serve. Although research into the use of ICTs to support health promotion, disease prevention, and chronic disease management is relatively new, it shows great promise. ICTs can also foster professional development for CHNs by providing access to communities of practice, online learning modules, and evidence-based materials to support practice.

KEY TERMS

information and communication technologies (ICTs)
e-health
nursing informatics
public health informatics
digital divide
Web Accessibility Initiative (WAI)
Web Content Accessibility Guidelines (WCAG)
accessible
HON code
readability
SMOG (Simple Measure of Gobbledygook) readability test
targeting
interactivity
tailoring
surveillance
communities of practice
NurseONE portal

STUDY QUESTIONS

1. Identify different ways that the "digital divide" has been conceptualized since the term first appeared.

2. Describe three tools that can be used to enhance internet accessibility for disabled populations.

3. What is HON code and what is its purpose?

4. Describe three online health promotion interventions that show promise.

5. Where can community health nurses get access to evidence-based information on the web to guide their decision making in practice?

6. What is the nursing role with respect to health information on the internet?

INDIVIDUAL CRITICAL THINKING EXERCISES

1. What criteria would you use to evaluate a health promotion intervention, such as a smoking-cessation website?

2. What would you need to consider when working as a community health nurse with a client who is visually impaired and wants to use the internet?

GROUP CRITICAL THINKING EXERCISES

1. Discuss the informatics core competencies you think a new graduate working in community health is required to have at a high level of proficiency. Use the Community Health Nurses Standards of Practice (Appendix A) to help you.

2. What trends do you anticipate in the use of the internet to promote health by youth, senior, new immigrant, and disabled populations?

3. Should nurses encourage their clients to join online social support groups? Why or why not?

REFERENCES

Adaptech Research Network. (2006). Adaptech. Dawson College. Retrieved April 24, 2007, from http://adaptech.dawsoncollege.qc.ca/.

Beich, A., Thorsen, T., & Rollnick, S. (2003). Screening in brief intervention trials targeting excessive drinkers in general practice: Systematic review and meta-analysis. *BMJ, 327*, 536–542.

Bensley, R., Brusk, J. J., Rivas, J., & Anderson, J. V. (2006). Impact of menu sequencing on internet-based education module selection. *International Electronic Journal of Health Education, 9*, 73–80.

Berger, M., Wagner, T. H., & Baker, L. C. (2005). Internet use and stigmatized illness. *Social Science & Medicine, 61,* 1821–1827.

Berland, G. K., Elliott, M. N., Morales, L., Algazy, J. I., Kravitz, R. L., Broder, M. S., et al. (2001). Health information on the internet: Accessibility, quality, and readability in English and Spanish. *Journal of American Medical Association, 285,* 2612–2621.

Bessell, T. L., McDonald, S., Silagy, C. A., Anderson, J. N., Hiller, J. E., & Sansom, L. N. (2002). Do internet interventions for consumers cause more harm than good? A systematic review. *Health Expectations, 5*(1), 28–37.

Boulos, M. N. K. (2005). British internet-derived patient information on diabetes mellitus: Is it readable? *Diabetes Technology & Therapeutics, 7,* 528–535.

Caldwell, B., Slatin, J., & Vanderheiden, G. (2006). *Web Content Accessibility Guidelines 2.0.* World Wide Web Consortium W3C. Retrieved April 24, 2007, from http://www.w3.org/TR/WCAG20/.

Canadian Council on Social Development. (2005). *Disability Information Sheet number 19* (Rep. No. 19). Retrieved October 4, 2007, from http://www.ccsd.ca/drip/research/drip19/index.htm.

Canadian Nurses Association. (2006). *NurseONE, The Canadian Nurses Portal.* Retrieved April 24, 2007, from http://www.nurseone-inf-fusion.ca/splash.html.

Canadian Nursing Informatics Association. (2003). *Educating tomorrow's nurses: Where's nursing informatics?* (Rep. No. G3-6B-DP1-0054).

Canadian Public Health Association. (1999). Plain Language Service. Canadian Public Health Association. Retrieved April 24, 2007, from http://www.pls.cpha.ca/.

Changrani, J., & Gany, F. (2005). Online cancer education and immigrants: Effecting culturally appropriate websites. *Journal of Cancer Education, 20,* 183–186.

Chisholm, W., Vanderheiden, G., & Jacobs, I. (1999). *Web Content Accessibility Guidelines.* W3C. Retrieved April 24, 2007, from http://www.w3.org/TR/WAI-WEBCONTENT/.

Community Health Nurses Association of Canada. (2003). *Canadian community health nursing standards of practice.* Retrieved October 4, 2007, from http://www.chnac.ca/.

Crump, B., & McIlroy, A. (2003). The digital divide: Why the "don't-want-tos" won't compute: Lessons from a New Zealand ICT project. *First Monday, 8.*

Cunningham, J. A., Humphreys, K., Kypri, K., & van Mierlo, T. (2006). Formative evaluation and three-month follow-up of an online personalized assessment feedback intervention for problem drinkers. *Journal of Medical Internet Research, 8.*

D'Alessandro, D. M., Kingsley, P., & Johnson-West, J. (2001). The readability of pediatric patient education materials on the World Wide Web. *Archives of Pediatrics & Adolescent Medicine, 155,* 807–812.

Dickerson, S. S. (2006). Women's use of the internet: What nurses need to know. *JOGNN-Journal of Obstetric Gynecologic and Neonatal Nursing, 35,* 151–156.

Dornan, B. A. & Oermann, M. H. (2006). Evaluation of breastfeeding Web sites for patient education. *MCN: American Journal of Maternal Child Nursing, 31,* 18–23.

Eakin, B. L., Brady, J. S., & Lusk, S. L. (2001). Creating a tailored, multimedia, computer-based intervention. *Computers in Nursing, 19,* 152–160.

Earl, L. (2004). Health information and internet use. *Innovation Analysis Bulletin (Statistics Canada), 6*(3). Retrieved October 4, 2007, from http://www.statcan.ca/bsolc/english/bsolc?catno=88-003-X20040037425.

Edwards, N. & Kothari, A. (2004). CHNET-Works! A networking infrastructure for community health nurse researchers and decision-makers. *Canadian Journal of Nursing Research, 36*(4), 203–207.

Escoffery, C., Milner, K. R., Adame, D. D., Butler, S., McCormick, L., & Mendell, E. (2005). Internet use for health information among college students. *Journal of American College Health, 53,* 183–188.

Etter, J. F. (2005). Comparing the efficacy of two internet-based, computer-tailored smoking cessation programs: A randomized trial. *Journal of Medical Internet Research, 7,* e2.

Etter, J. F. (2006). The internet and the industrial revolution in smoking cessation counselling. *Drug & Alcohol Review, 25*(1), 79–84.

Evers, K. E. (2006). eHealth promotion: The use of the internet for health promotion. *American Journal of Health Promotion, 20,* 1–7.

Eysenbach, G. (2001). What is e-health? *Journal of Medical Internet Research, 3,* e20.

Eysenbach, G., & Kohler, C. (2002). How do consumers search for and appraise health information on the world wide web? Qualitative study using focus groups, usability tests, and in-depth interviews. *British American Journal, 324,* 573–577.

Eysenbach, G., Powell, J., Englesakis, M., Rizo, C., & Stern, A. (2004). Health related virtual communities and electronic support groups: Systematic review of the effects of online peer to peer interactions. *BMJ, 328,* 1166.

Farvolden, P., McBride, C., Bagby, R. M., & Ravitz, P. (2003). A Web-based screening instrument for depression and anxiety disorders in primary care. *Journal of Medical Internet Research, 5*(3), e23.

Ferney, S. L., & Marshall, A. L. (2006). Website physical activity interventions: Preferences of potential users. *Health Education Research: Theory and Practice, 21,* 560–566.

Fichten, C. S., Barile, M., & Asuncion, J. (2003). Computer technologies and postsecondary students with disabilities: Implications of recent research for rehabilitation psychologists. *Rehabilitation Psychology, 48,* 207–214.

Fox, S. (2005). *Digital divisions: There are clear differences among those with broadband connections, dial-up connections, and no connections at all to the internet.* Pew Internet & American Life Project. Retrieved April 24, 2007, from http://www.pewinternet.org/PPF/r/165/report_display.asp.

Gagliardi, A., & Jadad, A. R. (2002). Examination of instruments used to rate the quality of health information on the internet: Chronicle of a voyage with an unclear destination. *British Medical Journal, 324,* 569–573.

Gaydos, C. A., Dwyer, K., Barnes, M., Rizzo-Price, P. A., Wood, B. J., Flemming, T., et al. (2006). Internet-based screening for *Chlamydia trachomatis* to reach non-clinic populations with mailed self-administered vaginal swabs. *Sexually Transmitted Diseases, 33,* 451–457.

Glasgow, R. E., & Bull, S. S. (2001). Making a difference with interactive technology: Considerations in using and evaluation computerized aids for diabetes self-management education. *Diabetes Spectrum, 14.*

Goldner, M. (2006). Using the internet and email for health purposes: The impact of health status. *Social Science Quarterly, 87,* 690–710.

Gottlieb, R., & Rogers, J. L. (2004). Readability of health sites on the internet. *International Electronic Journal of Health Education, 7,* 38–42.

Gray, N. J., & Klein, J. D. (2006). Adolescents and the internet: Health and sexuality information. *Current Opinion in Obstetrics and Gynecology, 18,* 519–524.

Greene, D. L., Appel, A. J., Reinert, S. E., & Palumbo, M. A. (2005). Lumbar disc herniation: Evaluation of information on the internet. *Spine, 30,* 826–829.

Grierson, T., van Dijk, M. W., Dozois, E., & Mascher, J. (2006). Policy and politics. Using the internet to build community capacity for healthy public policy. *Health Promotion Practice, 7,* 13–22.

Griffiths, F., Lindenmeyer, A., Powell, J., Lowe, P., & Thorogood, M. (2006). Why are health care interventions delivered over the internet? A systematic review of the published literature. *Journal of Medical Internet Research, 8.*

Health on the Net Foundation. (1997). *HON Code of Conduct (HONcode) for medical and health Web sites.* Health on the Net Foundation. Retrieved April 24, 2007, from http://www.hon.ch/HONcode/Conduct.html.

Health Summit Working Group. (2007). Information Quality Tool. Mitretek Systems. Retrieved April 24, 2007, from http://hitiweb.mitretek.org/iq/

Hesse, B. W., Nelson, D. E., Kreps, G. L., Croyle, R. T., Arora, N. K., Rimer, B. K., et al. (2005). Trust and sources of health information. *Archives of Internal Medicine, 165,* 2618–2624.

Houston, T. K., Cooper, L. A., Vu, H. T., Kahn, J., Toser, J., & Ford, D. E. (2001). Screening the public for depression through the internet. *Psychiatric Services, 52,* 362–367.

Jadad, A. R. & Gagliardi, A. (1998). Rating health information on the internet: Navigating to knowledge or to Babel? *Journal of American Medical Association, 279,* 611–614.

Jones, J. (2003). Patient education and the use of the World Wide Web. *Clinical Nurse Specialist, 17,* 281–283.

Kalichman, S. C., Cherry, C., Cain, D., Benotsch, E., Weinhardt, L. S., Pope, H., et al. (2006). Health information on the internet and people living with HIV/AIDS: Information evaluation and coping styles. *Health Psychology, 25,* 205–210.

Kaphingst, K. A., Zanfini, C. J., & Emmons, K. M. (2006). Accessibility of web sites containing colorectal cancer information to adults with limited literacy (United States). *Cancer Causes & Control, 17,* 147–151.

Kivits, J. (2006). A mediated context for consultations with health professionals. *Journal of Health Psychology, 11,* 382–385.

Korp, P. (2006). Health on the internet: Implications for health promotion. *Health Education Research, 21,* 78–86.

Kothari, A., Edwards, N., Brajtman, S., Campbell, B., Hamel, N., Legault, F., et al. (2005). Fostering interactions: The networking needs of community health nursing researchers and decision-makers. *Evidence and Policy, 1,* 291–304.

Kreuter, M. W., & Skinner, H. (2000). Tailoring: What's in a name? *Health Education Research, 15,* 4.

Kypri, K., & McAnally, H. M. (2005). Randomized controlled trial of a web-based primary care intervention for multiple health risk behaviors. *Preventive Medicine, 41,* 761–766.

Lenert, L., Munoz, R. F., Stoddard, J., Delucchi, K., Bansod, A., Skoczen, S., et al. (2003). Design and pilot evaluation of an internet smoking cessation program. *Journal of the American Medical Informatics Association, 10,* 16–20.

Lenert, L., Munoz, R. F., Perez, J. E., & Bansod, A. (2004). Automated e-mail messaging as a tool for improving quit rates in an internet smoking cessation intervention. *Journal of the American Medical Informatics Association, 11,* 235–240.

Lenhart, A., Horrigan, J., Rainie, L., Boyce, A., Madden, M., & O'Grady, E. (2003). *The ever-shifting internet population: A new look at internet access and the digital divide.* Washington: The Pew Internet and American Life Project.

Lin, C. A., & Hullman, G. A. (2005). Tobacco-prevention messages online: Social marketing via the Web. *Health Communication, 18,* 177–193.

Madge, C., & O'Connor, H. (2006). Parenting gone wired: Empowerment of new mothers on the internet? *Social & Cultural Geography, 7,* 199–220.

Maloney, S., Ilic, D., & Green, S. (2006). Accessibility, nature and quality of health information on the internet: A survey on osteoarthritis. *Rheumatology, 44,* 382–385.

Mathur, S., Shanti, N., Brkaric, M., Sood, V., Kubeck, J., Paulino, C., et al. (2005). Surfing for Scoliosis: The quality of information available on the internet. *Spine, 30,* 2695–2700.

McLaughlin, G. H. (1969). SMOG-grading: A new readability formula. *Journal of Reading, 12,* 639–646.

Mehra, B., Merkel, C., & Bishop, A. P. (2004). The internet for empowerment of minority and marginalized users. *New Media & Society, 66,* 781–802.

Milio, N. (1996). *Engines of empowerment: Using information technology to create healthy communities and challenge public policies.* Chicago: Health Administration Press.

Nagle, L. (2007). Informatics: Emerging concepts and issues. *Nursing Leadership, 20,* 30–32.

National Institute on Aging. (2002). *Making your website senior friendly.* Retrieved April 24, 2007, from http://www.nlm.nih.gov/pubs/checklist.pdf.

O'Carroll, P., & Public Health Informatics Competencies Working Group. (2002). *Informatics competencies for public health professionals.* University of Washington School of Public Health: Northwest Centre for Public Health Practice.

Parlove, A. E., Cowdery, J. E., & Hoerauf, M. S. (2004). Acceptability and appeal of a Web-based smoking prevention program for adolescents. *International Electronic Journal of Health Education, 7,* 1–8.

Pearce, L. C. (2004). Diabetes resources on the World Wide Web. *Home Healthcare Nurse, 22,* 502–506.

Public Health Agency of Canada. (2006). The Canadian Best Practices Portal for Health Promotion and Chronic Disease

Prevention: About the portal. Public Health Agency of Canada. Retrieved April 24, 2007, from http://cbpp-pcpe. phac-aspc.gc.ca/.

Purcell, G. P., Wilson, P., & Delamothe, T. (2002). The quality of health information on the internet. *British Medical Journal, 324,* 557–558.

Rice, R. E. (2006). Influences, usage, and outcomes of internet health information searching: Multivariate results from the Pew surveys. *International Journal of Medical Informatics, 75,* 8–28.

Roush, K. (2006). Two NIH Web sites on aging: One is for providers and the other is for older adults. *American Journal of Nursing, 106,* 17.

Saitz, R., Helmuth, E. D., Aromaa, S. E., Guard, A., Belanger, M., & Rosenbloom, D. L. (2004). Web-based screening and brief intervention for the spectrum of alcohol problems. *Preventive Medicine, 39*(5), 969–75.

Saunders, J. B., Aasland, O. G., Babor, T. F., de la Fuente, J. R., & Grant, M. (1993). Development of the Alcohol Use Disorders Identification Test (AUDIT): WHO Collaborative Project on Early Detection of Persons with Harmful Alcohol Consumption—II. *Addiction, 88,* 791–804.

Schon, D., Sanyal, B., & Mitchell, W. (1999). *High technology and low-income communities.* Cambridge, MA.

Seymour, W., & Lupton, D. (2004). Holding the line online: Exploring wired relationships for people with disabilities. *Disability & Society, 19,* 291–305.

Silence, E., Briggs, P., & Herxheimer, A. (2004). Personal experiences matter: What patients think about hypertension information online. *Health Information on the Internet, 42,* 3–5.

Silver, C. (2001, Winter). Older surfers. *Canadian Social Trends,* 9.

Skinner, H., Biscope, S., & Poland, B. (2003). Quality of internet access: Barrier behind internet use statistics. *Social Science & Medicine, 57,* 875–880.

Staggers, N., & Bagley Thompson, C. (2002). The evolution of definitions for nursing informatics: A critical analysis and revised definition. *Journal of the American Medical Informatics Association, 9,* 255–262.

Statistics Canada. (1997). Reading the Future: A Portrait of Literacy in Canada (Highlights). Retrieved April 24, 2007, from http://www.statcan.ca/bsolc/english/ bsolc?catno=89F0093X&CHROPG=1.

Statistics Canada. (2006). Characteristics of individuals using the internet. Retrieved April 24, 2007, from http:// www40.statcan.ca/l01/cst01/comm15.htm.

Stevenson, K. (2002, Autumn). Health information on the Net. *Canadian Social Trends,* 7.

Stout, P. A., Villegas, J., & Kim, H. (2001). Enhancing learning through the use of interactive tools on health-related websites. *Health Education Research, 16,* 721–733.

Summers, A. L., & Logsdon, M. C. (2005). Websites for postpartum depression. *MCN, 30,* 88–94.

Tapscott, D. (1998). The Digital Divide. In *Growing up digital: The rise of the net generation* (pp. 255–279). New York: McGraw-Hill.

Tate, D. F., Jackvony, E. H., & Wing, R. R. (2003). Effects of internet behavioural counselling on weight loss in adults at risk for type 2 diabetes. *JAMA: Journal of the American Medical Association, 289,* 1833–1836.

Treasury Board of Canada Secretariat. (2004). Common look and feel for the internet. Treasury Board of Canada. Retrieved April 24, 2007, from http://www.tbs-sct.gc.ca/ clf-nsi/index_e.asp?format=print.

Valaitis, R. K. (2005). Computers and the internet: Tools for youth empowerment. *Journal of Medical Internet Research, 7*(5), e51.

Valaitis, R., & O'Mara, L. (2005). Public health nurses' perceptions of mobile computing in a school program. *Computers, Informatics, Nursing: CIN, 23,* 153–160.

Valaitis, R. K. & Sword, W. A. (2005). Online discussions with pregnant and parenting adolescents: Perspectives and possibilities. *Health Promotion Practice, 6*(4), 464–71.

Voelker, R. (2005). Seniors seeking health information need help crossing "Digital Divide." *Journal of American Medical Association, 293,* 1310–1312.

W3C. (2006). *Web accessibility initiative (WAI).* World Wide Web Consortium W3C. Retrieved April 24, 2007, from http://www.w3.org/WAI/.

Wenger, E., McDermott, R., & Snyder, W. (2002). *A guide to managing knowledge: Cultivating communities of practice.* Boston: Harvard Business School Press.

West, D. M., & Miller, E. A. (2006). The digital divide in public e-health: Barriers to accessibility and privacy in state health department websites. *Journal of Health Care for the Poor & Underserved, 17*(3), 652–67.

Winett, R. A., Tate, D. F., Anderson, E. S., Wojcik, J. R., & Winett, S. G. (2005). Long-term weight gain prevention: A theoretically based internet approach. *Preventive Medicine, 41*(2), 629–41.

Woodruff, S. I., Edwards, C. C., Conway, T. L., & Elliott, S. P. (2001). Pilot test of an internet virtual world chat room for rural teen smokers. *Journal of Adolescent Health, 29,* 239–243.

WRAPIN. (2001). Worldwide online Reliable Advice to Patients and Individuals. European Project-IST-2001-33260. Retrieved April 24, 2007, from http://www.wrapin.org.

Yasnoff, W., O'Carroll, P., Koo, D., Linkins, R., & Kilbourne, E. (2000). Public health informatics: Improving and transforming public health in the information age. *Journal of Public Health Management Practice, 6,* 67–75.

Ybarra, M. L., & Eaton, W. W. (2005). Internet-based mental health interventions. *Mental Health Services Research, 7*(2), 75–87.

Zeng, X., & Parmanto, B. (2004). Web content accessibility of consumer health information web sites for people with disabilities: A cross sectional evaluation. *Journal of Medical Internet Research, 6*(2), e19.

About the Authors

Ruta Valaitis, RN, PhD, is an Associate Professor in the School of Nursing at McMaster University and was awarded the Dorothy C. Hall Chair in Primary Health Care Nursing in 2007. She has worked as a visiting nurse and a public health nurse and has had extensive experience as a clinical consultant for the Ontario Public Health Research Education and Development Program. Some of her past research has focused on the use of communication technologies to support health sciences education and public health nursing practice as well as e-health promotion for teen parents and rural youth. Currently, she is exploring the online communities of practice to support nursing and knowledge transfer.

Linda Ferguson, RN, PhD, is a Full Professor in the College of Nursing, University of Saskatchewan. Her undergraduate, master's, and PhD are in the field of nursing, and she has a Post-Graduate Diploma in Continuing Education. She has worked extensively in the field of faculty development within the College of Nursing and the University of Saskatchewan. She has taught educational methods courses at the undergraduate (nursing and physical therapy), post-registration, and master's levels for the past 17 years. Her research has focused on the continuing education needs of registered nurses in practice and precepting nurses, teaching excellence, inter-professional education, and the process of developing clinical judgment in nursing practice. She is currently the Director of the new Centre for the Advancement of the Study of Nursing Education and Inter-professional Education (CASNIE) within the College of Nursing at the University of Saskatchewan.

School Health

Yvette Laforêt-Fliesser, Carol MacDougall, and
Irene Buckland Foster

OBJECTIVES

After studying this chapter, you should be able to:

1. Understand the importance of the school years and identify major health concerns for the child and youth population.

2. Describe Canadian and international school-based health promotion models.

3. Understand the history of community health nurses' roles and contributions in Canadian schools.

4. Describe the roles and functions of community health nurses within the comprehensive school health approach.

5. Identify challenges and opportunities for the future development of community health nursing in school settings.

INTRODUCTION

While the 0 to 6 years age group has garnered much of the attention of policy makers and politicians in recent years, school-age children and youth need support in order to achieve important developmental and educational milestones. They also need good health to make the most of their opportunities for learning and growth. The academic success and optimal health and well-being of school-age children and youth will ultimately determine Canada's place in the world (Health Council of Canada, 2006). Today, more than 5 million Canadian children and adolescents attend school every day (Blouin, Courchesne, & Thony, 2006). Schools play a key role in child and youth development and therefore must figure prominently as partners in any health promotion effort (Kendall, 2003).

For more than a century, schools have been an important setting for community health nurses (CHNs) to provide health promotion services and programs. They are also a workplace for teachers and a place for students to learn and play. They act as a hub of a small town, a neighbourhood, or an ethnocultural community. In some communities, the school-based CHN may be the only health professional pro-

viding service on an ongoing basis. CHNs work within a primary health care model by offering a broad spectrum of services to promote and protect the health of individuals, families, groups, and aggregates within the school community.

Level of education attained and, in particular, literacy are significant determinants of long-term health and quality of life (Ronson & Rootman, 2004). While dropout rates are improving in Canada, more resources for non-involved, at-risk adolescents and teen parents would further decrease the dropout rate and increase return-to-school rates (Ungerleider & Burns, 2004). CHNs can enable students to complete their education by making a positive impact on access to health and social services, food, family support, and social inclusion. Examples can be seen in early identification and referral of students with mental health or other health concerns, programs that help pregnant and parenting teens stay in school, promotion of social inclusion through bullying prevention and programs that reach out to the many cultural groups in a community, parenting education programs, and initiation of school breakfast, lunch, or snack programs or cooking clubs for students or parents.

This chapter begins with an overview of growth and development in school-age children and youth and a discussion of some of the important health and social concerns in this population. Two socio-environmental frameworks for health promotion will be presented: comprehensive school health (CSH) and the health promoting school (HPS), followed by a brief historical perspective on school health. The diverse roles and functions of CHNs within school communities will then be examined within these frameworks.

THE IMPORTANCE OF THE SCHOOL YEARS

Healthy children and youth are an important predictor of a society's overall health. How children and adolescents negotiate the transitions from early to middle childhood, and from adolescence to adulthood, are important indicators of how healthy and well they will be as adults. Middle childhood extends from age 6 to the onset of puberty at 10 to 12 years, when children shift from seeing themselves as the centre of the world to realizing that the world is a complex place in which they must find a place (Davies, 2004). The transition to middle childhood is marked by entry into the formal education system, when children begin to move from home and their family into wider social contexts that strongly influence their development. During these years, the child is driven by basic needs to achieve competence, autonomy, and relationships with others. School-age children seek opportunities to master and demonstrate new skills, make independent decisions, control their own behaviour, and form good relationships with peers and adults outside the family. Nearing the end of this period, children who have successfully mastered these developmental tasks and not yet entered puberty are likely to appear confident, competent, reasonable, and composed. They are capable of reasoning, looking at situations from multiple perspectives, and using many adaptive strategies of self-regulation (Davies).

Just as early life experiences influence a child's readiness for school, success at school is associated with fewer health problems and greater success throughout life. To be happy, healthy, confident, and secure, children and youth need "love, nurturing, nutrition, security, stimulation and health care" (Health Council of Canada, 2006, p. 8). In most cases, the child's family will first meet this requirement; however, it is often the school setting where the child will experience nurturing and caring outside the family. A caring family together with an adequate income are the most important health determinants for children.

Adolescence begins with puberty and ends with the beginning of adulthood. The transition to this life stage involves a balance of school, extracurricular activities, and engagement in the workforce. The developmental tasks associated with adolescence include achieving independence, adjusting to sexual maturation, establishing cooperative relationships with peers, preparing for meaningful work or career, establishing intimate relationships, and developing a core set of values (Registered Nurses' Association of Ontario [RNAO], 2002). Other developmental outcomes related to successful transition to adulthood are "engagement with and participation in the community, empowerment to make healthy and responsible choices, and realistic hope for the future" (Canadian Institute for Health Information [CIHI], 2005, p. 21).

COMMON HEALTH CONCERNS

Almost one in six Canadian children and youth under 18 lives in poverty, with the plight being even worse for First Nations and off-reserve Aboriginal children—one in four, and two in five, respectively (Campaign 2000, 2006). Child poverty rates are also very high for new immigrants, visible minorities, and children with disabilities. Children and youth living in poverty are disadvantaged in almost every way and the health effects last a lifetime. They are more likely to live in unsafe neighbourhoods where exposure to violent and illegal activity occurs. These same conditions also create fewer opportunities for them to be physically and socially active (Ontario Public Health Association [OPHA], 2004). Approximately one in five Canadian children lives in small or rural areas that have limited access to public transportation, specialist services, and recreation opportunities (Health Council of Canada, 2006).

The health status of school-age children, in particular pre-teens and adolescents, is often described in terms of risky activities and problem behaviours. Health concerns commonly addressed in school settings include unintentional injuries, communicable diseases, inactivity and unhealthy eating, mental health, and risky behaviours (CIHI, 2005). The following section briefly outlines each of these health concerns in school-age children.

Unintentional Injuries

According to the Health Council of Canada (2006), unintentional injuries are "the leading cause of death and a major cause of hospitalization among children and youth" (p. 18). The unintentional injury death rate varies for children of different age groups, with the highest rate in male youth. Car crashes are the main cause of injury death among school-age children (Kidder, Stein, & Fraser, 2000). More than one in five adolescents age 12 to 19 years had an injury that limited their activities in 2000–2001 (Wilkins & Park, 2004); sports are a major cause of non-fatal injuries among all youth (Pickett, 2004). For children under the age of 10 in Canada, unintentional injury to the brain/skull resulted in the highest incidence of death or hospitalization (Smartrisk, 1998). Prevention initiatives have made a difference; for example, serious head injuries from bicycle crashes have dropped in regions where bicycle helmet legislation has been implemented (Macpherson et al., 2002).

Communicable Diseases

Immunization is often considered one of the most important public health achievements of the twentieth century. Just 100 years ago, infectious diseases were the leading cause of death around the world. Today, in Canada, they cause fewer than 5% of all deaths (Canadian Coalition for Immunization Awareness & Promotion, 2007). Immunization against vaccine-preventable communicable diseases is one of the most cost-effective public health interventions. Provincial health legislation allows public health units to collect and review immunization information on students relating to several diseases, such as measles, mumps, rubella, tetanus, diphtheria, and polio. Additional immunizations have been added over time in some jurisdictions, including hepatitis B and meningitis, as well as annual influenza immunization. Free universal vaccinations are available in most provinces and territories; however, not all children and youth have up-to-date immunizations due to such barriers as lack of transportation, transiency, and childcare problems (Health Council of Canada, 2006).

Inactivity and Unhealthy Eating

Overweight and obesity in Canadian 12- to 17-year-olds has more than doubled in the last 25 years (Shields, 2006) and is becoming a major health concern. The Health Council of Canada (2006) reports that more than 1 million young Canadians are overweight and another half million are obese.

Two major factors contributing to this health problem are lack of physical activity and poor food choices. Sedentary play and obesogenic environments have contributed to what many call an obesity epidemic. Fewer than half of Canadian children and youth participate in enough physical activity each day and eat sufficient fruits and vegetables.

Children living in lower socioeconomic situations are at increased risk of being overweight or obese than children living in higher socioeconomic groups (Health Council of Canada, 2006). Low-income families have much less choice when it comes to food and to opportunities for physical activity. Many rely on food banks for ongoing support. In 2003, 39% of Canadian food bank clients were children less than 18 years of age. Inadequate nutrition impacts a child's ability to learn, as well as develop physically (Ontario Ministry of Health and Long-Term Care, 2004).

Mental Health

According to the Health Council of Canada (2006), "an estimated 1.1 million—or 14 percent—of Canada's children under age 20 have mental health conditions that affect their lives at home, at school and in the community... In 2002, more than six per cent of youth and young adults experienced a major depressive episode in the previous year, six per cent reported suicidal thoughts, and five per cent had social anxiety disorder" (p. 20). Almost 29% of Canadian children 12 and under have developmental or behaviour problems that often persist into adulthood, thus seriously affecting their ability to lead happy, healthy lives (p. 20). Suicide rates decreased slightly between 2000 and 2003; however, suicide is still the cause for 9 percent of early adolescent deaths and 22 percent of older youth deaths (p. 20). Boys in Grade 6 (21%) and Grade 10 (25%) reported that they felt low at least weekly in the previous six months; 23% and 36% of girls in Grade 6 and 10, respectively, reported feeling low at least weekly in the previous six months (Boyce, 2004).

"In 1998–1999, males aged 15 to 19 years were more likely to complete their suicide attempts; hospitalization rates for suicide attempts were over two times higher among females aged 15 to 19 years" and "hospitalization rates for eating disorders in girls under age 15 increased by 34% from 1987 to 1999" (CIHI, 2005, p. 32). In some Aboriginal communities suicide is a grave concern, with rates for Aboriginal male youth being five times that of male national youth, and rates for female Aboriginal youth almost eight times that of female national youth (Kidder, et al., 2000). With early detection and intervention, most children can experience improvement in mental health conditions. Programs and services are more effective when they are part of a comprehensive approach for nurturing all children (Health Council of Canada, 2006).

Risky Behaviours

While risk-taking is a normal part of the growth and development of adolescents, in some cases it can be a symptom of deeper underlying issues. Risky behaviours can include alcohol and drug use, smoking habits, and unprotected sexual activity. Between 2000 and 2001, 31% of males and females aged 12 to 17 said they had tried marijuana, and 13% had tried other illicit drugs such as cocaine or crack. In 2002, the rate of weekly alcohol use increased from 3 to 23% between Grades 6 and 10 for girls and from 6 to 34% for boys; 16% of Grade 8 students reported having used alcohol to get drunk at least twice. By Grade 10, the proportion had increased to 44% (Boyce, 2004). In 2004, 62% of 15- to 17-year-olds and 91% of 18- to 19-year-olds drank alcohol (Adlaf, Begin, & Sawka, 2005). The Canadian Institute for Health Information (2005) reports that in 2003

smoking among teens declined to 18% from 22% in 2002, and more girls (20%) reported smoking than boys (17%). Between 1989 and 2002, the proportion of Grade 9 to 11 youth reporting having sex decreased; although those having sex said they did so more often. Boys (12%) and girls (13%) reported having had sex by ages 14 or 15, and, in 2003, 22% of 15 to 17 year olds and 33% of 18 to 19 year olds reported having had sex without a condom. Chlamydia cases in 15 to 19 year olds increased from 623 to 802 per 100,000 youth between 1991 and 2002. Between 1997 and 2001, pregnancy rates among 15 to 19 year old girls declined from 43 to 36 per 1,000 girls. (p. 32)

Experimentation in the above risky behaviours is mostly responsible for the morbidity and mortality in adolescence. There is strong evidence that teens who engage in one "risky behaviour" tend to engage in several other risk behaviours (RNAO, 2002). Many of the behaviours that begin during this time can continue into adulthood, with negative long-term health consequences. Thus, all known risk factors must be acknowledged and incorporated into a community's plan for prevention, protection, and health promotion with children and youth. Positive relationships with families, peers in schools, and community members may lessen the potential harm of these high-risk behaviours and encourage more health-enhancing behaviours (CIHI, 2005). Individual capacity and coping skills, such as personal competence and a sense of control over one's life, also play an important role in supporting mental and physical health (RNAO). Interventions that address both risky behaviours and positive child and youth development are more likely to be effective. Creating supportive environments and opportunities for connecting with caring, committed adults, engaging in age-appropriate decision making and problem solving, and meaningful youth participation can provide both prevention and health promotion benefits (Weare & Markham, 2005).

SCHOOL-BASED HEALTH PROMOTION MODELS

The term comprehensive school health (CSH) was coined in the 1980s to describe the socio-ecological approach to school-based health promotion in Canada and the United States. The American model evolved into the **Coordinated School Health Program (CSHP)**, which includes *eight components* to effectively address major health risks identified among the school-age population (Allensworth & Institute of Medicine, 1997; Marx, Wooley, & Northrop, 1998):

- health education;
- physical education;
- health services;
- nutrition services;
- health promotion for staff;
- counselling, psychological, and social services;
- healthy school environment (physical and psychosocial); and
- parent and community involvement.

The concept of the **health promoting school (HPS)** was born in Scotland in 1986 and provided the World Health Organization (WHO) with an opportunity to test the principles and strategies set out in the Ottawa Charter for Health Promotion. The HPS had three main elements: (a) formal curriculum time allocated to health-related issues in subjects such as biology, social education, health studies, and physical education; (b) the hidden curriculum, referring to the social and physical environment including staff/student relationships, relationships between the school and community, and school meals; and (c) health and caring services including screening, prevention, and child guidance (Young, 2005). Since that time, the HPS movement has further broadened and refined these initial ideas through the lens of a "settings approach," endorsed in the Jakarta Declaration on Health Promotion into the 21st Century (WHO, 1997). The settings where people live, work, play, and worship are considered ideal for promoting community development, participation, and partnership with other sectors.

The HPS movement has emphasized national policy formation, community mobilization, and inter-sectoral partnerships that are reflected in the *ten key principles* guiding the development of HPS: democracy, equity, empowerment and action competence, school environment, curriculum, teacher training, measuring success, collaboration, communities, and sustainability (Stewart Burgher, Barnekow Rasmussen, & Rivett, 1999). More recently, the International Union for Health Promotion and Education has produced protocols and guidelines for HPS based on evidence-based quality practices from around the world (St. Leger, 2005).

In Canada, CSH gained momentum following a national conference in 1990 that produced a consensus statement on CSH, subsequently endorsed by more than 20 national organizations (Canadian Association for School Health [CASH], 1991). In 2007, the consensus statement was revised to reflect a unifying vision for educators, health professionals, policy makers, parents, and youth. **Comprehensive school health (CSH)** is now defined as "a multifaceted approach that includes teaching health knowledge and skills in the classroom, creating health-enabling social and physical environments, and developing linkages with parents and the wider community to support optimal health and learning" (CASH, 2007). The four main components are (a) teaching and learning; (b) health and other support services; (c) supportive social environment; and (d) healthy physical environment. This approach emphasizes the creation of dynamic, collabora-tive partnerships among children and youth, parents, teachers, principals, school councils, and members of community agencies concerned about the health and learning of children (McCall, 1999).

Health Canada, CASH, and more recently the Public Health Agency of Canada (PHAC) have played an important role in promoting CSH through research, education, project development, and networking activities. An increasing emphasis on school improvement and school effectiveness has resulted in schools linking student health and academic success. In 2004, provincial and territorial deputy ministers of education and health and the PHAC formed the Joint Consortium on School Health to support federal–provincial/territorial cooperation and inter-ministerial coordination within jurisdictions.

In Canada, the terms HPS and CSH are essentially considered synonymous, and some regions use the term HPS; for clarity, we will use the term CSH in the remainder of this chapter. Table 16.1 outlines the key commonalities between the HPS and CSH models.

HISTORICAL PERSPECTIVES ON SCHOOL HEALTH NURSING IN CANADA

Community health nurses in Canada have a long history of working in school communities. With the emergence of public health nursing at the turn of the twentieth century, schools became one of the initial settings for the provision of health education and preventive programs. (See Chapter 1.) Medical inspection programs were initiated in most schools to counteract absenteeism of children due to communicable disease. Public health officials proposed that poor health inhibited a child's academic performance and could potentially have harmful effects on that child's future economic and social well-being. In several Canadian cities, boards of education initially established school health programs in which the CHNs moved between school and home providing preventive health teaching, screening, and counselling in addition to their primary role in communicable disease control.

For most of the twentieth century, CHNs in school settings primarily focused on individual and family counselling, classroom health teaching, screening, case finding programs, immunization programs, and advising school staff about student health problems. Interventions were based on a biomedical model where the emphasis was on the prevention and control of disease. Schools were one of the settings in a district or neighbourhood that received the services of the generalist CHN. District nursing created opportunities for the nurse to really know the community, where regular communication and collaboration with local family physicians, pharmacists, local businesses, and other health professionals occurred. School children and their families were often known to the nurse through home visiting or clinic work in the district (Falk-Rafael, 1999).

With the birth of health promotion in the mid-1970s, CHNs addressed lifestyle issues through health education, health communication campaigns, and individual or group

TABLE 16.1
Components of a Comprehensive School Health/Health Promoting Schools Approach

Teaching and Learning	K–12 Health and Physical Education **curriculum*** Relevant, high-quality teaching/learning materials Commitment to **teacher preparation**: pre-service and in-service training **Empowerment** approaches that consider individual and social contexts, promote **action competence,** and: • use active and cooperative learning techniques • develop health knowledge, attitudes, and behaviours	• emphasize generic skill development (e.g. information seeking, decision making, problem solving, refusal skills, critical thinking, media awareness, coping, personal goal setting, social skills, building relationships, conflict resolution) • encourage students to participate in local **community** action Cross-curriculum support for health
Services	Health services (e.g., physical, mental, public health) Guidance and career education Social work Psychology Child protection Police services Early identification, assessment, referral, treatment, and follow-up	Parks and recreation/Boys' and Girls' Clubs/YMCAs and YWCAs Access to community-based services "Healthy School" coordinators (provincial level, school board level, and local school level) Government, school board, and school policies/guidelines and funding facilitating access to services
Supportive Social Environment	Welcoming and positive environment Supportive relationships Clear expectations and limits Inclusive environment that celebrates diversity and ensures **equity** **Collaborative**, partnership approach with input from students, parents, administration, teachers, and local community agencies Establishment of **sustainable** structures and processes (e.g., school health committees/teams) to identify and address health issues and **measure success**	**Democracy**/involving students in decision-making/active student participation (e.g., in setting classroom rules, on a school health committee, on a student council, in peer leadership) High degree of staff participation Encouragement of staff and student autonomy Role-modelling by parents, teachers, peers Mentoring programs Universal, non-stigmatizing student nutrition/food programs Media reinforcing healthy behaviours Government, school board, and school policies/guidelines supporting health
Healthy Physical Environment	Clean and hygienic **environment** Acceptable air quality and ventilation Safe water Adequate lighting Low-allergen environment Safe playground equipment and injury prevention measures in the school	Smoke-free policy enforcement Availability of healthy food choices Safe food-handling practices Safe and healthy school policies/guidelines (e.g., prohibiting harassment, discrimination, violence, alcohol and drug use, as well as focusing on their prevention)

Note: *The words in bold refer to the 10 key principles of the Health Promoting School concept as identified at the First International Conference for Health Promoting Schools in Greece, 1997: 1. Democracy, 2. Equity, 3. Empowerment and Action Competence, 4. School Environment, 5. Curriculum, 6. Teacher Training, 7. Measuring Success, 8. Collaboration, 9. Communities, 10. Sustainability.

counselling in addition to the traditional screening and immunization programs. The 1986 Ottawa Charter introduced a new way of thinking about health promotion, including the important idea that health is created and maintained in the settings of people's lives: home and family, schools, workplaces, and community (Whitehead, 2006).

While CHNs across Canada have provided leadership in promoting the benefits of socio-environmental approaches for school-based health promotion, they have encountered a num-ber of challenges. In the last 15 years, significant reductions in the financing of health and social services eroded public health services across the country. Health services restructuring and changing public health mandates at the provincial/territorial level reduced or eliminated CHNs in schools or placed constraints on their practice (Falk-Rafael, Fox, & Bewick, 2005). The fragmentation of these programs into a restructured health service often contributed to the invisibility of PHNs and other staff (Meagher-Stewart & Aston, 2005).

Despite these challenges, CHNs in Canada have played an important role in advocating for school-based health promotion. In 1990, British Columbia was one of the first jurisdictions to adopt elements of a CSH framework for public health nursing in schools (British Columbia Ministry for Children and Families, 2003). During the 1990s, other pilot and demonstration projects appeared in Alberta, Northwest Territories, Ontario, and New Brunswick. A 2000 survey of 64 health units across Canada reported that the CHN was a key player for coordinating CSH programs in schools (Moore, 2000).

CHNs have made progress in articulating their health promotion and illness prevention roles within schools, in challenging the political forces that shape their practice, and in lobbying for the integration of CSH approaches into mandated public health programs and services (Mitchell & Laforêt-Fliesser, 2003; OPHA, 2005). CHN practice in school communities should be grounded in the principles and strategies of CSH/HPS and be consistent with the Community Health Nurses Association of Canada (CHNAC) standards of practice. A discussion of current and developing nursing roles and programs in relation to school-based practice will now be explored.

ROLES OF THE SCHOOL NURSE

Building Structures and Processes for Comprehensive School Health

The CSH process is, in essence, the community health nursing process applied in collaboration with a school community. Integral to this process is the development of effective working relationships with the community client. The core nursing skills of mutual respect, caring, listening, assessing, enabling, and empowering are critical to the CHN's work with school communities and school boards. A CHN's practice in school can be complex and challenging because relationships with school staff, parents, students, superintendents, or community partners occur within a complex, changing, and often ambiguous environment that may present conflicting circumstances for the CHN. Chapter 3 noted that CHNs practising in schools are often PHNs. They have specialized skills in working with groups and in population health promotion.

It is important to determine the school community's level of readiness and its areas of interest or concern. Some school communities may have a health champion who can easily facilitate the school's participation in health promotion activities. Other school communities may be immersed in their academic focus and the CHN has a role in assisting them to see the link between health and learning before any action is possible. Some school communities may be operating within a school board that has a strategic priority for promoting student health, while another board's emphasis may be focused on character-building. The formation of strong partnerships between boards of education and public health agencies at the local level enables sustainable implementation of CSH. Examples of effective partnerships include joint committees for curriculum and policy development, which support the health of students and the school environment (Laforêt-Fliesser & Mitchell, 2002). Joint development of a local comprehensive school health initiative or adoption of a provincial initiative greatly increases the commitment of principals and school staff, as their participation becomes part of expected school improvement efforts and is actively recognized by school board leaders. Central planning of in-services and networking and celebration events for school health committee representatives contributes greatly to building and maintaining momentum within schools and school boards. Today's schools are fast-paced, ever-changing environments, and CHNs need to work closely with school board superintendents, consultants, principals, and teachers to adapt the health agenda and their practice to fit with the reality of daily school life.

CSH is a flexible health promotion approach that empowers individuals and school communities to take action for health. This involves examining their strengths and implementing whole-school approaches to address health and social issues. A CHN can engage a school in reflecting on the following questions: How effective is the health, physical education, and other curriculum delivery? Is the school aware of and able to access support services from the board and local community to support the health of students, staff, and families in the school community? Does the school have a democratic and supportive social environment with shared decision making? Is the physical environment supportive of the health curriculum being taught in the classroom? (MacDougall, 2004a). The Quality School Health Checklist (Canadian Association for Health, Physical Education, Recreation and Dance [CAHPERD], n.d.) has been successfully used by a number of Canadian schools to measure their performance against 12 key elements. Other jurisdictions have developed their own assessment tools that foster discussion about the school's strengths and health issues and what it can do about them, including the Healthy School Profile (Middlesex-London Health Unit, 2004), the visioning approach used by British Columbia schools (British Columbia Ministry for Children and Families, 2003), and the HPS audit (St. Leger, 2005). Potential activities, services, and programs within the four components of the Comprehensive School Health approach are illustrated in Table 16.1.

CHNs play an important role in raising awareness among principals, teachers, students, and parents about "the possibility of addressing school health issues in a partnership structure" through school health committees or action teams (MacDougall, 2004b, p. 48). (See the box "The School Health Committee/Action Team".) It is critical to involve a diverse group of representatives, particularly people who may not be well-connected to the school community, so they can share their concerns about various aspects of school life that need to be improved. The CSH process is not about adults doing something to or for students, but rather about actively involving students and other members of the school community in a process leading to positive change (British Columbia Ministry for Children and Families, 2003). This broad participation and the active involvement of students have been identified as essential for the success of healthy school initiatives (Laforêt-Fliesser & Mitchell, 2002). Ideally, the chairperson should come from the school community itself to encourage local ownership of the health committee from the outset. PHNs could play a key role to facilitate the formation and development of such a committee.

The School Health Committee/Action Team

The School Health Committee/Action Team consists of a group of dedicated representatives or school champions including teachers, students, parents, and community members to lead and coordinate sustainable health promotion actions (St. Leger, 2005). Such a committee facilitates the entire school community living out the values of democracy, equitable access, and respect for all stakeholders within the school community. The committee can be a productive and permanent structure in a school, invites power sharing and mutual respect, intentionally builds caring communities, and tackles important topics on a school improvement agenda.

Canadian Research Box 16.1

MacDougall, C. A. (2004). School health committees: Making "healthy schools" happen. *Canadian Association for Health, Physical Education, Recreation and Dance Journal, 70*(2), 27–29.

This qualitative study sought to identify lessons learned from public health staff who have had experience working with school health committees. Five public health staff (four public health nurses and one health promoter) in three southern Ontario regions who had worked with a combined total of 35 school health committees (18 elementary and 17 secondary) were interviewed. The participants described how to mobilize a school health committee by first securing the support of the principal, and then by using personal contact by the principal to staff, by teachers to students, and through school newsletter notices or recruitment letters to parents. They emphasized the need to be truly representative of the school population, with continual recruitment to keep the committee inclusive and address normal member turnover. The process they followed was assessing strengths and needs of the school community, prioritizing issues, planning action, implementing the plan, evaluating outcomes, and celebrating successes. They suggested the need to respect input from all members, keep all other school committees and staff informed of activities, avoid power struggles, recruit students by offering course credits for committee members, minimize paperwork, and have students take ownership of the health action work.

Discussion Questions:

1. As a community health nurse assigned to work with a high school, describe possible ways you could support the establishment of a school health committee within that school community.

2. Visit three websites that deal with comprehensive school health or health promoting schools and describe how comprehensive school health/health promoting schools approaches contribute to youth empowerment.

Formulating Action Plans

The team structure creates a place to raise health concerns and plan appropriate action. When formulating a plan to address an identified health issue, the action team should identify strategies or activities within each of the four component areas to achieve a degree of comprehensiveness that is more likely to have a meaningful impact on the school community. For example, if student nutrition is the priority concern of the school, then the components of the plan might look like this:

1. *Teaching and learning*—In-service for teachers so they are better prepared to deliver the nutrition curriculum;

2. *Health and other support services*—Consult with a public health nutritionist, dietitian, or nurse to explore the many ways student nutrition could be addressed throughout the school or to suggest community agencies that could assist students who may have significant nutritional issues such as eating disorders or unhealthy weights;

3. *Supportive social environment*—Assist students to run a healthy tuck shop; establish healthy school nutrition policies that address foods offered at school events and for fundraising; encourage parents to reinforce healthy eating in the purchases they make for lunches and home meals;

4. *Healthy physical environment*—Establish universal student nutrition programs, such as breakfast, snack, or lunch programs; involve youth in advocacy for healthier high school cafeteria menus.

This planning process is carried out by the school health committee as a whole, with the CHN providing guidance and resource support as needed. The CHN can be instrumental in linking the school to a wide range of health-sector and community-based resources, including issue-specific public health resources (Mitchell & Laforêt-Fliesser, 2003).

Aggression between young people, which can take the form of physical, verbal, social, and electronic bullying, sexual harassment, and racial discrimination, is another prevalent issue in schools today (Craig, 2004; Ungerleider & Burns, 2004). Table 16.2 provides an example of a comprehensive approach to violence prevention in schools.

Providing Clinical Services

As mentioned earlier, restructuring of health services over the past 15 years has changed the nature of nurses' work in

FIGURE 16.1 A Healthy School's Approach to Violence Prevention

Component	
Teaching and learning (health education)	• Whole School Survey conducted to confirm bullying as an issue
	• "ABC" Anti-Bullying Crew raised money for the purchase of Anti-Bullying Integrated Resource Units for students from JK– Grade 8 from CAYRE (Community Alliance for York Region)
	• Classroom teaching of related curriculum for all grades facilitated by nursing students over a 3-month period
	• Grade-specific learning materials created to enhance curriculum
	• Taught students about the STAR problem-solving and decision-making model: Stop, Think, Act, and Reflect
	• Fridge magnets, personal badges, and bookmarks distributed to all students
	• Media invited to school "kick off" assembly
	• Evaluation of the project completed by nursing students
	• Newsletter inserts created to keep families informed about the initiative
Supportive social environment	• Anti-Bullying Pledge designed by students and signed by the entire school was plaqued and hung in the school entrance
	• Peer mediators took part in a workshop on defining and dealing with playground bullying
	• Increased reporting of harassment/bullying incidents on the playground helped to break the previous "code of silence," which was a barrier to help-seeking and bystander involvement
	• Posters were created by students and hung in the halls
Health and other support services	• Whole school assembly held to present new banner and highlight anti-bullying messages and activities from the CAYRE Program. School Board Director attended and affirmed these activities
	• OPP victim service workers and school social worker supported students as needed following a serious bullying incident at the school
	• Nursing students and their Public Health Nursing Preceptor worked closely with the school community to create and implement an action plan
	• Suggestion box placed in a private but accessible location and used for ongoing feedback from students
Healthy physical environment	• Large banner with "STAR" message made for the school
	• Health Walls posted relevant violence prevention information
	• Positive problem-solving messages posted throughout the school
	• Staff supervision around and behind portables
	• Time-out room set up to talk with students

Canadian schools. Today, clinical services provided by public health nurses may include immunization, sexual health services, vision and hearing screening, and health counselling and referral. CHNs are also employed by visiting nurse agencies or departments in regional health authorities and provide clinical services to support students with special needs. (See the case study on p. 271.)

Working with Individuals

CHNs working in school communities, especially high schools, will attest to the fact that the counselling role of the nurse is an important one. Dryfoos (1991) identified individual attention and counselling as one of the components that contributed to successful adolescent health programs, along with personal skill training in learning life and social skills and dealing with peer pressure and peer influences. CHNs are well prepared to provide this initial assessment, support, and referral as needed as they practise from a solution-based approach that optimizes the problem-solving and coping abilities of young people and families. However, individual counselling is rarely included within mandated public health services. Even in jurisdictions supportive of this CHN role, most CHNs are on-site only a few hours per week, so it is important that additional counselling services be provided by other professionals such as social workers, guidance counsellors, and psychologists. Collaborative partnerships between public health

Case Study

During the 1980s, most provincial and territorial ministries of education passed special legislation to integrate and accommodate exceptional children and youth in publicly funded schools. Prior to this time, many children with complex medical or developmental needs attended special residential or day schools. These schools were often part of the district PHN's caseload for targeted programs such as immunization. With integration of these students into public schools, many jurisdictions developed special services within their home care programs or community and social services to address the unique and often complex medical needs of this population. These nursing services continue today and include providing information and consultation about health issues relating to the special needs, planning of community care, providing treatments in the school setting or at home, and training of alternate caregivers. In a group of 4 to 6 students, discuss the following questions.

Discussion Questions

1. What role might a CHN who provides nursing support services in a school play in school-based health promotion?

2. Can you identify any advocacy issues that the visiting CHN and the PHN might address together?

3. Discuss how your jurisdictions currently support children and youth with special needs in schools.

departments, school boards, and community agencies can share responsibility for funding these types of support services in schools. For example, school boards with a significant rural population may enter into an agreement with the local public health unit for CHNs to offer counselling services to both elementary and secondary school students. Health unit CHNs may work with students on stress or coping-related issues, self-esteem, sexual health, and relationship difficulties with peers and parents (Perth District Health Unit & Avon Maitland District School Board, 2006). PHNs assist the students to recognize their strengths and explore options for handling the situations they are dealing with. They also link students and their families to other health and social services in the community. A survey of 773 parents in Perth County in Ontario indicated that 95.6% think all students should have access to a PHN at school (T. Allan-Koester, personal communication, November 13, 2006).

The school-based health clinic is another model that is gaining acceptance in many jurisdictions. Secondary-school Teen Health Clinics have been adopted as a model of care in various communities. Rural students often have limited access to community services, and urban students often have to take time out from classes to attend off-site medical appointments.

In 1989, the Wellington, Dufferin, and Guelph public health unit in Ontario worked with a number of community partners, including school police officers, physicians, and alcohol and drug service workers, to provide school-based comprehensive health services to high school youth. In a recent evaluation of this program, more than 95% of clients preferred to seek health services at school rather than at an off-site agency (Wellington-Dufferin-Guelph Health Unit, 2001).

In Nova Scotia, the Youth Health Centre (YHC) model offers a comprehensive range of services within a population health and youth-centred approach. In the Halifax region these centres often operate within high schools, where youth receive accessible, confidential, and non-judgmental programs and services, including health education, health assessment and intervention, referral, and support and follow-up by CHNs and other health providers (Halifax Regional School Board and Capital Health, 2005). Additionally, the YHC coordinators support student action teams, provide health curriculum support through classroom presentations, offer one-to-one consultation, and coordinate immunization clinics in the school. The Halifax model integrates individual-focused services, as well as opportunities for group work and peer-led student action teams that address whole-school issues.

Working with Small Groups

Group learning or group discussion is an effective approach to actively engage children and youth. The group setting can create a circle of peer support and learning on a variety of topics including smoking cessation, healthy relationships, sexual health, and parenting, to name a few. CHNs in schools are in an ideal position to offer their facilitation skills for group-oriented work. It may be a formal or informal program, for example an anger management program for boys, or Grade 5/6 girls discussing puberty at lunch hour in a question and answer format. It can involve the training of peer leaders to lead a variety of activities at recess or after school. It could consist of a 7-week Teen Esteem for Girls program where the CHN has prepared volunteer women from the community to lead lunch-hour discussions with Grade 7/8 girls related to growing up, careers, and life choices, and convey messages of valuing oneself and setting goals for the future (Perth District Health Unit, 2006). This work is particularly valuable because it enables a peer group as a whole to experience a shift in social norms, and collectively increase its awareness, knowledge, and critical-thinking skills.

Addressing Common Health Concerns

Health promotion programs in schools often focus on increasing the students' awareness about healthy eating, active living, safety issues, avoiding substance misuse, healthy sexuality, and developing healthy relationships, including violence prevention. For example, according to the RNAO's (2005) *Best Practice Guideline on the Primary Prevention of Childhood Obesity*, nurses must "promote healthy eating using Canada's Food Guide to Healthy Eating and focus on emphasizing fruits and vegetables"

(p. 11). Encouraging children to make healthy food choices necessitates creative interventions. CHNs working with elementary students can engage the whole school in campaigns such as Families are Munching to effect behaviour change. This campaign has been successful in encouraging students and a family member to eat 5 to 10 vegetables and fruits a day for one week. *Turn off the Screens* is example of a whole-school campaign designed to promote physical activity, encouraging school-age children and their families to turn off their televisions, video games, and computers for 5 days and enjoy activities together. The Canadian Best Practices Portal for Health Promotion and Chronic Disease Prevention (http://www.cbpp-pcpe.phac-aspc.gc.ca) is an excellent source of information on best practices in relation to a wide range of issues.

Research has also shown that an overarching focus on promoting young people's developmental assets or strengths, both internal and external, is another approach that is needed. Scales (1999) explains that "the more assets young people possess, the fewer risk behaviours they engage in—less violence, less problem alcohol and other drug use, less early sexual intercourse, less delinquency" (p. 113). Internal assets include items in the categories of having a commitment to learning, positive value system, social skills, and positive self-identity. External assets include items in the categories of support (for example, from family, adults, school, and neighbourhood), empowerment, clear boundaries and expectations, and opportunities for constructive use of time (Scales). School-wide programming that focuses on promoting these assets in all the children and youth, rather than just in the high-risk students, is the most recommended approach. Some specific targeted programs will still be needed, however, to support those with diagnosed concerns such as depression, eating disorders, sexually transmitted infections, and so on.

Researchers have identified general characteristics of programs/policies that may contribute to healthy youth development (CIHI, 2005):

1. Interventions that are comprehensive and address common factors associated with multiple behaviours (e.g., include policy initiatives, education, youth-focused media and marketing, skills training, peer support and community activities; address underlying factors such as influences of early childhood, family, school, community, and peers).

2. Approaches that support healthy youth development (e.g., instead of focusing on problem behaviours, focus on positive youth development through programs that promote a sense of belonging; bonding and connections to caring, committed adults; age-appropriate responsibility for decision making and problem solving; and leadership roles and activities that are youth friendly and encourage youth ownership and participation).

3. Approaches that engage youth (e.g., in meaningful structured activities such as sports, music, and community work).

The Health Council of Canada (2006) similarly identifies 10 key ingredients for effective child and youth health programs:

1. Act early, act often (e.g., build strengths from preconception and through pregnancy, through early child development programs, and promoting life skills through adolescence; act quickly to address problems that arise in children and youth).

2. Involve parents and families (e.g., promote good parenting and supportive positive relationships with parents).

3. Involve youth (e.g., engage young people to identify needs as well as plan and deliver services; promote youth leadership opportunities and peer-based approaches).

4. Harness the energy of the community (e.g., work closely with all relevant sectors and promote collaboration among community partners).

5. Use a variety of approaches (e.g., policy, legislation, regulation, education, and services).

6. Integrate policy and practice (e.g., reduce fragmented programs and promote integrated initiatives at the local, provincial, and federal levels).

7. Make programs accessible and equitable (e.g., remove barriers to accessing programs, such as income, distance, language, or lack of awareness).

8. Adapt programs to meet community needs (e.g., involve community members in tailoring and customizing child and youth programs to meet the needs and priorities of specific communities).

9. Modify programs based on what works (e.g., build mechanisms to share the growing body of knowledge about what works and plan interventions accordingly).

10. Maintain political commitment and sustain good programs (e.g., ensure sustainable funding from multiple ministries to widely support and adopt effective child and youth health initiatives).

Promoting mental health through schools is an excellent example of the application of these basic recommendations. The characteristics of effective mental health promotion programs in schools are that:

1. They provide a backdrop of universal provision to promote the mental health of all and then effectively target those with special needs.

2. They are multi-dimensional and coherent.

3. They create supportive climates that promote warmth, empathy, positive expectations, and clear boundaries.

4. They tackle mental health problems early when they first manifest themselves and then take a long-term, developmental approach that does not expect immediate answers.

5. They identify and target vulnerable and at-risk groups and help people acquire the skills and competencies that underlie mental health.

6. They involve end users and their families in ways that encourage a feeling of ownership and participation, and provide effective training for those who run the programs, including helping them to promote their own mental health (Weare & Markham, 2005, p. 118).

Summary

This chapter describes the importance of the school years and the evolution of the role of CHNs in promoting the healthy growth and development of children and youth in the school setting. It describes the international movement for healthy schools, including comprehensive school health, health promoting schools, and coordinated school health programs. This chapter illustrates the importance of building committee structures and processes within schools involving students, parents, teachers, administrators, CHNs, and other community partners. It also emphasizes the importance of central coordination between school boards and local public health agencies in order to ensure that a focus on health is incorporated in school improvement plans.

Numerous challenges will face community health nursing in the coming years. It will be essential to secure the ongoing commitment of various provincial/territorial ministries to the comprehensive school health approach. Within public health agencies, it will be essential to recognize the value of the community development and capacity-building role of CHNs within school communities.

School-based health promotion offers CHNs the opportunity to work within a broad scope of practice that is consistent with both a socio-environmental and a population health approach. Schools are unique settings in which CHNs can work collaboratively to optimize the health of young people, families, and school personnel. The comprehensive school health framework facilitates interventions on many levels: individual- or group-focused interventions, including one-to-one counselling in an office or school-based clinic; classroom education; small group facilitation; school-wide health promotion; and community-wide action. This framework, along with a comprehensive child health strategy, will ultimately improve both the health and academic success of Canada's children and youth.

KEY TERMS

Coordinated School Health Program (CSHP)
Health Promoting School (HPS)
Comprehensive School Health (CSH)

INDIVIDUAL CRITICAL THINKING EXERCISES

1. What are the main assumptions underlying comprehensive school health work, and in particular work with school health committees?

2. Think of a school you attended in your past, and identify an issue that you believe would have benefitted from a comprehensive school health approach.

3. How might a CHN in a school promote the health of families who have children in the school?

GROUP CRITICAL THINKING EXERCISES

1. Imagine a high school has a sudden increase in the number of teens becoming pregnant. Or imagine an elementary school is experiencing a high incidence of bullying. Describe how you would work with the school community to assist it to address this issue.

2. Review current provincial or territorial legislation to determine what health services are provided in schools.

3. What barriers exist for school-age children and youth with complex medical needs? How would you address these?

4. In developing a health profile for a school community, what assessment questions would you ask for each component of CSH? What methods might you use for various stakeholders: students, parents, teachers, administration, community members?

5. A high school administration wants to find ways to prevent substance use and abuse among its students. Identify five or six points that you would want to address with school staff, students, and parents.

REFERENCES

Adlaf, E. M., Begin, P., & Sawka, E. (Eds). (2005). *Canadian addiction survey: A national survey of Canadians' use of alcohol and other drugs: Prevalence of use and related harms.* Ottawa: Canadian Centre on Substance Abuse.

Allensworth, D. D., & Institute of Medicine (U.S.) Committee on Comprehensive School Health Programs. (1997). *Schools & health: Our nation's investment.* Washington, D.C.: National Academy Press.

Blouin, P., Courchesne, M-J., & Thony, I. (2006). *Summary Public School Indicators for the Provinces and Territories, 1997–1998 to 2003–2004.* Cat. No. 81-595-MIE No. 044. Ottawa: Statistics Canada.

Boyce, W. (Ed.). (2004). *Young people in Canada: Their health and well-being.* Ottawa: Health Canada.

British Columbia Ministry for Children and Families. (2003). *Healthy schools resource guide.* Retrieved April 20, 2007, from http://www.mcf.gov.bc.ca/publications/ecd/healthy_schools_website.pdf.

Campaign 2000. (2006). *Oh Canada! Too many children in poverty for too long: 2006 Report card on child and family poverty in Canada.* Retrieved April 18, 2007, from http://www.campaign2000.ca/rc/rc06/06_C2000NationalReportCard.pdf.

Canadian Association for Health, Physical Education, Recreation and Dance. (n.d.). *Quality school health checklist.* Retrieved April 20, 2007, from http://www.cahperd.ca/eng/health/qsh_checklist.cfm.

Canadian Association for School Health (CASH). (1991). *Comprehensive school health: A consensus statement.* Retrieved April 15, 2007, from http://www.schoolfile.com/cash/consensus.htm.

Canadian Association for School Health (CASH). (2007). *Comprehensive school health: Canadian consensus statement* (revised). Retrieved April 15, 2007, from http://www.safehealthyschools.org/CSH_Consensus_Statement2007.pdf.

Canadian Coalition for Immunization Awareness & Promotion. Immunization—the single most important public health triumph of the 20th century. (March 16, 2007). Retrieved October 4, 2007, from http://www. immunize.cpha.ca/english/index-e.htm.

Canadian Institute for Health Information. (2005). *Improving the health of young Canadians.* Ottawa: Author

Craig, W. (2004). Bullying and fighting. In Boyce, W. (Ed.). *Young people in Canada: Their health and well-being* (pp. 87–96). Ottawa: Health Canada.

Davies, D. (2004). *Child development: A practitioner's guide* (2nd ed.). New York: Guilford Press.

Dryfoos, J. G. (1991). Adolescents at risk: A summation of work in the field-programs and policies. *Journal of Adolescent Health, 12*(8), 630–637.

Falk-Rafael A. (1999). From rhetoric to reality: The changing face of public health nursing in southern Ontario. *Public Health Nursing 16*(1), 50–59.

Falk-Rafael, A., Fox, J., & Bewick, D. (2005). Report of a 1999 survey of public health nurses: Is public health restructuring in Ontario, Canada moving toward primary care? *Primary Health Care Research and Development 6*(2), 172–183.

Halifax Regional School Board and Capital Health. (2005). *The youth health centre model in Halifax regional municipality.* Unpublished manuscript.

Health Council of Canada. (2006). *Their future is now: Healthy choices for Canada's children & youth.* Retrieved April 20, 2007, from http://www.healthcouncilcanada.ca/docs/rpts/2006/HCC_ChildHealth_EN.pdf.

Kendall, P. R. W. (2003). *An ounce of prevention: A public health rationale for the school as a setting for health promotion: A report of the Provincial Health Officer.* Victoria, BC: Ministry of Health Planning.

Kidder, K., Stein, J. & Fraser, J. (2000). *The health of Canada's children: A CICH Profile* (3rd ed.). Ottawa: Canadian Institute of Child Health.

Laforêt-Fliesser, Y., & Mitchell, I. (2002). Healthy school communities: Collaborative approaches that work! *Physical Health and Education, 68*(2), 12–18.

MacDougall, C. A. (2004a). School health committees: Making "healthy schools" happen. *Canadian Association for Health Physical Education Recreation and Dance Journal, 70*(2), 27–29.

MacDougall, C. A. (2004b). *School health committees: Perceptions of public health staff.* Unpublished master's thesis, Ontario Institute for Studies in Education of the University of Toronto.

Macpherson, A. K., To, T. M., Macarthur, C., Chipman, M. L., Wright, J. G., & Parkin, P. C. (2002). Impact of mandatory helmet legislation on bicycle-related head injuries in children: A population-based study. *Pediatrics, 110*(5). Retrieved April 22, 2007, from http://pediatrics. aappublications.org/cgi/reprint/110/5/e60.

Marx, E., Wooley, S., & Northrop, D. (1998). *Health is academic: A guide to coordinated school health programs.* New York: Teachers College Press.

McCall, D. (1999). Comprehensive school health: Help for teachers from the community. *Canadian Association for Health Physical Education Recreation and Dance Journal, 65*(1), 4–9.

Meagher-Stewart, D., & Aston, M. (2005). *Fostering citizen participation and collaborative practice: Tapping the wisdom and voices of public health nurses in Nova Scotia.* Ottawa: Public Health Agency of Canada.

Middlesex-London Health Unit. (2004). *A guide to healthy schools.* Retrieved April 20, 2007, from http://www. healthunit.com/articlesPDF/10885.pdf.

Mitchell, I., & Laforêt-Fliesser, Y. (2003). Promoting healthy school communities. *Canadian Nurse, 99*(8), 21–24.

Moore, H. (2000). *Comprehensive school health: Looking at the role of public health.* Ottawa: Canadian Association for Health, Physical Education, Recreation and Dance.

Ontario Ministry of Health and Long-Term Care. (2004). *Healthy weights, healthy lives.* Chief Medical Officer of Health Report. Toronto: Author.

Ontario Public Health Association. (2004). *Public health responds to the challenge to reduce poverty and enhance resiliency in children and youth.* Toronto: Author.

Ontario Public Health Association. (2005). *Child and youth health: Strengthening interministerial integration.* Toronto: Author.

Perth District Health Unit & Avon Maitland District School Board. (2006). *School-based public health nurse support services: Statistics report for 2005–2006.* Retrieved April 15, 2007 from http://www.pdhu.on.ca/pdf/2007_01c17.pdf.

Perth District Health Unit. (2006). *Menu of school health services: Teen esteem.* Retrieved April 20, 2007, from http://www.pdhu.on.ca/pdf/menuschealth.pdf.

Pickett, W. (2004). Injuries. In Boyce, W. (Ed.). *Young people in Canada: Their health and well-being* (pp. 97–107). Ottawa: Health Canada.

Registered Nurses' Association of Ontario. (2002). *Nursing best practice guideline: Enhancing healthy adolescent development.* Toronto: RNAO. Retrieved April 20, 2007, from http://www.rnao.org/Storage/11/587_BPG_Adolescent.pdf.

Registered Nurses' Association of Ontario. (2005). *Nursing best practice guideline: Primary prevention of childhood obesity.* Toronto: RNAO. Retrieved April 20, 2007, from http://www.rnao.org/Storage/12/620_BPG_childhood_obesity.pdf.

Ronson, B., & Rootman, I. (2004). Literacy: One of the most important determinants of health today. In Raphael, D. (Ed.), *Social determinants of health: Canadian perspectives* (pp. 155–169). Toronto: Canadian Scholars' Press Inc.

Scales, P. C. (1999). Reducing risks and building developmental assets: Essential actions for promoting adolescent health. *Journal of School Health, 69*(3), 113–119.

Shields, M. (2006). Overweight and obesity among children and youth. *Health Reports* (Statistics Canada, Catalogue no. 82-003-XIE), *17*(3), 27–42.

Smartrisk. (1998). *The Economic Burden of Unintentional Injury in Canada.* Toronto: Author.

St. Leger, L. (2005). Protocols and guidelines for health promoting schools. *Promotion and Education, 12*(3–4), 145–147.

Stewart Burgher, M., Barnekow Rasmussen, V., & Rivett, D. (1999). *The European network of health promoting schools: The alliance of education and health.* International Planning Committee. Retrieved April 20, 2007, from http://www. euro.who.int/document/e62361.pdf.

Ungerleider, C., & Burns, T. (2004). The state and quality of Canadian public education. In Raphael, D. (Ed.), *Social determinants of health: Canadian perspectives* (pp. 139–153). Toronto: Canadian Scholars' Press Inc.

Weare, K., & Markham, W. (2005). What do we know about promoting mental health through schools? *Promotion & Education, 12*(3/4), 118–122.

Wellington-Dufferin-Guelph Health Unit. (2001). *Student health services study: Final report.* Unpublished manuscript.

Whitehead, D. (2006). The health-promoting school: What role for nursing? *Journal of Clinical Nursing, 15,* 264–271.

Wilkins, K., & Park, E. (2004). Injuries. *Health Reports* (Statistics Canada, Catalogue no. 82-003-XIE), *15*(3), 43–48.

World Health Organization. (1997). *Jakarta declaration on leading health promotion into the 21st Century.* Retrieved April 20, 2007, from http://www.who.int/hpr/NPH/docs/jakarta_declaration_en.pdf.

Young, I. (2005). Health Promotion in schools—A historical perspective. *Promotion & Education, 12*(3/4), 112–117.

ADDITIONAL RESOURCES

Websites

A National Assessment of Effects of School Experiences on Health Outcomes and Behaviours of Children
   www.phac-aspc.gc.ca/dca-dea/publications/pdf/schobc-esrcscj_e.pdf

Canadian Association for School Health
   www.cash-aces.ca

Canadian Joint Consortium on School Health
   www.jcsh-cces.ca

Communities and Schools Promoting Health
   www.safehealthyschools.org

European Network of Health Promoting Schools
   www.euro.who.int/eprise/main/WHO/Progs/ENHPS/Home

International School Health Network
   www.internationalschoolhealth.org

Public Health Agency of Canada/Health Canada: "Voices and Choices" Planning for School Health Assessment Tool
   www.phac-aspc.gc.ca/vc-ss/

School Health Research Network
   www.schoolhealthresearch.org

World Health Organization
   www.who.int/school_youth_health/resources/en/index.html

About the Authors

Yvette Laforêt-Fliesser, RN, BScN, MScN (University of Western Ontario), has worked in family and community health for more than 30 years. She is currently Manager of the Young Adult Program, Middlesex-London Health Unit, in London, Ontario. Her research and teaching interests include health promotion with families, communities, and schools. Yvette is a member of the Ontario Healthy Schools Coalition and is member of the Board of the Community Health Nurses Association of Canada. She is member of the Examination Committee and a Certification Mentor for CNA. Certification in Community Health Nursing.

Carol MacDougall, RN, BScN (McGill University), MA (Ontario Institute for Studies in Education, Department of Curriculum, Teaching and Learning, University of Toronto), has worked for 12 years as a Public Health Nurse in Toronto schools and 5 years as the School Health Consultant in Planning and Policy with Toronto Public Health, and is currently the Public Health Manager, School and Sexual Health, at the Perth District Health Unit in Stratford, Ontario. She has been involved in provincial advocacy for Comprehensive School Health since 1990, and is Co-Chair of the Ontario Healthy Schools Coalition.

Irene Buckland Foster, RN, BScN, MScN (University of Western Ontario), has worked as a PHN and clinical instructor in both college and university nursing programs. She is currently manager of the Child Health Team, which is responsible for providing health promotion and prevention programs in elementary schools and in implementing early identification initiatives in the preschool population. Irene participated in the School Health Benchmarking Project sponsored through the Ontario Teaching Health Units and is a member of the Ontario Healthy Schools Coalition.

Long-Term Care

Lori Schindel Martin

OBJECTIVES

After studying this chapter, you should be able to:

1. Recognize the need for long-term care services within the context of chronic illness.

2. Discuss the philosophy and goals of long-term care service delivery.

3. Distinguish the definitions and services related to chronic illness within the long-term care sector.

4. Discuss the issues and impact of societal viewpoints, government health policies, and political advocacy on the provision of long-term care services.

5. Discuss the roles of community health nurses in caring for long-term care clients.

INTRODUCTION

Community health nurses (CHNs) contribute to the overall health of Canadians through a variety of strategies, including the development and implementation of education, support, and wellness programs. Despite participation in various health promotion activities, many individuals will experience chronic illness that will compromise self-care potential. In addition to health promotion and disease prevention activities, CHNs must acquire competent knowledge and skills to care for persons with chronic illness so that they can experience life and living, and dying, with comfort, integrity, and connectedness.

During the course of a **chronic illness**, individuals may become compromised for self-care to the extent that they require access to services available within the *long-term care* sector. In this chapter, **long-term care (LTC)** is defined as those specialty services necessary for individuals who require extensive support to manage a health condition that represents a serious threat to integrity and self-care capacity. LTC includes a range of services that address the health care, personal care, and social needs of individuals who are living with a *disability* that results in some incapacity for self-care.

LTC services complement the care that is able to be provided by the family and may be delivered to the client in their own home or in an institutional setting. The LTC sector encompasses a vast range of services making entry to care a complex undertaking. CHNs can assist the client to navigate the health care system and identify both community-based and facility-based services that will enhance quality of life. The relationship between CHNs and people living with

chronic disease is longstanding as a result of the very fluctuant nature of ongoing health conditions. Thus, CHNs will play a significant role in assisting clients with accessing the appropriate services from among those available in their community that will enhance their quality of life and capacity for independence. Therefore, this chapter focuses on the services available for people with long-term health issues. Specifically, it describes the distinct levels of care available within the LTC sector, its related issues and challenges, and the roles of CHNs in caring for clients in LTC settings.

NEED FOR LONG-TERM CARE

It is estimated that more than half of Canadians, regardless of age or developmental stage, are experiencing one or more chronic health conditions. It is anticipated that this number will increase dramatically as the Canadian population ages and available medical technology and treatments make significant advances that sustain long-term survival (Canadian Nurses Association [CNA], 2005; World Health Organization [WHO], 2005). The need for the LTC sector has grown dramatically over the last two decades, representing a growing burden for the Canadian health care system. Premature loss of life, financial costs, family stress, and reduced quality of life are all consequences of chronic illness. While the three most prevalent chronic diseases in Canada that would require long-term care are cancer, cardiovascular disease, and diabetes, there are other chronic disease conditions that require intensive and ongoing input from an interdisciplinary health team; such conditions include, but are not limited to, arthritis, asthma, chronic mental illness, Parkinson's disease, multiple sclerosis, renal disease, and cognitive impairment due to Alzheimer's disease and related dementias. The critical issue is that persons living with chronic illness will experience disabilities that result in significant *dependence* on others in order to complete basic self-care activities. Consequently, many of these individuals will require the services of the long-term care sector.

It is difficult to get a precise account of the extensive requirements for LTC in Canada from a statistical sense, given that prevalence and financial data are often analyzed in the context of specific disease conditions. Suffice it to say that the LTC sector represents a significant cost to Canadian society, both in terms of treatments costs and lost productivity. The management of cardiovascular disease alone is estimated to cost $28 billion per year (CNA, 2005), which is only one small portion of the entire LTC sector. This is significant given that chronic conditions such as cardiovascular disease pose a threat to independence. For example, individuals affected by stroke are highly likely to become dependent as a result of disabling outcomes such as paralysis, muscle tone loss, speech difficulties, confusion, and memory loss. In addition, people living with diabetes and bronchitis/emphysema and heart disease have a high probability of becoming dependent (Martel, Belanger, & Berthelot, 2002).

It is not clear as to the number of Canadians who receive services as clients of the LTC sector. In 1996, an estimated 532 000 older adults with a long-term disability were living at home and requiring help with such activities as housework, grocery shopping, meal preparation, and personal care. Disabilities affecting these individuals included immobility (61%), chronic pain (48%), cognitive impairment (46%), and communication problems (29%). It is significant to note that dependent older adults who remain in their homes receive most of the help they need from nonprofessional sources such as family, friends, and neighbours (Lafreniere, Carriere, Marten, & Belanger, 2003). However, for some individuals with disabilities, it becomes impossible for them to continue to be managed at home. In addition, Canadians who require long-term care include younger adults with developmental disabilities and chronic illnesses whose conditions necessitate ongoing monitoring and assistance to maintain self-care activities.

In 2003/2004, there were approximately 4185 residential care facilities in Canada serving 219 472 residents. These individuals include both young adults and seniors who are living with a range of chronic illnesses that must involve professional services on a daily basis. This figure does not include those individuals who are cared for by hospital-based chronic care facilities or apartment-type dwellings where professional teams provide support for residents. Activity in residential care facilities generated $11.6 billion in revenues and expenditures (Statistics Canada, 2006). It is estimated that in Ontario for the time period 2004/2005 those with chronic illness living in hospital-based LTC were 23 787 residents (Canadian Institute for Health Information, 2006). Clearly, adults living with chronic illness receiving care in the home or in institutional settings represent a significant segment of the Canadian population who require health care and financial and social supports.

PHILOSOPHY OF LONG-TERM CARE

One of the primary philosophical tenets of LTC is one that embraces respect for the individual experiencing a chronic illness. It is imperative that CHNs seek to understand each unique individual's life story and the experience of chronic illness within this context. While an appreciation of ethical principles such as *autonomy* is necessary for compassionate practice, no single concept is more important than the recognition and honouring of the *personhood* of the individual since denial of this is crippling and contributes to suffering. In the LTC sector, health concerns are longstanding. If the primary focus of life becomes preoccupation with the illness, the richness and meaning of life may be lost (Buzzell & Gibbon,

1991; Grant, Reimer, & Bannatyne, 1996). By uncovering the individual's life history, hopes, fears, frustrations, pleasures, strengths, beliefs, and personal goals, CHNs will be able to develop a relationship of trust that is grounded in the context of unconditional positive regard for the person. They can assist the individual in living life as fully as possible within the constraints of the chronic health condition.

A complementary philosophical tenet is the concept of *maximization of remaining strengths*. Often, both young adults and seniors who require LTC services have experienced many losses. It is imperative that the CHN identify and maximize the remaining strengths of the individual, rather than focusing on the inherent disabilities associated with the chronic illness. CHNs can assist their LTC clients to adapt to living within the parameters of maximum wellness in their living environment that are possible within the limitations of their illness and the available resources (Paterson, 2001a; Sullivan, Weinert, & Cudney, 2003).

An additional complementary philosophical tenet is the concept of *partnership*. The clients of an LTC service should be involved in their care as active partners rather than as passive recipients of care. CHNs act as facilitators of services to empower the clients and their family members to navigate the system, and to engage them in decision making and self-management strategies wherever possible (Gallant, 2003; Paterson, 2001b).

GOALS OF LONG-TERM CARE

Considering the complex issues inherent in long-term care, and the extended duration of most chronic illnesses, it is critical that CHNs understand that the goals of the LTC sector may not always include discharge from services given that the requirements for care may continue for the lifespan of the individual. The type of LTC service will alter as the needs of the individual become more extensive or change as the chronic disease progresses. In addition, nursing care for LTC clients may involve:

- Management of the impact of the chronic illness on the psychological/spiritual context of the individual (e.g., pain and symptom management, anxiety, depression, stress, spiritual health, coping).
- Exploration of the impact of the chronic illness on the self-esteem of the individual (e.g., self-image, body image, sick role, family role, employability, disability).
- Positive transition of the client into the care delivery experience (e.g., adaptation to the relational and environmental context of the LTC setting or agency).
- Management of the underlying chronic illness experienced by the individual (e.g., cancer, cardiovascular disease, diabetes, chronic obstructive lung disease, arthritis, chronic renal disease).
- Management of the end-stages of the underlying chronic illness (e.g., end-of-life care, palliative care).

It is important to provide LTC services that will be responsive to clients' needs. The main *goal of LTC services* is to provide a wide range of accessible community services to people in their own homes and community settings as well as those available in the institutional setting. Specifically, this involves (Ontario Ministry of Health and Long-term Care, 1994):

- Providing support and relief to caregivers who provide care for a person at home;
- Promoting the health and well-being of persons requiring such services, and respecting their ethnic, spiritual, linguistic, familial, and cultural orientations;
- Integrating health and social community services in order to facilitate support and deliver seamless and equitable care; and
- Encouraging local community involvement, including the involvement of volunteers, in planning, coordinating, integrating, and delivering community services and in governing the agencies that deliver community services.

TYPES OF LONG-TERM CARE SERVICES

At the turn of the twentieth century, chronic illness was measured in terms of weeks or months, not as it is currently, in terms of years. LTC services can be provided in the client's own home or community. If the requirements for care extend to too many hours and involve the input of multiple members of the interdisciplinary team, the services may need to be provided in a residential care setting such as a supportive housing complex, a retirement home, a nursing home facility, or a chronic care facility/hospital.

LTC services are not publicly insured under the Canada Health Act. In addition, the federal government endorses provincial autonomy in the implementation and regulation of long-term care services. Consequently, there is great variety and range of services and associated funding across the country, and these services are subject to governance by provincial and territorial legislation (Crichton, 1997; Health Canada, 2005). In most Canadian communities, access to any level of long-term care is facilitated through a single point of entry and features some type of case management system. This might be offered through a Regional Health Authority or a Community Care Access Centre. In the case of Ontario, the Long-Term Care Act of 1994 (Ontario Ministry of Health and Long-Term Care, 1994) ensures that health care services are equitably available to people in their own homes as an alternative to facility-based care within a framework of multi-service agencies that apply consistent and uniform assessment criteria. The following section describes the two main components of LTC services: home and community support services and residential care. It is important to note here that each territory and province in Canada uses terminology that is unique to their own region; however, the main focus of each component is the same.

Home and Community Support Services

A number of home and community support services are available to adults experiencing chronic illness that will assist the client to manage their own care while living at home. Most regions of Canada have the following main categories of home and community support services available:

Professional Services   **Professional services** include nursing services, occupational therapy services, physiotherapy services, social work services, speech–language pathology services, and dietetics services. Visits are made to the home of the client by registered health care professionals to assess health care needs, plan care requirements, and tender out provision of care to a contracted service provider. For example, a visiting registered nurse care provider may be contracted to provide consultation and care related to management of wounds, preventing falls, promoting continence, delivery of personal care, pain management, or palliative and hospice care. Supplies and equipment related to these service requirements may also be made available, although depending on the regional funding arrangements costs of these supplies may be absorbed by the client or reimbursed to the client through private insurance.

Personal Care and Support   Personal care and support services are available in many regions of Canada through a contracted service provider. *Personal care attendants* are trained to assist the client with a variety of daily living activities such as bathing, grooming, dressing, toileting, and eating. These attendants are typically non-regulated and deliver services under the supervision of a registered nurse. In some regions of Canada, these attendants also assume the duties described under the homemaking section below.

Homemaking   *Homemaking services* assist the client with routine household activities and may include light housekeeping, menu planning, child care, laundry, banking, paying bills, grocery shopping, meal preparation, and the making of and accompaniment to health care appointments such as visits to the doctor or dentist.

Community Support Services   The *community support services* available in many communities are wide and varied. These services facilitate easy access for both young and older disabled adults and can assist these clients to remain in the home, living with greater independence for as long as possible. The community support services available in the typical community would be delivery of prepared meals, subsidized adapted transportation, adult day programs, day attendance respite services, social and recreational services, and security and emergency response services. Many communities have expanded these services to include specialty services such as wheelchair and seating assessment clinics, fall prevention clinics, wound management clinics, swallowing assessment clinics, palliative care and chronic pain consultation teams, diabetic management clinics, foot care services, continence assessment clinics, and many more. In addition, a variety of community support groups are facilitated that are designed to offer education and information around particular chronic disease experiences. In some communities, these support services are utilized by clients living in residential care facilities in addition to those living in their own homes.

Private Home Care Services   Private pay services are becoming increasingly available to assist individuals with chronic illness who are living in their own homes. These include the hiring of paid companions and paid home shopping services that are not regulated by local communities or government bodies.

Long-Term Facility-Based Care

Long-term care facilities provide accommodation and on-site 24 hours a day/7 days a week supervised care. The services include a wide range of professional health services, personal care, and services such as meals, laundry, and housekeeping. The care is governed by provincial and territorial legislation (Health Canada, 2005).

Long-term facility-based care service providers enable people to move to an environment that provides accommodations with the corresponding level of professional and health care support needed to maximize quality of life. The type and funding of services will vary between communities across the country but can be summarized in the following main categories of residential care. Any of these residential care service providers may offer services on a temporary or "respite" basis for those families who need a break from ongoing caregiving activities in the home. CHNs can help support families through the decision-making process as they consider the options available for care for their loved ones.

Supportive Housing and Group Homes   *Supportive housing accommodations* are for adults who require minimal to moderate levels of personal care and support to live independently. Many communities have subsidies available that allow rent to be geared to income. Supportive housing and group homes are also available for persons living with developmental disabilities, mental health issues, and other non-elderly adults who require minimum to moderate levels of care for independent living.

Retirement Homes   *Retirement homes*, sometimes called "*care homes*" or "*assisted living residences*," are rental accommodations for individuals who require minimal to moderate levels of personal care and support to live independently. Retirement homes are either privately or publicly owned facilities that are often not subsidized by governmental funding; rather, it is typical that the resident and/or his or her family pay a considerable fee in order to live in the home. In some regions of Canada rent increases are controlled through tenancy protection legislation. In most cases, services include meals, social and recreational programs, emergency response, supervision of medications, and some assistance with bathing and grooming. Monitoring of health care needs and nursing services is not necessarily provided unless there is a tenant agreement that specifies this.

Nursing Homes   *Nursing homes* are designed for people who need the availability of 24-hour care, at a high level that requires assessment and intervention by skilled nursing staff. It is often the case that a person must meet a minimum threshold of care needs to be eligible for admission. Nursing homes are sometimes referred to as "intermediate care" or "extended care" homes. These homes are typically inspected and regulated by government. They may be charitable or operated by regional government (not-for-profit) or privately owned and operated (for-profit). The persons residing in such facilities typically live with several chronic illnesses. In addition, some nursing homes specialize in such issues as hospice/end-of-life care, dialysis treatments, dementia care, or convalescence/rehabilitation. The residents living in such facilities typically pay for a percentage of the costs associated with accommodation and care delivery, but in many regions of Canada, the care may be subsidized, at least in part, by government. The majority of persons living in nursing homes will remain there through their final journey with chronic illness until the end of their lives.

Hospice   While many community-based agencies and nursing homes offer quality palliative care to those experiencing chronic illnesses, the *hospice* setting is a facility that specializes in delivery of end-of-life care. Hospice organizations offer emotional, psychological, and spiritual support to individuals and families who are experiencing a life-threatening illness. Services include pain and symptom management in additional to other concerns related to death, dying, and grief.

Chronic Care Facilities   Some regions of Canada offer complex, continuing care in a setting that is often funded by government. Individuals who live in such a setting are living with concomitant chronic illnesses that require intensive skilled care from an advanced-practice, interdisciplinary team. They may require ventilation, artificial feeding, dialysis, and other intensive ongoing support to maximize quality of life.

ROLE OF THE COMMUNITY HEALTH NURSE

CHNs provide continuity in assessment and follow-up when an individual is living through the experience of a chronic illness. The CHN is an essential link between the patient and family and other members of the interdisciplinary health care team(s). The CHN identifies service gaps and needs arising that may have medical, social, or spiritual implications. This section discusses some of the key activities that CHNs are engaged in.

Integrating Specialized Knowledge

The evidence-based conceptual knowledge of the CHN working or providing consultation in LTC is extensive. Some of the critical knowledge that is essential for exemplary care of the older adult living with chronic illness includes the following: advanced care planning; ethics and legalities; competency and cognitive impairment; risk (e.g., falls, fire, elder abuse, restraint use, neglect, poverty); delirium; depression and other chronic mental health disorders; behavioural disorders; addiction and substance abuse; pain and symptom management; adherence/compliance;

end-of-life care; culture, ethnicity, and diversity; nutrition; poly-pharmacy; infection control; wound management; family systems; local, provincial/territorial government LTC standards; leadership; advocacy; and completing related assessments.

CHNs in the LTC sector must develop skill in the implementation and interpretation of assessments related to functional status and daily activity performance, cognitive screening, risk assessment, and pain assessment, to name a few. These skills enable the nurse to identify the potential exacerbation of symptoms related to the disease of concern, and plan for comprehensive, interdisciplinary care necessary to manage a changing disease state. For example, the CHN's identification of a swallowing difficulty may indicate the need to work in an interdisciplinary partnership with a *speech-language pathologist* and a *nutritionist* in order to plan for the nutritional and self-feeding requirements of an individual who has experienced a stroke.

Providing Patient/Family Education and Support

A primary role of the CHN is to use effective listening skills to provide emotional and educational support to the client and family. CHNs can reinforce interventions prescribed by other members of the health care team through ongoing education and follow-up. They serve as a sounding board as clients and their families experience stress and coping in response to the impact of chronic illness. CHNs also play a critical role in advanced care planning for the individual who will experience progressive and debilitating changes associated with chronic illness. (See Canadian Research Box 17.1.) Their involvement minimizes the strain of repeated exacerbations of illness, hospital admissions and discharges, inevitable fluctuations in health status, and the emotional trauma often associated with admission to a long-term care facility (Ryan, 2002). (See Photo 17.1.)

Canadian Research Box 17.1

Jonas-Simpson, C., Mitchell, G., Fisher, A., Jones, G., & Linscot, J. (2006). The experience of being listened to: A qualitative study of older adults in long-term-care settings. *Journal of Gerontological Nursing, 32*(1), 46–53.

The data in this qualitative study were collected through researcher–participant interviews that were semi-structured, with open-ended questions. The final sample included 19 residents recruited from two LTC facilities that provided complex continuing care to a large urban area of Canada. The participants were between the ages of 70 and 90 and were experiencing a range of physical and cognitive disabilities requiring complex health interventions. Thematic content analysis resulted in three themes that revealed the participants' experiences of being listened to: *nurturing contentment, vital genuine connections,* and *deference triumphs mediocrity.* The results support that when residents in long-term care are listened to with the intent to understand, they engage in an experience that is nurturing and unburdening and its genuine connectedness can strengthen the nurse–resident relationship and enhance quality of life.

Discussion Questions:

1. What implications do the results of this study have for the way a CHN puts the role of interdisciplinary team member into practice?

2. Discuss strategies and barriers through which the CHN engages in active listening. How could these strategies be taught to non-regulated staff of a community health team that the CHN supervises?

Photo 17.1

Caring for a frail elderly client in the home.

Credit: Jim West/Alamy

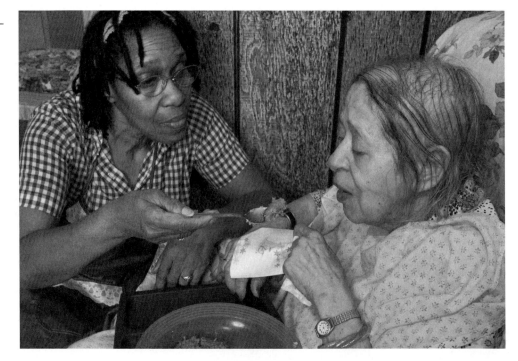

Providing Educational and Clinical Support to Other LTC Providers

The needs of the client within the long-term care sector are often relentlessly overwhelming to care providers. Consequently, the CHN is in a unique position to assist with the professional development of other care providers in the sector. The CHN may also act in the role of a clinical supervisor to non-regulated staff in a community practice. In such a supervisory role, the CHN will provide direction, guidance, and feedback to the front-line caregiver.

Making Referrals and Establishing Community Provider Partnerships

The role of the CHN includes assessment and referral to community partners within and outside the health care system. CHNs must have extensive knowledge with respect to the resources available in the immediate community and beyond. They work with a cadre of **interdisciplinary team partners**, which may include homemakers, recreational therapists, chaplains or pastoral care workers, social workers, occupational therapists, physiotherapists, speech-language pathologists, pharmacists, and other complementary therapists providing massage, reflexology, Reiki, therapeutic touch, and music therapy. In many instances CHNs will be required to act as advocates for those clients who may be at risk for abuse or exploitation. Therefore, CHNs will also need to establish excellent working relationships with law enforcement providers such as seniors' community police and protection services.

Actively Participating in Research

The role of the CHN includes being aware of resources to assist with continuing to develop an evidence-based practice and building knowledge in the area of LTC. Consequently, the CHN will often be in a position to disseminate and engage in research in the practice setting. For example, a CHN with a specialty in continence management may conduct a systematic review to develop the best practice guidelines to care for older adults living in the nursing home.

ISSUES, TRENDS, AND CHALLENGES IN LONG-TERM CARE

The multifaceted nature of care delivered in the long-term care sector requires commitment, energy, compassion, and creativity. The LTC sector, whether community- or facility-based, is not funded to the degree that every service requirement is readily available in sufficient quantity to effectively manage chronic illness and disability (Wilson & Truman, 2005). Consequently, there is a great deal of uncertainty with respect to ongoing funding levels that will be made available to publicly funded community services (Aronson, 2002; Cloutier-Fisher & Joseph, 2000). In addition, many myths are associated with the level of expertise required in the LTC

sector, possibly because the complexity of care and the capacity for autonomous practice is not well understood by practising nurses. Because the acute care sector is represented as "exciting" in the media, nursing shortages in LTC are of concern. The many care levels available in the LTC sector lead clients and their families to be confused about appropriate resources, therefore it is necessary to develop a seamless and integrated service system between and across the sectors that represents a true continuum of care.

Some of the ongoing issues that represent significant challenges and opportunities for improvement within the LTC sector include:

- staffing shortages,
- ineffective use of professional skills,
- high client-to-staff ratios,
- insufficient funding,
- limited research-based literature that supports best practice initiatives and the development and implementation of clinical practice guidelines,
- inadequate servicing of rural communities, and
- silo of services with limited access to client information.

Several encouraging trends have arisen that suggest at least some of these issues will be addressed. Many of the provincial governing bodies that legislate health care are becoming increasingly invested in the development, implementation, and evaluation of care models that involve algorithms, templates, care maps, or health assessment tools. For example, British Columbia has based its Expanded Chronic Care Model on a prototype developed by the MacColl Institute for Healthcare Innovation in Washington State (Government of British Columbia, 2005).

Several provinces in Canada are investigating the efficacy of systems such as the Resident Assessment Instrument 2.0/ Minimum Data Set 2.0 to assist with planning, delivery, evaluation, and funding in the long-term care sector (Atherley, 2006; Hirdes, 2006). In addition, scholars, clinicians, and researchers are forming collaborative investigator teams to build knowledge in the areas of improved health outcomes, application of clinical practice guidelines, and cost-effective expenditures that directly applies to the long-term care sector (Harrison, Browne, Roberts, Graham, & Gafni, 1999). In order to support an evidence-based approach to long-term care many communities are in the process of building virtual library resources that allow clinicians in the field to access research literature, thereby enhancing quality practice (Brazil, Royle, Montemuro, Blythe, & Church, 2004; Wilkins, McKey, & Schindel Martin, 2003).

However, of continued deep concern is the lack of public and political will to ensure that disenfranchised adults living with chronic illness, who are frail, disabled, and/or cognitively impaired, are deemed entitled to support and care. As the demographic of the population changes to reflect an aging society that includes individuals with multiple concomitant chronic illnesses, it may become necessary to revisit the ethical and moral obligation that society has to care for its more vulnerable members. It is critical to address the issue of recommitment to care given that it is estimated chronic illnesses such as heart disease, diabetes, depression, obesity, and cancer account for 46% of the global burden of disease (WHO, 2006). Indeed, piecing together a comprehensive long-term care program for an individual living with an ongoing illness in Canada is a prime concern for CHNs and requires political advocacy to ensure that dollars are made available to support those who are chronically ill and require ongoing access to quality health care.

Case Study

Helen is a 37-year-old woman who lives with her 49-year-old brother, Henry. Helen has a developmental disability that prevented her from attending school. She also has a limited functional capacity and uses a walker. Helen has a cat that she loves dearly. The day program Helen attends three days a week has contacted the family doctor with concerns about Helen's nutritional and hygiene status. The community nursing agency receives a referral to assess the situation. Henry's daughter lives across the country and is concerned that her father's health status is failing and that Helen's care is being compromised. As the CHN making an assessment visit, you notice there are piles of magazines and newspapers scattered through the home. Helen's appearance is dishevelled, and she appears very thin. The siblings both have an avid interest in trains and locomotives; Henry has strung a model train throughout the whole downstairs of the home and is preoccupied with stringing new track across the floor. His dogs bark at the trains as they chug along the track.

There is little food in the refrigerator, and Henry's and Helen's medications have been poured, all together, into a bowl in the centre of the kitchen table. Henry, who is a visually impaired diabetic, has already experienced several small strokes, and is afflicted with a chronic ulcer on his right great toe that he treats himself by spraying on "Bactine," which he thinks is a cure-all. He is having problems managing his insulin, and has taken to instructing Helen to draw it up so that he can self-inject. He also seems to be having trouble navigating the stairs to the upper level where his bedroom is. He tells you loudly, "I don't trust doctors. You will have to take me out of this place in a pine box because I'm not going to an old age home like you probably think I should! I'm too young and who would look after Helen and the dogs!?"

Discussion Questions

1. Outline your assessment of Helen and Henry's health care requirements.

2. What long-term care resources would be available in your community to assist Helen and Henry to maintain independence at home, or to assist them to transition into a LTC facility?

3. What specific features of personhood would be able to be utilized by the CHN in order to establish a relationship of trust?

Summary

This chapter presented the various services available within the long-term care sector that are useful resources for CHNs caring for adults living with chronic illness. The main challenge to CHNs working in LTC settings is to further develop services and interventions despite economic constraints and political/societal deterrents. While the federal government is sponsoring activity to move these services forward, and provincial governments and health care legislators are recognizing an urgent need for quality improvements, there are many competing health priorities that limit success. CHNs are challenged to harness public and political interest to encourage forward momentum for a growing population demographic experiencing chronic illness. They must take an active role in advocacy, working in collaborative fashion with the recipients of care, broader communities, and other practice disciplines, using evidence-based data sources to steer health care policy and service delivery in the area of long-term care toward a positive, equitable, and integrated whole. Persons with chronic health diseases will continue to be a primary concern for considerable time to come; consequently, it will be essential that committed, articulate, passionate, research-informed CHNs with political savvy help their clients plot a course through the future.

KEY TERMS

chronic illness
long-term care (LTC)
professional services
interdisciplinary team partners

INDIVIDUAL CRITICAL THINKING EXERCISES

1. Discuss what types of preventive programs could be designed and implemented by CHNs to reduce the risk of chronic illnesses such as heart disease and diabetes.

2. Identify several key health policies that could be developed in order to promote general public health in this area.

GROUP CRITICAL THINKING EXERCISES

The regional/municipal government of your community has decided to reduce funding by 50% for many home support programs that are offered to adults with chronic illness, for example homemaking services, subsidized housing, and transportation.

1. Discuss your concerns with respect to the impact that such reduced funding will have on the members of your community who rely on these services.

2 How will you bring this to the attention of municipal councillors and policy makers?

REFERENCES

Aronson, J. (2002). Elderly people's account of home care rationing: Missing voices in the long-term care policy debates. *Aging & Society, 22,* 399–418.

Atherley, G. (2006). The long-term care homes common assessment project: Is it justifiable? *Long-term Care, 16*(2), 10–11.

Brazil, K., Royle, J., Montemuro, M., Blythe, J., & Church, A. (2004). Moving to evidence-based practice in long-term care: The role of a best practice resource centre in two long-term care settings. *Journal of Gerontological Nursing, 30*(3), 14–19.

Buzzell, M., & Gibbon, M. (1991). Personhood: What's the point of long-term care if the person doesn't feel cared for? *The Canadian Nurse, 87*(6), 32–33.

Canadian Institute for Health Information. (2006). *Facility-based continuing care in Canada, 2004–2005.* Retrieved August 25, 2006, from http://secure.cihi.ca/cihiweb/dispPage.jsp?cw_page=AR_103_E.

Canadian Nurses Association. (2005). *Chronic disease and nursing: A summary of the issues.* Retrieved August 10, 2006, from http://www.cna-aiic.ca.

Crichton, A. (1997). Long-term care in Canada. *Health Care Manag, 3*(1), 115–124.

Cloutier-Fisher, D., & Joseph, A. E. (2000). Long-term care restructuring in rural Ontario: Retrieving community service user and provider narratives. *Soc Sci Med, 50*(7), 1037–1045.

Gallant, M. (2003). The influence of social support on chronic illness self-management: A review and directions for research. *Health Education and Behaviour, 30*(2), 170–195.

Government of British Columbia, Ministry of Health. (2005). *Chronic Disease Management.* Retrieved November 16, 2006, from http://www.healthservices.gov.bc.ca/cdm/cdminbc/chronic_care_model.html.

Grant, N. K., Reimer, M., & Bannatyne, J. (1996). Indicators of quality in long-term care facilities. *Int J Nurs Stud, 33*(5), 469–478.

Harrison, M., Browne, G., Roberts, J., Graham, I., & Gafni, A. (1999). Understanding continuity of care and how to bridge the intersectoral gaps: A planning and evaluation framework. *National Academies of Practice Forum, 1*(4), 315–326.

Health Canada. (2005). *Health care system: long-term facilities-based care.* Retrieved April 26, 2006, from http://www.hc-sc.gc.ca/hcs-sss/home-domicile/longdur/index_e.html.

Hirdes, J. (2006). Addressing the health needs of frail elderly people: Ontario's experience with an integrated health information system. *Age and Aging, 35,* 329–331.

Lafreniere, S., Carriere, Y., Martel, L., & Belanger, A. (2003). Dependent seniors at home—Formal and informal help. Statistics Canada, *Health Report, 14*(4), 31–40.

Martel, L., Belanger, A., & Berthelot, J.M. (2002). Loss and recovery of independence among seniors. Statistics Canada, *Health Reports, 13*(4), 35–48.

Ontario Ministry of Health and Long-term Care. (1994). *Long Term Care Act,* S.O. 1994, Chapter 26. Retrieved April 26, 2007, from http://www.e-laws.gov.on.ca/DBLaws/Statutes/English/94l26_e.htm.

Paterson, B. (2001a). The shifting perspectives model of chronic illness. *Journal of Nursing Scholarship, 33*(21), 21.

Paterson, B. (2001b). Myth of empowerment in chronic illness. *Journal of Advanced Nursing, 34*(5), 574–581.

Ryan, A. (2002). Transitions in care: Family caregivers' experiences of nursing home placement. *NT Research, 7*(5), 324–334.

Statistics Canada. (2006). *Residential care facilities, 2003/2004.* Catalogue no. 83-237-XIE. Retrieved August 25, 2006 from http://www.statcan.ca/english/freepub/83-237-XIE/83-237-XIE2006001.htm.

Sullivan, T., Weinert, C., & Cudney S. (2003). Management of chronic illness: Voices of rural women. *Journal of Advanced Nursing, 44*(6), 566–574.

World Health Organization. (2005). *Facing the facts: The impact of chronic disease in Canada.* Retrieved August 17, 2006 from http://www.who.int/chp/chronic_disease_report/media/CANADA.pdf.

World Health Organization. (2006). *Global strategy on diet, physical activity and health. Facts related to chronic diseases.* Retrieved October 11, 2006 from http://www.who.int/dietphysicalactivity/publications/facts/chronic/en.

Wilkins, S., McKey, C., & Schindel Martin, L. (2003). Supporting clinical and program decision-making: A long-term care resource center. *Long-term Care, 13*(4), 13–19.

Wilson, D., & Truman, C. (2005). Comparing the health services utilization of long-term-care residents, home-care recipients, and the well elderly. *CJNR, 37*(4), 138–154.

ADDITIONAL RESOURCES

Websites

Improving Chronic Illness Care
www.improvingchroniccare.org

Info Long-Term Care
http://infoLtc.blogspot.com

Ministry of Health, Government of British Columbia
www.healthservices.gov.bc.ca

Ministry of Health and Long-Term Care, Ontario
www.health.gov.on.ca

Statistics Canada: Disability Among Persons Aged 65 and Over
www.statcan.ca/english/freepub/89-577-XIE/seniors.htm

World Health Organization: Preventing Chronic Diseases
www.who.int/chp/chronic_disease_report/en/

Readings

Canadian Institute for Health Information. (2006). *Facility-based continuing care in Canada, 2004–2005: An emerging portrait of the continuum.* Ottawa: Author.

Fallon, M., & Hanks, G. (Eds.). (2006). *ABC of palliative care* (2nd ed.). Oxford, UK: Blackwell Pub.

About the Author

Lori Schindel Martin, RN, BA (Guelph), BScN (McMaster), MScCHN (D'Youville, NY), PhD (McMaster), is an Associate Professor at Ryerson University, School of Nursing, Faculty of Community Health Services, Toronto. Her research focuses on the educational and professional development of clinicians caring for older adults living with cognitive impairment. She is interested in enhancing staff resilience and creativity in the management of responsive behaviours associated with dementia such as aggression, sexual expression, and resistance to bathing. She is co-author of the Gentle Persuasive Approaches in Dementia™ curriculum, which focuses on training interdisciplinary team members to respond respectfully and with tenderness to catastrophic behaviour in the long-term care sector.

Dr. Schindel Martin wishes to acknowledge the assistance of Shannon Buckley, Library Technician with the Long-term Care Resource Centre at St. Peter's Hospital in Hamilton, Ontario, in acquiring articles used for the preparation of this chapter.

Clients in the Community Mental Health System

Elaine Mordoch

OBJECTIVES

After studying this chapter, you should be able to:

1. Understand the historical context and challenges surrounding mental health and illness in Canadian society.

2. Analyze the effectiveness and adequacy of community mental health services.

3. Discuss the effects, impact, and risk factors for mental illness and how they affect the vulnerable populations.

4. Examine the causes of suicide, the at-risk groups, and related assessment, intervention, and prevention strategies.

5. Explain mental health legislation in relation to the provision of services for people with mental illness.

6. Discuss the organization of services in the mental health system and selected models of care.

7. Discuss the role of the community mental health nurse.

8. Discuss the future directions in community mental health and their implications for nursing.

INTRODUCTION

Mental illness (MI) affects the potential life trajectory of individuals, significantly disrupts family processes, and impacts communities and society with lost productivity and costly treatment. Stigma and discrimination continue to influence the identification and treatment of people with MI and their families. Resources and services are often not timely or adequate to facilitate recovery from MI. With the realization that community services must incorporate rehabilitation, treatment, prevention, and mental health promotion strategies, community mental health nurses (CMHNs) have the potential to establish best practices with this population. Mental health can impact the ability of all people, with or without MI, to enjoy life and deal with its challenges. This chapter discusses challenges facing persons with MI, available services, and strategies to promote mental health within Canadian society.

HISTORICAL CONTEXT AND CHALLENGES

Historically, mental health care in Canada has taken place within a context of culture, gender, and social-political attitudes. Beliefs surrounding the etiology of MI have decreed the treatment of people with MI. Formal management of people with MI began in poor houses and jails that provided little but containment. In the mid-nineteenth century large institutional hospitals or asylums were built with the intent of providing more humane care to persons with MI. Hospitals were first built in Quebec, New Brunswick, Nova Scotia, Manitoba, British Columbia, and Prince Edward Island, followed by Saskatchewan and Alberta (Sussman, 1998). Although physically isolated from their homes and families, people with MI were believed to be in safe healing environments where they followed structured therapeutic routines (Sussman).

In 1846 the term "psychiatry" was first used and the *Journal of Mental Science* was published. Efforts to define psychiatry and to find a cure for the illnesses prevailed. When the expectations that patients would return to the community proved unrealistic, the asylums became increasingly overcrowded and difficult to staff, deteriorating to little more than warehouses for people with MI (Nolan, 1993). The resultant inhumane care evoked public outcry and demanded more humane treatment for residents and education for caregivers.

Beginning in the 1960s, a philosophical shift proposed that more humane treatment would be best achieved in the community. This, in combination with the discovery of the psychotropic medications chlorpromazine and lithium, and cost containment measures related to maintenance of large institutions, contributed to **deinstitutionalization**, wherein long-stay hospitals were depopulated and people with schizophrenia and other major mental illnesses were placed in the community hospitals and other community facilities (Eaton, 2001).

The process of deinstitutionalization resulted in a decrease in bed capacity in provincial mental hospitals from 47 633 beds in 1960 to 15 011 beds in 1976, and a rise in general hospital psychiatric beds from 844 to 5836 (Goering, Wasylenki, & Durbin, 2000). Unfortunately, the level of resources that former residents needed to live in the community was underestimated. Many of the people discharged from the institutions now were marginalized and vulnerable in the community, with families not having the resources to assist them (Canadian Mental Health Association, 2001; Davis, 2006).

Several additional trends continue to influence psychiatric/mental health services: the consumer and family movements, and the current rehabilitative recovery model. Through lobbying efforts, the consumer and family movements have advanced more holistic services such as respite for families, rehabilitative resources for patients, and efforts toward health promotion (Davis, 2006). The **recovery model of rehabilitation** identifies life beyond symptom management. It is based upon a collaborative, consumer-driven process that challenges previous conceptions of the goals of intervention (Anthony, 1993, 2000). Consumers of mental health services may expect active collaboration with their health care providers rather than passive participation in dictated treatment. There is a growing body of consumer survivor literature and consumer-driven journals such as the *Schizophrenia Bulletin* (Davis; Hinshaw, 2004). These trends, while not wholly accepted by the status quo, have influenced changes within the Mental Health Act, service delivery, the direction of research, policy development, and the relationship between service providers and people with mental illness and their families (Anthony; Davis).

Despite societal efforts to address mental health and illness in the community, stigma and discrimination continue to be a reality facing people with MI (Health Canada, 2002; Kirby & Keon, 2006). Throughout history, society has viewed persons with MI as being different. Cultural beliefs, superstitions, and poor understanding of MI contribute to fear, stereotyping, and avoidance of persons with MI. This stigmatism causes many persons to conceal their illness and delay or refuse treatment and follow-up care (Kirby & Keon).

While most people with MI live and receive mental health services and supports within their own communities, poor integration of services, isolation of psychiatric hospitals, general hospitals, community mental health programs, and private practitioners fragment service delivery (Latimer, 2005). A significant population in rural and remote areas does not have access to appropriate or timely mental health services. Universally, a **basket of community services** with comprehensive services that address socioeconomic factors such as housing, income, and supportive resources to facilitate people living in the community is needed to assist people and families of persons with MI in their daily lives (Kirby & Keon, 2006). Increased recognition of the social determinants of health, the need for consumer involvement at the policy level, the value of self-help groups and peer consultations, and the importance of policy based on a recovery model will assist people with MI to live more satisfying, hopeful, and productive lives. Current recommendations suggest that a national Mental Health Transition Fund be developed to aid the provinces in the transition to more comprehensive community services to offset the downsizing of the institutional sector (Kirby & Keon).

There is ongoing debate regarding the language used to describe people with mental illness. As language is embedded with underlying assumptions and biases inferring diverse connotations, careful consideration of the language used is warranted. Currently in psychiatry, "consumer" and "survivor" are frequently used. **Consumer** describes people with mental illness who are actively choosing care from a more critical stance of the available treatment. **Survivor** describes people who actively resist and challenge care and labels that they do not find helpful or relevant in their recovery process. Survivors actively challenge status quo treatments and advocate for alternative treatments and social changes (Speed, 2006). Nurses need to be cognizant of the terminology that they use in their practice and respectful of the language that people with mental illness prefer.

CANADIAN MENTAL HEALTH ORGANIZATIONS

The provision of community mental health services in Canada is the responsibility of provincial ministries of health. In most provinces, mental health services are governed by regional health authorities with no national strategy in place (Davis, 2006). In addition, many community organizations exist that have been involved in the consumer, recovery, and family movements.

Community mental health programs such the Canadian Mental Health Association operate under the provincial mental health division. The **Canadian Mental Health Association (CMHA)** is an umbrella organization founded in 1918 to fight MI, prevent MI, and promote mental health of residents living in their own communities. (See the CMHA website, listed in Additional Resources.) Today, the CMHA is a tri-level enterprise with a national office, provincial divisions, and local community-based branches within each province. Local branches provide resources, mental health programs, and other human services to individuals, families, and groups within their communities. This is accomplished through self-help, generic community resources and services, and the support of family, friends, and neighbours. These services are tied to factors that determine health and wellness, such as housing, income, education, leisure opportunities, employment, peer and social supports, and self-esteem (Bezzina, 1996).

Other community groups such as the Anxiety Disorders Association of Canada, the Mood Disorders Society of Canada, and the Schizophrenia Society of Canada (see websites listed in Additional Resources) have emerged to address concerns within the mental health system. These organizations advocate for rehabilitative services, research, validation for family experiences and knowledge, and public education to reduce the stigma shrouding MI. Other organizations, such as the Native Mental Health Association, Psychosocial Rehabilitation Canada, and Canadian National Committee for Police/Mental Health Liaison, augment formal services for consumers and families and highlight concerns and solutions to issues affecting people and families living with MI.

MENTAL ILLNESS AND ITS EFFECTS

Mental illness (MI) refers to a group of diagnosable diseases or disabilities of the mind described as some combination of altered thinking, mood, behaviour, or will that can be linked with distress or impaired functioning (Mental Health Act, 1990, amended 2002).

Mental health is the capacity to think, feel, and act in ways that enhance the enjoyment of life and ability to face life's challenges. "It is a positive sense of emotional and spiritual well being that respects the importance of culture, equity, social justice interconnections and personal dignity" (Government of Canada, 2006, p. 2). Having an MI does not preclude the importance of nurturing mental health.

Each year, 3% of the Canadian population experience serious MI with another 18% experiencing mild to moderate MI (Kirby & Keon, 2006). One in five Canadian adults will require mental health services or support at some point in their lifetime (Statistics Canada, 2002). In Canada, the *Diagnostic and Statistical Manual,* 4th edition with text revisions (*DSM-IV TR*) is the standard used to diagnose MI. The *DSM-IV* has been criticized for gender bias, cultural insensitivity, and reliance on non-empirical evidence. Efforts to address these biases are ongoing (Davis, 2006; Eaton, 2001). (See Table 18.1.)

MAJOR MENTAL ILLNESSES

Mood disorders encompass depression, bipolar disorders, dysthymia and cyclothymias, with depression the most prevalent with rates of 4.2% for men and 6.3% for women in Canada in the past 12 months (Government of Canada, 2006). Physical illnesses, such as heart disease, thyroid conditions, and diabetes, often potentate depression. The utmost concern for people with depression is risk of suicide. Ongoing assessment of suicide risk is necessary and must be followed by appropriate intervention. Family members are affected by the depressive episodes and require peer support, education, and resource information.

Bipolar illness has a population prevalence of 2.4% and is increasingly recognized in children and adolescents (Government of Canada, 2006). Children may suffer from co-morbidity, most commonly attention deficit disorder and conduct disorder (Kowatch & DelBello, 2005). Adults who suffer with bipolar disorder often place themselves and their families at risk. Grandiosity, poor judgment, impulsivity, and expansive mood may lead to social and financial indiscretions, increasing the visibility of the MI and shame related to stigma associated with MI.

Anxiety disorders are the most common of all psychiatric disorders and consist of generalized anxiety disorder, specific phobia, post-traumatic stress disorder, social phobias, obsessive compulsive disorder, panic disorder, and agoraphobia. Lifetime prevalence rates are estimated at 10%, with anxiety disorders being the most commonly treated MI in children with a rate comparable to asthma (Castellanos & Hunter, 2000). Substance abuse and depression may develop secondary to anxiety.

Schizophrenia, affecting 1% of the population, is a serious MI characterized by delusions, hallucinations, social withdrawal, and lack of insight. The associated costs are high in terms of treatment, management, lost potential, and suffering of people with schizophrenia and their families. Hospitalization is required in acute illness, with schizophrenia being the most common diagnosis of involuntary patients (Government of Canada, 2006). To ensure their family members' well-being, families absorb much of the burden of care in the community. Disproportionate numbers of people with schizophrenia are found in homeless and prison populations. People with schizophrenia require adequate health services to promote their physical health and to monitor medications

---

TABLE 18.1

Twelve-Month Prevalence of Mental Disorders and Substance Dependence Measured in the 2002 Mental Health and Well-Being Survey (CCHS 1.2), Canada

Mental Disorder or Substance Dependence	Total**		Men		Women	
	Number	%	Number	%	Number	%
Any measured mood disorder, anxiety disorder, or substance dependence*	**2 660 000**	**11.0**	**1 220 000**	**10.2**	**1 440 000**	**11.7**
Any mood	1 310 000	5.3	510 000	4.2	800 000	6.3
• Major depressioin	1 200 000	4.8	450 000	3.7	740 000	5.9
• Bipolar disorder	240 000	1.0	120 000	1.0	120 000	1.0
Any anxiety	1 160 000	4.8	430 000	3.6	730 000	5.9
• Panic disorder	380 000	1.5	130 000	1.0	250 000	2.0
• Agoraphobia	180 000	0.7	40 000	0.4	140 000	1.1
• Social anxiety disorder (Social phobia)	750 000	3.0	310 000	2.6	430 000	3.4
Any substance dependence	760 000	3.1	550 000	4.5	210 000	1.7
• Alcohol dependence	640 000	2.6	470 000	3.9	170 000	1.3
• Illicit drug dependence	190 000	0.8	130 000	1.1	60 000	0.5
Eating Attitude Problems	**430 000**	**1.7**	**60 000**	**0.5**	**360 000**	**2.9**
Moderate Risk for/or Problem Gambling	**490 000**	**2.0**	**320 000**	**2.6**	**170 000**	**0.5**
• Problem Gambling	120 000	0.5	70 000	0.6	50 000	0.4
• Moderate Risk for Problem Gambling	370 000	1.5	250 000	2.0	130 000	0.1

Source: Statistics Canada, Canadian Community Health Survey, 2002, Mental Health and Well-being, Cycle 1.2.

* Respondents could have reported symptoms that met the criteria for more than one condition.

** Numbers have been rounded to the nearest 10 000.

and complications such as diabetes and cardiovascular problems. To promote mental health and recovery, comprehensive services for housing, vocational, recreational, and treatment of co-occurring substance abuse problems are needed. Integration of these diverse services and supportive government policies is needed to promote recovery and basic well being (Kirby & Keon, 2006).

Serious mental illness (SMI) refers to MI that has compromised a person's level of competence and quality of life. SMI generally refers to schizophrenia or bipolar disorder, which are manifested by bizarre behaviours, extreme thought disorder, and problems with social and occupational functioning that make the person highly visible (Davis, 2006). *Serious and persistent MI* (SPMI) refers to the chronic or enduring nature of a person's MI. Currently, 3% of Canadians suffer from SMI causing significant financial and social hardship (Kirby & Keon, 2006).

Less visible mental illnesses, such as depression and anxiety disorders (obsessive compulsive disorder, generalized anxiety disorders, agoraphobia, post-traumatic stress disorders), cause subjective distress and social and occupational difficulties (Government of Canada, 2006). Anxiety disorders, although affecting 12% of the population, are underserviced within the publicly funded mental health system (Davis, 2006; Health Canada, 2002). Personality disorders, wherein people have developed maladaptive ways of responding and interacting that prevent them from functioning in society, are difficult to effectively treat. People with borderline personality disorder frequently use emergency rooms and require hospitalization and ongoing psychotherapy (Government of Canada). Both children and the elderly suffer from particular mental illness (depression, substance abuse, anxiety, eating disorders, attention deficit disorder), with estimates of 15% of children afflicted with MI and 15% to 30% of the elderly suffering with dementia and Alzheimer's disease (Southern Alberta Geriatric Mental Health Working Group, 2003; Waddell & Sheppard, 2002).

THE IMPACT OF MENTAL ILLNESS

Disability and burden related to MI are significant. The World Health Organization (WHO) states that 5 of the 10 leading causes of disability are related to mental disorders and predicts that within 20 years depression will be the second leading cause of worldwide disability and the first in developed countries (World Health Organization, 1999, 2001).

Disability related to MI places persons at risk for poverty due to underemployment and unemployment (National Council of Welfare, 2006). People who are unable to maintain adequate employment and live in poverty are forced to live in conditions that are unsafe, demoralizing, and perpetuate stigma (Wilton, 2003). People with MI are disproportionately represented in the homeless and prison populations (Allen 2002; Hall, 2001). These disproportionate numbers suggest that social systems and treatment options are inadequate to support this vulnerable population.

People with MI are at risk for accidents, suicide, and premature deaths from treatable medical conditions (Hall, 2001). In a follow-up study of patients with psychiatric diagnoses who were discharged from hospital, these patients were found to be at six times the risk for mortality (British Columbia Ministry of Health Services, 2003; Health Canada, 2002). People with MI are subject to an increased incidence of physical health concerns, in particular diabetes, HIV, chronic obstructive pulmonary disease, gastrointestinal disorders, and cardiovascular disorders. Co-occurring disorders, wherein there is a diagnosable MI and an addiction, place people at further risk for health problems (Jones et al., 2004). People with MI smoke more than the general population, placing them at risk for health concerns and consuming a substantial amount of their income (Wilton, 2003).

RISK FACTORS

The etiology of MI is not fully understood, with links between specific brain dysfunction and specific disorders remaining unclear. At best, psychiatric illness is explained as a combination of complex interactions between genetics, environment, biology, and personality (Health Canada, 2002). In the recent report *The Human Face of MI in Canada* (Government of Canada, 2006), the etiology of MI is discussed under three categories: genetics, poverty, and violence. (See Table 18.2.)

Genetics links are more complex than originally presumed, with more than one gene being implicated. Genetic and heredity influences in the etiology of schizophrenia, autism, and bipolar illness were supported by considerable research and the push for biological evidence in the 1990s, the Decade of the Brain (Rutter, Pickles, Murray, & Eaves, 2001). Neuro-imaging techniques identifying minute neurological and anatomical abnormalities have generated new explanations of MI and strengthened the biomedical explanation.

Conversely, the *effects of poverty* on mental health and the development of MI are complex. Poverty, when combined with a genetic predisposition, can cause MI due to the ongoing stress, despair, and anger that may accompany it. However, the effects of MI may cause the individual to "drift" downward into poverty. A significant number of people with disabilities and substance abuse problems are on welfare as they face multiple barriers to compete successfully in the job market (National Council of Welfare, 2006).

Childhood sexual abuse (CSA), with a global prevalence of 6% to 11% for girls and 2% for boys, increases the risk of mental disorders in adulthood. Victims of CSA are at increased risk for depression, panic disorder, alcohol and drug abuse, post-traumatic stress disorder, and suicide (WHO, 2002). Complex trauma reactions, resulting from multiple and ongoing violence, have been identified in children who have been exposed to maltreatment and traumatic experiences (Cook et al., 2005).

TABLE 18.2

Risk Factors Potentially Influencing the Development of Mental Health Problems and Mental Disorders in Individuals

Individual factors	Family/social factors	School context	Life events and situations	Community and cultural factors
▪ prenatal brain damage ▪ prematurity ▪ birth injury ▪ low birth weight, birth complications ▪ physical and intellectual disability ▪ poor health in infancy ▪ insecure attachment in infant/child ▪ low intelligence ▪ difficult temperament ▪ chronic illness ▪ poor social skills ▪ low self-esteem ▪ alienation ▪ impulsivity	▪ having a teenage mother ▪ having a single parent ▪ absence of father in childhood ▪ large family size ▪ antisocial role models (in childhood) ▪ family violence and disharmony ▪ marital discord in parents ▪ poor supervision and monitoring of child ▪ low parental involvement in child's activities ▪ neglect in childhood ▪ long-term parent unemployment ▪ criminality in parent ▪ parent substance misuse ▪ parental mental disorder ▪ harsh or inconsistent discipline style ▪ social isolation ▪ experiencing rejection ▪ lack of warmth and affection	▪ bullying ▪ peer rejection ▪ poor attachment to school ▪ inadequate behaviour management ▪ deviant peer group ▪ school failure	▪ physical, sexual and emotional abuse ▪ school transitions ▪ divorce and family breakup ▪ death of family member ▪ physical illness/impairment ▪ unemployment, homelessness ▪ incarceration ▪ poverty/economic insecurity ▪ job insecurity ▪ unsatisfactory workplace relationships ▪ workplace accident/injury ▪ caring for someone with an illness/disability ▪ living in a nursing home or aged care hostel ▪ war or natural disasters	▪ socioeconomic disadvantage ▪ social or cultural discrimination ▪ isolation ▪ neighbourhood violence and crime ▪ population density and housing conditions ▪ lack of support services including transport, shopping, recreational facilities

* Many of these factors are specific to particular stages of the lifespan, particularly childhood; others have an impact across the lifespan, for example socioeconomic disadvantage.

Source: Australia. Promotion, prevention and early intervention for mental health (monograph on the Internet). Retrieved March 7, 2000, from http://www.ausienet.flinders.edu.au/files/resources/other/monograph.pdf. Copyright Commonwealth of Australia reproduced by permission.

Studies report that 83% of women in a psychiatric hospital had experienced CSA, while 80% of young adults who experienced childhood abuse met the criteria for a *DSM-IV* disorder (Government of Canada, 2006). *Violence,* experienced as bullying and domestic violence, contributes to MI. Many women experience multiple traumas that affect their mental and physical health. The trauma of CSA and the psychological effects of violence contribute to the development of depression, anxiety, and suicidal behaviours (Martsolf & Draucker, 2005). For women who are socially marginalized, poor, and have SMI, the effects of violence are compounded (Government of Canada). Social barriers influencing MI include limited opportunities for personal development, relocation, family dysfunction, violence, social isolation, stigmatization, homelessness, and inadequate health and human services within the community (Pevalin & Goldberg, 2003).

The *risk/vulnerability model* offers an alternative explanation. The degree of exposure to environmental stress and the resultant stress vulnerability interaction influence mental heath and illness. Within the stress vulnerability model, the person who is genetically susceptible to low stress tolerance when met with stressors will become ill, while the person with a higher stress tolerance will not. Protective factors such as medications, social supports, and stress management reduce vulnerabilities. This model has limited application to change socioeconomic variables that impact on people's lives and relies on medication as the first line of intervention underscoring the need for social change (Davis, 2006).

In Canada, the impact of colonialism, the political domination of one nation over the other, and the ensuing decolonization process has contributed to the MI problems of Aboriginal people. Forced assimilation, residential schools, and loss of language and traditional lifestyles have influenced the mental well being of individuals, families, and communities (Government of Canada, 2006).

Universally, chronic medical conditions such as diabetes, hypertension, malignancies, and HIV/AIDS predispose people to MI, particularly depression. Depression hinders the person's ability to comply with medical treatment. Also, behavioural lifestyle choices altered by mental illness predispose the individual to many communicable diseases (WHO, 2001).

VULNERABLE POPULATIONS

Children

The prevalence of MI causing significant distress and impairment in children is estimated at 15% of the Canadian population (BC Partners for Mental Health and Addictions Information, 2006; Waddell, McEwan, Hau, & Shepherd, 2002). Children suffer from a variety of mental disorders such as anxiety, mood disorders leading to suicidal thoughts and actions, conduct disorder, attention deficit disorder, developmental delays, substance abuse, and eating disorders. Youth suicide is of particular concern in some First Nations communities (Davis, 2006; Government of Canada, 2006). Services for children are scarce, with only 1% of children receiving assistance (Ministry of Children and Family Development, 2003). This is important in that diagnosis and treatment are critical to prevent the worsening of symptoms that increases the likelihood of the disorders in adulthood. For example, 90% of people who suffer from co-occurring substance abuse and mental disorders developed the first symptoms at the average age of 11 years (Ministry of Children and Family Development). The lack of mental health professionals specializing in children, the stigma of having an MI, and the difficulty of diagnosing children's behaviour over their growth and developmental lifespans contribute to inadequate treatment. Causative factors for MI in children are varied; genetic and hereditary influences, traumatic and abusive experiences, social pressures, and low self-esteem. (See the text box "Signs of Mental Illness in Children and Youth".)

A multifaceted approach, inclusive of programs that promote mental health for all children and programs and services for children at risk and with severe disorders, is urgently required (Waddell & Sheppard, 2002). At risk are children of parents with an MI. These children are at three times the risk to develop emotional and/or behavioural problems (Warner, Weismann, Fendrich, Wickramaratne, & Moreau, 1992). Despite their being identified in the literature as at an at-risk population, services for these children are not well integrated into the mental health system (Mordoch & Hall, 2002).

Signs of Mental Illness in Children and Youth

Changes in behaviour: for example, an active child becomes quiet and withdrawn or a good student suddenly starts getting poor grades

Changes in feelings: for example, a child may show signs of feeling unhappy, worried, guilty, angry, fearful, hopeless, or rejected

Physical symptoms: frequent headaches, stomach or back aches, problems eating or sleeping, a general lack of energy

Changes in thoughts: for example, a child may begin saying things that indicate low self-esteem, self-blame, or thoughts about suicide

Abuse of alcohol and/or drugs

Difficulty coping with regular activities and everyday problems

Consistent violations of the rights of others: e.g. thefts and vandalism

Intense fear of becoming fat with no relationship to the child's actual body weight

Odd or repetitive movements beyond regular playing such as spinning, hand-flapping, or head banging

Unusual ways of speaking or private language that no one else can understand

Source: Canadian Mental Health Association.

Refugees and Immigrants

Eighteen percent of people living in Canada are immigrants. A significant number (30%) live in poverty for the first ten years of their lives in Canada, which may predispose them to developing mental health problems or MI. Refugees may be at increased risk for post-traumatic stress disorder related to their past experiences (Government of Canada, 2006). There is growing recognition of the need for culturally sensitive and language-appropriate services in the mental health field (Kirby & Keon, 2006).

Prison Inmates

Prison inmates have elevated rates of mental disorders and substance abuse, with 1% to 2% of this population having an intellectual disability. In the maximum-security settings up to 69% to 78.3% of women and 41% to 51% of men have problems with alcohol and drug addictions. In addition, 43% of inmates have a diagnosable mental disorder. Most inmates are male (97%) and under the age of 50 years (Government of Canada, 2006). Mental health services are often inadequate and inaccessible (Kirby & Keon, 2006). It is likely that MI is underdiagnosed.

Canadian Research Box 18.1

Valiakalayil, A., Paulson, L. A., & Tibbo, P. (2004). Burden in adolescent children of parents with schizophrenia: The Edmonton High Risk Project. *Social Psychiatry Psychiatric Epidemiology, 39,* 528–535.

The qualitative study was designed to determine the impact of burden related to having a parent with schizophrenia. Thirteen adolescent children—9 females and 4 males between ages 13 and 18—who had a parent diagnosed with schizophrenia were interviewed in a pilot study. They completed the Global Assessment Scale of Functioning, the Modified Pre-morbid Adjustment Scale, the Diagnostic Interview for Children and Adolescents, and Hollingshead's Scale for Socio-economic Status. Results suggest that adolescents feel that their lives are impacted by having a parent with schizophrenia. Adolescents identified that they required more information about the illness of schizophrenia; that they attributed the illness to something "bad" the parent had done in the past; and that they experienced strong emotional reactions to their parent's illness, often experiencing grief, sadness, anger, fear, and resentment. While able to identify coping skills that helped them to manage their circumstances, the adolescents often felt that they were left alone to deal with their problems. Positive aspects of their relationships with their parents are that the experience of MI had drawn them closer to their parents, and that they had a stronger sense of self and an increased tolerance for others with disabilities. The findings demonstrate the need to assist adolescent children with managing their circumstances by giving them emotional support, practical skills, and access to information. There is a need to ensure adequate follow-up for these children, particularly when their parents are hospitalized and also for long-term monitoring.

Discussion Questions:

1. How would you work with the adolescent children and their parents to help children learn about schizophrenia?

2. How would you implement mental health promotion strategies with adolescent children whose parents have schizophrenia?

3. How can CMHNs decrease stigma around MI?

4. What other research questions might arise from this study?

Co-occurring Disorders

Co-occurring disorders refers to the existence of a psychiatric diagnosis and an additional diagnosis of substance abuse. People with MI frequently self-medicate by using alcohol and other drugs. In the past, addictions and MI were treated by two distinct systems, psychiatry and addiction services, each with its separate philosophy on treatment and causes. As this strategy has not worked well, there is current interest in treating both disorders in an integrated manner (Kirby & Keon, 2006).

SUICIDE IN CANADA

Suicide is a public health concern affecting all ages and socioeconomic classes of Canadian society. The prevalence of suicide in Canada is at the mid to high range, with 18.7% of men and 5.2% of women completing suicide. Suicide is the fifth leading cause of death in Canada, the leading cause of death for men aged 25 to 29 years and 40 to 49 years, and the second leading cause of death in youth 10 to 24 years of age (Health Canada, 2003). Due to the stigma surrounding suicide, the number of deaths by suicide is unknown. Deaths may be labelled as "undetermined" and accidental and if confirmed a suicide are not registered as such (Government of Canada, 2006). Canadian society does not condone suicide. This prevents populations at risk and their families from seeking help and discussing suicide. Survivors of suicide often feel isolated and experience complex emotions in dealing with a family member's suicide. Survivors of suicide may need encouragement to attend self-help groups, where they may benefit from discussion with other group members who have experienced suicide deaths (Government of Canada, 2006).

Contributing Factors to Suicidal Behaviour

According to the Canadian Mental Health Survey: Mental Health and Well-Being Survey (Statistics Canada, 2002), suicidal behaviour may be classified as suicidal ideation, suicide attempt, and completed suicide. Suicidal ideation refers to thoughts about suicide; 13.4% of people had seriously thought about suicide during their lifetime. As suicide attempts are not always reported, the incidence of attempts is difficult to determine. Statistics indicate that 3.1% of the population over 15 years of age has attempted suicide in their lifetime, with a larger percentage of women attempting than men. Hospitalization rates were higher for women, peaking between the ages of 15 and 19 and then again in mid-life. Completed suicides demonstrate a mortality rate 4 times higher among men than women. Men have historically chosen more fatal means for completing suicide and have been reluctant to seek help. This trend is changing as more women are choosing lethal methods for suicide.

Youth are particularly vulnerable to suicidal thoughts and attempts. Developmental crisis, impulsivity, and lack of life experiences contribute toward suicidal behaviours. Aboriginal youth between the ages of 15 and 24 years of age are at increased risk, with boys being at 5 times the risk and girls being at 7 times the risk when compared with the general Canadian population. Seniors face multiple losses of friends and family, health problems, and diminished capacity, and in facing their own mortality may choose to end life (Government of Canada, 2006). Due to the stigma associated with their sexual identity, gay, lesbian, bisexual, and transgender (GLBT) youth are identified as at risk for suicide (Russell & Joyner, 2001). People who come out may face increased harassment, while not coming out may lead to extreme isolation (Morrison & L'Heureux, 2001). Thus, GLBT youth require sensitive assessment in order to determine their suicide risk.

First Nations Communities

First Nations communities have a suicide rate twice the national average. Although the suicide rate varies among communities, it has shown little change since 1979. Inuit have the highest rate of suicide, particularly among young males, with Nunavut having one of the highest suicide rates in the world. This rate continues to rise, particularly among youth. The high incidence of youth suicide in First Nations communities represents a significant loss of potential years of life. Addictions and depression, both factors in increasing the risk of suicide, are disproportionately represented in the First Nations population (Government of Canada, 2006; Kirby & Keon, 2006). (See Table 18.3.)

Prompt and accurate assessment of suicide lethality is crucial, with safety of the individual paramount. To assess sui-

cide lethality, all nurses must be comfortable with asking directly about suicidal ideation, the suicide plan, the means, and if the person has access to the means. Ropes, firearms, and medications should be removed until the person has received treatment and is able to keep himself or herself safe. Acutely suicidal people need to be under suicidal observation in a safe environment. Survivors of suicide often feel isolated and emotionally overwhelmed. As such they require specific resources to manage their grief and to promote their mental health. Suicide prevention efforts at the provincial, territorial, and national levels must be both population-wide and target at-risk populations. Efforts to reduce stigma, increase pubic awareness of suicidal behaviours, restrict access to lethal means (guns, access to bridges, quantities of over the counter medications), and incorporate universal mental health promotion in public policy are needed to address the problem of suicide in Canada (Government of Canada, 2006).

CARING FOR MENTAL HEALTH CLIENTS IN THE COMMUNITY

CMHNs work with individuals, families, and populations affected by the major mental illnesses (mood disorders, anxiety disorders, and schizophrenia) in addition to childhood MI and personality, eating, and trauma-related disorders. CMHNs implement specific target-group interventions and contribute to population-wide interventions that have the potential to influence population incidence. Currently, recommendations for a more comprehensive inter-sectoral delivery of mental health services and a national strategy for mental health promotion are under discussion (Kirby & Keon, 2006). How these recommendations are implemented will affect the CMHN's future practice.

TABLE 18.3
Contributing Factors to Suicidal Behaviour among Canadians

Predisposing Factors	Precipitating Factors	Protective Factors
MI (depression, bipolar, schizophrenia)	Physical illness	Tolerance for frustration
Substance abuse	Substance abuse	Adaptive coping skills
Previous suicide attempt	Isolation	Positive expectations for the future
Male	Suicide of a friend	One healthy relationship with a confidante
Aboriginal	Early loss	
Losses: divorce, job, relationships, stature	Sexual identity issues	
	Difficulty with peers, in society social supports, unstable family, family history of suicide	
	Risk taking, self-destructive behaviour	

Source: Adapted from Government of Canada. (2006). The face of mental illness in Canada: Suicide assessment, intervention and prevention. *Ottawa. Reproduced with the permission of the Minister of Public Works and Government Services Canada.*

Case Study

Gloria is a 27-year-old Cree woman recently admitted to the hospital from a remote reserve. She is admitted for depression with suicidal thoughts. Recently, Gloria lost her infant daughter as the result of sudden infant death syndrome. Since then she has had continual thoughts of harming herself and difficulty sleeping. She describes her husband as a good man who sometimes drinks and beats her. Gloria has experienced both physical and sexual abuse as a child. She states that she has forgiven the people who hurt her. Gloria has been unable to look after her older daughter (age 4). Her daughter is now living with her grandparents in Gloria's home community several hundred kilometres away from Gloria's present community. Gloria feels isolated and has no one with whom she can talk in the community. When asked about her life, she states she lives in a shack and everything is wrong. She is unkempt and requires dental care. Gloria is put on a trial of antidepressant medication. The plan is to return her to the reserve when she is stable. There are limited mental health resources on the reserve.

You are the primary nurse who will be looking after Gloria while she is in the hospital. You will be responsible for discharge planning upon her return to the reserve.

Discussion Questions

1. What do you assess as the personal issues in Gloria's situation that contribute to her depression?

2. How can you implement care with Gloria around these issues?

3. What are the systemic issues that impact on Gloria's situation?

4. How will you plan for discharge in order to help Gloria remain safe?

Community Mental Health Service Delivery

The **Mental Health Act** is a legal document that attempts to provide humane and just care to people with MI while protecting society and individuals with MI from harm. It is evoked when acute treatment services are needed on an involuntarily basis. People with mental illness and family members often have diverse opinions when an involuntary admission is enacted, with people with mental illness feeling that their rights are violated and family members expressing concerns that their loved ones are not receiving needed treatment. Mental health acts across Canada vary in the wording of each act and focus on the criteria for curtailing the freedom of an individual. Most declare self-harm or harm to others as criteria for involuntary admission, with some provinces adding the criteria of potential physical and mental deterioration (Davis, 2006). While the mental health act covers multiple details related to the rights of people with MI, this discussion will focus on two central issues: committal and compulsory treatment orders.

Committal While each province and territory will have specific wording to the law detailing when a person may be involuntarily admitted, there is general consensus that harm to others or self are key deciding factors. Manitoba, Alberta, and British Columbia include potential of physical and mental deterioration, while Ontario has specified this may be a criterion only when there is evidence of past successful psychiatric treatment (Davis, 2006). CMHNs need to be familiar with the basic components of the Mental Health Act and the issues that arise related to the unique concerns of people with mental illness, of their families, and of the public.

Compulsory Treatment Orders **Compulsory treatment orders** decree that persons with MI be compliant with treatment or they will be returned to the hospital. The laws on compulsory treatment orders vary from province to province, with Saskatchewan, Ontario, and British Columbia having statutes for compulsory treatment orders. There appears to be a trend toward this type of legislation (Davis, 2006). Alberta is currently considering including compulsory treatment orders within the Alberta mental health system (Libin, 2007).

SERVICE ORIENTATION

Discussion is ongoing regarding how to allocate resources for an adequate balance of mental health services in the institutional care and community sectors. While the focus on community has been underway for some time, service reorganization has not yet provided adequate and comprehensive supports to enable recovery from MI or to implement national, population-based mental health promotion strategies. Practising CMHNs will be aware of the continuing need for improvement in mental health services.

Three main problems affecting service orientation warrant consideration. First, while the move from institutions to comprehensive inter-sectoral community services is expected to ultimately reduce costs, currently both systems must be operated with continued investment in community services. An institutional bias requiring public funding of physician and hospital services disadvantages people with limited incomes to obtain alternative services. People living with MI do not always have adequate access to mental health services, particularly in remote and rural regions. Second, comprehensive services must be intersectoral and address the basic determinants of health to enable people with MI in their recovery from MI. For example, housing is a major problem, with 27% of people with MI unable to find and afford adequate housing (Kirby & Keon, 2006). Third, stigma and discrimination continue to be formidable barriers for people living with MI, preventing people from accessing services. The principles of recovery, which challenge society's assumptions regarding MI, are in the beginning stages of implementation into policy and service delivery (Government of Canada, 2006; Kirby & Keon).

Resources for mental health are organized around primary, secondary, and tertiary services. Primary intervention aims to reduce the number of new cases or to slow the development of mental disorders. It occurs through case finding of at-risk individuals and mental health promotion intervention. Key strategies are to promote healthy growth and development of individuals and resourcefulness of the family and the community. The goal is to reduce the number of new cases and the rate of development of mental disorder in the community. Currently there is continuing discussion on how best to integrate mental health services within primary health care services. Secondary intervention focuses on the early treatment of people living with MI, healing strategies, and the health promotion of individuals, families, and communities. The goal is to reduce episodes of acute distress and the prevalence of MI in the community.

Tertiary intervention focuses on the case management of people with MI with emphasis on rehabilitation and recovery. It is accomplished through tangible resources, psychoeducation, and rehabilitative strategies. The goal of tertiary intervention is to reduce the severity of the illness and associated disability and to assist people in recovery from MI.

Organization of Services in the Mental Health System

Emergency Services   Emergency services, consisting of admissions to hospitals and crisis stabilization units, are frequently initiated through the emergency wards of general hospitals, where services are organized around medical emergencies, not psychiatric emergencies. General or psychiatric hospitals provide services for more serious acute illness, while crisis stabilization units provide services to less acutely ill people, generally judged by indicators of self-harm or homicide (Mordoch, 1995). Additional services include 24-hour mobile crisis response teams and professional and peer support telephone crisis lines.

Outpatient clinics and specialized programs, for example, eating disorder programs and child and adolescent treatment clinics, may be offered as follow-up services in the form of day hospitals, day treatment, and daycare settings. Community mental health workers follow people with MI in the community but often carry large caseloads that leave little time for consistent intervention.

Case Management   Case management has been identified as a best-practice model to provide assistance to people with mental illness and families in negotiating the mental health system (Clarke Institute, 1997). Case managers coordinate holistic care over the long term, providing and negotiating services for a wide variety of needs, some of which include physical health, leisure, education, and housing. Case management fosters continuity and coordination of care (Commission on the Future of Health Care, 2002).

Assertive Community Treatment   Assertive community treatment (ACT) is a comprehensive, long-term, intensive case management approach to treating persons who have a SPMI, functional impairment, and are "intensive users of the health care system" (British Columbia Minister of Health, 2003). Functional impairment refers to an inability to look after hygiene, nutritional needs, and finances and to develop or sustain support systems. Services are organized on an outreach basis and attempt to decrease hospitalizations by addressing compliance issues and improving the quality of community life (British Columbia Minister of Health). Programs exist in many areas of Canada and are noted in best-practice documents as vital to coordination of services for this difficult-to-serve population (McEwan & Goldner, 2001).

**Primary Health Care Services   The first point of contact in primary health care services is often a general practitioner who does not have expertise in mental health or time to spend with clients. This can result in overprescribing of medications and fewer people being seen by mental health specialists. In order to integrate mental health practitioners with primary health care providers, shared care where general practitioners would work in tandem with mental health service providers has been suggested. Shared care could involve telephone access to psychiatrists or on-site psychiatrists at clinics (Davis, 2006).

Acute Home Treatment   Acute home treatment is proposed as an alternative to hospitalization and involves service providers in the home until the person is stabilized. While not common in Canada, several programs have been trialed with promising results noted from people with mental illness. This approach has also proved favourable in terms of family satisfaction and as a cost-constraint measure (Commission on the Future of Health Care, 2002).

Early Intervention Programs   Early intervention programs arose in response to treatment delays and in an attempt to intervene prior to a full-blown episode of MI with the goal of decreasing the effects of the illness. One such program is Early Psychosis Intervention (EPI). This program attempts to address stigma and demoralization associated with an MI, supports the engagement of family, and actively seeks timely treatment and follow-up (Lines, 2000). Research related to such EPI programs is currently being conducted in several Canadian cities.

**Co-occurring Disorder Programs   Currently there is interest in co-occurring disorders and intervention to address both the MI and the addiction. People with anxiety disorders and depression have higher rates of substance dependence than the general population. Acceptance of both addictions and MI as conditions requiring treatment that may be long-term, inclusive of relapse, is crucial (Davis, 2006).

**Self-Help and Peer Support   Self-help programs are recognized as an integral part of services for people with MI and their families. Recommendations to fund these programs from public funding attest to their value. Current discussion suggests increasing the number of paid peer support helpers and peer counsellors. Research in this area is new but shows promise for innovation (Kirby & Keon, 2006).

Mental Health Promotion   Mental health promotion emphasizes positive mental health and the personal, social, economic, and environmental factors that are thought to contribute to mental health. Efforts are directed to the population and attempt to alter determinants that are amenable to change (Kirby & Keon, 2006). Mental health promotion is becoming increasingly prominent in the mental health and public health system. Recommendations to include mental health promotion in a Pan-Canadian Healthy Living Strategy and the development of a Canadian Mental Health Guide demonstrate the growing trend to incorporate mental health promotion at a policy level. Suicide prevention efforts inclusive of a national policy to implement mental health promotion efforts to decrease suicidal behaviour and completed suicides in Canada are under discussion. Currently there are holistic programs, such as *Promoting Good Mental Health in Labrador,* which blends traditional and Western knowledge, policy changes affecting service delivery, and a range of multisectoral approaches to deliver mental health promotion efforts (Kirby & Keon).

Models of Mental Health Service Delivery

The Recovery Model and the Tidal Model are current philosophies in use and under discussion in the implementation of mental health services.

The Recovery Model   The model of recovery from MI arose from the writings of people with mental illnesses who were in the mental health system. These writings challenged professional attitudes that suggested that MI irrevocably led to deterioration and diminished lives (Anthony, 2000). In consultation with the Boston University Center for Psychiatric Rehabilitation, the recovery model has been implemented in parts of the mental health system. The assumptions of recovery challenged and continue to challenge the status quo in psychiatric mental health service delivery (see Table 18.4). Essential services proposed by the **recovery model** include crisis intervention, case management, rehabilitation, enrichment, rights protection, basic support, self-help, and wellness/prevention (Anthony). In Canada, inroads to organize services concurrent with recovery principles are evident. Current interest and a growing body of evidence posit that service and policy recommendations incorporate recovery principles (Government of Canada, 2006; Kirby & Keon, 2006).

The Tidal Model of Mental Health Recovery   The **Tidal Model of Mental Health Recovery** has been developed as an alternative way to frame services and professional relationships within psychiatric/mental health nursing. The model focuses on the development of an understanding of the person's needs through a collaborative relationship built on empowerment principles. People with MI are encouraged to tell their stories in their own language and the nurse becomes the apprentice within the relationship. The model helps the nurse to understand what mental health might mean for the person. It is guided by the principles of curiosity as to what might help the person, resourcefulness of the individual, respect for the person's wishes, recognizing crisis as an opportunity, thinking small goals versus the end point of care, and elegance, depicting the most simple intervention to experience change

TABLE 18.4
Assumptions about Recovery

Factors	Reasons
Can occur without professionals	Consumers hold the key to recovery
Consumers must have people to believe in them and stand by them	Someone to be there in time of need
Recovery is not based on a theory of causation of MI	There is hope for the future
Recovery can occur even though symptoms reoccur	Recovery occurs within MI
Recovery is unique	There is no one path
Recovery means choices	That one has options is important
Recovery from the consequences of the illness is difficult	Stigma, discrimination, segregation, effects of treatment

Source: Adapted from Anthony, W. (2000). A recovery oriented service system: Setting some service level standards. Psychiatric Rehabilitation Journal, *24(2), 159–168.*

(Brookes, 2006). The Tidal Model Care Continuum is based on 10 principles known as commitments (see Table 18.5 and Figure 18.1). Nursing is viewed as a social construct wherein nurses "care with" people and assist them to tell their narrative stories (Brookes).

TABLE 18.5
Ten Commitments of the Tidal Model of Mental Health Recovery

Commitment	Meaning
Value	The person's story, voice of experience
Respecting the language	People own the most powerful language
Curiosity	Genuine interest in the storyteller
Be the apprentice	Storyteller is the expert
Reveal personal wisdom	Help the storyteller reveal wisdom
Be transparent	Help the person focus on understanding what is being done and why
Use the available toolkit	Story represents what has worked in the past, what might work now
Craft the step beyond	What needs to be done now
Give the gift of time	Time is the midwife of change
Know change is constant	Change is inevitable; use change for recovery

Source: Brookes, N. (2006). Tidal model of mental health recovery. In A. Marriner-Tomey & M. Raile-Alligood (Eds.), Nursing theorists and their work (6th ed.) (p. 22). St. Louis, MO: Elsevier-Mosby.

FIGURE 18.1 Tidal Model Care Continuum

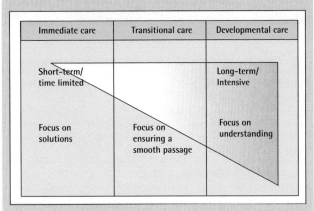

Immediate care	Transitional care	Developmental care
Short-term/time limited		Long-term/Intensive
Focus on solutions	Focus on ensuring a smooth passage	Focus on understanding

Source: Brookes, N. (2006). Tidal model of mental health recovery. In A. Marriner-Tomey & M. Raile-Alligood (Eds.), Nursing theorists and their work (6th ed.) (pp. 696–725). St. Louis, MO: Elsevier-Mosby.

ROLE OF COMMUNITY HEALTH NURSES

When working with individuals, families, and populations, CMHNs attempt to promote mental health, prevent MI, assess dysfunction, assist people to improve their coping abilities, and prevent further disability. The Canadian Federation of Mental Health Nurses strives to examine and influence national policy on mental health and illness (Canadian Federation of Mental Health Nurses, 2005).

Epidemiological Base for Decision Making

CMHNs contribute to and use epidemiological databases to make informed decisions on how best to respond to a community's needs. They use data to investigate the prevalence and incidence of mental disorders in the community and to identify known and suspected risk factors. The results of these analyses determine the health needs of individuals, families, and communities.

Case Finding and Referral

Early identification and treatment of MI reduces its severity and promotes quicker recovery. For example, early identification and timely referral can decrease secondary problems of substance abuse and depression commonly associated with anxiety disorders. CMHNs providing mental health promotion programs will have opportunities to assess people who may be at risk for the development of MI or who are not receiving appropriate services. CMHNs play an important role in screening for physical health problems and adherence

to medical treatment regimes in the SMI population who are at risk for the development of physical disorders and the inability to adhere to treatment plans (Jones et al., 2004). From a family nursing perspective, CMHNs can assess children who are living with a parent with MI and ensure that their needs are adequately met. CMHNs may also refer parents to parenting programs to ensure that they are adequately supported in their efforts as parents (Nicholson & Biebel, 2002). CMHNs play a key role in early identification and referral for assessment and treatment of MI.

Advocacy is often needed to negotiate the mental health system (Kirby & Keon, 2006). Finding services when one is unfamiliar and stressed is difficult. CMHNs ease this tension for people with MI and their families, ensuring their rights are protected and they have access to appropriate services. CMHNs analyze what services are needed to assist consumers and families to participate optimally in their communities. CMHNs advocate for funding to develop new community programs based on needs and best practice evidence; are pivotal in advocating for mental health care services in rural and remote settings; and serve on advisory boards and lobby groups to influence healthy public policy such as mental health promotion. With the current development of the Mental Health Commission of Canada and the impetus for change within mental health services, CMHNs have a critical opportunity to ensure that client and family concerns are accurately represented and managed. Within mental health promotion, CMHNs have a significant role to play in advocating for the reduction of social inequities that create barriers toward achieving mental health and recovery from MI.

Education and Counselling

CMHNs provide education to the general public, to specific targeted groups, and to individuals and families. The Tidal Model of Mental Health Recovery provides a framework for developing therapeutic relationships honouring the person's experience (Brookes, 2006). Within this therapeutic relationship, CMHNs work with individuals and groups to promote self-care, develop people's abilities to cope with MI, and foster social support networks. Nurses work with clients and families in crisis assisting them to find appropriate resources. Individual and group educational counselling promotes discussion of the signs of MI, medication, treatment options, and the recovery model. CMHNs support peer and self-help recovery-based programs; facilitate cognitive behavioural therapy groups; and organize educational programs for the general public to promote mental health and reduce risk factors associated with mental illness. Programs that inform schools and children of ways to protect children from childhood sexual abuse help to reduce the risk of such abuse, a precursor to mental health problems. Programs can offer information on specific illnesses, stigma, and suicide prevention. CMHNs can develop creative educational programs that will decrease the stigma associated with having an MI and increase public awareness of the issues surrounding MI and mental health (Kenny, 2001).

FUTURE DIRECTIONS IN COMMUNITY MENTAL HEALTH

Reports on mental health services in Canada have identified the need for continued support for people with MI and their families and have called for integrated comprehensive services from diverse sectors, such as income and housing (Commission on the Future of Health Care, 2002; Davis, 2006; Kirby & Keon, 2006). As of November 2005, the Canadian federal government has initiated the Mental Health Commission of Canada (2007). The Commission is mandated:

- to serve as a catalyst to reform mental health policies and improve service delivery,
- to facilitate a national approach to mental health issues,
- to diminish the stigma and discrimination associated with mental illness, and
- to disseminate evidence-based information on mental health and mental illness to governments, stakeholders, and the public.

The Commission will undertake three strategic initiatives:

- a systematic 10-year anti-stigma campaign aimed at changing public attitudes toward mental illness,
- in collaboration with all members of the mental health community, develop a national strategy to address mental illness, and
- the development of a knowledge exchange centre to facilitate access to evidence-based information and to encourage collaborative activities across Canada.

CMHNs are well positioned to contribute to these initiatives. CMHNs have the capacity to encourage and support clients and families to become actively involved in the work of the Commission. Within collaborative efforts with the mental health community, nurses can be involved in the planning and delivery of anti-stigma initiatives. As CMHNs are well grounded in the realities that clients and families face, they can also advocate for specific services and collaborative efforts to improve outcomes for clients and their families. CMHNs can contribute to the knowledge exchange centre by engaging in pertinent research and facilitating dissemination and knowledge translation of research findings in order that the research will be utilized within meaningful strategies.

Increased recognition of peer support programs, self-help, and the principles of recovery have the potential to change the way services are delivered. The family is gaining increasing recognition for their efforts in sustaining family members with MI. These changes challenge the philosophical underpinnings of current modes of service delivery. Nurses will face challenges in service reorganization. Specific populations are at risk for mental health problems and MI; children and adolescents, First Nations people, inmates, refugees, and immigrants. Co-occurring disorders, both of which require intervention, are common with people with MI. Mental health promotion is increasingly recognized as an important health strategy for the Canadian population. Innovative programs are expected in mental health promotion with policy changes at the national level. Efforts to decrease stigma toward people with MI are essential to mental health promotion efforts.

IMPLICATIONS FOR NURSING

Current reports have advocated for significant change in the underlying philosophies affecting service delivery and for more comprehensive funding to address the macro societal barriers that influence people living with MI. Target populations that appear vulnerable, such as children, adolescents, First Nations people, inmates, and people with co-occurring disorders, will require specific intervention and health promotion strategies to promote their optimal mental well being.

Nurses have the opportunity to prepare themselves to address the gaps in mental health services. The serious lack of child/adolescent mental health professionals presents such an opportunity. Nurses also play a key role in facilitating peer programs, self-help groups, and family advocacy and support groups. The Recovery Model and the Tidal Model of Mental Health outline respectful and validating approaches to working with people with MI. The Recovery Model acknowledges the macro support structures that people require to live successfully in the community. Future directions in mental health service delivery require increased nursing efforts to affect policy and services that will attain the essentials of successful community living for people with MI. With increasing recognition of the wisdom of mental health promotion, new opportunities will arise, opportunities in which nurses will participate to affect the mental health of the Canadian population.

Summary

When working with people with MI, their families, and their communities, nurses are practising in a system that is undergoing change. New models of direct nursing care propose reconfigurations of care that honour personal narratives and change the nurse/person relationship. These changes will challenge nursing to examine its practice and nursing's openness to innovations. Population data sets will assist nurses to identify vulnerable groups and direct health promotion efforts toward them. As colonialism's effects are recognized in the development of mental health problems in First Nations communities, nurses are now challenged to advocate for policies that promote healing within the strengths and the challenges of First Nations communities. As cultural diversity increases within Canadian society, nurses will consider alternative ways of understanding MI. Perhaps most importantly, the Recovery Model will help nurses to focus on consumers' abilities to build meaningful lives and strengthen nurses' resolve to change the inequities that influence the mental well being of people living with MI. In conjunction with the newly formed Mental Health Commission of Canada, CMHNs can work towards increased national awareness of mental health issues and improved health and social outcomes for people and families living with mental illness.

KEY TERMS

deinstitutionalization
recovery model of rehabilitation
basket of community services
consumer
survivor
Canadian Mental Health Association (CMHA)
mental illness (MI)
mental health
mood disorders
bipolar illness
anxiety disorder
schizophrenia
serious mental illness (SMI)
co-occurring disorders
Mental Health Act
compulsory treatment orders
emergency services
case management
assertive community treatment (ACT)
acute home treatment
early intervention programs
mental health promotion
recovery model
Tidal Model of Mental Health Recovery
advocacy

INDIVIDUAL CRITICAL THINKING EXERCISES

1. What strategies might a community mental health nurse use to promote the mental health of elementary-school-age children?

2. How would a community mental health nurse implement the Tidal Model of Mental Health Recovery with a depressed client and his or her family?

3. Why do you think "people first" language (i.e., a person with schizophrenia rather than schizophrenic) is important?

GROUP CRITICAL THINKING EXERCISES

1. How might CMHNs ensure that the physical and mental health needs of people with MI are met within a primary health care clinic?

2. How might CMHNs influence and develop a national suicide prevention strategy?

3. How can the principles of recovery be implemented and researched within the mental health system?

REFERENCES

Allen, T. (2000). *Someone to talk to: Care and control of the homeless.* Halifax: Fernwood.

Anthony, W. A. (1993). Recovery from mental illness. The guiding vision of the mental health service system in the 1990s. *Psychiatric Rehabilitation Journal, 16*(4), 11–23.

Anthony, W. A. (2000). A recovery service system: Setting some systems level standards. *Psychiatric Rehabilitation Journal, 24*(2), 160–166.

Bezzina, A. (1996). *ACCESS: A framework for a community based mental health system.* Toronto: Canadian Mental Health Association, Ontario Division.

BC Partners for Mental Health and Addictions Information. (2006). Children, youth and mental disorders. *The Primer, 2006.* Retrieved May 23, 2007, from http://www. heretohelp.bc.ca/publications/factsheets/child_youth_ mentaldisorders.shtml.

British Columbia Ministry of Health. (2003). *Historical perspective: Mental health resource utilization in British Columbia (1997/98 to 1999/00). Prior to health authority restructuring in 2001.* Victoria: B.C. Ministry of Health Services.

Brookes, N. (2006). Tidal model of mental health recovery. In A. Marriner-Tomey & M. Raile-Alligood (Eds.), *Nursing theorists and their work* (6th ed.; pp. 696–725). St. Louis, MO: Elsevier-Mosby.

Canadian Mental Health Association. (2001). *Submission to the Commission on the Future of Health Care in Canada.* Retrieved May 23, 2007, from http://www.ontario.cmha. ca/content/reading_room/submissions.asp?cID=2590.

Canadian Federation of Mental Health Nurses. (2005). *Canadian standards of psychiatric and mental health nursing practice* (3rd ed.), Standards Committee of the Canadian Federation of Mental Health Nurses. Retrieved May 23, 2007, from http://www.cfmhn.ca/about_us.html.

Castellanos, D., & Hunter, T. (2000). Anxiety disorders in children and adolescents. *Southern Medical Journal, 92*(10), 946–954.

Clarke Institute of Psychiatry. (1997). *Best practices in mental health reform: Discussion paper.* Report prepared for the Federal/Provincial/Territorial Advisory Network on Mental Health.

Commission on the Future of Health Care in Canada. (2002). *Building on values: The future of health care in Canada.* Saskatoon: Commission on the Future of Health Care in Canada.

Cook, A., Spinazzola, J., Ford, J., Lanktree, C., Blaustein, M., Cloitre, M., et al. (2005). Complex trauma in children and adolescents. *Psychiatric Annals, 35*(6), 390–396.

Davis, S. (2006). *Community mental health in Canada: Policy, theory, practice.* Vancouver: University of British Columbia.

Eaton, W. (2001). *The sociology of mental disorders* (3rd ed.). Westport, CT: Praeger.

Goering, P., Wasylenki, D., & Durbin, J. (2000). Canada's mental health system. *International Journal of Law and Psychiatry, 23*(3–4), 345–359.

Government of Canada. (2006). *The human face of mental health and mental illness in Canada 2006.* Minister of Public Works and Government Services Canada, Cat. No. HP5-19/2006E. Retrieved May 23, 2007, from http:// www.phac-aspc.c.ca.

Hall, N. (2001). *Growing the problem: The second annual report of the mental health advocate of British Columbia.* Vancouver: Office of the Mental Health Advocate of British Columbia.

Health Canada. (2002). *A report on mental illness in Canada.* Ottawa: Health Canada.

Health Canada. (2003). *Acting on what we know: Preventing youth suicide in First Nations.* Retrieved May 23, 2007, from http://www.hc-sc.gc.ca/fnih-spni/pubs/suicide/prev_youth-jeunes/index_e.html.

Hinshaw, S. P. (2004). Parental mental disorder and children's functioning: Silence and communication, stigma and resilience. *Journal of Clinical Child and Adolescent Psychology, 33*(2), 400–411.

Jones, D. R., Macias, C., Barriers, P. J., Fisher, W. H., Hargreaves, W. A., & Harding, C. M. (2004). Prevalence, severity, and co-occurrence of chronic physical health problems of persons with serious mental illness. *Psychiatric Services, 55*(11), 1250–57.

Kenny, J. E. (2001). Mental illness: Cloaked in secrecy and shame. *Canadian Nurse, 97*(1), 20–24.

Kirby, M. J., & Keon, W. J. (2006). *Out of the shadows at last: Highlights and recommendations.* Senate, Final Report of the Standing Senate Committee on Social Affairs, Science and Technology.

Kowatch, R. A., & DelBello, M. P. (2005). Pharmacotherapy of children and adolescents with bipolar disorder. *Psychiatric Clinics of North America, 28*(2), 385–397.

Latimer, E. (2005). Organization implications of promotion effective evidence based interventions for people with severe MI. *Canadian Public Policy, 31,* Supplement: S47–S52.

Libin, K. (2007). March 7. All eyes on mandatory care for mentally ill. *The National Citizen,* p. 7.

Lines, E. (2000). *An introduction to early psychosis intervention: Some relevant findings and emerging practices.* Retrieved May 23, 2007 from http://www.cmha.ca/data/1/rec_docs/162_introdoc.pdf.

Mental Health Act. (2002). *RSO 1990 Chapter M7.* Retrieved May 23, 2007, from http://www.e-laws.gov.on.ca/DBLaws/Statutes/English/90m07_e.htm.

Martsolf, D. S., & Draucker, C. B. (2005). *Issues in Mental Health Nursing, 26,* 801–825.

McEwan, K., & Goldner, E. (2001). *Accountability and Performance indicators for mental health sciences and supports: A resource kit.* Ottawa: Health Canada.

Mental Health Act. (2002). *RSO 1990 Chapter M7.* Retrieved May 23, 2007, from http://www.e-laws.gov.on.ca/DBLaws/Statutes/English/90m07_e.htm.

Mental Health Commission of Canada. (2007). *The Mental Health Commission of Canada.* Retrieved July 19, 2007, from http://www.mentalhealthcommission.ca/mhcc.html.

Ministry of Children and Family Development. (2003). *News release: New Children's Mental Health Plan First in Canada.*

Mordoch, E. (1995). *Cope: Care of psychiatric emergencies. A short term emergency project.* Unpublished report.

Mordoch, E., & Hall, W. (2002). Children living with a parent who has a MI: A critical analysis of the literature and research implications. *Archives of Psychiatric Nursing, XVI*(5), 208–216.

Morrison, I. L., & L'Heureux. (2001). Suicide and gay, lesbian and bisexual youth. Implications for clinicians. *Journal of Adolescence, 24,* 39–49.

National Council of Welfare. (2006). *Welfare incomes* 2005. Retrieved October 5, 2007, from http://dsp-psd.pwgsc.gc.ca/Collection/SD25-2-2005E.pdf.

Nicholson, J., & Biebel, K. (2002). Commentary on "Community mental health care for women with severe mental illness who are parents": The tragedy of missed opportunities: What providers can do. *Community Mental Health Journal, 38*(2), 167–172.

Nolan, P. W. (1993). A history of the training of asylum nurses. *Journal of Advanced Nursing, 18*(8), 1193–201.

Pevalin, D. J., & Goldberg, D. P. (2003). Social precursors of onset and recovery from episodes of common mental illness. *Psychological Medicine, 33*(2), 299–306.

Russel, S. T., & Joyner, K. (2001). Adolescent sexual orientation and suicide risk. Evidence from a nation study. *American Journal of Public Health, 9*(8), 1276–1281.

Rutter, M., Pickles, A., Murray, R., & Eaves, L. (2001). Testing hypotheses on specific environmental causal effects on behavior. *Psychological Bulletin, 127,* 291–324.

Southern Alberta Geriatric Mental Health Working Group. (2003). *Summary report of the Southern Alberta Geriatric Mental Health Working Group.* Calgary, Alberta, 1–12.

Speed, E. (2006) Patients, consumers and survivors: A case study of mental health service user discourses. *Social Science and Medicine, 62,* 28–38.

Statistics Canada. (2002). *Canadian Community Health Survey: Mental health and well-being.* Retrieved July 6, 2007, from http://www.statcan.ca/bsolc/english/bsolc?catno=82-617-X&CHROPG=1.

Sussman, S. (1998). The first asylums in Canada: A response to neglectful community care and current trends. *Canadian Journal of Psychiatry, 43,* 260–264.

Waddell, C., McEwan, K., Hau, J., & Shepherd, C. (2002). *Child and youth mental health: Population health and clinical service considerations.* Vancouver: Mental Health Evaluation and Community Consultation Unit, British Columbia.

Waddell, C., & Sheppard, C. (2002). *Prevalence of mental disorders in children and youth.* Mental Health Evaluation and Community Consultation Unit, University of British Columbia.

Warner, V., Weissman, M., Fendrich, M., Wickmarante, P., & Moreau, D. (1992). The course of major depression in the offspring of depressed parents, Incidence, recurrence and recovery. *Archives of General Psychiatry, 49,* 795–801.

Wilton, R. (2003). Poverty and mental health: A qualitative study of residential care facility clients. *Canadian Journal of Community Mental Health, 39,* 139–156.

World Health Organization. (1999). *The world health report 1999: Chapter 2.* Geneva, Switzerland: Author. Retrieved May 23, 2007, from http://www.who.int/whr/1999/en/index.html

World Health Organization. (2001). *The world health report 2001. Mental health: New understanding, new hope.* Retrieved May 23, 2007, from http://www.who.int/whr/2001/en/index.html.

World Health Organization. (2002). *The world health report 2002. Reducing risks, promoting health life.* Retrieved May 23, 2007, from http://www.who.int/whr/2002/en/index.html.

ADDITIONAL RESOURCES

Film

The Interventionist: Chronicles of a Mental Health Crisis Team. (2006). National Film Board of Canada.

Websites

Anxiety Disorders Association of Canada
www.anxietycanada.ca

Canadian Federation of Mental Health Nurses
www.cfmhn.ca

Canadian Mental Health Association
www.cmha.ca

Canadian Psychiatric Research Foundation
www.cprf.ca

Health Canada, Mental Health
www.hc-sc.gc.ca/hl-vs/mental/index_e.html

Mental Health Commission of Canada
www.mentalhealthcommission.ca

Mood Disorders Society of Canada
www.mooddisorderscanada.ca

National Network for Mental Health
www.nnmh.ca

Schizophrenia Society of Canada
www.schizophrenia.ca

About the Author

Elaine Mordoch, RN, PhD (University of Manitoba), has been passionate about psychiatric/mental health nursing throughout her nursing career. She has practised as a primary nurse in acute psychiatry and facilitated groups for the well elderly living with depression and women identifying abuse in their relationships. She has developed and managed COPE (Care of Psychiatric Emergencies) for a tertiary hospital general emergency unit with a focus on family care and intermediate follow-up services. Her dissertation topic was Perceptions of Children Living with a Parent with a Mental Illness, a grounded theory study on how children perceived and managed living with a parent with an MI. She is also interested in the long-term effects of childhood sexual abuse on adult survivors. Currently she teaches psychiatric/mental health nursing and counselling skills in the Faculty of Nursing and in the Aboriginal Focus Programs at the University of Manitoba.

Judith Kulig, Martha MacLeod, Norma Stewart, and Roger Pitblado

OBJECTIVES

After studying this chapter, you should be able to:

1. Define and describe the meaning of rural in a Canadian context.

2. Investigate the impact of the rural context on the health status and access to care experienced by rural residents.

3. Identify the challenges associated with being a community resident in rural Canada.

4. Understand the context of rural nursing practice and its interrelationship with the care of clients in rural areas.

INTRODUCTION

This chapter introduces concepts relevant to caring for clients in rural areas. The character of rural and remote Canada is delineated, with an emphasis on diversity. The discussion provides a contextual understanding of clients who live in these areas and some of the practice characteristics of rural nurses. The rewards and challenges of rural nursing, including the key features of this practice, are identified and explained in depth. Sample questions enable opportunities for discussion and application of the materials presented.

THE CHARACTER OF RURAL/ REMOTE CANADA

Definitions

Approximately 95% of Canada's land mass, or 9.5 million square kilometres, consists of rural and remote areas (Public Health Agency of Canada, 2002). However, longstanding debate exists about the definitions of key terms including rural, remote, northern, and isolated. Pitblado (2005) has noted two main ways to define rural: technical and social.

Technical approaches to the definition of rural include locators or geographic regions, like the location of hospitals, roads, or specific political areas (i.e., provinces, counties). Statistics Canada (du Plessis, Beshiri, & Bollman, 2001) has examined six possible ways to define rural, with each emphasizing different criteria such as population size, population density, and settlement or labour market contexts. One example is the definition of "census rural," which refers to "individuals living in the countryside outside centres of 1000 or more population" (du Plessis et al., 2001, p. 6). Another example, from the Organisation of Economic Co-operation

and Development (OECD), is the definition of "rural communities" that include "individuals in communities with less than 150 persons per square kilometre" (du Plessis et al., p. 6).

Other technical definitions focus on distances and interrelated features to define rural. In practice disciplines such as nursing and medicine, a common application of this approach is to use degrees of rurality for the purposes of financial reimbursement for working in isolated locations. For example, the First Nations and Inuit Health Branch (FNIHB) within Health Canada (2005a) uses the following designations for that purpose:

1. *Non-isolated community* includes communities with road access less than 90 kilometres to physician services;

2. *Semi-isolated community* includes communities with road access greater than 90 kilometres to physician services;

3. *Isolated community* refers to communities with good telephone service, scheduled air transportation flights but no roads; and

4. *Remote, isolated community* means the communities have no scheduled air flights, minimal telephone or radio access, and no roads.

Examination of the FNIHB designations highlights the importance of access to services and the types of locally available health services. Transportation and communication limitations are important factors in their differentiation. A wide variety of indices of rurality exist, such as the Canadian General Practice Rurality Index (Leduc, 1997) or the Rurality Index of Ontario (Kralj, 2001). Many of these indices are based on point systems that give various weights to characteristics such as the number of family physicians in a community, availability of physician specialists, presence and characteristics of the nearest hospital, availability of ambulance services, and so on. Many of these indices of rurality are of theoretical value as they have never been put into operation. And almost all of them have been designed with physicians in mind—not nurses.

Defining "north" and "remote" is equally complicated because there has been an assumption that these terms are naturally equated with the 50th parallel, with no rationale for its selection. However, there is considerable variation in this definition as well. For example, one of the national research funding organizations refers to northern as "north of the southern limit of sporadic discontinuous permafrost" (Northern Research Development Program, 2006, n.p.). This definition is not equivalent with the 50th parallel, but instead represents a jagged line that varies by province while including the three territories (Atlas of Canada, 2006).

Social approaches to define rural refer to the nature of the rural community, with such features as specific services that are normally associated with larger population sizes (e.g., specific types of stores or restaurants) (Pitblado, 2005). Although this social nature of place in defining rural is relevant to health care service delivery, particularly the recruitment and retention of health professionals including registered nurses (RNs), there has been limited work done on examination of its specific meaning.

The population that Statistics Canada designates as "rural and small town" refers to those "individuals in towns or municipalities outside the commuting zone of larger urban centres" (du Plessis et al., 2001, p. 6). Using this definition, 20% of Canadians are rural and live in communities with populations of less than 10 000 people. This is the definition of rural employed in this chapter. It was selected because of its growing use in studies of a wide variety of rural issues in Canada, including the determinants of health and the delivery of health care.

Diversity of Rural

Rural economies vary by the specific geographic features of the land itself. Hence, rural communities may be dependent upon natural resources that permit oil exploration, forestry, fishing, or farming activities. Of late, some rural communities are becoming increasingly dependent upon alternative economic ventures such as tourism because of changes in the local economy and the inability to financially survive solely on natural resources, the prices of which are highly influenced by global markets. Rural Canada is not homogenous. Therefore, this chapter provides examples from a variety of natural-resource rural communities rather than generalizing to one type of rural community. It is incumbent on nurses to determine the socioeconomic context of the rural community within which they work.

The geographic **diversity of rural** communities influences the types of services available (i.e., ability to access roads, telephones, satellite transmission), while the economy of the rural community has an impact on the cycle of activities within the community. Thus, during seeding and harvest within an agricultural community, there is less opportunity for RNs to work with groups or the entire community on health promotion activities. The type of natural resource base emphasized in the community will also influence health status. For example, in 2001 there were 346 000 farm operators across Canada (Statistics Canada, 2004b). Of this total, the most common reported injuries were fractures (21%), followed by open wounds (19%) and nerve or spinal cord injuries (14.7%) (Statistics Canada, 2003). Operators on medium-sized farms had the highest incidence of injury because they worked the longest hours without reliance on hired help in comparison to those on the largest farms (Statistics Canada, 2003).

Being Rural

Although there has been some discussion about whether there is a "type" of rural person, emphasizing such notions can lead to generalizations and inaccurate descriptions of the variety of people who live in rural settings. It is more useful for nursing practice to discuss the intersection between living rural and the meanings of health and health status.

Rural residents have been the focus of studies examining the meaning of health. Some of the original research conducted among both women and men in different rural geographic locations in the United States has indicated that good health is associated with being able to work and perform one's expected duties (Long, 1993). More recent research that focused on the health beliefs of rural Canadians in two western provinces found that being healthy was defined as having a holistic relationship among mental, social, physical, and spiritual aspects (Thomlinson, McDonagh, Baird Crooks, & Lees, 2004). The participants differentiated sickness as a curable and short-term condition, whereas illness was chronic and life-threatening. Practitioners were encouraged to build a trusting relationship with rural residents and examine their health complaints in a holistic manner.

Other research with rural residents focuses specifically on their health status, examining differences in disease patterns and occurrences. For example, one study found a lower proportion of those living in small-town regions, rural regions, and northern regions who rate their health as excellent. Specific conditions such as arthritis are higher than the national average among rural regions and those in northern regions had a higher prevalence of hypertension (Mitura & Bollman, 2003). Another recent study (DesMeules et al., 2006) that examined health status and health determinants among the rural population found that:

- Rural areas reported higher proportions of people with low income and less than secondary education level. On the other hand, a strong sense of community belonging was reported by rural residents in greater proportions than by their urban counterparts.
- Health-related factors, such as the prevalence of smoking and obesity, were elevated in rural Canada, while analyses of other health influences, such as dietary practices and leisure-time physical activity, indicated lower practice levels in rural areas.
- Life expectancy at birth was significantly higher in urban areas.
- Higher overall mortality risks among rural communities appear to be driven by higher death rates from such causes as circulatory diseases, injuries, and suicide; residents of the most rural areas are often at highest risk.
- Incidence rates of most cause-specific cancers were lower in rural areas.
- Respiratory disease mortality risks were for the most part significantly higher among rural residents.
- Women living in the most rural areas had higher risks of dying from diabetes.
- The importance of disease prevention and health promotion is well recognized in public health and clinical settings. What is less clear is whether conventional strategies, mostly developed by urban program planners for urban residents, are equally effective in rural settings.

Unique Groups of People in Rural Areas

In addition to unique geographic features that affect the livelihood and everyday life cycle of rural residents, a number of **unique groups** of people live in rural areas. For many of these groups, challenges are inherent in being diverse and living in a rural environment. Thus, some may feel excluded, whereas others want to live separate from larger society and prefer rural living where they can co-exist with other groups but not be expected to interact with others. It is part of the role for nurses to assess the rural community within which they live to determine its diversity and the strengths or needs that arise from such diversity. Many groups could be included for further discussion in this chapter; however, the emphasis is on Aboriginal people and unique religious groups, including the Amish, Hutterites, Mennonites, and Conservative Dutch. Discussing these groups in some detail provides the opportunity to examine the intersection between diversity and living rural with implications for nursing practice, while also providing examples of how to work with other diverse groups. General principles in relation to assessing and caring for multicultural clients are identified in Chapter 20. Other diverse groups live in rural settings, but this chapter will not discuss them in detail. For example, individuals with alternative lifestyles or sexual orientations may experience challenges when living in rural settings. The complexity of their situations is beyond the scope of this chapter but needs to be considered by rural nurses who may encounter such individuals in their practice.

Identifying unique groups in rural areas is important for the development and implementation of appropriate nursing care. However, accurate statistics regarding the number of these groups living in rural areas are usually not available. In general, few databases exist that provide community-specific demographic profiles of rural populations. Thus, an accurate picture of rural residents, including their health status, is often not readily available. Although precise statistics may be lacking, it is essential for rural nurses to be aware of the diversity of the rural population and the implications it has for health status and provision of health services.

Aboriginal People Aboriginal people includes First Nations, Métis, and Inuit groups. (See Chapter 21.) In 2001, there were 976 305 Aboriginal people in Canada (Statistics Canada, 2004a). Aboriginal people are increasingly becoming urban dwellers, with projections of 457 000 living in urban settings by 2016 (Statistics Canada, 2005). Despite these projections, many continue, and will continue, to live in rural settings on or off-reserve. For example, 43% of First Nations communities have fewer than 500 residents, and only 11% have more than 2000 residents. Consequently, in order to provide appropriate care nurses working in such settings need to understand the historical context of Aboriginal people; their health care issues; the policy context of health care delivery, including the transfer of health services to local control (Kulig et al., 2003); and the challenges and rewards of working with Aboriginal

people. In addition, the strategic initiatives to increase the numbers of Aboriginal RNs in Canada provide an opportunity for non-Aboriginal RNs to learn about working with Aboriginal people (McBride & Gregory, 2005).

Aboriginal people have a number of specific health issues related to the social determinants of health (i.e., inadequate housing and water; lack of infrastructure supports on-reserve; and inadequate social supports within family units). Highlights of their health status include:

- Life expectancy at birth for Registered Indians is 68.9 years for males and 76.6 for females (Health Canada, 2005b);
- First Nations birth rate (23.4%) is twice as high as the Canadian rate, with 1 out of 5 births involving teenage First Nations mothers (Health Canada, 2005b);
- The most common causes of death among First Nations aged 1 to 44 years are injury and poisoning (Health Canada, 2006);
- Suicide and self-injury remain the leading causes of death for youth (aged 15–24) and adults (aged 25–64) (Health Canada, 2005b);
- Type 2 diabetes occurrence is 2 to 3 times higher, and tuberculosis infections are 8 to 10 times higher, among First Nations (Health Canada, 2006).

Unique Religious Groups Unique religious populations who live predominantly in rural communities include the Anabaptist groups, specifically the Amish, Hutterites, and Mennonites. Each of these three groups has its own particular lifestyle based upon the desire to have the freedom to live according to religious principles with no interference by governmental intervention. All three live by the principles of adult baptism, pacifism, and separation from the physical world. In addition, they also emphasize a literal interpretation of the Bible. Most of the members of these groups work in the agricultural sector. Hutterites in Canada number 28 020 (Statistics Canada, 2005), with the majority residing in Alberta, Manitoba, and Saskatchewan, respectively. The Hutterites live a communal lifestyle with each member contributing through specific duties such as cooking or animal husbandry. Conservative Mennonites in Canada number 57 000 (Janzen, 2004). This group is more often referred to as the Low-German-Speaking Mennonites; they represent individuals and families whose ancestors lived in Canada but moved to Mexico and other Central and South American countries in the 1920s (Bensen, 1998; DeLuca & Krahn, 1998; Sawatzky, 1971). For religious and economic reasons they are now returning to Canada, mainly Alberta, Manitoba, and Ontario, where many of them live according to a strict interpretation of the Bible (dictating that, for example, they cannot use devices such as radios). Their religious beliefs impact their health knowledge and behaviours, including the silence surrounding child bearing that prohibits the sharing of information about this important life transition (Kulig, Babcock, Wall, & Hill, 2006) and the belief that alcoholism is a spiritual illness caused by a straying away from God (Kulig & Hall, 2004). Another unique religious group is the Conservative Dutch, who are also predominantly agricultural-based and live according to a traditional interpretation of the Bible. Variations within all of these groups exist and thus it would not be appropriate to generalize from one Hutterite, Mennonite, or Conservative Dutch family to another. However, generally speaking, literacy levels can be low among these groups and hence specifically targeted health teaching approaches need to be developed to ensure concepts are understood and can be applied. There are also specific health issues that are more common in each of these groups. Among Hutterites heart disease is common due to their high-fat and -caloric diet; genetic disorders are also not uncommon among them because of the close relationship between spouses (Brunt, 1998). Such diseases as diabetes, autoimmune disorders (i.e., rheumatoid arthritis), and congenital malformations (i.e., inborn errors of metabolism) have been found as disease clusters among Conservative Mennonites because of their close genetic relationships (Jaworski et al., 1988). Immunization is not accepted among many Conservative Dutch families because they believe that immunizations challenge the will of God, who is ultimately responsible for a child's life (Kulig, Meyer, Hill, Handley, Lichtenberger, & Myck, 2002).

The Challenges Experienced by Rural Communities

Several challenges are faced by rural communities and their residents in Canada. It is commonly acknowledged that the population of rural Canada is increasing only in predominantly rural regions that are within commuting distance of large urban areas (du Plessis et al., 2001). Thus, many more-distant rural areas are experiencing an out-migration of all age groups (Rothwell, Bollman, Tremblay, & Marshall, 2002). Generally speaking, there are fewer individuals to contribute to the functioning of the community. Youth migration out of rural communities has escalated, thus further decreasing the community's future workers and residents (Tremblay, 2001). There is less infrastructure in rural communities, thus resources such as retail businesses and health care delivery services are more limited. Rural communities are more often dependent upon a limited range of economic opportunities; boom and bust cycles play into this, leading to an overall decreased availability of employment for individuals. Finally, there is a perception of a loss of political voice within the rural regions of Canada, decreasing the sense of independence and autonomy for which rural residents are often known (Government of Canada, 1998).

All of these challenges have impacts on health status in general and on health care delivery in particular. For example, the loss of youth and economic opportunities in rural communities leads to fewer individuals available to provide care to elderly parents and other relatives. In communities that are dependent on oil and gas extraction, there may be many single men or young families with few supports. Therefore, nursing practice needs to be designed to specifically address the particular situation in each rural community.

THE REALITIES OF RURAL NURSING PRACTICE

Although all graduates of nursing programs in Canada are prepared for a generalist role, working with clients in rural communities as a nurse stretches the meaning of being a generalist. Primarily, this is due to the wide range of practice demands on nurses in small communities. It is compounded by the statistical profile of rural RNs discussed below. However, it is also due to several key issues that are particularly at play for rural RNs. These issues include **leadership, quality work environments, education for rural settings,** and **policy issues for rural environments.** Each of these is subsequently discussed in depth.

Statistics

Recent analyses (Canadian Institute for Health Information [CIHI], 2002; MacLeod, Kulig, Stewart, Pitblado, & Knock, 2004; Pitblado, 2005) of the Registered Nurses Database (RNDB) reveal that there were 41 500 RNs working in rural Canada in 2000, a 2% decline from 1994. While the absolute numbers of rural RNs has declined, the population of rural Canada in absolute terms has increased. The majority were female (95.6%), with 50.3% working full time. Like their urban counterparts, rural RNs are aging. The average age of a rural RN in 2000 was 42.9 years, representing an increase since 1994 when it was 40.6 years. In 2000, 9.2% of rural RNs graduated with a bachelor's degree. However, 18.5% of rural RNs have achieved this degree as their highest level of education. When comparing rural and urban RNs, rural RNs have achieved lower levels of education at entry to practice and throughout their nursing careers.

Nurse-to-client ratios vary by rural region, but on average there were 62 nurses per 10 000 in rural Canada compared to 78 per 10 000 in urban Canada. There is also an east to west trend, with higher nurse-to-population ratios in Eastern Canada. One hundred and sixty-nine rural communities were identified as being served by only one RN (CIHI, 2002). In 54 of these communities, the nurse was under 30 years of age with limited experience in nursing. Higher proportions of rural RNs are employed in community settings (12.7%) compared with their urban counterparts (7.8%).

The national survey on nursing practice in rural and remote Canada had a 69% response rate ($N = 3933$) from RNs working in rural and remote regions across Canada (Stewart et al., 2005a). The demographic findings from the survey revealed that the majority of the sample were female (94.8%), between the ages of 35 and 54 (66.6%), married or living with a partner (81%), and living with one or more dependent child or relative (58%) (Stewart, D'Arcy, Pitblado, Forbes, et al., 2005b). Just over 5% ($n = 210$) of RN respondents indicated they were of First Nations or Métis ancestry (Stewart, Kulig, Penz, et al., 2006). In this 2001–2002 survey, 27% of rural RNs had a bachelor's degree in nursing, compared to 18% rural (23.8% urban) in 2000 and 12.5% rural (17.6% urban) in 1994 (CIHI, 2002). Their primary areas of nursing practice were acute care (39%), long term care (17%), community health (14%), home care (8%), and primary care (7%), and another 16% were in other areas such as administration, education, research, and government. Although 34% of RN respondents in the survey thought of their role as advanced nursing practice, only 4.3% were in nurse practitioner positions (Stewart & MacLeod, 2005).

Key Features of Rural Nursing

Regardless of primary work setting, all rural nurses are faced with the issues discussed below, which impact the care of rural clients. The context of rural communities plays a role in these issues because there is greater professional isolation, the need for nurses to take on multiple roles, a blurring of professional and personal boundaries, and the challenges of contending with a lack of infrastructure and resources, including a limited range of available transportation and communication services. In addition, unlike their urban counterparts in acute care settings, rural nurses care for clients of all ages with a variety of health concerns (Bushy, 2000).

Leadership In the narrative component of the study "The Nature of Nursing Practice in Rural and Remote Canada," almost all nurses talked about issues related to nursing leadership (MacLeod & Ulrich, 2005). Issues included finding ways of working through conflicting priorities, coping with having leaders at a distance, and creating support networks. Leadership was more effective when leaders set up possibilities for quality practice, even in situations of few resources. When leaders planned for the realities of rural practice, nurses felt supported. For nursing leaders, providing the appropriate support at a distance was a challenge; for nurses, seeking and accepting that support was equally challenging. Both nursing managers and nurses needed to work creatively within organizations that did not always understand the realities of their practice.

Quality Work Environments Creating quality work environments in rural practice settings is particularly challenging. A central challenge is that many nurses in rural settings work alone all the time (Andrews, Stewart, Pitblado, Morgan Forbes, & D'Arcy, 2005) or with few colleagues during much of their everyday work. Thorough orientations that include discussion about working alone and safety issues when entering homes or travelling on isolated roads also need to be conducted. A strategy for developing a quality work environment in rural or remote practice includes developing consistent expectations and approaches among managers and nurses to address practice issues at the site level. This includes relevant rural practice standards; policies and practices that support rural nurses' scope of practice; practice-driven, rural-focused nursing education programs; rural reality–based preceptorship and mentorship programs; and the development of sustained processes for direct rural nursing involvement in local and regional planning (Ulrich & MacLeod, 2005).

Nursing Education for Rural/Remote Environments Few documents address the unique educational needs that would assist nurses to work in rural communities. Some of the documents that are available automatically equate remote practice with First Nations health issues or with the need for advanced nursing practice (i.e., nurse practitioners). Although First Nations communities often are in rural or remote areas, it is inappropriate to assume that such locations do not include other groups of people who have unique health needs due to their geographic location. For example, many agricultural and mining communities exist in rural and remote areas, where individuals experience occupational health problems, such as lung disorders, that require health professionals who understand the specific disease processes and the challenges of providing care despite the limited resources in the community. Still other documents emphasize the nursing standards but leave them in a generic format without specific comments about implementing the standards in a rural environment (Manitoba Association of Registered Nurses [MARN], 2000).

In the past, some documents that discussed nursing education focused on addressing accessibility to nursing education by reducing geographic barriers (College of Nurses of Ontario, as cited in Nursing Association of New Brunswick [NANB], 1997) rather than specifically highlighting the need for nurses who can address the challenges of rural nursing practice.

A few nursing programs in Canada are rural-focused due to their geographic location. Examples include the University of Lethbridge, the University of Northern British Columbia, and the University of Saskatchewan, which include rural placements and theoretical content related to rural nursing. Other programs include Aurora College in the Northwest Territories and the Nunavut Arctic College, which partners with Dalhousie University to offer a four-year collaborative degree program. All of these nursing programs are locally available, addressing the geographic barriers for those who wish to pursue an education experience. However, these programs also incorporate information that is specifically pertinent to providing care in their locale.

Canadian Research Box 19.1

MacLeod, M., Kulig, J., Stewart, N., Pitblado, R., Knock, M. (2004). The nature of nursing practice in rural and remote Canada. *The Canadian Nurse, 100*(6), 27–31.

A three-year multiple-method study was conducted to examine the nature of nursing practice in rural and remote Canada (MacLeod et al., 2004; MacLeod, Kulig, Stewart, & Pitblado, 2004). A research team of four co-principal investigators, 13 co-investigators, and 27 advisory team

→

members received funding from more than 20 funders to examine and articulate the nature of registered nursing practice in primary care, acute care, community health, continuing care (home care), and long term care settings within rural and remote Canada.

Four complementary research approaches were simultaneously employed in the study. The analysis of the Registered Nurses Database (RNDB) provided a demographic profile of rural RNs for the first time for the individual provinces and territories and for Canada as a whole (CIHI, 2002). A documentary analysis of 159 administrative and policy documents allowed for a critical analysis of the policy context within which rural RNs work (Kulig et al., 2003). A national survey of 3933 rural RNs collected information on variables such as the quality of their work life, satisfaction with their community life, and intent to pursue additional education or employment (Stewart et al., 2005b). Finally, narratives were generated from 152 nurses who provided in-depth discussion about being a rural nurse in a variety of practice settings and geographic areas across Canada. The data from each of these research approaches were analyzed and provide an in-depth understanding of rural and remote nursing practice.

Major findings from the study include: (1) there is a need for further analysis of the meaning of the terms rural and remote—the reliance on technical definitions for these terms does not adequately depict the experience of being a rural RN; (2) the supply of rural RNs does not match the demands of this particular geographic setting; (3) there is limited attention paid to the unique educational needs for practising in rural areas; (4) the complexity of rural nursing practice is poorly understood and acknowledged; (5) out-migration has a dramatic negative impact on the supply of RNs in many rural communities (Pitblado, Medves, & Stewart, 2005). Some implications include (1) the need for a rural lens to assist in the development and implementation of relevant policies and programs; (2) creation of undergraduate and postgraduate education programs to prepare RNs to work in rural settings; (3) development of interprofessional models of practice to support rural communities; and (4) creation of recruitment and retention strategies that address work and community satisfaction concerns identified by rural RNs.

Discussion Questions:

1. As a rural nurse, what are some strategies you could put in place to deal with the realities of working in a smaller facility?

2. What are the challenges of developing and implementing interprofessional models of practice for health professionals who work in rural communities?

Research with rural nurses has provided some direction about the specific needs for nurses who want to work in rural communities (MacLeod et al., 2004). Two themes exist: (1) program curriculum issues including the use of reality-based cases that highlight rural health and offer at least part of the curriculum in rural settings, and (2) infrastructure program supports including incorporating telehealth education into universities to help prepare nurses to work in this mode of delivery; additional financial support for educational institutions that prepare rural nurses and mentoring programs in the workplace that help with the transition of new graduates in rural and remote communities (MacLeod et al., 2004). Other studies among rural health care professionals in Canada (Curran, Fleet, & Kirby, 2006; Penz, D'Arcy, Stewart, Kosteniuk, Morgan, & Smith, 2007) and New Zealand (Janes, Arrol, Buetow, Coster, McCormick, & Hague, 2005) acknowledge workplace issues including lack of access to computers as a barrier to continuing education and learning.

Although the internet is commonly thought of as a solution for continuing education for individuals who live in rural communities, one recent Canadian study has shown that internet use is not common among rural nurses as an avenue to locate information (Kosteniuk, D'Arcy, Stewart, & Smith, 2006). Rural and remote RNs were more likely to use information sources central to their own work environment (e.g., colleagues, in-service) than peripheral sources such as the internet or library. This study also found, however, that nurses who had more recently graduated and were in positions of authority or in multiple positions that required ongoing research use, and who had been employed fewer than five years, had significantly greater odds of using the internet (Kosteniuk et al.). We can therefore anticipate that more recent graduates of nursing programs who are employed by workplaces that emphasize the need for evidence-based practice and provide infrastructure support for technology would be more amenable to accessing continuing education over the internet.

Case Study

The Gibbons family lives on their family farm 90 km east of a small city (population 68 000). After completing high school at the local community school, Nancy and John were married in the Anglican Church. Nancy is now 45 and John is 46. Nancy has been an active mother, raising their three sons while also volunteering in the community. John and his son Peter work on the farm together, which has been in the family for two generations. The older two sons, Jack and Ian, live and work in cities that are 3 hours and 5 hours, respectively, from the family farm. Both Jack and Ian are married and have children. Their jobs, family life, and other responsibilities mean that they are not able to visit on the farm very often.

Nancy has had an uneventful health history; she had regular physical examinations and three normal pregnancies. A few years ago she had a hysterectomy, and from a health perspective was expecting to enjoy retirement with her husband and their sons, daughters-in-law, and grandchildren. About a year ago, Nancy began to feel "unwell." She was tired, shaky, and having difficulties sleeping. Four months ago, tests revealed that she had amyotrophic lateral sclerosis (ALS), a terminal condition for which there is no cure.

She was referred to home care for assessment, but John refused to have them in the home and instead has provided all care to Nancy. The ALS Society was notified by home care about Nancy's diagnosis and has called and offered to visit and assist in any way possible. John would agree only after Peter convinced his mother and father that it could be helpful. While the ALS Society was at the home, John expressed his frustration at his wife's deteriorating condition and related he was unsure if he could continue providing care by himself. Nancy is now dependent upon John to bathe her, assist her with feeding, and transfer her to the toilet. She is also frequently in pain, and due to the muscle weakness is at risk for falls. Depression has set in and Nancy has said that "life is not worth living." At the same time, she wants to die peacefully at the farm and does not want to be moved into the city hospital. John is increasingly upset about his wife's condition and appears overwhelmed and bewildered; he realizes he needs support to continue to care for Nancy in their home.

It takes some time but John finally agrees to have a home care nurse return, do another assessment, and set up equipment resources such as oxygen and personal care aides on a routine basis. The home care nurse also refers the family to the palliative care nurse. Peter calls his brothers and asks that they come home to visit their mother as soon as possible.

Discussion Questions

1. Describe the roles and responsibilities of a home care and palliative care nurse in this case study.

2. Identify three factors related to living in a rural setting that provide challenges in the delivery of nursing care for Nancy Gibbons. Identify how a home care nurse could address these factors.

3. Identify three rural community factors that could provide assistance to the Gibbons family. Identify how a home care nurse could incorporate these factors into a care plan for Nancy.

Source: This case study is a modified version from the Nursing Education in Southern Alberta (NESA) problem-based curriculum used by the collaborative partners The University of Lethbridge and Lethbridge Community College.

Policy Issues in Rural/Remote Environments Most policies in Canada, with health policies being no exception, are based upon an urban perspective with little consideration of their applicability in rural environments. In order for this situation to be changed, the following key issues need to be addressed:

- Having a specific individual champion in Canada that focuses on the importance of addressing the unique situation experienced by rural residents would be beneficial.

- Few RNs are educationally prepared for work in the policy arena (Kulig, Nahachewsky, Thomlinson, MacLeod, & Curran, 2004), and although nurse educators have been encouraged to include information about the policy cycle and its application in their curriculum (Murphy, 1999) it will be some time before any change is realized.

- Relevant information about the nature of rural communities, including the number and location of rural residents and their health issues, is not readily available. Some organizations are lobbying to have this altered (e.g., Canadian Rural Health Research Society).

- The perspectives of rural residents and their involvement in setting the policy agenda, even at their local level, needs to be acknowledged and respected as a key component of rural development (Morton, Glasgow, & Johnson, 2004). Rural RNs have a key role in helping this to transpire (Kulig et al., 2004).

Summary

This chapter has focused on the unique nature of caring for clients in rural areas. Precise definitions of rural are lacking and need to include both technical and social characteristics. Rural residents experience challenges including depopulation, distance to services, and the need to develop local initiatives. Nurses who practise in rural areas would benefit from educational supports including continuing education by distance and the development of appropriate work expectations given the rural settings. Many diverse groups within rural Canada offer opportunities for a rewarding nursing practice.

KEY TERMS

technical approaches
social approaches
diversity of rural
unique groups
leadership
quality work environments
education for rural settings
policy issues for rural environments

INDIVIDUAL CRITICAL THINKING EXERCISES

1. Examine the provincial or territorial nursing standards related to professional boundaries and identify three challenges in the provision of care within rural communities. As a professional registered nurse, how would you address the challenges without jeopardizing ethical standards and professional boundaries?

2. Jacob Hofer is a 56-year-old Hutterite colony boss who is experiencing chest pains and fatigue. Consider his unique religious background and lifestyle as well as his rural

agricultural setting and outline three nursing strategies that can be implemented in his care plan. One of these strategies needs to reflect an interprofessional practice perspective.

GROUP CRITICAL THINKING EXERCISES

1. You work part-time as a public health nurse in a two-nurse office in a rural community. The other nurse works full time. You are both responsible for implementing the full range of public health programs. Because of the difficulty in finding casual replacements over the last two months, you deferred your vacation and have worked more than full time. You have just received a call that the full-time nurse has gone on sick leave. As your manager, who works 200 km away, tells you this, she adds that the Medical Health Officer has identified two TB cases in your community. Your manager asks you to work overtime again. You are debating what your answer should be. As a group:

   a. Identify the personal and professional concerns you would face in this situation.

   b. Identify the dilemmas being faced by the public health administration.

   c. Identify the potential impacts on client and community safety.

   d. Identify strategies, including ones that reflect interprofessional practice, to address the above concerns.

2. You are the new community nurse in an outpost setting on a transferred Aboriginal reserve. Two other nurses are stationed at the centre but they are from the community and live with their spouses away from the station. You are the only nurse who works at the outpost accommodation. This particular community (population of 545) is fly-in only with interruptions of flight service due to inclement weather. As a group:

a. Identify the priorities you would engage in as the new nurse.

b. Identify the process you would use to assess the community.

c. Identify how you would develop a relationship with the other nurses and community residents.

REFERENCES

Andrews, M. E., Stewart, N. J., Pitblado, J. R., Morgan, D. G., Forbes, D., & D'Arcy, C. (2005). Registered nurses working alone in rural and remote Canada. *Canadian Journal of Nursing Research, 37*(1), 14–33.

Atlas of Canada, Natural Resources Canada. (2006). Retrieved July 27, 2006, from http://atlas.nrcan.gc.ca/site/english/maps/environment/land/permafrost.

Bensen, J. (1998). Protective retreat: Mexico's Mennonites consider a new migration. *World and I, 13*(8), 1–6.

Brunt, H. (1998). Canadian Hutterites. In R. E. Davidhizar & J. N. Giger (Eds.), *Canadian transcultural nursing* (pp. 230–245). Toronto: Mosby.

Bushy, A. (2000). Analysis of rural nursing: Australia, Canada, United States. In A. Bushy (Ed.). *Orientation to nursing in the rural community* (pp. 233–242). Thousand Oaks, CA: Sage.

Canadian Rural Health Research Society. About Us. Retrieved October 8, 2007, from http://crhrs-scrsr.usask.ca/eng/aboutus/index.php.

Canadian Institute of Health Information. (2002). *Supply and distribution of registered nurses in rural and small town Canada, 2000.* Ottawa: Author.

Curran, V., Fleet, L., & Kirby, F. (2006). Factors influencing rural health care professionals' access to continuing professional education. *Australian Journal of Rural Health, 14*(2), 51–5.

DeLuca, S. A., & Krahn, M. A. (1998). Old Colony Mexican–Canadian Mennonites. In R. E. Davidhizar & J. N. Giger (Eds.), *Canadian transcultural nursing* (pp. 343–358). Toronto: Mosby.

DesMeules, M., Pong, R., Lagacé, C., Heng, D., Manuel, D., Pitblado, Bollman, R., Guernsey, J., Kazanjian A., & Koren, I. (2006). *How healthy are rural Canadians? An assessment of their health status and health determinants.* Ottawa: Canadian Population Initiative, Canadian Institute for Health Information.

du Plessis, V., Beshiri, & Bollman, R. (2001). Definitions of rural. *Rural and Small Town Analysis Bulletin, 3*(3) 1–17. #21-006-XIE. Ottawa: Statistics Canada. Available at stat-can.ca.

Government of Canada (1998). Rural Solutions to Rural Concerns. National Rural Workshop Final Report. Retrieved October 4, 2007, from http://www.rural.gc.ca/nrw/final_e.html.

Health Canada. (2005a). *Ten years of health transfer First Nation and Inuit control.* First Nations and Inuit Health Branch. Retrieved September 11, 2006, from http://www.hc-sc.gc.ca/fnih-spni/pubs/agree-accord/10_years_ans_trans/5_agreement-entente_e.html.

Health Canada. (2005b). *Statistical profile on the health of First Nations in Canada.* Retrieved September 7, 2006, from http://www.hc-sc.gc.ca/fnih-spni/pubs/gen/stats_profil_e.html.

Health Canada. (2006). *Diseases and health conditions.* Retrieved September 7, 2006, from http://www.hc-sc.gc.ca/fnih-spni/diseases-maladies/index_e.html.

Janes, R., Arroll, B., Buetow, S., Coster, G., McCormick, R., & Hague, I. (2005). Rural New Zealand health professionals' perceived barriers to greater use of the internet for learning. *Rural and Remote Health, 5*(4). Online. 11 pages.

Janzen, W. (2004). Welcoming the returning 'Kanadier' Mennonites from Mexico. *Journal of Mennonite Studies, 22,* 11-22.

Jaworski, M. A., Slater, J. D., Severini, A., Hennig, K. R., Mansour, G., Mehta, J. G., Jeske, R., Schlaut, J., Pak, C. Y., & Yoon, J.-W. (1998). Unusual clustering of diseases in a Canadian Old Colony (Chortitza) Mennonite kindred and community. *CMAJ, 138,* 1017–1025.

Kosteniuk, J., D'Arcy, Stewart, N., & Smith, B. (2006). Central and peripheral information source use among rural and remote Registered Nurses. *Journal of Advanced Nursing, 55*(1), 100–114.

Kralj, B. (2001). Measuring "rurality" for purposes of health-care planning: An empirical measure for Ontario. *Ontario Medical Review,* October, 33–52.

Kulig, J., Meyer, C., Hill, S., Handley, C., Lichtenberger, S., & Myck, S. (2002). Refusals and delay of immunization within southwest Alberta. *Canadian Journal of Public Health, 93*(2), 109–112 .

Kulig, J., Thomlinson, E., Curran, F., Nahachewsky, D., MacLeod, M., Stewart, N., & Pitblado, R. (2003). *Rural and Remote Nursing Practice: An Analysis of Policy Documents.* Lethbridge, AB: University of Lethbridge. R03–2003.

Kulig, J., & Hall, B. (2004). Health and illness beliefs among southern Alberta Kanadier Mennonites. *Journal of Mennonite Studies, 22,* 185–204.

Kulig, J., Nahachewsky, D., Thomlinson, E., MacLeod, M., & Curran, F. (2004). Maximizing the involvement of rural nurses in policy. *Nursing Leadership, 17*(1), 88–96.

Kulig, J., Babcock, R., Wall, M., Hill, S. (2006). *Growing up as a woman: The health perspectives of low-German-speaking Mennonite women.* Lethbridge, AB: University of Lethbridge.

Leduc, E. (1997). Defining rurality: A general practice rurality index for Canada. *Canadian Journal of Rural Medicine, 2*(2), 125–134.

Long, K. (1993). The concept of health: Rural perspectives. *Nursing Clinics of North America, 28*(1), 123–130 .

MacLeod, M., & Ulrich, C. (2005). *Nursing leadership at a distance: Addressing the experience of rural and remote nurses.* Proceedings of the National Nursing Leadership Conference, Ottawa, February 13–15, 2005.

MacLeod, M., Kulig, J., Stewart, N., Pitblado, R., Knock, M. (2004). The nature of nursing practice in rural and remote Canada. *The Canadian Nurse, 100*(6), 27–31.

MacLeod, M., Kulig, J., Stewart, N., & Pitblado, R. (2004). *Nursing Practice in Rural and Remote Canada.* Canadian Health Services Research Foundation. www.chsrf.ca.

Manitoba Association of Registered Nurses. (2000). *Entry level competencies for registered nurses in Manitoba 2000–2006.* Winnipeg: Author.

McBride, W., & Gregory, D. (2005). Aboriginal health human resources initiatives: Towards the development of a strategic framework. *Canadian Journal of Nursing Research, 37*(4), 89–94.

Mitura, V., & Bollman, R. (2003). The health of rural Canadians: A rural–urban comparison of health indicators. *Rural and Small Town Analysis Bulletin,4*(6)1–23. #21-006-XIE. Ottawa: Statistics Canada. Available at statcan.ca.

Morton, L., Glasgow, N., & Johnson, N. (2004). Reaching the goal: Less disparity, better rural health. In N. Glasgow, L. Morton, & N. Johnson (Eds.), *Critical Issues in Rural Health* (pp. 283–291). Iowa: Blackwell Publishing.

Murphy, N. (1999). A survey of health policy content in Canadian graduate programs in nursing. *Journal of Nursing Education.* 38(2), 88-91.

Northern Research Development Program, Social Sciences and Humanities Research Council. (2006). Retrieved July 27, 2006, from http://www.sshrc.ca/web/apply/program_descriptions/northern_e.asp.

Nurses Association of New Brunswick. (1997). *Standards for nursing education in New Brunswick.* Retrieved June 25, 2001, from http://www.nanb.nb.ca/english/nursed.html.

Penz, K., D'Arcy, C., Stewart, N., Kosteniuk, J., Morgan, D., & Smith, B. (2007). Barriers to participation in continuing education among rural and remote nurses: Results from a national survey. *The Journal of Continuing Education in Nursing, 38*(2) 58–68.

Pitblado, J. R. (2005). So, what do we mean by "rural," "remote," and "northern"? *Canadian Journal of Nursing Research,37*(1), 163–168.

Pitblado, J. R., Medves, J., & Stewart, N. J., (2005). For work and for school: Internal migration of Canada's rural nurses. *Canadian Journal of Nursing Research,37*(1), 102–121.

Public Health Agency of Canada. (2002). *Rural health in rural hands: Strategic directions for rural, remote, northern and Aboriginal communities.* Retrieved September 11, 2006, from http://www.phac-aspc.gc.ca/rh-sr/pdf/rural_hands.pdf.

Rothwell, N., Bollman, R., Tremblay, J., & Marshall, J. (2002). Migration to and from rural and small town Canada. *Rural and Small Town Analysis Bulletin, 3*(6), 2–22. #21-006-XIE. Ottawa: Statistics Canada. Available at statcan.ca.

Sawatzky, H. L. (1971). *They sought a country: Mennonite colonization in Mexico.* Berkley, CA: University of California Press.

Statistics Canada. (2003). *Injured parties.* Retrieved April 2, 2007, from http://www.statcan.ca/english/agcensus2001/first/profiles/10injured.htm.

Statistics Canada. (2004a). *Aboriginal identity population, 2001 Counts.* Retrieved July 20, 2006, from www12.statcan./ca/English/census01/products/highlight/Aboriginal/Page.cfm?Lang=English.htm.

Statistics Canada. (2004b). *Labour force, farm operators by country of birth, by province* (2001 Censuses of Agriculture and Population). Retrieved April 2, 2007, from http://www40.statcan.ca/l01/cst01/agrc44a.htm?sdi=agriculture.

Statistics Canada. (2005). *Population in collective dwellings, by province and territory (2001 census).* Retrieved July 7, 2006, from http://www40.statcan.ca/l01/cst01/famil62b.htm.

Stewart, N., Kulig, J., Penz, K., Andrews, M. E., Houshmand, S., Morgan, D., MacLeod, M., Pitblado, J. R., & D'Arcy, C. (2006). *Aboriginal registered nurses in rural & remote Canada: Results from a national survey.* Saskatoon: University of Saskatchewan. R06-2006.

Stewart, N., D'Arcy, C., Pitblado, R., Morgan, D., Forbes, D., Remus, G., Smith, B., Andrews, M. E., Kosteniuk, J., Kulig, J., & MacLeod, M. (2005a). A profile of registered nurses in rural and remote Canada. *Canadian Journal of Nursing Research, 37*(1), 122–145 .

Stewart, N., D'Arcy, C., Pitblado, J. R., Forbes, D., Morgan, D., Remus, G., Smith, B., & Kosteniuk, J. (2005b). *Report of the national survey of nursing practice in rural and remote Canada.* Saskatoon: University of Saskatchewan, College of Nursing and Applied Research/Psychiatry. R05-2005.

Stewart, N., & MacLeod, M. (2005, August). RNs in nurse practitioner positions in rural and remote Canada. *The Nature of Rural & Remote Nursing, 3.* Retrieved October 8, 2007, from http://www.ruralnursing.unbc.ca/factsheets/factsheet3.pdf.

Thomlinson, E., McDonagh, M., Baird Crooks, K., & Lees, M., (2004). Health beliefs of rural Canadians: Implications for rural practice. *Australian Journal of RuralHealth, 12,* 258–263.

Tremblay, J. (2001). Rural youth migration between 1971 and 1996. *Rural and Small Town Analysis Bulletin, 2*(3) 1–10. #21-006-XIE. Ottawa: Statistics Canada. Available at statcan.ca.

Ulrich, C., & MacLeod, M. (2005). *Overcoming distance and accommodating diversity: Creating a practical northern nursing strategy.* Proceedings of the National Nursing Leadership Conference, Ottawa, February 13–15, 2005.

ADDITIONAL RESOURCES

Websites

British Columbia Rural & Remote Health Research Network
  www.bcrrhrn.ca

Canadian Association for Rural & Remote Nursing
  www.carrn.com

Canadian Rural Health Research Society
  http://crhrs-scrsr.usask.ca

Canadian Rural Revitalization Foundation
  www.crrf.ca

Centre for Rural and Northern Health Research
  www.cranhr.ca

Rural Policy Research Institute
  http://rupri.org

Readings

Hegney, D., Pearson, A., & McCarthy, A. (1997). *The role and function of the rural nurse in Australia.* Canberra: Royal College of Australia.

Kulig, J., Macleod, M., & Lavoie, J. (2007, February). Nurses and First Nations and Inuit community-managed primary health services. *The Nature of Rural and Remote Nursing, 5.* Retrieved from http://www.ruralnursing.unbc.ca/factsheets/factsheet5.pdf.

Phillips, C., & McLeroy, K. (Eds.). (2004). Special issue on rural health. *American Journal of Public Health, 94*(10), 1660–1812 .

Ramp, W., Kulig, J., Townshend, I., & McGowan, V. (Eds.). (1999). *Health in rural settings: Contexts for action.* Lethbridge: University of Lethbridge.

About the Authors

All four authors were co-principal investigators for the study "The Nature of Nursing Practice in Rural and Remote Canada."

Judith C. Kulig, RN, DNSc (University of California San Francisco), is a Professor in the Nursing Program in the School of Health Sciences at the University of Lethbridge. She conducts a research program related to rural health that focuses on community resiliency of rural communities, unique populations in rural communities, and nursing practice in rural communities.

Martha L. P. MacLeod, RN, PhD (University of Edinburgh), is Associate Professor in Nursing and Community Health Sciences Programs at the University of Northern British Columbia. Her research program is on rural and northern practice and its development.

Norma J. Stewart, RN, PhD (University of British Columbia), is a Professor and Associate Dean in the College of Nursing at the University of Saskatchewan. Her research program has focused on dementia care and rural health services.

Roger Pitblado, PhD, is a Senior Research Fellow in the Centre for Rural and Northern Health Research at Laurentian University. His research deals with geographical variations in health status and the relative locations of health human resources, with a particular emphasis on rural Canada.

Multicultural Clients

Kathryn Edmunds and Elizabeth Kinnaird-Iler

OBJECTIVES

After studying this chapter, you should be able to:

1. Define and explain culture and multiculturalism.

2. Discuss the relationship of culture and health.

3. Discuss the common experiences of newcomers and migrant workers and the implications for community health nurses.

4. Describe how cultural values shape clients and nurses and their interactions.

5. Apply transcultural nursing principles to community health nursing practice and describe the knowledge, attitudes, sensitivity, and skills that are needed to provide culturally competent care.

INTRODUCTION

Canadian nurses have a long history of providing care to all people and communities, where and when it was required, while adapting to local contexts, resources, and circumstances. The Canadian Nurses Association (CNA) (2004) recognizes that in order for optimum patient outcomes to occur for increasingly diverse clients, nurses must provide care that is culturally competent as outlined in the Code of Ethics. Competencies include "demonstrating consideration for client diversity; providing culturally sensitive care (e.g., openness, sensitivity, and recognizing culturally based practices and values); and incorporating cultural practices into health promotion activities" (CNA, 2000, p. 1). Valuing multiple ways of knowing, engaging in reflective practice, facilitating access and equity, empowering clients through negotiation, and providing culturally appropriate care in multiple settings are all expectations in the standards of practice of the Community Health Nurses Association of Canada (CHNAC, 2003). The College of Nurses of Ontario (CNO, 1999) has also developed standards of practice for providing culturally sensitive care.

Diversity refers to variety and differences of attributes among and between groups. We all have attributes that give us membership in certain groups, yet we can be diverse in many ways that are fluid. Diversity can refer to both the preservation and value of heritage, and adaptation leading to creativity and innovation. In this chapter, we will discuss the meaning and characteristics of culture, and how cultural values shape nurse–client interactions. Some of the issues associated with Canadian multiculturalism will be discussed, as will some of the common experiences of newcomers. The population of federally sponsored seasonal agricultural workers will be discussed in order to illustrate some of the current systems issues in displacement related to economic policies and globalization. Implications for community health nursing practice and the development of cultural competence will be described.

CULTURE

Madeline Leininger, the founder of the field of transcultural nursing and the Sunrise Model (Figure 20.1), defines **culture** as "the learned, shared, and transmitted knowledge of values, beliefs, and lifeways of a particular group that are transmitted intergenerationally and influence thinking, decisions, and actions in patterned or in certain ways" (Leininger & McFarland, 2002, p. 47). Culture is learned, shared, and transmitted over time. It also encompasses all aspects of our lives. What we have learned to value underlies our assumptions about how to perceive, think, and behave in acceptable, appropriate, and meaningful ways.

The underlying assumptions to the provision of culturally competent care that is centred on the unique and individual culture of each client (person, family, community, or institution) (CNO, 1999, p. 3) are as follows:

- *Everyone* has a culture.
- Culture is individual. Individual assessments are necessary to identify relevant cultural factors within the context of each situation for each client.
- An individual's culture is influenced by many factors such as race, gender, religion, ethnicity, socioeconomic status, sexual orientation, and life experience. The extent to which particular factors influence a person will vary.
- Culture is dynamic. It changes and evolves over time as individuals change over time.
- Reactions to cultural differences are automatic, often subconscious, and influence the dynamics of the relationship.
- A nurse's culture is influenced by personal beliefs as well as nursing's professional values. The values of the nursing profession are upheld by all nurses.
- The nurse is responsible for assessing the client's cultural expectations and needs.

These assumptions shape our understanding of what "makes up" culture. Five characteristics are shared by all cultures (Allender & Spradley, 2005):

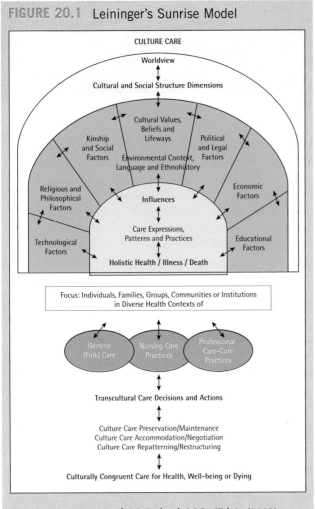

FIGURE 20.1 Leininger's Sunrise Model

Source: Leininger, M., & McFarland, M.R. (Eds.). (2002). Transcultural nursing: concepts, theories, research & practice (3rd ed.). Sudbury, MA: Jones and Bartlett Publishers, http://www.jbpub.com. Reprinted with permission.

- *Culture is learned.* Cultural norms, behaviours, and values are acquired through socialization within the family and community. However, socialization is interpreted and shaped individually. Behaviours that the nurse may assume are universal can differ across *and within* cultures.
- *Culture is an integrated system.* Beliefs and health care practices are usually consistent with the overall paradigms that are used to make sense out of the world. For example, an individual or a community may value treatment from traditional healers whose care is based on that culture's holistic or spiritual world view rather than a biomedical model of disease and illness.
- *Culture is shared.* Beliefs that have meanings, either positive or negative, and are shared by a group are called **cultural values**. These values are transmitted within a group and transmitted over time. Values shared by people form cultural stability and security. They become a standard for behaviour to guide members about what to believe and how to act.
- *Culture is largely implicit and tacit.* This means it shapes us at an unconscious level. Most of the time we do not

stop to consider the assumptions and expectations that ground our behaviours and decisions. Culture becomes the way we do things in our daily living.

- *Culture is dynamic.* Culture is always adapting and changing. Consider the changes to Canadian culture that have occurred since your grandparents were young adults. Minority cultures are certainly influenced by the dominant culture; however, increasing diversity has influenced the dominant culture in return.

Shared characteristics and patterns can be used to identify cultural groups; however, individual experiences and meanings vary as everyone participates in multiple cultures, has many layers of identity, and is influenced by the dominant social order. Generalizations can be useful in providing background information about meanings of care and health practices, but must be used with caution and sensitivity (Masi, 1993). Clients, whether individuals, families, or communities, may or may not share or value generalizations about their culture that are known to the nurse. Therefore, a *cultural assessment* is necessary with each client. (See the text box "A Guide to Transcultural Nursing Assessment" and Chapter 10.)

Culture is a socially constructed reality that is constantly being renewed, affirmed, and adapted. A nurse learning about the lifeways of people and what is meaningful to them should realize that culture is a phenomenon that is created (Allen, 1996) and needs to be described appropriately. Part of that process is distinguishing between etic and emic perspectives. An **etic** perspective is from an outsider's point of view, and often uses an outsider's classification system (e.g., a nursing diagnosis that is made for a client). An **emic** perspective is the insider's point of view, the experience of that culture from someone who is of that culture (e.g., a nurse describing nursing). Both perspectives are useful; however, if outsiders impose their views on a culture without critical reflection of their own assumptions and perceptions, it can perpetuate misinterpretations, judging of "the others," and inaccurate conclusions that perpetuate social inequities.

Multiculturalism

Cultural diversity has always existed in Canada. However, formal recognition for language rights and different legal systems was restricted to the English and French at the time of Confederation in 1867. Treaty rights, which were negotiated with some First Nations, took place in the context of colonization and were largely motivated by land and resource acquisition. Multiculturalism was based on European, Christian, and colonial perspectives (Joy, 1995), with layers and separations based on class, race, gender, formal education, and ability to speak English (Lee, 1995). People who look different because of their skin colour, ethnicity, or race may always be considered as "visible minorities" in the mainstream society. In 1971, federal multiculturalism policy recognized cultural pluralism and acknowledged this as a contribution to Canadian culture. More recently still, debate about the assumptions, benefits, and barriers of multiculturalism has been articulated.

A Guide to Transcultural Nursing Assessment

Cultural Affiliation

1. Can you tell me about your cultural group and its heritage?
2. How long have you or your parents/your family been in this country?
3. Do you have close social relationships with people from your cultural group?

Family Relationships

1. How important is family in your culture?
2. Can you tell me how your family members communicate with one another?
3. Who has the authority to make the major and final decisions in your family, and how? Please give examples.
4. What are the roles and responsibilities of mothers, fathers, sons, and daughters in your culture? i.e., what are their duties in the family?
5. Can you tell me about your views of parenting? What do parents expect from their children when they are children and when they are adults?
6. How do families in your culture view marriage, single parenthood, divorce, separation, and unemployment?
7. Can you tell me about your views of caregiving? Who takes care of the young children? Who takes care of the aging parents?

Health Beliefs and Practices

1. What does health mean to you?
2. What do you do to stay healthy?
3. What are the common health beliefs and practices for the following life events and their significance?
   a. pregnancy   d. marriage
   b. birth   e. middle years
   c. adolescence   f. old age
4. How important is it for you to have regular health care follow-up and why? for example immunization, dental care, regular physical examinations, and screening.
5. Who plays the major role in keeping the family healthy, and how?

Illness Beliefs and Practices

1. What does being sick or ill mean to you?
2. What do you do when you are feeling ill?
3. Can you tell me about your beliefs regarding why people become ill in your culture?
4. What are the common health beliefs and practices for the following?
   a. a major illness   d. a terminal illness
      or disability   e. death
   b. an accident   f. other (please describe)
   c. a chronic illness

5. Who would usually be involved in caring for the ill family member? Why? What would this person do?
6. In your culture, what traditional healing do you practice, if any? Please describe your experiences with traditional healing practitioners/practices.
7. Please describe your experiences with health professionals. How would you describe a caring/non-caring health professional?
8. How do you determine when to use traditional healers or when to seek care from health professionals?

Religious and Spiritual Practices

1. Describe your religious and spiritual beliefs?
2. What are the customs and beliefs for special religious and spiritual days in your culture?
3. Who in the family usually ensures that these religious and spiritual practices are being followed?
4. Can you tell me your beliefs about life and death?
5. How important are religious and spiritual supports for someone who is healthy/someone who is ill?

World Views

1. Describe how you see your life in relation to the world around you.
2. What is most important in your life?
3. How important do you view education, technology, politics, economic, and legal matters in your life?
4. If you are new to the country, have your world views changed since your arrival? Why? How?

Socialization

1. What is the language that you speak and write?
2. What languages are spoken in your home? Why? How do you feel about this?
3. What do you do to socialize with your families and friends?
4. What are the "do's" and "don't's" when teaching children to be successful in life?
5. If you are new to this country, what barriers/difficulties did you experience while adapting to the new country? What helped you to adapt to the new country?
6. If you are from an immigrant family, tell me how you relate your expectations for your parents and/or children to what you were taught in your own culture?
7. To what extent do you practice or observe the customs and traditions that you learned in your culture? and in the new country?

Yiu, L., & Edmunds, K. (2007). A Guide to Transcultural Nursing Assessment. (Revised) Unpublished guide, University of Windsor, Windsor, Ontario.

Multiculturalism can be defined as the notion of cultural diversity as a valuable resource that should be preserved, extended, and strengthened (Locke, 1992). This is seen to benefit the entire population. The Canadian Multiculturalism Act of 1988 states:

> The Constitution of Canada … recognizes the importance of preserving and enhancing the multicultural heritage of Canadians …; [and] the government of Canada recognizes the diversity of Canadians as regards to race, national or ethnic origin, colour and religion as a fundamental characteristic of Canadian society and is committed to a policy of multiculturalism designed to preserve and enhance the multicultural heritage of Canadians while working to achieve the equality of all Canadians in the economic, social, cultural and political life of Canada. (As cited in James, 2003, p. 208.)

Ethnicity is a way of describing social identity with a group that is based on a shared history and social structure (James, 2003). The dominant culture tends not to define itself in terms of ethnicity; it is usually minority groups that are viewed as ethnic. **Race** is often thought of as an objective biological distinction (usually based on visible differences such as skin colour). However, historically the concept of race has been socially constructed and used to maintain the dominant social order; this continues to occur today. "Race is significant as long as groups are determined by their physical traits, and attributes are assigned as a result of these traits. It is significant as long as groups and individuals suffer consequences because of race" (p. 40). The social construction of both ethnicity and race can often result in prejudice, racism, and discrimination.

Acculturation refers to the adaptation that occurs when cultures are in contact. Culture is dynamic, with inevitable change and adjustment; groups who immigrate to Canada and value retaining their culture also acculturate to living in a new country. The dominant culture acculturates as well but may not recognize this. **Assimilation** refers to total integration into the dominant culture. Kymlicka and Norman (2000) state that one needs to distinguish between assimilation and multicultural integration (acculturation). Both involve a new identity and both seek to integrate people from diverse backgrounds into common social and political institutions. However, assimilation has the intent of eliminating cultural differences. In contrast, multiculturalism "accepts that ethnocultural identities matter to citizens, will endure over time, and must be recognized and accommodated within these common institutions. The hope is that citizens from different backgrounds can all recognize themselves, and feel at home, within these common institutions" (p. 14). However, there are issues of power inherent in multiculturalism, and community health nurses should not assume that all Canadians perceive multiculturalism in such a constructive and beneficial light.

The meaning of multiculturalism has gone through phases and changes of interpretation (Srivastava, 2007). Currently, the focus of multiculturalism is the integration of practices of diversity, tolerance, and respect for multiple ways of knowing and being, with issues of equity and social justice. International movement in immigration means that racial, ethnic, religious, and linguistic diversity will continue to increase and that multiculturalism will continue to dynamically influence the Canadian identity (Padolsky, 2000).

NEWCOMERS IN CANADA

Newcomers may include "refugees, immigrants, legal or illegal aliens, migrants, international adoptees and others" (Smith, 2001, p. 53). Newcomers may share some similarities (e.g., language barriers, cultural adaptation), but like all groups of people, there are significant differences both within and across cultures. In 2001, Canadian Census data (Statistics Canada, 2003) showed that 5.4 million people (18.4% of the total population) were born outside the country, the highest proportion in 70 years. Since 1901, 13.4 million immigrants have come to Canada. The decade with the highest number of immigrants in the past 100 years was the 1990s, when 1.8 million immigrants were welcomed. Between 1900 and 1961, immigrants to Canada were primarily from European countries. (See Table 20.1.) However, since then most immigrants have been from Asia. Factors that caused this shift include changes to federal immigration policies and changes in the international movement of immigrants and refugees. Between July 1, 2006, and June 30, 2007, Canada received 238,100 immigrants (Statistics Canada, 2007b). Immigration has a significant impact on the growth and diversity of Canada's population. However, since immigrants arrive at an average age of 30, this does not slow our population's overall aging (Statistics Canada, 2007c).

Most immigrants settled in Canada's largest cities: Toronto, Vancouver, and Montreal. Newcomers were younger (46% between the ages of 25–44) than the rest of the population (31% between the ages of 25–44), and nearly one in five (17%) school-age children in Toronto and Vancouver in the last decade was an immigrant (Statistics Canada, 2003). Four million Canadians (13.4% of the population) now identify themselves as visible minorities, a three-fold increase since 1981. "Visible minorities are defined by the Employment Equity Act as 'persons, other than Aboriginal peoples, who are non-Caucasian in race or non-white in colour'" (Statistics Canada, 2003, p. 10).

Canadian Research Box 20.1

Ruppenthal, L., Tuck, J., & Gagnon, A. (2005). Enhancing research with migrant women through focus groups. *Western Journal of Nursing Research, 27*(6), 735–754.

The purpose of this research was to explore the use and process of focus groups with migrant women in order to advance the validity of measurement strategies and the quality of research with this target population. Comment from multilingual and multiethnic women on the suitability and relevance of proposed research tools and protocols was elicited.

Participants were refugee women recently arrived in Canada, able to speak English or French, and with a mix of backgrounds, including ethnicity, education, religion, family situation, migration, and current employment sta-

TABLE 20.1
Top 10 Countries of Birth, Canada, 2001

Immigrated before 1961	Number	%	Immigrated 1991–2001[1]	Number	%
Total immigrants	**894 465**	**100.0**	**Total immigrants**	**1 830 680**	**100.0**
United Kingdom	217 175	24.3	China	197 360	10.8
Italy	147 320	16.5	India	156 120	8.5
Germany	96 770	10.8	Philippines	122 010	6.7
Netherlands	79 170	8.9	Hong Kong		
Poland	44 340	5.0	Special Administrative Region	118 385	6.5
United States	34 810	3.9	Sri Lanka	62 590	3.4
Hungary	27 425	3.1	Pakistan	57 990	3.2
Ukraine	21 240	2.4	Taiwan	53 755	2.9
Greece	20 755	2.3	United States	51 440	2.8
China	15 850	1.8	Iran	47 080	2.6
			Poland	43 370	2.4

[1] *Includes data up to May 2001.*

Source: Top 10 countries of birth, Canada, 2001 *from the Statistics Canada publication* Canada's Ethnocultural Portrait: The Changing Mosaic, *2001 Census: Analysis Series. Catalogue 96F0030XIE2001008. Released January 21, 2003, page 39: http://www12.statcan.ca/ english/census01/products/analytic/companion/etoimm/pdf/96F0030XIE2001008.pdf.*

tus, Eleven women participated in three different groups in Montreal. Each group of two to four participants met twice for four-hour sessions conducted in English or French. Participants were given questionnaires and research protocols to review and were asked to share concerns and possible resolutions. Recommendations by the women were made in relation to consent and interpretation procedures, development of trust in the research process, home visits after birth, approaches to sensitive topics, discrimination as an area of inquiry, and compensation for participants.

Because of their diversity, participants gave more detailed cultural information and their responses were more explicit. The absence of other members from their personal ethnic groups meant the women could discuss sensitive topics while safeguarding their anonymity. Areas of consensus strengthened research validity with diverse groups; differences alerted the researchers to issues where they could experience difficulties.

Discussion Questions:

1. What are some of the strengths of this study?

2. What are some of the limitations?

3. How would you determine if your area of inquiry was best served by homogeneous or heterogeneous focus groups? Which factors would make a group similar or diverse? How important would ethnicity be in determining this?

While most new immigrants have positive opinions about Canada's social and political environment, their most significant difficulties after living in Canada for four years relate to finding appropriate and adequate employment, and learning a new language (Statistics Canada, 2007a). Language is a signif-

icant barrier to seeking and gaining access to health care, and community health nurses must understand issues related to translation and working with interpreters. For convenience, an English-speaking family member may be considered an interpreter, but this choice has inherent problems. The family member may not understand the information given and may not know specific terminology used by the nurse. The use of a family member may also inhibit frank discussion of sensitive topics. Children are frequently the first to learn English in a family. However, using children as interpreters is not recommended since the child may no longer recognize the parent in the role of family leader when they are seen as dependent on the child for communication (Anderson et al., 2005).

Newcomers bring significant strengths such as diversity, determination, and resilience (DeSantis & Thomas, 1997), yet their health often becomes at risk due to barriers that exist at many levels (Yiu Matuk, 1995). An often-low standard of living, language barriers, adjusting to the dominant culture, and the possibility of working in unsafe conditions all contribute to increased health risks for the newcomer. It is often difficult to find a family doctor, meaning that primary care services may be limited to episodic treatment rather than comprehensive care. Stress associated with immigration alone can put an individual at risk for poor health outcomes. Refugees (who may have been in refugee camps for many years), older people, individuals separated from their families, and those with limited or nonexistent support in the host country are at particular risk.

MIGRANT WORKERS

According to Clark (2000), it is estimated that there are 200 000 to 300 000 "visa workers" in Canada. Foreign and *migrant workers* without permanent residence who are authorized for employment include people in the Live-in Caregiver Program (someone who provides care to children, the elderly, or the disabled in a private household), some refused refugee claimants, and those with limited-term work visas, including seasonal farm workers. Most foreign workers in federally sponsored caregiver and agricultural programs are adults who have left their families behind in their home countries. Migrant workers can also include Canadian citizens who travel in search of work.

Canada ranks fourth in the world for exporting food or food products to other countries, with agriculture contributing $90 billion yearly to the Canadian economy (Gibb, 2006). Farmers must compete in global markets where large agri-business companies increasingly dominate. The Canadian Seasonal Agricultural Workers Program (SAWP) was introduced by the federal government in 1966 to address a long-standing shortage of farm workers (Basok, 2000).

Originally, 264 agricultural workers from the Caribbean were allowed to participate in SAWP (Basok, 2000); beginning in 1974, workers from Mexico were also included. The demand for offshore workers has steadily increased. In 2005, a total of 18 887 seasonal agricultural workers were approved by Human Services Canada (North-South Institute, 2006). Workers are overwhelmingly male, and 80% of workers in this program find placement on farms and greenhouses in Ontario. Criteria for acceptance into SAWP include prior agricultural experience; lower levels of education; and limited means of earning an income in one's own country. Participants with family obligations in their country of origin are preferred. Labour migration provides an economic opportunity not available in the home country and becomes a strategy to attain individual and family goals.

The structure of SAWP limits and constrains full participation in Canadian society. Workers sign a "named" contract with one employer. While in Canada, workers are assigned to that employer and remain on that farm or greenhouse operation for the eight months of their stay. Basok (2000) interviewed agricultural employers who highly supported SAWP, as they perceived seasonal workers to be a reliable and dependable source of labour. Employers must provide private health insurance and register employees with the relevant Workers' Compensation Board. However, many workers are not aware of their rights to claim benefits (Gibb, 2006). Workers must contribute to the federal Employment Insurance (EI) program, though they are not allowed to claim regular EI benefits. Workers often do not understand Canada's immigration laws, federal and provincial laws that are applicable, and the rules that apply to SAWP (Gibb). Agricultural workers in Ontario do not have the right to belong to a union and, until June of 2006, were exempt from provincial health and safety legislation. Housing is provided by the employer, usually on site, leaving workers geographically isolated from the local community and dependent on the employer for transportation requiring automobiles (e.g., to obtain groceries).

In her research with more than 300 Mexican agricultural workers, conducted in Leamington, Ontario, and in the workers' home communities in Mexico, Basok (2000, 2002)

identified workers' perceptions of pressure to participate in SAWP due to lack of economic opportunities at home, worker and family stress related to the long absences, marginalization and isolation of the workers in Canada, and fear of reporting substandard or unsafe living and working environments. Loneliness, anxiety and/or depression, fear of being sent home, language barriers, difficulty in gaining access to health care due to long hours at work, and hazardous working conditions result in complex health problems and unmet physical and psychological needs (Cooper et al., 2006; Grzywacz et al., 2006).

CULTURE AND HEALTH

Determinants of health such as culture, income, education, social support, and access to health care are relevant for all individuals, families, and communities. As culture is individually and collectively defined and expressed, so is health. Many immigrants define health, health care, and health promotion very differently from the dominant culture, which can lead to the perception on the part of health care providers that immigrants "don't care" about their health or the health of their families. Newcomers and migrant workers will continue to utilize health care practices from within their culture and may have no reason to trust that the Canadian health care system will be understanding or responsive in a way that is meaningful to them (Waxler-Morrison & Anderson, 2005). As Canadians welcome ever-increasing cultural diversity, community health nurses must be willing to accept the responsibility of responding to individual, family, and community health care needs with cultural sensitivity and competence.

Implications for Community Health Nursing Practice

Since the passing of the Canadian Multiculturalism Act of 1988, much emphasis has been placed on cultural awareness and sensitivity. Cultural competence requires more attention. The concept of **cultural competence** integrates the knowledge, attitudes, and skills that the nurse would use to plan effective and appropriate interventions (Andrews & Boyle, 2003). It is a process that "includes a genuine passion to be open and flexible with others, to accept differences and build on similarities, and to be willing to learn from others as cultural informants" (Camphina-Bacote, 2002, p. 183). Becoming a culturally competent community health nurse requires reflection of oneself, openness to the discovery of different realities, and the opportunity to practise assessment and collaborative skills. Camphina-Bacote describes five constructs, the intersection of which informs the process of cultural competence: cultural awareness (self-examination), cultural knowledge, cultural skill (collecting and assessing data), cultural encounters (the process of relationships), and cultural desire (motivation of the health care provider). In addition to these individual resources and skills of the nurse, it is also important to recognize the role of institutional resources (such as interpreters, continuing education, and policies) that support culturally competent practices (Srivastrava, 2007). An example of culturally competent organizational expectations and guidelines can be found in the Nova Scotia Department of Health weblink in the Additional Resources section at the end of this chapter.

There is always interplay between making use of background information the nurse may have and checking that information with every client. Background information that is never checked with the client and assumed to be true for all becomes a **stereotype**. What must also be assessed is how important an intervention is to the client and how the concept of "care" is perceived, expressed, and demonstrated.

Clients bring multiple cultures to their interactions with nurses. They too are shaped by their personal culture, professional values, and unique life experiences. The key to understanding lies in being open to and appreciating the diversity within each individual. Influences such as power, economic migration because of poverty, and the effects of dominant cultures also need to be integrated in any assessment (Swendson & Windsor, 1996).

Although the literature is replete with calls for cultural competency, little work has been done focusing on the dimensions of culturally competent care from the perspective of the client. In her research with Mexican American participants, Warda (2000) discovered that positive and enabling health care relationships and experiences were congruent with the clients' cultural values of being respected, valued, communicated with in Spanish, and having a health care provider who was familiar with their culture. Experiences that discounted the clients' perceptions, blamed clients, and included barriers to access were incongruent with their cultural values and were clearly identified by the participants as negative. Being open to and aware of multiple ways of knowing and experiencing the world leads to the recognition that decisions can take place in different moral contexts (Baker, 1997). Characteristics of culture can lead to **ethnocentrism**, which is the belief that one's own culture is the best or most desirable. Nurses who believe that the culture and practices of nursing are the only or "best" way to interpret what the client is expressing and to achieve improvements in health are being ethnocentric.

Knowledge of every culture is impossible and unnecessary (Waxler-Morrison & Anderson, 2005). Community health nurses need to have the assessment, interviewing, and collaborative skills in order to be open to the discovery and reflection required for providing effective care. These skills are needed not only with clients but also with interpreters and community agencies. Leininger's transcultural care decisions and actions (Leininger & McFarland, 2006) provide a framework for planning nursing interventions with individuals, families, and communities. These professional decisions and actions are:

- cultural care preservation/maintenance,
- cultural care accommodation/negotiation, and
- cultural care repatterning/restructuring.

These actions help clients maintain and preserve relevant health care values and practices, accommodate and adapt for beneficial health outcomes, and help clients modify or change existing health care patterns while respecting the values of both the client and the nurse. (See case study.)

The concept of cultural safety arose in New Zealand in response to issues raised by Maori nurses. It has much in common with cultural competence making explicit issues of power (Anderson et al., 2003). The concept of **cultural safety** is defined as effective nursing practice with a client from another culture; whether the practice is effective or not is determined by that client. The emphasis is on the experience of the client receiving nursing care, the capacity of clients to shape and contribute to their health experiences and outcomes, and the recognition of the context of power relations. "Unsafe cultural practice comprises any action which diminishes, demeans or disempowers the cultural identity and wellbeing of an individual" (Nursing Council of New Zealand, 2005, p. 4).

Case Study

You have just accepted a position as a community health nurse in a small town 50 km from the city where you grew up and went to school. You assume you are familiar with the geographic area and the values and needs of the residents. You have been asked to speak to a community group about caring for the elderly at home. This is a topic that is near and dear to your heart because your grandmother lives with your parents, and geriatrics was of special interest to you as a nursing student. People in the audience look like "regular" people, and you give your presentation, emphasizing access to resources in the city, the decline of mental status in the elderly, and safety concerns in the home for the elderly when they are left alone. The audience listens to you quietly and there are few questions.

Discussion Questions

1. You as the nurse used caring behaviours from your professional and personal cultures. What strengths and limitations did this have?

2. How could the nursing care have been more culturally competent?

3. How would you conduct a community cultural assessment?

Summary

This chapter has introduced the concept of culture, the Canadian experience of multiculturalism, the experiences of newcomers and migrant workers, and the development of a culturally competent community health nursing practice. Community health nurses need to bring the same set of skills, behaviours, and expertise to every encounter, whether the person looks the same as or different from them. A culturally competent approach requires commitment to personal reflection and growth, an understanding of the layers of cultural identity that shape us all, and the development of knowledge and skills so that in every interaction the nurse strives to discover the values and meanings of health for the client. "For community health nurses, real cultural competence is the extent to which they are effective in building community capacity—for example, assisting communities to identify, enhance, and deploy their cultural capital" (Dreher, Shapiro, & Asselin, 2006, p. 8). As community health nurses, we must nurture our common humanity and social responsibilities while also addressing systemic inequities.

KEY TERMS

diversity
culture
cultural values
etic
emic
multiculturalism
ethnicity
race
acculturation
assimilation
newcomers
cultural competence
stereotype
ethnocentrism
cultural safety

INDIVIDUAL CRITICAL THINKING EXERCISES

1. What is the difference between healthy cultural identification and ethnocentrism?

2. How would you assess whether the nursing model or theory you are using is helping you deliver culturally competent care?

GROUP CRITICAL THINKING EXERCISES

1. How would you go about gaining and demonstrating the skills and behaviours needed for culturally competent practice?

2. In pairs, do cultural assessment (A Guide to Transcultural Nursing Assessment). What have you learned about your own culture? What have you learned about your partner's culture? What did you discover about the process?

3. Are the members of your nursing class representative of your community's population? Why or why not?

REFERENCES

Allen, D. G. (1996). Knowledge, politics, culture, and gender: A discourse perspective. *Canadian Journal of Nursing Research, 28*(1), 95–102.

Allender, J. A., & Spradley, B. W. (2005). *Community health nursing: Promoting and protecting the public's health* (6th ed.). Philadelphia: Lippincott Williams and Wilkins.

Anderson, J., Perry, J., Blue, C., Browne, A., Henderson, A., Basu Khan, K., Reimer Kirkham, S., Lynam, J., Semeniuk, P., & Smye, V. (2003). "Rewriting" cultural safety within the postcolonial and postnational feminist project: Towards new epistemologies of healing. *Advances in Nursing Science, 26*(3), 196–214.

Anderson, J., Reimer Kirkham, S., Waxler-Morrison, N., Herbert, C., Murphy, M., & Richardson, E. (2005). Conclusion: Delivering culturally responsive health care. In N. Waxler-Morrison, J. Anderson, E. Richardson & N. Chambers (Eds.), *Cross-cultural caring: A handbook for health professionals* (2nd ed.; pp. 323–352). Vancouver: UBC Press.

Andrews, M. M., & Boyle, J. S. (2003). *Transcultural concepts in nursing care* (4th ed.). Philadelphia: Lippincott.

Baker, C. (1997). Cultural relativism and cultural diversity: Implications for nursing practice. *Advances in Nursing Science, 20*(1), 3–11.

Basok, T. (2000). Migration of Mexican seasonal farm workers to Canada and development: Obstacles to productive investment. *International Migration Review, 34*(1), 79–97.

Basok, T. (2002). *Tortillas and tomatoes: Transmigrant Mexican harvesters in Canada.* Montreal: McGill–Queen's University Press.

Camphina-Bacote, J. (2002). The process of cultural competence in the delivery of healthcare services: A model of care. *Journal of Transcultural Nursing, 13*(3), 181–184.

Canadian Nurses Association. (2000). Cultural diversity—Changes and challenges. *Nursing Now: Issues and Trends in Canadian Nursing, February* (7), 1–6.

Canadian Nurses Association. (2004). *Position statement: Promoting culturally competent care.* Ottawa: Author

Clark, T. (2000). *Migrant workers in Canada.* Retrieved November 14, 2006, from http://www.december18.net/web/docpapers/doc626.pdf.

College of Nurses of Ontario. (1999). *Standards of practice: A guide to nurses for providing culturally sensitive care.* Toronto: Author.

Community Health Nurses Association of Canada. (2003). *Canadian community health nursing standards of practice.* Ottawa: Author.

Cooper, S. P., Burau, K. E., Frankowski, R., Shipp, E. M., Del Junco, D. J., Whitworth, R. E., Sweeney, A. M., Macnaughton, N., Weller, N. F., & Hanis, C. L. (2006). A cohort study of injuries in migrant farm worker families in south Texas. *Annals of Epidemiology, 16*(4), 313–320.

DeSantis, L., & Thomas, J. (1997). Building healthy communities with immigrants and refugees. *Journal of Transcultural Nursing, 9*(1), 20–31.

Dreher, M., Shapiro, D., & Asselin, M. (2006). *Healthy places healthy people: A handbook for culturally competent community nursing practice.* Indianapolis: Sigma Theta Tau International.

Gibb, H. (2006). *Farmworkers from afar: Results from an international study of seasonal farmworkers from Mexico and the Caribbean working on Ontario farms.* Ottawa: The North-South Institute.

Grzywacz, J. G., Quandt, S. A., Early, J., Tapia, J., Graham, C. N., & Arcury, T. A. (2006). Leaving family for work: Ambivalence and mental health among Mexican migrant farmworker men. *Journal of Migration and Minority Health, 8*(1), 85–97.

James, C. E. (2003). *Seeing ourselves: Exploring race, ethnicity and culture* (3rd ed.). Toronto: Thompson Educational Publishing.

Joy, M. (1995). Multiculturalism and margins of intolerance. In C. Pizanias & J. S. Friederes (Eds.), *Freedom within the margins: The politics of exclusion* (pp. 3–13). Calgary, AB: Detselig Enterprises.

Kymlicka, W., & Norman, W. (2000). Citizenship in culturally diverse societies: Issues, contexts, concepts. In W. Kymlicka & W. Norman (Eds.). *Citizenship in diverse societies* (pp. 1–32). Oxford: Oxford University Press.

Lee, J. (1995). Community development with immigrant women: Theory and practice. In C. Pizanias & J. S. Friederes (Eds.). *Freedom within the margins: The politics of exclusion* (pp. 87–109). Calgary: Detselig Enterprises.

Leininger, M., & McFarland, M. R. (Eds.) (2002). *Transcultural nursing: Concepts, theories, research & practice* (3rd ed.). New York: McGraw-Hill.

Leininger, M., & McFarland, M. (Eds.) (2006). *Culture care diversity and universality: A worldwide nursing theory* (2nd ed.). Boston: Jones and Bartlett.

Locke, D. C. (1992). *Increasing multicultural understanding: A comprehensive model.* Newbury Park: Sage.

Masi, R. (1993). Multicultural health: Principles and policies. In R. Masi, L. Mensah, & K. McLeod (Eds.), *Health and cultures: Exploring the relationships: Vol. I. Policies, professional practice and education* (pp.11–31). Oakville: Mosaic Press.

North-South Institute. (2006). *Migrant workers in Canada: A review of the Canadian Seasonal Agricultural Workers Program.* Ottawa: Author. Retrieved November 14, 2006, from http://www.nsi-ins.ca/english/pdf/MigrantWorkers_Eng_Web.pdf.

Nursing Council of New Zealand. (2005). *Guidelines for cultural safety, the Treaty of Waitangi and Maori health in nursing education and practice.* Wellington: Author. Retrieved November 14, 2006, from http://www.nursingcouncil.org.nz/Cultural%20Safety.pdf.

Padolsky, E. (2000). Multiculturalism at the Millennium. *Journal of Canadian Studies, 35*(1), 138–160.

Smith, L. S. (2001). Health of America's newcomers. *Journal of Community Health Nursing, 18*(1), 53–68.

Srivastava, R. (2007). *The health care professional's guide to clinical cultural competence.* Toronto: Mosby.

Statistics Canada. (2003). *2001 census: Analysis series. Canada's ethnocultural portrait: The changing mosaic.* Ottawa: Author.

Statistics Canada. (2007a). *Canadian social trends. Immigrant's perspectives on their first four years in Canada: Highlights from three waves of the longitudinal survey of immigrants to Canada.* Ottawa: Author. Retrieved September 27, 2007, from http://www.statcan.ca/english/freepub/11-008-XIE/2007000/pdf/11-008-XIE20070009627.pdf.

Statistics Canada. (2007b). The daily: Canada's population estimates. Ottawa: Author. Retrieved September 27, 2007, from http://www.statcan.ca/Daily/English/070927/d070927a.htm.

Statistics Canada. (2007c). *Portrait of the Canadian population in 2006, by age and sex, 2006 census.* Ottawa: Author. Retrieved September 27, 2007, from http://www12.statcan.ca/english/census06/analysis/agesex/pdf/97-551-XIE2006001.pdf.

Swendson, C., & Windsor, C. (1996). Rethinking cultural sensitivity. *Nursing Inquiry, 3,* 3–10.

Warda, M. R. (2000). Mexican Americans' perception of culturally competent care. *Western Journal of Nursing Research, 22,* 203–224.

Waxler-Morrison, N., & Anderson, J. (2005). Introduction: The need for culturally sensitive care. In N. Waxler-Morrison, J. Anderson, E. Richardson, & N. Chambers (Eds.), *Cross-cultural caring: A handbook for health professionals* (2nd ed.; pp. 1–10). Vancouver: UBC Press.

Yiu Matuk, L. (1995). Health promotion surveys for multicultural clients. In M. Stewart (Ed.), *Community nursing: Promoting Canadian's health* (2nd ed.; pp. 267–281). Toronto: W.B. Saunders.

ADDITIONAL RESOURCES

Websites

Cultural Diversity in Nursing
www.culturediversity.org

Government of Canada: Multiculturalism
http://canada.gc.ca/acanada/ViewCategory.htm?lang=eng&font=0&categoryId=70

Transcultural Nursing Society
www.tcns.org

Readings

Canadian Heritage. (2004). *What is multiculturalism?* Retrieved May 14, 2007, from http://www.pch.gc.ca/progs/multi/what-multi_e.cfm.

Hrycak, N., & Jakubec, S. (2006). Cultural awareness: Listening to different voices. *Canadian Nurse, 102*(b), 24–28.

Nova Scotia Department of Health. (2006). *A cultural competence guide for primary health care professionals.* Retrieved on May 14, 2007, from http://www.gov.ns.ca/health/primaryhealthcare/pubs/Cultural_Competence_guide_for_Primary_Health_Care_Professionals.pdf.

About the Authors

Kathryn Edmunds, RN, BN (University of Manitoba), MSN (Wayne State University with a specialization in transcultural nursing), is currently a doctoral student in the School of Nursing at the University of Western Ontario. She has been a faculty member in nursing at the University of Windsor and has extensive experience as a public health nurse with the Windsor-Essex County Health Unit, working in rural southwestern Ontario. Current theoretical and research interests include the effects of uprootedness, displacement, and marginalization on culture and health.

Elizabeth Kinnaird-Iler, RN, BScN, and MSc (University of Windsor) is a manager in the Healthy Babies Healthy Children program at the Windsor-Essex County Health Unit. She provides direct supervision to public health nurses and family home visitors who visit new mothers and young families from a variety of cultural backgrounds. Her interests include areas of women's health, program evaluation, health promotion, and transcultural health.

Aboriginal Clients

Rhonda J. King Blood and Rose Alene Roberts

OBJECTIVES

After studying this chapter, you should be able to:

1. Identify culturally appropriate nursing practice for Aboriginal communities.

2. Describe Aboriginal health care delivery.

3. Describe how Aboriginal health care systems obtain funding.

4. Describe how culture and policy can impact on the health of Aboriginal communities.

5. Identify health care issues that are important in Aboriginal communities.

INTRODUCTION

This chapter is a broad overview of community health nursing in Canadian Aboriginal communities. Waldram, Herring, & Young (2006) state, "Currently, the Indian, Inuit, and Métis peoples are recognized as '**Aboriginal** peoples' under Section 35 of the Constitution, and their 'existing Aboriginal and treaty rights [are] recognized and affirmed.' While the courts and politicians continue to wrangle about the legal implication of this section, clearly the Constitution establishes the Aboriginal peoples as unique, with special status within Canada" (p. 12). The Indian and Inuit communities may also be called First Nations communities. The term **First Nations** typically excludes the Métis, who are also recognized as one of the founding nations in the Canadian constitution. First Nations and Métis peoples have been made **vulnerable populations**, who are more likely than other populations to have adverse health outcomes (Flaskerud & Winslow, 1998). This has occurred not only through colonization, but also by the culture of poverty superimposed on their societies. Community health nurses (CHNs) need to adapt knowledge and skills to provide meaningful community health nursing care to Aboriginal communities. Nurses who choose to practise in Aboriginal communities must come prepared to deal with complex issues in health and nursing.

In this chapter, the history of Aboriginal people is outlined from **pre-European contact** (prior to exploration and settlement by Europeans) to contemporary populations. The historical context is important in order to provide culturally appropriate community health care to Aboriginal populations. Deagle (1999) contends that Canada's health care system is a three-tier system, with the Aboriginal populations on the last tier. Here, the third tier is described in order to enhance the CHN's understanding that health care is delivered to the First Nations and Inuit by a distinctly different system, whereas health care is delivered to the Métis in typically the same method as to non-Aboriginals. Included is the description of the funding of First Nations health care systems. Finally, cultural, policy, and health issues important to the Aboriginal people of Canada in the modern context are discussed. The CHN can influence changes to improve the health of the descendants of Canada's First Peoples.

FIRST NATIONS HISTORY

Pre-European Contact

North America's Aboriginal peoples have maintained that they were the original inhabitants of the Americas. That fact is not questioned; however, the date and path of the arrival of humans to this continent are still being debated (Dickason, 2002a). Most tribes have a version of a creation story of being the original inhabitants of North America. Unearthed artifacts prove that humans arrived and resided in the Americas during the later Ice Ages. The first inhabitants of the Americas arrived with the necessary skills to survive in harsh environments (Ricciuti, 1990). Despite the hardships, cultures developed and adapted to the locale (Ballantine & Ballantine, 1993). However, the lives of Aboriginal people were profoundly altered by colonization. Mann (2005) presents somewhat controversial theories, based on research, of the possibility that the Americas may have been more densely populated as many as twenty thousand or thirty thousand years earlier than history accepts.

Before the arrival of the Europeans on this continent, an estimated 18 million inhabitants and more than 2200 languages flourished. First Nations peoples of Canada had an oral history (Dickason, 2002a). Aboriginal languages evolved into dialects spoken in different areas of a region, leading to the following linguistic and cultural groupings: Arctic, Western Subarctic, Eastern Subarctic, Northeastern Woodlands, Plains, Plateau, and Northwest Coast (Waldram et al., 2006). These cultures were based on the resources of the area that the people inhabited. For example, the Plains people were hunter-gatherers who provisioned their **bands** or **tribes** by hunting and harvesting the fauna and flora of the prairies (Schultz, 1962). The Haudenosaunee (Six Nations) in the Ontario regions grew up to 80% of their food requirements, while the tribes along the Northwest Coast met their needs from the abundance in the oceans (Dickason, 2002a). Thus, cultural and historical diversity of Aboriginal people of Canada clearly existed before the arrival of the immigrants.

Childcare and education were the responsibility of the extended family (Sherman, 1996). The adults provided for themselves and the community. Methods of food preservation were devised to store food for less plentiful seasons. Housing materials included animal hides or the trees of the woodlands. Any less fortunate members of the band were provided sustenance by the whole group. Sharing of resources among the group was expected and ensured the survival of the community; for example, among the Northwest Coast tribes, the potlatch was a method of redistributing resources. Transgression by anyone was dealt with according to custom law. The culture of the group included the spirituality that was a characteristic of most Aboriginal people. Life, if not ideal, was valued, and individuals knew their roles and purpose (Fleet, 1997).

Aboriginal communities had traditional beliefs about health. Shamans and herbalists held the knowledge of curing illness. Mothers or grandmothers practised folk medicine to care for their families. The medicine wheel philosophy, which encompassed all nature, was extensively used by numerous tribes, with regional variability.

European Contact

Initial contact with Europeans was on Canada's east coast and extended over a significant period of time. Explorers and fur traders from England and France began to explore and to harvest the plentiful animals for the fur trade. Missionaries made their way westward to bring Christian doctrine. The newcomers brought diseases such as smallpox, tuberculosis, and measles, which decimated the population by the thousands. For example, Mann (2005) cites research that the initial Aboriginal population's small homogeneous gene pool made them more susceptible to European diseases. Biochemistry research of measles vaccine responses of an Aboriginal group concluded that "virgin-soil Indians" were more susceptible to European diseases, while "virgin-soil Europeans" had acquired immunity. The result was the devastation and fragmenting of Aboriginal cultures. Further, resources that had supplied Aboriginal livelihoods, such as the buffalo, became scarce. The establishment of Canada as a country brought settlers from Europe into virtually all areas of the country. The process of establishing colonies and settlements in Canada required treaty negotiations with the original inhabitants. The establishment of reserves created further problems, including malnutrition, starvation, and death. At the time of European contact, Canada was estimated to have 50 to 60 languages. Many of those languages became extinct, and the rest continued to dwindle over time (Waldram et al., 2006), further contributing to the decimation of Aboriginal culture (Chrisjohn, Young, & Maraun, 1994).

Post-European Contact

Even though there were about 500 distinct tribes in the early 1600s, the land was legally considered empty and therefore claimable (Fleet, 1997). Britain developed the **treaty** method with the Indians to claim land that the Aboriginal people occupied. The British North America Act of 1867 gave Canada its birth as a country, but The Royal Proclamation specified that only the British government could buy Indian lands or negotiate treaties. Private individuals or other nations (including Canada) could not go into Indian communities to buy land directly (Dickason, 2002b). The **Indian Act** of 1876 was passed to ensure that the terms of the treaties were observed.

As a result of the treaties, First Nations were relegated to living on **reserves**. Aboriginal people who came from agrarian cultures had lived their entire lives in villages; hunter-gatherers travelled within their territories for their sustenance. Now their territories were reduced to small plots of land, some as small as a few acres, and in many cases the land was of no economic value. The Indian reserves were governed by the federal government under the Indian Act (Venne, 2002). The **Department of Indian Affairs and Northern Development** was and continues to be the government department responsible for managing the reserves and the treaty Indians. (More recently, an Office of the Interlocutor was developed within the Department of Indian Affairs to oversee the Métis.) Individuals called **Indian agents** were assigned to carry out the terms of the treaty. Once accustomed to having freedom, Indians found that they now required written permission from the Indian agent to leave the reserve. Indians became dependent on the Indian agent for all aspects of their sustenance (Canada, Department of Indian & Northern Affairs, 1997).

The Residential School Legacy

Residential schools were first established by the missionaries in the late 1800s in various locations of Canada. The federal government took over the administration of some residential schools as a response to the treaty right to education. Leaders of First Nations communities wanted schools built on the reserves. However, the federal government decided that residential schools would be cheaper; furthermore, a similar system in the United States was showing promise in assimilating the American Indian children into the white society. Approximately 135 residential schools were operated through an agreement between the federal government and the Roman Catholic Church, the Church of England, the Methodist Church, and the Presbyterian Church between 1892 and 1969 (Aboriginal Healing Foundation, 1999). After the withdrawal of the federal government, some residential schools continued to operate into the 1970s, 1980s, and 1990s. The vast majority of residential schools were in the western provinces. The number of children sent to residential schools has been estimated to be more than 150 000, and the Assembly of First Nations estimates that there are more than 105 000 survivors still alive today (Aboriginal Healing Foundation, 1999).

The premise of the residential schools was to assimilate the children through a process of education, religious and otherwise, as well as cultural degradation—teaching the children to be ashamed of their heritage in order to facilitate the assimilation process. Parents were legally required to send their children to residential schools. Physical, emotional, and sexual abuse was rampant in the schools, and little was done to stop it or to punish the abusers. Living conditions were often far below acceptable levels in modern-day society's terms. Children often went hungry; children report their parents bringing them food on their weekend visits to supplement their substandard diet (Aboriginal Healing Foundation, 1999). Some children report being forced to steal food from the kitchens. The education they received was also substandard. As late as the 1950s, more than 40% of the teaching staff at the schools had no professional training (Aboriginal Healing Foundation, 1999). Cultural degradation practices included physical and emotional abuse for speaking a traditional language, cutting of hair (hair has strong cultural and spiritual implications), imposing foreign religious practices, and intentional separation from visiting parents. The residential school experiences of Aboriginal peoples continue to have a detrimental impact on Aboriginal communities. High rates of suicide, addictions, and abuse plague Aboriginal communities. The intergenerational impact of loss of parenting skills is being felt by today's children. Aboriginal communities are striving to reweave the strands of their social, cultural, and spiritual worlds. Federally funded programs such as the Aboriginal Healing Foundation have helped the healing process in some communities. Compensation for survivors has been ongoing since the findings of the Royal Commission on Aboriginal Peoples were published in 1996.

Treaty Status

An understanding of how Aboriginal status is acquired and defined is indispensable to understanding the health care of Aboriginal people. The status of being a First Nations person in Canada is not only acquired by birth but also legislated by the Indian Act. Prior to 1985, the definition of an Indian was any *male* person of Indian blood belonging to a recognized band, any child of such a person, and any woman legally married to such a person (Furi & Wherrett, 1996). A **registered** or **status Indian** is recognized under the Indian Act and has a unique registration number called a treaty number. Non-status Indians are culturally Indians, but because their tribe did not sign a treaty they are not recognized as Status Indians by the federal government. One of the main goals of the Indian Act was assimilation. There were several ways one could lose treaty status, otherwise known as enfranchisement, such as entering the armed forces, obtaining a university education, becoming a Christian minister, gaining access to vote, or, for a woman, marrying a non-status man. There was an amendment to the Indian Act in 1985; many of the issues relating to loss of treaty status were intended to be resolved through the passing of **Bill C-31**. For example, a status woman who marries a non-status man no longer loses her treaty status, and neither do her children. Furthermore, individuals who had lost their status could apply for its return. However, the assimilative intent of the Indian Act remains in Bill C-31, because there are limitations on how far treaty status can be passed on generationally. In two generations of

intermarriage, whether the non-status spouse is male or female, the children lose their treaty status. There have been several court challenges to this aspect of Bill C-31; however, no definitive changes or decisions have been made since it was enacted in 1985 (Furi & Wherrett, 1996). **Inuit** are in a separate category, because no treaties were signed in the far north, but they are treated in the same manner as registered Indians by the federal government (Waldram et al., 2006). The **Métis**, who were the mixed-blood children born of marriages between Aboriginal and non-Aboriginal parents, are legally considered the same as non-status Indians. The Métis are considered Aboriginal peoples of Canada and are acquiring rights, such as hunting. Métis acquire services through the Office of the Interlocutor.

CONTEMPORARY ABORIGINALS

A White Paper was written in 1969 (Health Canada-FNIHB, 2005) for the purpose of abolishing the treaties and the Indian Act and disassembling the government departments responsible for reserves and treaty Indians. Generally, a White Paper is a government report on an investigation into a given topic. Often, a White Paper offers recommendations that become policy or law. However, this White Paper never became policy or legislation (Canada, Department of Indian & Northern Affairs, 1997), because of an unprecedented show of force and unity among Aboriginal communities. Though the White Paper did not succeed in terminating the First Nations and Inuit relationship with the federal government, its very attempt appears to have created a resurgence in the culture of Canada's Aboriginal people (Schouls, 2002). Today, there is increasing interest in speaking the languages of the remaining 11 language families: Algonquian, Athapaskan, Eskimo-Aleut, Haida, Tlingit, Siouan, Tsimshian, Wakashan, Salishan, Kutenai, and Iroquoian.

Canada's Aboriginal peoples' rights were given recognition in the Canadian Constitution. Several attempts have been made to define the treaty rights. The federal government attempted to clarify governance issues through its First Nations Governance Act (FNGA) The FNGA would allow effective self-governance for Aboriginal people (Canada, Department of Indian & Northern Affairs, 2002). However, once again, Aboriginal communities, political bodies, and community groups acted in unity to prevent this act being passed by parliament into law.

First Nations on Reserves

First Nations reserves are located in all of Canada's provinces, but not in the territories. Some reserves are adjacent to or located within urban centres. The reserves located in the south are easily accessible. Farther north, most reserves are remote and isolated unless they are located near an urban centre. Inuit live in settlements throughout the far north. Most reserves are governed by an elected chief and council for two to four terms of office. There are also Métis settlements; most are found in the western prairie provinces.

The existence of reserves continues to exclude First Nations people from participating in and enjoying a place in Canadian society. The lack of opportunity on reserves is evident. Some residents seek opportunities in urban centres, but because family and social support networks are absent, the result is similar to living on the reserve. Modern housing, taken for granted by other Canadians, is only a dream for too many Aboriginal people. Lack of childcare, low educational achievement, high unemployment, and lack of food security for children in particular are serious concerns for Aboriginal communities, both on and off reserve. Health and social indicators of Aboriginals highlight the grim statistics relative to health, the justice system, education, and the social and child welfare system. But the resilience of individuals can result in their being educated and participating as members of mainstream Canadian society (Mercredi & Turpel, 1993).

Urban Aboriginals

Aboriginal people are moving to urban communities in increasing numbers, often to seek a better life for their children. However, the same problems that plague rural and reserve communities can also be apparent for urban Aboriginals. Those problems present themselves as unemployment; inadequate housing; social exclusion; lack of childcare, food insecurity, and lack of transportation; and intermittent access to health care. Depending on the resilience of the individuals, poverty may be temporary until they obtain an education or job training.

The picture is not all bleak. Aboriginal people are adapting to Western society and are represented in all occupations including education, health, justice, business, and the trades. Some individuals receive a Western-based education and return to work and live in their communities, while others elect to remain in urban settings. The National Aboriginal Achievement Awards showcase the talent in the Canadian Aboriginal community. It is important to become aware of the positive aspects of being Aboriginal. It counteracts the negative stereotyping of Aboriginal people.

The national profile of First Nations communities and their health status highlights the dire need for change. The relatively new health determinants have emphasized the health needs of the Canadian Aboriginal people. The change has to be made to the social determinants of health, such as income, to overcome the poverty and third-world conditions present in too many Aboriginal communities.

HEALTH STATUS OF ABORIGINAL WOMEN

Several reports have stated that Aboriginal women continue to be overrepresented in statistics relating to poverty, violence, abuse, and overall health status (Dion-Stout, Kipling, & Stout, 2001; Royal Commission on Aboriginal Peoples [RCAP] 1996; Saskatchewan Women's Secretariat, 1999). While it is important to present epidemiological evidence in order to provide an overview of health and illness within a population, the authors wish to offer the following cautionary note to the reader. Aboriginal communities and peoples have repeatedly stated that they have been over-researched, and the research has consistently portrayed primarily negative health status; this runs the risk of creating institutional and health professional biases and perpetuating the negative stereotypes. This concept is no different when it comes to Aboriginal women.

It is difficult to obtain population-level health indicators for Métis populations, as has previously been stated. One source that provides inclusive information is the Census. According to the Canadian 2001 Census, Aboriginal women compose 1.7% of the Canadian population (n = 499 605) (Statistics Canada, 2002). When compared with Aboriginal males, females are more likely to be married, separated, divorced, or widowed. Women are more likely to have attained higher education levels, including high school, trades, and postsecondary education. However, they earn less overall income, work more part-time jobs, and depend on government sources more than men do (Statistics Canada, 2002).

The 2002/2003 First Nations Regional Longitudinal Health Survey (RHS) reports similar findings, which is not surprising considering that the RHS is run concurrently with the Census, but the RHS does provide data on a wider array of health indicators. In regard to First Nations women living on reserves, 56% live in smoke-free homes, which is positive as women are more likely to live with children under the age of 15 (National Aboriginal Health Organization [NAHO], 2006). Women reported less use of alcohol and marijuana as well as receiving fewer alcohol and drug treatment programs than men. In terms of preventive and screening services, women were more likely to have accessed such services. Coincidentally, women also reported more barriers and problems accessing health care services. First Nations women are being diagnosed earlier with diabetes (20–34 age group) and they also are more likely to be obese or morbidly obese. They also report higher rates of arthritis, allergies, hypertension, asthma, stomach/intestinal problems, rheumatism, and osteoporosis. First Nations women were also more likely to report feeling blue, sad, or depressed for two weeks or more in the previous year, as well as to having ever attempted suicide. Furthermore, 20% reported they had attended residential school and they believed this affected their health negatively. However, women also reported they had support systems in place when they needed to talk to someone. An interesting finding is that 70% of respondents stated they talked to family and friends, compared with only 29% who talked to their family physician (NAHO, 2006).

Health care practitioners need to be aware of the colonialistic history of Canada and Aboriginal peoples, and the effect this has on health-seeking behaviours. A study of Mi'kmaq patients reported favourable encounters with the health system when there was compassion and a non-discriminatory attitude among health care workers (Baker & Daigle, 2000). The avoidance of health systems that are not culturally safe does little to acknowledge patterns of individual or institutional discrimination (Browne & Fiske, 2001). Examples of negative encounters included dismissal by health care providers, negative stereotypes including lack of parenting skills, marginalization, situations of vulnerability, and disregard for personal circumstances. Positive or affirming encounters were situations where the women were active participants in health care decisions, received exceptional care, received affirmation of personal and cultural identity, and developed a long-term relationship with health care providers (Browne & Fiske, 2001).

This brief synopsis of the health status of Aboriginal women is not intended to be the complete picture. Health determinants are intended to be guidelines to assess equality among communities and populations; the reader must remain aware that these guidelines have been drawn up by the dominant society. Community initiatives such as *Naspici Miyomahcihowin (Continuous Good Health): A Community-Based Research Project Examining the Health Needs of Aboriginal Women in Saskatoon* encourages Aboriginal women to determine their own health requirements, incorporating their cultural values and beliefs throughout the process (Saskatoon Aboriginal Women's Health Research Committee, 2004). Aboriginal communities are continuing to strive for improvement in health outcomes, and more often than not the leaders are women.

FIRST NATIONS HEALTH CARE

A component of working with First Nations communities is knowing the larger health care system that enacts policy to establish the practice and standards for First Nations health care systems. Health care for First Nations and Inuit is considered a treaty right. Government policy states that health care provided to First Nations is benevolence by the federal government. The federal government, through its Health Minister and department and the **First Nations and Inuit Health Branch (FNIHB)** (formerly Medical Services Branch of Health Canada), provides the health services and support for First Nations and Inuit living on reserves. First Nations are increasingly assuming local control through the transfer of health services. (See Appendix 2A.) Health services for the Métis are provided by the provincial health care systems. Furthermore, First Nations and Inuit living off reserve get their health care services provided within the provincial health care system, and then the province asks for reimbursement from the federal government. The territories assume responsibility for their Aboriginal populations through their agreements with Ottawa. The FNIHB is based in Ottawa, where policy is planned. The First Nations and Inuit health policy is administered by the regional branches in each province, headed by a regional director.

Part of the politics of First Nations, Métis, and Inuit are the national organizations that represent their interests in Ottawa. For example, the Assembly of First Nations elects a Grand Chief, who negotiates with federal officials for program funding of First Nations health care; The Inuit Tapiriit Kanatami represents Inuit, and the Métis National Council represents the Métis.

Why do CHNs need to know about government and its functions? The answer is that it affects how health care is delivered to First Nations on a daily basis. It is advantageous to know and understand policies, thereby increasing the effectiveness of health care practitioners. When the governing party changes, often the agreements that have been in place are altered, deleted, or replaced by new legislation.

Much has changed in the health care field since Marc Lalonde, Minister of National Health and Welfare, produced the document *A New Perspective on the Health of Canadians: A Working Document* (1974). In it, he spoke about environmental and behavioural threats to health. He stated that the economy affects the health status of Canadians. Little has changed since the Lalonde Report in the socioeconomic status of Aboriginal Canadians to produce improvement in the health and social indicators. The majority of reserve residents are dependent on social services for their subsistence. Considerable economic development must be made to improve the economy of First Nations. First Nations must have the same opportunities as other Canadians; after all, Canada was established on First Nations signing treaties to share land base with the newcomers.

For acute care services, First Nations health care systems interface with the greater Canadian health care system, primarily because hospitals are a provincial responsibility. The degree of interfacing required with the surrounding communities depends on the type and scope of health services that exist on the reserves. The more remote and isolated the reserve, the more likely it is that the health care services include comprehensive care, including short-term acute care services. The federal government operated Indian hospitals but has been divesting itself of this responsibility.

The process for community-based health services is different. The governance for health services is derived from the chief and council, the governing authority for First Nations. Once the band council resolution is signed, a health committee or health board can be formed to begin the process of exploring community-based health services for its membership. First Nations health authorities were established to prepare for the transfer of control of health services to First Nations. Various types of funding arrangements are available to First Nations groups seeking to administer their own health programs. (See Appendix 2A.)

Cultural Issues in Community Health Nursing in Aboriginal Communities

First Nations' health care systems are varied in scope and practice. The nurse may practise in a large health care system that utilizes nursing skills in a limited scope. In contrast, the nurse may arrive in a remote northern community where the expectation is that all of the nursing roles will be met by one individual (Cradduck, 1995). Giger and Davidhizar's (1998) conceptual framework states that there are six key cultural phenomena in all cultures: communication, space, time, social organization, environmental control, and biological variations. The Giger and Davidhizar transcultural assessment model is one tool that can be utilized in assessing Aboriginal populations to develop culturally appropriate community health nursing care.

Development of competent, culturally appropriate nursing care (Andrews & Boyle, 1999) for Aboriginal clients requires the CHN to keep in mind the historical, cultural, and changing clinical and health care delivery system. As noted earlier, the traditional lifestyles of Canada's Aboriginals profoundly changed because of colonization. Reserves effectively excluded First Nations from participation in mainstream Canadian society (McMurray, 1999).

Aboriginal populations continue to remain a distinct cultural segment of Canadian society. Traditional holistic health beliefs, traditional medicine, and herbal medicine are deemed acceptable alternatives to Western medicine by some Aboriginals. First Nations communities are societies in themselves. Based on a culture continuum, the society may have different members who are traditionalists, traditionalists/ modernists, and modernists. Each group's strengths and challenges present for interesting nurse practice. The CHN must learn protocol for communicating with the traditionalists, who may possess cultural manners, diet, and health beliefs contrary to nursing knowledge and skills (Holland & Hogg, 2001). For example, some individuals believe that bear grease is the best treatment for abrasions and wounds. The CHN must respect the client's health beliefs, yet attempt to maintain sterile wound care. The outcome is establishing sufficient trust with the client so that the wound heals without infection and the client continues to seek the required health care.

Rumbold (1999) states that ethics provides a framework for dealing with issues, problems, and dilemmas. An understanding of ethical or moral theories helps a person decide on an appropriate line of action, although it may not necessarily provide the answer. Nurses need to study ethics because they often have to deal with moral or ethical problems. Nurses need to examine their own beliefs and values. Rumbold makes the case that nurses who move from one culture to another need to be informed of the values and norms of the society to which they are moving. It does not mean that they should abandon their own ethical values (Rumbold, 1999). Aboriginal communities can present dilemmas in which it is crucial that CHNs make wise choices. Dilemmas may be related to childcare, family violence, or geriatric abuse (Dumont-Smith, 2001). Aboriginal nurses working with First Nations communities may find different challenges, such as a personal tension between cultural practices and their knowledge of health science. Clients may assume a belief system (e.g., traditional medicine) that is not included in the nurse's practice. The Aboriginal Nurses Association of Canada (ANAC) which was formed in 1975, is an organization that provides support to Aboriginal and non-Aboriginal nurses practising in First Nations communities.

Nurses contemplating employment with FNIHB or a First Nations health authority should prepare by doing prior research on the tribe's culture, language, geographic location, education, economy, and health care system. CHNs require excellent skills for assessment, planning, implementing, and evaluating community health programs. (See Chapters 11 and 13.) Knowing your client, whether it is the individual, family, or community, facilitates evidence-based decision making. The nurses should be genuinely interested in the health of the Aboriginal clients requiring community health nursing. Required skill sets include the ability to remain objective and to resist stereotyping the community and its residents. Often nurses arrive in an Aboriginal community having already drawn conclusions from media and other sources. The person who wishes to become familiar with the health status of the First Nations populations could begin by reviewing the First Nations Regional Longitudinal Health Survey (RHS). The RHS describes Canada's First Peoples' health, using the cultural framework. Adult, youth, and children's results are available as national and regional reports.

Health personnel must continually be recruited, and nurses often must relocate to remote or isolated First Nations communities (Tarlier, Johnson, & Whyte, 2003). Retention of health personnel for only short lengths of time can result in some communities becoming distrustful of new nurses. This can provide another challenge to the nurse's communication skills (Sundeen, Stuart, Rankin, & Cohen, 1998).

Formal and informal leadership in First Nations communities can be difficult to grasp. CHNs require the skills to assess the community and outline the health priorities and health issues of the population. They have to decide on the course of action in consultation with the community. Historically, First Nations people made decisions on a consensus basis; some communities continue to make decisions in this way (Cookfair, 1991). CHNs have to find roles that can be filled by a non-member health professional, perhaps as a consultant who provides information the community can use to make its best decision. Alternatively, the nurse may be seen as the individual who makes the decisions. The nurse must rely on community-development knowledge and allow the community to make its own decisions over time. It is easy to assume control of the decision making if you are seen as the individual with the best health knowledge. However, it is important to consult with leaders, whether they are the elected leaders or the administrators of the health care system (McMurray, 1999). Elders are traditionally seen as the knowledge keepers of communities, and as such they can be important allies and sources of knowledge.

Policy Issues Affecting Community Health Nursing in Aboriginal Communities

Unlike public health nursing in urban communities, First Nations and Inuit health care systems vary in size and services offered. Nurses who seek employment in an Aboriginal community must establish a network of colleagues who can assist with information when required. Health professionals establish liaisons with other service agencies or professional organizations such as the ANAC to promote the population health approach.

CHNs must also be aware of competing policies. For instance, the federal government is responsible for the health care of Aboriginal people; thus, nursing services are provided for home care clients by FNIHB. However, the Department of Indian Affairs is responsible for funding personal care and home support services. The nurse must be innovative in coordinating the home care services for clients from two service agencies. In addition, the CHN may be requested to supervise staff responsible for personal care, homemaking, and transportation.

Health Issues in Community Health Nursing with Aboriginal People

In addition to the cultural disorganization caused by colonization are the issues from the culture of poverty (Bartlett, 2003). Because reserves effectively excluded Aboriginal people from mainstream Canadian society, poverty became permanent (Allender & Spradley, 2001). A people made powerless have no hope. Risk factors, accumulated over generations, affect health; this is demonstrated in the high rates of mortality and morbidity from injury and trauma, chronic illness, depression, and family violence (Sebastian, 2000). The effects of the residential school on individuals, family, and community have only begun to be addressed by the state and the churches. Illnesses such as tuberculosis remain a health threat, while preventable conditions such as fetal alcohol spectrum disorders and HIV/AIDS are on the increase. Other lifestyle illnesses caused by drug and alcohol abuse continue to be commonplace afflictions for Aboriginal people.

Trauma and injury, whether accidental or intentional, are high on the list of health issues besetting Aboriginal communities. The communities that practise a hunting and gathering culture may be prone to injuries from firearms or other hunting equipment. Vehicle safety is another area of health education that the nurse must contend with frequently. Perhaps the community is a fly-in community with different modes of transportation such as all-terrain vehicles, boats, and snowmobiles, all of which have their own safety issues. Burns caused by fires are another area of concern. Housing in these communities may be substandard by Canadian standards, and smoke alarms are not mandatory in such homes. Utilities that are considered essential in urban homes, such as electricity, heating, and indoor plumbing, are not always available to all First Nations community homes. Health determinants cite environment as one of the factors that determine the health of individuals in a community. The nurse must be an advocate for clients and community to improve housing standards and safety for the Aboriginal community.

Diabetes has reached epidemic proportions in Aboriginal communities. Mortality rates from diabetes for Aboriginal women living in First Nations communities are five times higher than the national average. Diabetes is also being diagnosed at a younger age. Rates of amputation, blindness, and kidney failure are higher among Aboriginal populations. Nurses must understand the health promotion and health education needed to change the lifestyle of those affected by diabetes (McMurray, 1999). Canadian Research Box 21.1 gives an example of research with Aboriginal people living with diabetes.

Recollections of Nursing—Jennie Nielsen, Aboriginal Registered Nurse

"I remember my mother interpreted for the doctor on his rounds on the Blood Reserve. My first contact with nursing was with two nurses at St. Paul's Anglican Residential School. I completed my high school in Sault Ste. Marie, Ontario. One day, while walking by the hospital, I decided to become a nurse. The director of nurses encouraged me to apply. It was three years of hard, rewarding work. I first worked near home, at the Cardston General Hospital. Next, I left for Bermuda with an adventurous friend to experience nursing in another country. Later, I was a community health nurse for 17 1/2 years on the Blood Reserve. We tried to meet the immense health needs of our community. Today, community health nursing is provided by Aboriginal nurses with baccalaureate degrees. There have been enormous changes to nursing since I graduated in 1949."

Source: J. Nielsen, personal communication, 2003.

Canadian Research Box 21.1

Iwasaki, Y., Bartlett, J., O'Neil, J. (2005). Coping with stress among Aboriginal women and men with diabetes in Winnipeg, Canada. *Social Science and Medicine, 60*(5), 977–988.

The purpose of this phenomenological study was to examine how First Nations and Métis women and men with diabetes coped with stress. Focus groups were used as the data collection method to enable participants to express themselves in their own words. The 26 participants ranged in age from 26 to 69.

Within the analysis, several themes were identified: interdependence/connectedness, spirituality/transcendence, enculturation/facilitation of Aboriginal cultural identity, self-control/self-determination/self-expression, and leisure as a means of coping with stress and healing. Participants identified activities and practices such as support from family and friends, church-based support groups, participating in sweat lodges, meditation, burning a smudge, participating in pow-wows, having a positive attitude toward life, keeping a journal, and using physical activity, laughter, and humour.

The researchers concluded that identification and utilization of the strengths of individuals and groups was very important. As well, healing must be balanced or holistic. Finally, coping with stress can result in a transformative experience, which strengthens the quality of life of the individuals, families, and communities.

Discussion Questions:

1. How might a new CHN begin to facilitate coping with stress and healing with an Aboriginal community?

2. How might a CHN apply the findings of this research in the development of a community-based diabetes health project?

Grace (2003) cites the grim health outlook for Aboriginal women, particularly Ontario Aboriginal women, who are more prone to heart disease, diabetes, suicide, depression, substance use, and family violence compared with their non-Aboriginal counterparts. Though cervical cancer rates are higher in Ontario Aboriginal women, rates for other types of cancer are lower. The types of cancer studied include colon, breast, uterine, and lymphoma.

Health education and promotion are part of the everyday contact with communities and groups. CHNs need to make the effort to make these activities culturally appropriate. The medicine wheel framework is an excellent teaching tool and, because of its diversity, can be adapted to virtually any health issue. Medicine wheels are found in the United States and southern Canada, mostly in Alberta and Saskatchewan; they are made of stone and small boulders set in various circular patterns. However, their origins and meaning have been lost in time. Some say they are for navigation by using the stars or to mark events such as the solstice. Whatever significance they had for the original inhabitants of North America, they still influence the thinking and lives of Canadian Aboriginal people today. Not unlike other Aboriginal cultures in the world, Canadian Aboriginals have a holistic belief about life.

Traditional world views of Aboriginal peoples emphasize the interconnectedness of all things, and this concept is the basis of the medicine wheel framework. Most First Nations in Canada have holistic beliefs, yet not all believe in the medicine wheel philosophy. The present significance of the medicine wheel is that it provides a framework for the holistic beliefs of the descendents of those original inhabitants of Canada.

The medicine wheel usually represents four quadrants of the emotional, physical, mental, and spiritual aspects of health and wellness. (See Figure 21.1.)

It is said that a balance has to be maintained in the four aspects for an individual to maintain optimal health. On first glance, the medicine wheel model can be simple; however, the concepts it represents are complex. The four directions are represented, just as the races of humankind are represented. The different teachings of how one can lead a purposeful life are also represented. The four life stages of infancy, childhood, adulthood, and the elder are also represented. The four components of our human-ness are the physical, the intellectual, the spiritual, and the emotional. Colours, animals, and characteristics such as strength, humility, and illumination are also assigned to their respective quadrants. Today, the medicine wheel philosophy still is being taught by elders to the youth in Aboriginal populations across North America. Examples can be found online where communities have adapted the medicine wheel to issues including HIV/AIDS, diabetes, family violence, and addictions.

An alternative framework can be found in the First Nations cultural framework of the national First Nations and Inuit Regional Longitudinal Health Survey (NAHO 2005). The two are similar but cannot be deemed to be the same.

FIGURE 21.1 A Medicine Wheel

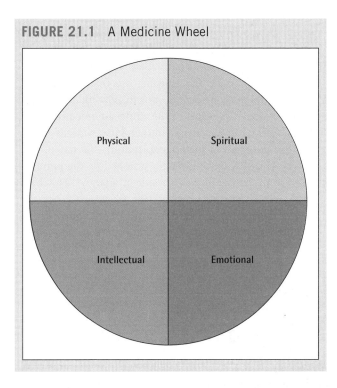

Case Study

A First Nations community has a total population of 3200. Two thousand members live on the reserve and 1200 members live off-reserve. The community is located near a mid-size city. The unemployment level is consistently at 70%. Most families rely on social services for their subsistence. Sixty percent of the population is 18 years of age or less. The education level is at the junior-to high-school range. The community is governed by an elected chief and eight councillors.

Most homes are 25 to 35 years old and have indoor plumbing, central heating, and electricity. However, potable water is delivered by water trucks. Sewage disposal is the community sewage system, but rural homes have a septic tank sewage disposal system. The climate is temperate, with cold winters and dry summers.

The community-controlled school system goes from Kindergarten to Grade 6, and six of the ten teachers are Aboriginal. The community no longer practises its Aboriginal beliefs, and fewer than 5% of the school children speak their language. High school students are bused for an hour each way to attend school in the nearby city. Most families end up being single-parent households.

The economy is based on school transportation, employment with the band administration, the band-controlled school, and two privately owned gas stations/convenience stores. The school principal has initiated a

→

good recreation program for the students, and Aboriginal teacher assistants keep the students interested in being physically active. Parents participate in the school activities. However, once the students are bused to attend school in the city, parents do not display much interest in school activities. Most of the adults attended the residential school at the neighbouring First Nations community, and most of them completed middle school.

The Health Centre is readily accessed by the population for all the community health programs. The Chief and Council transferred control of the health programs five years ago to a health administrator hired from another First Nations community. Immunization levels are at 55% for all ages. Chronic disease rates for diabetes, arthritis, and circulatory diseases have not been assessed since prior to the health program transfer. The First Nations and Inuit Health Branch continue to provide support for the CHN. During your orientation at the Regional FNIHB office, the zone nurse manager informs you that one of the priorities is the immunization program because the *Canada Disease Weekly* has reported pertussis in the area. On weekends, parents leave the community to shop in the nearby city. They frequent the bars to drink alcohol and gamble on the video lottery terminals. Children are often left in the care of elderly grandparents or alone at home to fend for themselves until their parents return.

There have been disturbing developments in the community in the last five years. Family violence, child neglect, and an increased number of motor vehicle accidents and house fires are causing concern for the various community agencies. The frequency of fetal alcohol spectrum disorder is not known. In the last five months, five teenagers have attempted suicide.

You are the new nurse. When you arrive, a lone community health representative is there to welcome you to the Health Centre. She seems to know the community very well, as people greet her warmly on the way to the Health Centre. The people that you meet appear very glad that you have arrived at the community. They greet you heartily and make you feel welcome.

Discussion Questions

1. How would you, as the CHN, use the nursing process to begin planning to improve the population health?

2. Whom would you ask to help you familiarize yourself with the community?

3. List the resiliency factors of the community.

4. What factors make this First Nations community a vulnerable community?

5. Describe how you will begin to work on the immunization program.

Part of the community health nursing practice in Aboriginal communities is the evaluation component of health programs. Nurses should recognize that nursing standards of practice can be maintained through continuous quality improvement. First Nations health systems are becoming members of the Canadian Council on Health Services Accreditation.

Summary

The chapter outlined the complexities of working with Aboriginal populations. Nurses working in First Nations communities must understand First Nations status, because it affects nursing services delivery. The employers of nurses working in First Nations communities can be the federal, provincial, or local health authorities, each with its own organizational complexities.

Aboriginal populations have immense health challenges that nurses must assess in order to plan health services. Nurses may be responsible for the implementation of health services and programs, and should have the skills to evaluate the efficacy of health programs for Aboriginal communities. In addition, nurses must have the communication skills to allow effective interaction with First Nations leadership and other service agency personnel. Advance preparation for working with First Nations should be a priority for nurses contemplating employment in First Nations communities to lessen the possible effects of culture shock. Nurses working with Canadian Aboriginals face complex challenges in a rewarding practice setting.

KEY TERMS

Aboriginal
First Nations
vulnerable populations
pre-European contact
bands
tribes
treaty
Indian Act
reserves
Department of Indian Affairs and Northern Development
Indian agents
registered Indian
status Indian
Bill C-31
Inuit
Métis
First Nations and Inuit Health Branch (FNIHB)

INDIVIDUAL CRITICAL THINKING EXERCISE

The Chief of the First Nations community that employs you has just asked to see the chart of one of the clients in your care. How would you handle the situation? How do you maintain security for client records?

GROUP CRITICAL THINKING EXERCISE

The routine water sample of the First Nations community indicates heavy growth of E. coli. As the nurse manager, how would you deal with this threat to public health? Whom would you contact?

REFERENCES

Aboriginal Healing Foundation. (1999). *Annual Report 1999.* Retrieved January 31, 2007, from http://www.ahf.ca/newsite/english/pdf/annual_report_1999.pdf.

Allender, J. A., & Spradley, B. W. (2001). *Community health nursing: Concepts and practice.* (5th ed.). Toronto: Lippincott.

Andrews, M. M., & Boyle, J. S. (1999). *Transcultural concepts in nursing* (3rd ed.). Philadelphia, PA: Lippincott.

Baker, C., & Daigle, M. C. (2000). Cross-cultural hospital care as experienced by Mi'kmaq clients. *Western Journal of Nursing Research, 22*(1), 8–28.

Ballantine, B., & Ballantine, I. (Eds.). (1993). *Native Americans: An illustrated history.* Atlanta, GA: Time.

Bartlett, J. G. (2003). Involuntary cultural change, stress phenomenon and Aboriginal health status. *Canadian Journal of Public Health, 94,* 165–167.

Browne, A. J., & Fiske, J. (2001). First Nations women's encounters with mainstream health care services. *Western Journal of Nursing Research, 23*(2), 126–147.

Canada, Department of Indian & Northern Affairs. (1997). *First Nations in Canada.* Ottawa: Author.

Canada, Department of Indian & Northern Affairs. (2002). *A summary of the First Nations Governance Act.* Ottawa: Author.

Chrisjohn, R. D., Young, S. L., & Maraun, M. (1994). *The circle game: Shadows and substance in the residential school experience in Canada: A report to the Royal Commission on Aboriginal Peoples.* Published 1997. Penticton, BC: Theytus.

Cookfair, J. M. (1991). *Nursing process and practice in the community.* Toronto: Mosby.

Cradduck, G. R. (1995). Primary health care practice. In M. J. Stewart (Ed.), *Community nursing: Promoting Canadians' health* (pp. 454–471). Toronto: Saunders.

Deagle, G. (1999). The three-tier system. [Editorial]. *Canadian Family Physician, 45,* 247–249.

Dickason, O. P. (2002a). Reclaiming stolen land. In J. Bird, L. Land, & M. Macadam (Eds.), *Nation to nation: Aboriginal sovereignty and the future of Canada* (pp. 34–42). Toronto: Irwin.

Dickason, O. P. (2002b). *Canada's First Nations: A history of founding peoples from earliest times* (3rd ed.). Don Mills: Oxford.

Dion-Stout, M., Kipling, G. D., & Stout, R. (2001). Aboriginal women's health research synthesis project. Ottawa: Women's Health Bureau.

Dumont-Smith, C. (2001). *Exposure to violence in the home: Effects on Aboriginal children.* Ottawa: Aboriginal Nurses Association of Canada.

Flaskerud, J. H., & Winslow, B. J. (1998). Conceptualizing vulnerable populations health-related research. *Nursing Research, 51*(2), 69–78.

Fleet, C. (1997). Introduction. In C. Fleet (Ed.), *First Nations firsthand: A history of five hundred years of encounter, war, and peace inspired by the eyewitnesses* (pp. 7–9). Edison: Chartwell.

Furi, M., & Wherrett, J. (1996). *Indian status and band membership issues.* Retrieved on January 31, 2007, http://www.parl.gc.ca/information/library/PRBpubs/bp410-e.htm.

Giger, J. N., & Davidhizar, R. E. (1998). *Canadian transcultural nursing assessment and intervention.* Toronto: Mosby.

Grace, L. S. (2003). Hepatitis A among residents of First Nations reserves in British Columbia, 1991–1996. *Canadian Journal of Public Health, 94,* 173–175.

Health Canada-FNIHB. (2005). *Indian health policy 1979.* Retrieved April 23, 2007, http://www.hc-sc.gc.ca/fnih-spni/services/indi_health-sante_poli_e.html.

Holland, K., & Hogg, C. (2001). *Cultural awareness in nursing and health care: An introductory text.* New York: Oxford University Press.

Lalonde, M. (1974). *A new perspective on the health of Canadians: A working document.* Ottawa: Canada, National Health and Welfare.

Mann, Charles C. (2005). *1491: New Revelations of the Americas Before Columbus.* New York: Vintage Books.

McMurray, A. (1999). *Community health and wellness: A sociological approach.* Toronto: Mosby.

Mercredi, O., & Turpel, M. E. (1993). *In the rapids: Navigating the future of First Nations.* New York: Penguin.

National Aboriginal Health Organization (NAHO) First Nations Centre. (2006). *First Nations Regional Longitudinal Health Survey (RHS) 2002/03: Report on selected indicators by gender.* Retrieved April 23, 2007, http://rhs-ers.ca/english/pdf/rhs2002-03reports/rhs2002-03-report_on_selected_indicators_by_gender.pdf.

Ricciuti, E. (1990). *The natural history of North America.* New York: Gallery.

Rumbold, G. (1999). *Ethics in nursing practice* (3rd ed.). Toronto: Bailliere Tindall.

Royal Commission on Aboriginal Peoples (RCAP). (1996). *Report of the Royal Commission on Aboriginal Peoples: Perspectives and realities. Vol. 4.* Ottawa: The Commission.

Saskatchewan Women's Secretariat. (1999). *Profile of Aboriginal women in Saskatchewan.* Regina: Saskatchewan Women's Secretariat.

Saskatoon Aboriginal Women's Health Research Committee. (2004). *Naspici miyomahcihowin (continuous good health): A community-based research project examining the health needs of Aboriginal women in Saskatoon.* Winnipeg: The Prairie Women's Health Centre of Excellence.

Schouls, T. (2002). The basic dilemma: Sovereignty or assimilation. In J. Bird, L. Land, & M. Macadam (Eds.), *Nation to nation: Aboriginal sovereignty and the future of Canada* (pp. 34–42). Toronto: Irwin.

Schultz, J. W. (1962). *Blackfeet and buffalo: Memories of life among the Indians.* Norman: University of Oklahoma Press.

Sherman, J. (1996). *Indian tribes of North America.* New York: Todri Productions.

Sebastian, J. G. (2000). Vulnerability and vulnerable populations: An overview. In M. Stanhope & J. Lancaster (Eds.), *Community & public health nursing* (5th ed.; pp. 638–661). Toronto: Mosby.

Statistics Canada. (2002). *2001 Census Aboriginal population profiles*. Retrieved April 23, 2007, http://www.12statcan.ca/english/Profil01/AP01/Index.cfm?Lang=E.

Sundeen, S. J., Stuart, G. W., Rankin, A. D., & Cohen, S. A. (1998). *Nurse–client interaction: Implementing the nursing process* (6th ed.). Toronto: Mosby.

Tarlier, D. S., Johnson, J. L., & Whyte, N. B. (2003). Voices from the wilderness: An interpretive study describing the role and practice of outpost nurses. *Canadian Journal of Public Health, 94,* 180–184.

Venne, S. (2002). Treaty-making with the Crown. In J. Bird, L. Land, & M. Macadam (Eds.), *Nation to nation: Aboriginal sovereignty and the future of Canada* (pp. 45–52). Toronto: Irwin.

Waldram, J. B., Herring, D. A., & Young, T. K. (2006). *Aboriginal health in Canada: Historical, cultural and epidemiological perspectives.* Toronto: University of Toronto Press.

ADDITIONAL RESOURCES

Websites

Aboriginal AIDS Network
    www.caan.ca

Aboriginal Nurses Association of Canada (ANAC)
    www.anac.on.ca

First Nations and Inuit Health Branch
    www.hc-sc.gc.ca/fnihb-dgspni

National Aboriginal Health Organization (NAHO)
    www.naho.ca

Population Health Approach
    www.phac-aspc.gc.ca/ph-sp/phdd

About the Authors

Rhonda J. King Blood, daughter of the late Raymond and Isabella King of the Blood Tribe, is married to Charles Sr. She is the mother to Pamelynn, Cameron Todd, Charles Jr., and a proud grandmother to Cherilynn. Educated at Blood Reserve, Magrath and Lethbridge schools, Rhonda obtained a registered nurse diploma and subsequently a Bachelor of Nursing in 1982. She graduated with a Master of Arts (Honours) from Gonzaga University, Spokane, Washington, in 1997. Employed by Health Canada, she worked primarily as a community health nurse manager among Alberta's First Nations for more than 20 years. Rhonda was also employed at the Canadian Council on Health Services Accreditation in Ottawa. Rhonda is a past Vice President and Board Member for the Aboriginal Nurses Association of Canada and a member of the College and Association of Registered Nurses of Alberta. Rhonda is employed in Lethbridge, Alberta, as a Health Promotions Specialist with the Urban Aboriginal Mental Health Program, Population Health Department, Chinook Health.

Dr. Rose Alene Roberts is a member of the Lac La Ronge Indian Band and is originally from the community of Stanley Mission, Saskatchewan. She has an undergraduate degree in nursing, and master's and doctoral degrees in Community Health and Epidemiology, all from the University of Saskatchewan. Dr. Roberts currently holds a faculty position of Assistant Professor at the College of Nursing, University of Saskatchewan. Her research interests include cancer in Aboriginal populations, alternative healing modalities, residential school survivorship, and autoimmune diseases.

CHAPTER 22

Clients in the Correctional Setting

Joanne Shaw, Cindy Peternelj-Taylor, and Phil Woods

OBJECTIVES

After studying this chapter, you should be able to:

1. Examine challenges and opportunities for nursing interventions in correctional environments.

2. Identify correctional nurses' professional and ethical responsibilities for health care.

3. Consider the most common health challenges seen in correctional settings.

4. Understand the role of the nurse in the provision of health care and client advocacy.

5. Reflect on ongoing education, research, and practice developments relative to the correctional setting.

INTRODUCTION

Nurses working in correctional settings are primarily responsible for providing health care services to a large and diverse population. Through their use of clinical assessment and triage skills, they engage in primary, secondary, and tertiary intervention strategies including early case finding, infection control, treatment and medication administration, health promotion and illness prevention, as well as rehabilitative services and end-of-life care. As per the Corrections and Conditional Release Act (CCRA), and various provincial corrections acts, clients incarcerated in correctional facilities are entitled to physical and mental health care in accordance with professional and community standards (Canadian Public Health Association [CPHA], 2004). Nurses represent the largest group of health care professionals working with incarcerated individuals, and as such they have a significant role to play. Timely identification, treatment, and management of health care concerns not only contribute to the health of the individual client but also further contribute to the health and safety of other inmates, facility staff, and the community at large.

And although correctional facilities are not generally considered part of the traditional health care system, by default they are responsible for the provision of health care services to a diverse group of individuals who have come into conflict with the law, including those who are remanded in custody while awaiting trial (charged but not yet sentenced), and those found guilty and sentenced by the courts to various periods of time in custody. Generally, individuals receiving a sentence of two years less a day are incarcerated within **provincial correctional centres**, while those sentenced to two years or

greater serve their sentence within **federal correctional institutions**, operated by the **Correctional Service Canada (CSC)**. Those on remand tend to have greater and more complex health care needs than sentenced inmates, who may have had these issues addressed during the remand period.

On an average day in 2004/2005, approximately 152 600 adults were under custodial or community supervision; approximately 32 100 adults were in provincial/territorial or federal custody in Canada; approximately 120 500 were under community supervision; while an additional 9600 (approximately) adults were held on remand. While the majority of those in custody are male, females accounted for 10% of provincial and 5% of federal admissions sentenced to custody, and 11% of all remand admissions (Beattie, 2006). On any given day in 2003/2004 there were approximately 23 400 young persons either in custody or under probation in Canada; of this group, a daily average of 1340 youth were in sentenced custody; 740 were held on remand; while the majority were on probation. Females accounted for 13% of those sentenced in custody and 18% of remand admissions (Calverley, 2006). The health and psychosocial issues experienced by this large captive group are extremely complex and contribute to treatment challenges during incarceration and upon release from custody.

PRACTICE SETTING

The effects of the correctional environment can be particularly severe, given the interpersonal climate, organizational culture, and social context. The incarceration experience represents a significant, stressful life event, as separation from family and friends, limitations on privacy, overcrowding, and the fear of assault, can severely impact the offender's health status and quality of life. Furthermore, power, control, and implicit authority are manifested in the physical and interpersonal environments of correctional systems and can be incompatible with the achievement of health-related treatment goals (Peternelj-Taylor, 2008).

Access to clients can be difficult depending on the mandate of the institution and the clients' specific health care needs. For instance, in many correctional facilities, inmates are housed in units with two-person cells and a common day area. They are allowed out of their cells 12 hours per day, and health care must be provided within this time frame. In some settings, for example, in Ontario, assessment of health concerns and provision of minor interventions is provided in the living unit, and more complex care is provided in a centralized ambulatory health care clinic. In many facilities a correctional officer accompanies the nurse and supervises the inmate for every inmate contact, and this officer must maintain visual contact of the inmate at all times. And although the nurse respects the officer's security responsibilities, the nurse must maintain client confidentiality while providing health care and eliciting health-related information.

The priorities of the correctional system centre on confinement and security, and matters of security will often take precedence over nursing care. It is not uncommon for nurses to have to wait while the officer completes security-related tasks. And although nurses, as employees of correctional facilities, must abide by the correctional policies that govern all correctional employees, correctional nurses often find themselves in a "catch 22" position as they attempt to juggle the expectations and philosophies of security, their profession, and the clients in their care. For example, how do nurses refer to the recipients of nursing care? Is the incarcerated individual an inmate or a client? (Maroney, 2005). To be successful, correctional nurses have to confront their own reactions to inmates' alleged offences or crimes for which they have been sentenced. In order to develop therapeutic relationships and provide professional and ethical care, it is important that they not get caught up in the sensationalism that surrounds a particular offender, or the setting in which nursing practice takes place.

While professional autonomy in practice has often been described as a factor related to job satisfaction in correctional nursing in general (Smith, 2005), in practice this often means working alone, and professional isolation is a concern for some correctional nurses (LaMarre, 2006). In some instances, there may only be one registered nurse for as many 200 inmates, on the day and evening shifts. This large caseload results in nurses having to set priorities based on assessment of individual client needs. In other settings, nursing practice may reflect a more traditional approach to health care, for instance in secure treatment facilities operated by provincial and federal correctional agencies.

Regardless of the setting, however, the therapeutic treatment needs of clients must always be considered within the context of maintaining security. For instance, nurses need to be ever vigilant regarding security awareness, including **static security**, the structural environmental features common to correctional facilities (e.g., video monitoring, internal barriers, perimeter fences or walls, personal protection alarms, staffing patterns, policies related to counting inmates, and counting equipment), and **dynamic security**, which addresses such things as institutional policies and procedures related to interpersonal security, including developing professional relationships, "knowing" the client in one's care, managing professional boundaries, and methods of operation. Nurses must be attentive to the materials left with clients, as many could be fashioned into weapons; for example, in some settings, dental floss may be used (and disposed after use) only in the health care clinic, rather than being allowed in the client's living area. Nurses working in a community setting certainly understand the need for innovation; nurses working in a correctional setting require similar "thinking outside the box."

HEATH CARE CHALLENGES

Historically, those who are incarcerated have experienced limited and inconsistent exposure to our health care system; while they may experience many of the same age and gender specific health care concerns common to the general population, morbidity and mortality data suggest higher rates of disease and disability when compared with non-incarcerated populations (CPHA, 2004). For many individuals, health care received while incarcerated may be the first real opportunity that they have had to address their health care needs. Numerous opportunities exist for correctional nurses to provide leadership in the provision of health promotion and illness prevention, especially if individuals are motivated to make lifestyle changes that would improve their overall health status.

The correctional system provides care for inmates with all types of acute and chronic illnesses (CPHA, 2004). The lifestyle of many inmates includes substance abuse, which gives rise to various drug and alcohol withdrawal syndromes, diverse infectious diseases, and the need for long-term treatment interventions. Crowded living conditions can result in higher exposure to infectious diseases, a concern of public health officials worldwide, as most clients eventually return to the community (Thomas, 2005). Furthermore, the "deinstitutionalization movement" that began in Canada in the 1960s and continues today has frequently been blamed for the **criminalization of the mentally ill**. In a recent editorial, White and Whiteford (2006) refer to prisons as the mental health institutions of the twenty-first century—a sad but true reality. Finally, it is not uncommon for nurses to care for clients who have experienced multiple traumas such as sexual assaults, stabbings, and/or beatings.

Provincial correctional facilities admit extremely large numbers of inmates on a daily basis; clearly, the volume, turnover, and lengths of stay (which can range from a few hours to years) definitely affect what nurses can do. Daily admissions to federal correctional facilities are minimal compared to provincial correctional facilities, so the care they are able to provide is different. Clients presenting with acute health care problems are assessed and triaged by nurses, and those requiring acute emergency care are normally transferred to a local community general hospital for further assessment and treatment. Nursing staff, in collaboration with the facility physician, manage other less urgent issues. Nurses frequently assist the clients to bring chronic conditions under better control, by attending to treatment protocols, assessing for complications, preventing recurrence of problems, health teaching, and preparing for eventual discharge to the community.

Special Populations in Correctional Settings

While it could be argued that all individuals who are incarcerated have special needs requiring the attention of correctional nurses, the unique needs of the mentally ill, the elderly, women, and youth are highlighted here to draw attention to the disparities experienced by inmates with mental illness when compared with the community standard, and overall gender and developmental health related concerns.

The Mentally Ill in Corrections
Deinstitutionalization has resulted in an influx to correctional facilities of individuals with serious mental illness. Prior to this, police would transport individuals exhibiting bizarre behaviours in public to a mental health facility; now they have few choices but to remand the individual in custody in a local jail or remand centre.

In *Out of the Shadows at Last: Transforming Mental Health, Mental Illness, and Addiction Services in Canada,* the final report of the Standing Senate Committee on Social Affairs, Science and Technology (2006), a mother whose son has bipolar disorder poignantly shared her concerns regarding the lack of mental health beds within the health care system:

> [I]ncarcerating mentally ill people in jails and prisons, is cruel, unjust and ineffective. Prisons do not have adequate or appropriate facility resources or medical care to deal with the mentally ill. Poorly trained staff is unable to handle the difficulties of mental illness. The mentally ill suffer from illogical thinking, delusions, auditory hallucinations, paranoia, and severe mood swings. They do not always comprehend the rules of jails and prisons. They are highly vulnerable and prone to bizarre behavior that prison staff must deal with and inmates must tolerate. (p. 300)

The CPHA (2004) reports that epidemiological studies in the CSC have found high prevalence of mental disorder in inmates, often with two or more coexisting disorders, and higher rates of psychosis, depression, anxiety, and personality disorder when compared to the Canadian population. Over the past ten years, the number of those with significant mental health problems has doubled in federal correctional institutions. According to the CSC (2006), one of the major challenges they currently have with the changing offender profile is that more than one out of ten male offenders, and one out of four female offenders, are identified at admission as presenting with mental health problems. Between March 1997 and March 2006 they saw a growth rate of 71% in men, 117% in Aboriginal men, and 67% in women. In a prevalence study of mental illness in inmates in Ontario correctional facilities, the prevalence of schizophrenia was 4.5%, depression 5.6%, bipolar 5.2%, antisocial personality disorder 4.1%, adjustment disorder 3.4%, anxiety 1.9%, and attention deficit hyperactive disorder 1.5% (total 20%) (Brown, Girard, & Mathias, 2006). Although these figures are somewhat lower than those identified by the CSC, the discrepancy is most likely due to how mentally ill inmates are assessed and labelled in Ontario facilities. Similar high prevalence rates are reported in other countries. In a survey of psychiatric morbidity among prisoners in England and Wales, Singleton, Meltzer, Gatward, Coid, & Deasy (1998) report a high prevalence of mental illness and personality disorder in both remanded and sentenced males and females. A more recent study by the U.S. Department of Justice reported that 64% of local jail inmates, 56% of state prisoners, and 45% of federal prisoners have symptoms of serious mental illness (James & Glaze, 2006).

Generally, correctional facilities are not in a position to provide mental health care at the same standard as that found within community mental health systems. Indeed, the Office of the Correctional Investigator (OCI, 2006) emphasizes that treatment within federal facilities is often non-existent, or unsatisfactory, when compared to the community standard. Furthermore, the CPHA (2004) highlights the need for more proactive standardized mental health intake assessments rather than reactive, crisis-oriented services. However, the CPHA (2004) also notes that promoting mental health in a correctional setting is challenging at best, as the environment is coercive by definition.

Correctional nurses must conduct mental health assessments on all new admissions, and, moreover, be astute to assessing those who may become mentally ill while incarcerated. Often, those with a mental illness are withdrawn, non-communicative, and suicidal. The nurse requires highly developed assessment and communication skills to elicit data necessary to identify those with mental illness (or mental health problems) and to ensure their safety. It is very important that those with psychosis, or those who have decompensated, are housed in an area where they can be protected from predatory inmates, as those with mental illness can be victimized and/or physically bullied for their medications. Those with mental illness are especially vulnerable within correctional systems, due to the pecking order that exists within the prison subculture.

Although policies vary across the country and across jurisdictions, individuals presenting as mentally ill at the time of remand require an advocate to ensure that they move through the justice system as quickly as possible and that appropriate transitional discharge plans are in place. Specifically, the advocate ensures that court-ordered assessments and court reports are completed, informs court support services of an inmate with mental illness, and develops a joint care plan with court support services. Often those with a mental illness do not have their own lawyers and instead use duty counsel. Consequently, the advocate role falls to the correctional nurse. There is a great opportunity for nurses to work with external community-based organizations in order to meet the treatment and release needs of this vulnerable group. Collaboration with various community agencies can assist correctional nurses with the provision of mental health services while the client is in custody and provide the link to their home community upon release. Increasingly, court diversion schemes are being embraced as a way of diverting those with mental illness from the criminal justice system. In Canada, diversion can occur with the police, upon arrival at court, or upon initial incarceration (Statistics Canada, 2003). Such schemes hold promise for humane treatment and reduced recidivism among this population.

All inmates are assessed for suicidal thoughts and plans on admission and as indicated throughout their incarceration. Suicide may be viewed by inmates as the only way to cope with their charges (and/or their sentence), family responsibilities that cannot be met, fear of the actions of fellow inmates, and the living conditions within the correctional facility. For the mentally ill, severity of current psychotic symptoms is related to current risk of suicide (Tandon & Jibson, 2003). Inmates may be placed on a suicide watch if assessment indicates, and referred to a psychiatrist for further assessment, medication, other treatments, and admission to hospital as necessary.

In most settings, mentally ill inmates are generally supervised 24 hours per day by correctional staff. The security training and experience varies among this group; minimal training in mental health theory and practice is often the norm. Clearly, suitable educational programs should be an integral part of the training of all front-line staff (OCI, 2006). It is important that correctional staff have the necessary skills to identify those with mental health problems, to provide appropriate supervision, and to make referrals to health care accordingly. And, although Appelbaum, Hickey, & Packer (2001) conclude that correctional officers have important responsibilities when working with this vulnerable group, collectively as a group correctional nurses should be advocating for mental health care that is consistent with the community standard. Correctional officers cannot, and should not, be replacing nurses.

The Aging Offender Unfortunately, for an increasing number of elderly Canadians, growing old in prison is a harsh reality; a trend also experienced in other Western countries. Individuals over the age of 50 years are among the fastest-growing subgroup found within correctional environments. On average, correctional clients are thought to be 10 to 12 years older physiologically when compared with their chronological age (Beckett, Peternelj-Taylor, & Johnson, 2003).

Common physical health care needs experienced by this population include cardiovascular disease, pulmonary disorders, diabetes, arthritis, cancer, and Alzheimer's disease and other dementias. The mental health issues most evident in this group include stress, social isolation, depression, and suicide (CPHA, 2004).

Prisons and correctional facilities were never designed for an aging population; subsequently, the increased "greying population" in many facilities has resulted in the need for significant improvements in relation to accommodation planning, program development, palliative care, and reintegration options (OCI, 2006). For many elderly and infirm correctional clients, the fear of dying while imprisoned is a terse reality.

And although the CCRA and various pieces of provincial legislation provide for *parole or release by exception,* also known as *compassionate release* (often to community-based long term care facilities), it is rarely utilized, as ongoing fears about community safety, acute bed shortages in long term care, and the stigma associated with incarceration are factors impacting on placement. The public in general is not interested in having convicted criminals residing in long term care facilities (regardless of their health status). As a result, correctional nurses are responsible for developing and providing services geared specifically to the elderly, including palliative care services (Beckett et al., 2003; Duggleby, 2005).

Women's Issues Women most likely to be incarcerated have grown up in poor communities, have limited education and job skills, are victims as well as perpetrators of crime, and are the primary caregivers for dependent children (Pate, 2003). And, like "free" women, they are likely to experience multiple roles such as mother, daughter, wife, sister, and friend (Harner, 2004) and to be responsible for the emotional maintenance of the family unit, even when they are not with their families. The fear of losing custody of their children is an ever-present reality (Canadian Centre on Substance Abuse [CCSA], 2006).

Studies indicate that 50% to 70% of female inmates report physical and/or sexual abuse (Heney & Kristiansen, 2002). Common health concerns experienced by incarcerated women include substance abuse and related sequelae; infectious diseases, including HIV, AIDS, and hepatitis B (HBV) and C (HCV); pregnancy-related concerns; gynecological problems; urinary incontinence (especially within the aging population); obesity; and chronic health disorders (Maeve, 2003). Common mental health concerns include diagnoses of personality disorder (particularly borderline personality disorder and self-injurious behaviour); anxiety-related disorders (including post-traumatic stress disorder); serious mental illness (e.g., schizophrenia and depression); and poor overall cognitive functioning (McDonagh, Noël, & Wichmann, 2002; Roth & Pressé, 2003). Langner, Barton, McDonagh, Noël, and Bouchard (2002) found that 87% of federal female inmates have orders for medication. Of these, 42% had an order for psychotropic medication.

The development of "healthy" relationships impacts on a woman's ability to adapt to incarceration, engage in treatment, and foster rehabilitative efforts. Correctional nurses are in key positions to help women develop safe and meaningful relationships with others including family members, volunteers, and peers (Harner, 2004).

Reproductive issues require considerable attention for women who are pregnant and incarcerated, and nurses are often thrust into a counselling role regarding the woman's choice and decision making surrounding pregnancy. Nurse-to-nurse collaboration with local hospitals is critical, as hospital nurses are often unaware of the extra security precautions that are required during medical transfers. For example, labour and delivery nurses are not generally accustomed to working with women who are in shackles and accompanied by correctional officers. Following delivery, special provisions must be made so the woman has contact with her child in order to facilitate normal mother–child bonding (Fogel & Belyea, 2001). The mother may require help with parenting skills, and community agencies are often called upon to assist with these skills while the mother is in custody and upon her release. If there is a prior history of child abuse, the newborn may be taken into care as per the authority of provincial child protection services. In such cases, women may need additional support in relation to the grieving process over the loss of their child. Pregnant women who are addicted to opiates and/or are involved in a methadone maintenance program will need to have this program either initiated or continued to prevent damage to the fetus from opiate withdrawal.

Women who are incarcerated are often interested in learning more about their health, including family-planning services. Nurses in Ontario correctional centres have developed a prenatal, birth, and postpartum care program and are piloting a mental health program for women who are incarcerated. Federally, nurses have been actively involved in the development and implementation of a number of programs related to self-harming behaviours (Roth & Pressé, 2003); gender-specific substance abuse treatment (Hume, 2004); and the use of storytelling to enhance health promotion among Aboriginal women (Rowan, Auger, Toto, Simpson, & McNab, 2004).

Youth   Youth ages 12 to 17 residing in youth centres and youth and adult shared facilities are sentenced under the authority of the Youth Criminal Justice Act (YCJA).

More often than not, youth in custody present with a variety of symptoms consistent with schizophrenia, anxiety disorders, depression, and behavioural disorders, although they may never have had a formal diagnosis as such (Shelton, 2004). The first episode of schizophrenia may be seen in this age group and needs to be considered by nurses when conducting mental health assessments. Symptom presentation is often more subtle in this age group. For example, the youth may be withdrawn, display an abnormal affect, and demonstrate a minor thought disorder. A suicide assessment of every youth is also necessary since studies have found that 11% of non-incarcerated people with a first episode of psychosis have attempted suicide (Tandon & Jibson, 2003). In addition, youth in custody often experience higher rates of fetal alcohol spectrum disorder, significant substance abuse issues, self-harming, suicidal ideation, and high rates of physical, sexual, and emotional abuse, and many are involved with a child protection agency at the time of their arrest (Latimer & Fosse, 2004).

Canada has the reputation of incarcerating more youth per capita than any other Western country, even though the YCJA mandates that alternatives to incarceration be considered. Changes in incarceration rates are being realized. In Ontario alone, the number of youth sentenced in custody between 2002/2003 and 2004/2005 dropped by one-third (J. Underwood, personal communication, 2006). Aboriginal youth are almost eight times as likely to be in custody as compared with their non-Aboriginal counterparts. These figures are particularly distressing when one considers that Aboriginal youth represent approximately 5% of the Canadian population, yet 33% of the youth sentenced in custody (Latimer & Fosse, 2004).

Youth require life skills and substance abuse programs plus education in prevention of sexually transmitted infections, family planning, and parenting skills. A recent study on the prevalence of HIV and HCV in youth in secure custody found 0% prevalence of HIV and 0.4% of HCV. However, many youth reported engaging in risky behaviours: 33.3% injected drugs with a used needle, and 78% engaged in vaginal or anal intercourse without a condom (Calzavara et al., 2006). Nurses have to be aware of treatment boundaries and the power inherent within their professional roles. A participant in Shelton's (2003) study lamented that "the big problem is when patients get attached to staff. For some kids, this is as good as it gets. In many ways you're the parent this kid wished he had" (p. 49).

Cultural Diversity

The ethnic diversity of Canada as a whole is reflected in the demographic profile of Canadian correctional facilities. As in other Western societies, people of colour are disproportionately represented in most correctional facilities in Canada. Aboriginal offenders are overrepresented in all levels of Canada's correctional facilities, and even though they compose only 2% of Canada's adult population they represent approximately 17% of the federally incarcerated population (CPHA, 2004; CSC, 2005).

The overrepresentation of Aboriginal people within the criminal justice system represents the commingling of a number of complex factors including rapid culture change, cultural oppression, marginalization, and the long-term effects of the residential schools (Kirmayer, Brass, & Tait, 2000), which together have contributed to high rates of poverty, substance abuse, and victimization within families and communities of origin (CSC, 2005). The OCI (2006) is particularly critical of the federal government's response to Aboriginal offenders, citing evidence of systematic discrimination against Aboriginal inmates within Canada's prisons.

There has been a growing awareness in recent years of the need to provide culturally competent care in all areas of health care (Srivastava, 2007); the same can be said for provincial and correctional systems. Increasingly, specific cultural practices are incorporated into programming offered within correctional facilities. For example, in collaboration with First Nations and Métis communities, as part of the rehabilitation process elders, healers, and community leaders often lead traditional activities, including sweet grass ceremonies, smudging, and sweat lodges.

Substance Abuse

Substance abuse, including alcohol, nicotine, cocaine, opiates, benzodiazepines, cannabis products, and hallucinogens, is a major problem within correctional systems worldwide, and this problem is no different in Canada, although different levels of the problem are reported. The CPHA (2004) has reported that the majority of federally incarcerated inmates meet criteria for substance or alcohol abuse disorders. Likewise, the CSC (2006) reports that there continues to be a high prevalence of substance abuse within its correctional facilities (80% overall, 95% Aboriginal men, 77% women). The Ontario correctional system has reported that 7.1% of inmates have a definite substance abuse diagnosis (Brown et al., 2006). However, 85% have a substance abuse note on their correctional files, and the severity of withdrawal syndromes varies, requiring nurses to be astute in their assessments and observations regarding how withdrawal is manifested.

Harm reduction is the most widely accepted approach for dealing with substance abuse in many correctional institutions worldwide (Thomas, 2005, p. 1). These strategies are controversial, and debate regarding the introduction of needle exchange programs within correctional facilities is ongoing.

From a public health perspective, the OCI (2006), together with other advocacy groups, including the Canadian HIV/AIDS Legal Network, recommends their immediate introduction. To date, no correctional facility in Canada has adopted this recommendation. Instead, bleach kits, for the purposes of decontaminating injection equipment, are available in some jurisdictions. Although bleach may provide a high level of disinfection, it does not kill all viruses such as HBV and HCV (Thomas, 2005).

Methadone maintenance treatment (MMT) programs are in place in most facilities in Canada and, like other harm-reduction strategies, are controversial. Staff members' lack of understanding contributes to the belief that methadone administration simply gives offenders a drug that replaces the illicit drug they were taking prior to arrest. On the other side of this issue, the Prisoner AIDS Support Action Network (PASAN) has pressed for more liberal continuation, and initiation, of MMT for substance abusers dependent upon opiates. By 2002, most Canadian correctional facilities had adopted polices that allowed the continuation of MMT for those placed in custody while in treatment; however, fewer jurisdictions allow for the initiation of MMT for those already in custody (CCSA, 2006). Correctional officers' concerns often stem from the fact that methadone is a highly valued commodity within correctional systems, and there are many inmate attempts to divert the drug and to bully/muscle other inmates for it. Consequently, the procedure for administration of methadone is tightly supervised and time consuming. Nurses have to be alert for drug-seeking attempts and differentiate those who are simply trying to manipulate the system from those who legitimately require medications for health-related problems.

Infectious Diseases

The prevalence of blood borne infections such HIV, AIDS, and HBV and HCV are higher in the incarcerated population, primarily as a result of the high-risk behaviours demonstrated by inmates before and during incarceration such as tattooing, ear and body piercing, intravenous drug use, and risky sexual activity (which also leads to increased presentation of sexually transmitted infections such as chlamydia and gonorrhea).

A CSC study found that in 2000 and 2001 the number of reported infections of hepatitis B in the federal facilities was 13 and 43, respectively. This corresponded to 0.1% of the inmate population in 2000 and 0.3% in 2001. The rate in the general population was estimated to be between 0.5% and 1.0% in 2000 (De, 2002). The prevalence of HCV in an Ontario study during 2003 to 2004 was 17.6%. HCV prevalence was 15.9% in adult males and 30.2% in adult females, while HIV prevalence was reported to be 2% (Calzavara et al., 2006). In Ontario, HIV antibody prevalence in provincially held adult female inmates was 1.8%, and 2% in males held provincially. The study concluded that, based on 52 876 admissions per year, one could expect a projected 1097 HIV-positive inmates and 9208 HCV-positive inmates.

The HIV infection rate in federal facilities is 1.7% for males and 4.7% for females (CSC, 2003). However, as in the Canadian population, true prevalence rates are unknown because screening for HIV and other blood borne infections is voluntary. It is estimated that up to 70% of federal inmates remain unscreened. Across the country, incarcerated women have a rate of infection 2.5 times that of men, which raises the question: Is this difference due to an actual higher infection rate, or do women request testing more often than men?

In 2001, 0.18% of federal inmates had genital chlamydia and 0.10% had gonorrhea. The general population rate of chlamydia infection was estimated at 0.15%, and gonorrhea was 0.02% (De, 2002). Harm-reduction strategies such as condoms, dental dams, and water-based lubricants are available to inmates who request such products. However, sexual activity between inmates can result in a citation for misconduct. Consequently, inmates are ambivalent about requesting these products. On one hand, they are being responsible by using a coping mechanism to prevent spread of disease; on the other hand, by merely requesting these products they are risking a misconduct. PASAN and other advocacy groups such as the Canadian HIV/AIDS Legal Network further recommend that bleach be freely available and that correctional centres introduce needle exchange programs (Lines, 2002). However, many inmates have charges of drug possession and/or trafficking, and governments are loath to be seen as condoning criminal behaviour. Such harm-reduction programs, although endorsed by the health care community and advocacy groups alike, continue to be deemed controversial and subject to the political whim of governments, as was illustrated in the cancellation of the safe tattooing project being piloted in select federal correctional facilities. This is another example where correctional policies (e.g., custody) and health care interventions (e.g., caring) often collide.

The prevalence of tuberculosis (TB) infections in previously TB skin test naive or negative inmates in Ontario was 7.5% for the 12 months ending March 2006. Of these, one inmate was diagnosed with active TB (Ferris, personal communication, 2006). TB in crowded correctional settings represents a public health challenge worldwide (CPHA, 2004; Centers for Disease Control and Prevention, 2006).

Nurses are often the first health care providers to assess inmates for infectious disease. This assessment is important in case finding and subsequent medical treatment. Nurses also implement infection-control precautions to prevent subsequent infection of staff and other inmates. Health education for inmates and staff on the prevention of infection transmission is a good example of a primary prevention strategy.

When the Ontario government declared a provincial emergency because of severe acute respiratory syndrome (SARS), nurses working in Ontario correctional centres saw a potential for massive risk to inmates and staff working in correctional facilities. At that time, not much was known about the disease and its control or treatment. The strategy from the beginning was to prevent an inmate or staff member with symptoms of SARS from entering the facilities, and inmate visits in the greater Toronto area were stopped where SARS cases had been reported.

A group of senior nurse leaders developed a screening tool to screen all people entering a facility and/or transferring to another facility. Approximately 6000 inmates were screened in the Toronto area in an eight-week period. This tool was later adopted for screening in many other sectors in Ontario, and adapted as new information became available. (See Figure 9.2 in Chapter 9.)

Using this screening tool, Ontario correctional nurses identified several inmates who required voluntary quarantine as directed by the local public health unit. These inmates were isolated in the province's correctional facilities. Several other inmates, identified with SARS-like symptoms, were sent to hospital and returned to the facility once SARS had been ruled out. As well, several staff members were advised to leave work and consult with public health, Telehealth Ontario, or their family physicians. Ontario correctional nurses worked very closely with nurses in their local public health units to determine who should be in voluntary isolation and what should be done with inmates with SARS-like symptoms. Their efforts were successful in finding symptomatic inmates and in allaying some of the anxiety felt by inmates and staff over this new infectious disease.

Correctional Staff and Infectious Diseases   Nurses function within a very narrow margin when addressing staff members' "need to know" and inmates' confidentiality. Nurses cannot provide confidential information regarding diagnoses. However, they must educate and inform correctional staff of infection control and other health care procedures. The pressure from staff for confidential health care information will continue, as will the need for nurses to protect that confidentiality. Most nurses do find a way to provide health education to correctional staff and alleviate some of their work-related stress. For example, nurses can instruct correctional officers regarding the principles of harm reduction; the use of standard practices; airborne, droplet, and direct-contact isolation procedures; and the need for confidentiality in health-related matters.

COMMUNITY CONNECTION

Increasingly, correctional facilities are being identified as a "public health opportunity" (CSC, 2003). From a public health perspective, the health of the incarcerated population is a reflection of the state of the health of the community at large. Harm-reduction strategies as discussed are recommended for disease prevention and control within correctional facilities, and have direct implications for the community at large, as the majority of those in custody will eventually reintegrate into the community. Attending to the comprehensive needs of this population requires interdisciplinary and intersectoral collaboration between health care, criminal justice, education, social services, non-governmental organizations, and the voluntary sector. Such partnerships need to be established, nurtured, and evaluated (Peternelj-Taylor, 2008).

Freudenberg (2001) challenges practitioners, researchers, and policy makers to ask new research questions, develop new policies, and implement new programs that improve health and social services, emphasize community reintegration efforts, and support alternatives to incarceration. Correctional

environments are being selected more frequently as community health placements for nursing students. Recognition of correctional nursing as a specialized area of nursing practice is critical to ongoing growth and development of this specialty area. In 2005, a Registered Nurses Association of Ontario (RNAO) Correctional Nurses' Interest Group was established by correctional nurses, the first such group in Canada.

POLICY CHANGES

Nurses are especially well situated to influence, develop, and change correctional health care policies. For example, nurses have played a huge role in initiating and implementing non-smoking policies in many correctional facilities across the country. In Ontario alone, the correctional system has been completely non-smoking since the year 2000. And although many observers predicted riots and assaults upon implementation of this policy, in actuality it was a non-event from a security perspective. However, through the implementation of this public health initiative, healthier living and work environments have been created for all concerned. Nurses have also been staunch advocates for policy development and change, including the development of infection control courses for delivery in local and regional facilities; prenatal and postnatal program development in women's institutions; resource management (including staffing and scheduling patterns); the introduction of telemedicine and automated external defibrillators; and policies regarding palliative care and end-of-life care.

The SARS outbreak of 2003 saw nurses—in Ontario and British Columbia in particular—develop policies directly related to inmate and staff screening. For many, this was a wake-up call of sorts, and correctional nurses are now at the forefront of policy development in relation to pandemic planning.

Nurses have been involved in developing policies related to mental health care delivery in secure mental health treatment units. Such mental health facilities, operated under provincial corrections, can be found in Ontario and Nova Scotia. Ontario currently has a 100-bed secure treatment unit affiliated with a hospital, and plans are in place for another mental health facility.

RESEARCH IN CORRECTIONAL NURSING

The ongoing evolution of correctional nursing as a specialty is dependent on the establishment of a nursing culture that supports and nurtures the development of nursing research. And although correctional nursing has undergone significant transformations in professional role development in recent years, the professional literature remains largely anecdotal as correctional environments have attracted very few nurse researchers (Peternelj-Taylor, 2005). This has resulted in a severe scarcity of research in correctional nursing in Canada and elsewhere, even though a goldmine of research opportunities exists within correctional environments.

Nursing has a pivotal research role to play in the correctional milieu, both in the translation and interpretation of research relevant to incarcerated populations and in the identification of important nursing research questions that emerge from practice. There are unique research issues with this population, for example ensuring that consent is free, informed, and given without expectation of special favours. Therefore, guidelines are in place that clearly prevent the offer of privileges, early release, or favourable parole assessments in return for participation in a research study during incarceration.

While published research is sparse in Canada, some projects are underway. For example, the Ontario Ministry of Community Safety and Correctional Services is proceeding with a program evaluation of nurses providing discharge planning to remanded inmates with mental illness, is developing an operational definition of the discharge-planning program, and will soon start to study the effects of the program on inmates. Embracing a research agenda with incarcerated populations will provide new insights into nursing practice in this domain (Peternelj-Taylor, 2005). Canadian Research Box 22.1 highlights a recent Canadian project.

Since 1989, the College of Nursing, University of Saskatchewan, in collaboration with the Regional Psychiatric Centre (Prairies), Correctional Service of Canada, has sponsored a biennial nursing conference that showcases the unique contributions nurses make to health care within the criminal justice system. This international forum provides opportunities for clinical practitioners, educators, administrators, researchers, and policy makers to learn about matters of interest to correctional nurses.

Canadian Research Box 22.1

Schafer, P. E., & Peternelj-Taylor, C. (2003). Therapeutic relationships and boundary maintenance: The perspective of forensic patients enrolled in a treatment program for violent offenders. *Issues in Mental Heath Nursing, 24,* 605–625.

These authors wanted to describe the relationships, as described by the clients, between nurses and clients in a correctional treatment setting. The clients were referred to the treatment program from their parent correctional facilities. Twelve male clients volunteered to participate in the study and each was interviewed at least three times. The data were the verbatim transcripts of the interviews. Themes that emerged from the data were set in the analogy of a house and included:

- adjusting to the house (transition from parent institution);
- knowing the fundamental structures of the house (influential contextual factors);
- evaluating the primary therapist as a guide (is the therapist "for them or against them"?);
- experiences that promote or hinder the relationship; and
- ways of being with the primary therapist: head, head and heart, heart, and wallet (four types of relationships identified by the clients).

Though the authors note that the themes are interrelated, they present them individually, supported by quotes from the data. As the authors state, "This research indicates that therapeutic relationships, gender relations, power, patterns of interacting, and self-awareness are among the essential concepts to guide forensic mental health nurses in establishing therapeutic relationships and maintaining boundaries" (p. 622).

Discussion Questions:

1. Inmates are considered a vulnerable population. Are there other vulnerable populations to which this research may apply? Why?

2. How might a nurse use the information gleaned from this study in establishing and maintaining therapeutic relationships with clients who are incarcerated?

Case Study

An 18-year-old male is admitted to a local detention centre, charged with the sexual assault of a child. On assessment, you find that he is quiet, has difficulty establishing eye contact, and simply answers "yes" or "no" to most questions asked. His affect is incongruent with the topic under discussion. He tells you he has been consuming three cannabis cigarettes per day for the last year. The police call and want to know his HIV, HBV, and HCV status, as the victim's family wants their child treated if such a risk is present.

Discussion Questions

1. What are your thoughts and feelings about this young man? the child? the child's family?

2. What might you do to work through your feelings in order to provide care for your client?

3. What might your working nursing diagnosis be? What other data would you need to collect?

4. How would you respond to the request for information regarding the inmate's HIV, HBV, and HCV status?

Summary

Correctional nursing, as a specialty area of practice, has undergone significant transformations in role development in recent years. And although accepting the challenge to provide nursing care in environments where health care delivery is not the primary goal can lead to myriad personal and professional issues for nurses, correctional nursing is collaborative and interdisciplinary by its very nature; the most successful health care outcomes are achieved when nurses and correctional officers share a common vision, one of professionalism in the provision of security and quality nursing care to those in custody (Hufft & Kite, 2003).

KEY TERMS

provincial correctional centres
federal correctional institutions
Correctional Service Canada (CSC)
static security
dynamic security
criminalization of the mentally ill

INDIVIDUAL CRITICAL THINKING EXERCISES

1. What types of assessment tools would you need to assess inmates for their most prevalent health problems?

2. What information would you give to a correctional officer when asked what an inmate's positive TB skin test means?

3. Define "vulnerability" within the context of nursing research. How is this definition relevant to individuals who are incarcerated? What guidelines exist to protect correctional clients as research participants?

GROUP CRITICAL THINKING EXERCISES

1. What issues need to be considered when implementing harm-reduction strategies, such as needle exchanges and accessible bleach in correctional facilities?

2. What is the role of the nurse in advocating for individuals with mental illness who find themselves in conflict with the justice system?

3. In comparison with other Western countries, Canadian statistics regarding youth incarceration, especially youth of Aboriginal ancestry, are particularly alarming. What factors contribute to this phenomenon in Canada?

REFERENCES

Appelbaum, K. L., Hickey, J. M., & Packer, I. (2001). The role of correctional officers in multidisciplinary mental health care in prisons. *Psychiatric Services, 52*(10), 1343–1347.

Beattie, K. (2006). Adult correctional services in Canada, 2004/2005. *Juristat, 26*(5), (Catalogue No: 85-002 XIE). Ottawa: Canadian Centre for Justice Statistics.

Beckett, J., Peternelj-Taylor, C., & Johnson, R. (2003). Growing old in the correctional system. *Journal of Psychosocial Nursingand Mental Health Services, 41*(9), 12–18.

Brown, G., Girard, L., Mathias, K. (2006, June). *Identifying the psychiatric care needs of adult offenders in the Ontario correctional system.* Paper presented at the 20th Annual Mental Health Centre, Penetanguishene Forensic Conference: Mentally disordered offenders: What have we learned in 20 years? Penetanguishene, ON.

Calverley, D. (2006). Youth custody and community services in Canada, 2003/04. *Juristat, 26*(2), (Statistics Canada Catalogue No. 85-002 XPE). Ottawa: Canadian Centre for Justice Statistics.

Calzavara, L., Burchell, A., Meyers, T., Swantee, C., Feron, M., Ford, P., et al. (2006). *Prevalence and risk factors for HIV and hepatitis C in Ontario's jails and detention centres (2003–2004).* Toronto: University of Toronto Press.

Canadian Centre on Substance Abuse. (2006). *Fact sheet: Self harm among criminalized women.* Retrieved December 4, 2006, from http://www.ccsa.ca/NR/rdonlyres/6EC2EA26-D953-4E82-AC09-A1B9BEF7DAC1/0/ccsa0113382006e.pdf.

Canadian Public Health Association. (2004). A health care needs assessment of federal inmates. *Canadian Journal of Public Health, 95*(supplement 1), S1–S63.

Centers for Disease Control and Prevention. (2006, July). Prevention and control of tuberculosis in correctional and detention facilities: Recommendations from CDC. *Morbidity and Mortality Weekly Report, 55*(RR-9), 1–64.

Correctional Service Canada. (2003). *Infectious diseases prevention and control in Canadian federal penitentiaries 2000–01*(Cat. No. 0-662-67144-9). Ottawa: Author.

Correctional Service Canada. (2005, February). *Issues and challenges facing CSC.* Retrieved January 12, 2007, from http://www.csc-scc.gc.ca/text/pblct/guideorateur/pdf/sec6_e.pdf.

Correctional Service Canada. (2006). *2006–2007 estimates: Part III—Report on plan and priorities.* (Catalogue No. BT31-2/2007-III-44). Ottawa: Minister of Public Works and Government Services.

De, P. (2002). Infectious diseases in Canadian federal penitentiaries. *Forum on Corrections Research, 14*(2), 15–19.

Duggleby, W. (2005). Fostering hope in incarcerated older adults. *Journal of Psychosocial Nursing and Mental Health Services, 43*(9), 15–20.

Fogel, C. I., & Belyea, M. (2001). Psychosocial risk factors in pregnant inmates: A challenge for nursing. *American Journal of Maternal Child Nursing, 26*(1), 10–16.

Freudenberg, N. (2001). Jails, prisons, and the health of urban populations: A review of the impact of the correctional system on community health. *Journal of Urban Health: Bulletin of the New York Academy of Medicine, 78*(2), 214–235.

Harner, H. M. (2004). Relationships between incarcerated women: Moving beyond stereotypes. *Journal of Psychosocial Nursing, 42*(1), 38–46.

Heney, J., & Kristiansen, C. (2002). *Working with women in conflict with the law: A trainers' guide.* Toronto: Ministry of Public Safety and Security.

Hufft, A., & Kite, M. M. (2003). Vulnerable and cultural perspectives for nursing care in correctional systems. *The Journal of Multicultural Nursing & Health, 9*(1), 18–26.

Hume, L. (2004). A gender specific substance abuse program for federally sentenced women. *Forum on Corrections Research, 16*(1), 40–41.

James, D. J., & Glaze, L. E. (2006, September). *Mental health problems of prison and jail inmates. Bureau of Justice Statistics Special Report.* U.S. Department of Justice, Office of Justice Programs. Retrieved December 5, 2006, from http://www.ojp.usdoj.gov/bjs/pub/pdf/mhppji.pdf.

Kirmayer, L. J., Brass, G. M., & Tait, C. L. (2000). The mental health of Aboriginal peoples: Transformations of identity and community. Canadian Journal of Psychiatry, 45(7), 607–616.

LaMarre, M. (2006). Nursing role and practice in correctional facilities. In M. Puisis (Ed.), *Clinical practice in correctional medicine* (2nd ed.; pp. 417–418). Philadelphia: Mosby Elsevier.

Langner, N., Barton, J., McDonagh, D., Noël, C., & Bouchard, F. (2002). Rates of prescribed medication use by women in prisons. *Forum on Corrections Research, 14*(2), 10–13.

Latimer, J., & Fosse, L. C. (2004, February). *A one-day snapshot of aboriginal youth in custody across Canada: Phase II,* Department of Justice Canada. Retrieved February 18, 2006, from http://www.justice.gc.ca/en/ps/rs/rep/2004/snap2/index.html.

Lines, R. (2002). *Action on HIV/AIDS in prisons: Too little, too late. A report card.* Ottawa: Canadian HIV/AIDS Legal Network.

Maeve, K. M. (2003). Nursing care partnerships with women leaving jail: Effects on health and crime. *Journal of Psychosocial Nursing and Mental Health Services, 41*(9), 30–40.

Maroney, M. K. (2005). Caring and custody: Two faces of the same reality. *Journal of Correctional Health Care, 11*(2), 157–169.

McDonagh, D., Noël, C., & Wichmann, C. (2002). Mental health needs of women offenders: Needs analysis for the development of the intensive intervention strategy. *Forum on Corrections Research, 14*(2), 32–35.

Office of the Correctional Investigator. (2006). *Annual report of the Office of the Correctional Investigator 2005–2006 (No. PS100-2006).* Ottawa: Minister of Public Works and Government Services Canada. Retrieved December 22, 2006, from http://www.oci-bec.gc.ca/reports/AR200506_download_e.asp.

Pate, K. (2003, September). *Prisons: The latest solution to poverty, homelessness and mental illness.* Paper presented at Women Speak Series, Calgary. Retrieved November 15, 2006, from http://www.elizabethfry.ca/confernc/prison/1.htm.

Peternelj-Taylor, C. (2005). Conceptualizing nursing research with offenders: Another look at vulnerability. *International Journal of Law and Psychiatry, 28,* 348–359.

Peternelj-Taylor, C. (2008). Forensic psychiatric and mental health nursing. In W. Austin & M. A. Boyd (Eds.). *Psychiatric nursing for Canadian practice* (pp. 791–804). Philadelphia: Lippincott, Williams & Wilkins.

Roth, B., & Pressé, L. (2003). Nursing interventions for para-suicidal behaviors in female offenders. *Journal of Psychosocial Nursing and Mental Health Services, 41*(9), 20–29.

Rowan, J., Auger, S., Toto, H., Simpson, S., & McNab, C. (2004). The use of stories for healing interventions with women. *Forum on Corrections Research, 16*(1), 42–44.

Shelton, D. (2003). The clinical practice of juvenile forensic psychiatric nurses. *Journal of Psychosocial Nursing and Mental Health Services, 41*(9), 43–53.

Shelton, D. (2004). Experiences of detained young offenders in need of mental health care. *Journal of Nursing Scholarship, 36*(2), 129–133.

Singleton, N., Meltzer, H., Gatward, R., Coid, J., & Deasy, D. (1998) *Psychiatric morbidity among prisoners in England and Wales.* London: The Stationery Office.

Smith, S. (2005, February). Stepping through the looking glass: Professional autonomy in correctional nursing. *Corrections Today,* pp 54–56, 70.

Srivastava, R. H. (2007). Understanding cultural competence in health care. In R. H. Srivastava (Ed.), *The healthcare professional's guide to clinical cultural competence* (pp. 3–27). Toronto: Mosby Elsevier.

Standing Senate Committee on Social Affairs, Science and Technology. (2006, May). *Out of the shadows at last: Transforming mental health, mental illness and addiction services in Canada.* Retrieved January 5, 2007, from http://www.parl.gc.ca/39/1/parlbus/commbus/senate/com-e/soci-e/rep-e/rep02may06-e.htm.

Statistics Canada. (2003). *Special study on mentally disordered accused and the criminal justice system.* Canadian Centre for Justice Studies (No. 85-559-XIE). Ottawa: Ministry of Industry. Retrieved December 1, 2005, from http://www.statcan.ca/english/freepub/85-559-XIE/85-559-XIE2002001.pdf.

Thomas, G. (2005). *Harm reduction policies and programs for persons involved in the criminal justice system. Harm reduction for special populations in Canada.* Canadian Centre on Substance Abuse. Retrieved December 4, 2006, from http://www.ccsa.ca/NR/rdonlyres/B092A5D6-C627-4503-8F21-8A1AB8923B3A/0/ccsa0039002005.pdf.

Tandon, R., & Jibson, M. D. (2003). Suicidal behavior in schizophrenia: Diagnosis, neurobiology and treatment implications. *Current Opinion in Psychiatry, 16*(2), 193–197.

White, P., & Whiteford, H. (2006). Prisons: Mental health institutions of the 21st century. *The Medical Journal of Australia, 185*(6), 302–303.

ADDITIONAL RESOURCES

Websites

Canadian Association of Elizabeth Fry Societies
www.elizabethfry.ca

Children and Youth: Crime Prevention through Social Development
www.ccsd.ca/cpsd/ccsd/index.htm

Correctional Service Canada
www.csc-scc.gc.ca

Custody and Caring: International Conference on the Nurse's Role in the Criminal Justice System
www.usask.ca/nursing/custodycaring/index.htm

Human Rights Watch
www.hrw.org

John Howard Society of Canada
www.johnhoward.ca

Ministry of Community Safety and Correctional Services (Ontario)
www.mcscs.jus.gov.on.ca/English/english_default.html

National Commission on Correctional Health Care
www.ncchc.org

Prisoners' HIV/AIDS Support Action Network
  www.pasan.org
Registered Nurses' Association of Ontario Correctional
Nurses' Interest Group
  **www.rnao.org/Page.asp?PageID=122&ContentID=
  1452&SiteNodeID=113&BL_ExpandID=**

About the Authors

Joanne Shaw, RN, BN, retired in April 2007 as the Manager, Corporate Health Care Services, Ministry of Community Safety and Corrections Services, Government of Ontario. She graduated from the Saint John General Hospital School of Nursing and the University of New Brunswick. In the early part of her career, she worked as a general duty nurse and an infection control nurse. Later, she worked at the Clinical Institute of the Addiction Research Foundation, Toronto. She then moved to the mental health field, working at two large psychiatric hospitals in Ontario. One of these hospitals was the Oak Ridge Division of the Mental Health Centre in Penetanguishene, a maximum-security facility for the assessment and treatment of men with a serious mental illness that put them in conflict with the justice system. Joanne worked for two years at the Registered Nurses' Association of Ontario, where she was the staff resource to the entry-to-practice project. In 1997, Joanne became the coordinator of health care services at a mid-size detention centre in Toronto and then moved to corporate office.

Cindy Peternelj-Taylor, RN, MSc (University of Saskatchewan), is a Professor with the College of Nursing, University of Saskatchewan. She is a graduate of Lakehead University and the University of Saskatchewan and is currently completing doctoral studies with the University of Alberta. Much of Cindy's career has focused on professional role development for nurses who work with vulnerable populations in forensic psychiatric and correctional settings. She is a member of the Editorial Board of the *Journal of Psychiatric and Mental Health Nursing* and is an Associate Editor of the *Journal of Forensic Nursing.* She has presented at numerous national and international conferences, and her publications can be found in peer-reviewed nursing journals and textbooks.

Phil Woods, RPN, PhD (Anglia Polytechnic University), is an Associate Professor with the College of Nursing, University of Saskatchewan. He trained as a mental health nurse in the United Kingdom and is a registered psychiatric nurse in Saskatchewan. Phil has a PhD in Nursing Studies. He has an extensive personal portfolio of forensic-related research and is a well-known author of mental health and forensic nursing articles and books. His specific research interests are risk assessment and management, violence prediction, and developing mental health and forensic mental health practice. Phil is currently undertaking research projects involving Saskatchewan psychiatric acute units, forensic units, and correctional institutions in relation to violence prediction and risk assessment and management.

Gay, Lesbian, Bisexual, and Transgender Clients

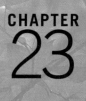

Anne Katz

OBJECTIVES

After studying this chapter, you should be able to:

1. Understand the societal attitudes and health care risks confronting gay, lesbian, bisexual, and transgender clients in communities and health care settings.

2. Relate the meaning of disclosing homophobia and heterosexism.

3. Identify strategies to reduce challenges of access in the Canadian health care system for gay, lesbian, bisexual, and transgender clients.

INTRODUCTION

Conservative estimates suggest that 2% to 3% of the North American population self-identify as gay (homosexual) or lesbian (Blank, 2005), and less commonly as bisexual or transgender. **Homosexuality** refers to people whose sexual and emotional attraction is to persons of the same sex. While **homosexual** refers to both men and women, most women prefer to be called **lesbians** and many men prefer to be called **gay**; this removes the word "sexual" from the descriptor and is thought to be more politically correct. Aboriginal or First Nations people may prefer the term "two-spirited," which refers to the duality of the male and female in one person. A **bisexual** person is one who is attracted to both men and women. **Transgenders** are men or women who believe that their physical body and sexual characteristics do not match their self-concept (a man's mind in a woman's body or vice versa). These individuals will often dress and act the way they feel rather than according to their sexual characteristics and may choose to undergo sexual reassignment surgery where their physical sex organs are surgically altered. Acknowledging one's sexual orientation to the self and others is termed **coming out**. There are various theories about the nature of homosexuality and bisexuality; some claim this is genetically determined and cannot be altered, while others maintain this is a lifestyle choice that can be controlled, denied, or accepted.

Most nurses can expect to encounter at least some gay, lesbian, bisexual, and, less commonly, transgender clients, in all age groups from adolescents to older adults. These numbers will reflect regional variation, with large metropolitan cities having more gay/lesbian/bisexual/transgender residents than smaller cities or rural towns. The purpose of this chapter is to describe the factors in Canadian society that contribute to ill health in gays, lesbians, and bisexual individuals, and to identify strategies that community health nurses can use to mitigate these influences.

SOCIETAL ATTITUDES

Some gay/lesbian/bisexual clients choose to not disclose their sexual orientation, or limit disclosure to a limited group that they trust. This reluctance to disclose or fear of the consequences of disclosure relate to two essential concepts: homophobia and heterosexism. **Homophobia** describes a fear, often irrational, of gay men and lesbian women on the part of heterosexuals. This fear is not usually based on experience or knowledge of gays and lesbians but rather on myths and assumptions. It is often manifested in derogatory language, jokes, and discriminatory treatment of those individuals perceived or known to be gay or lesbian. At its very worst, it may involve extreme violence (gay bashing) toward those perceived to be homosexual. More often it is manifested as bullying in schools and social situations when young persons are seen to be "different" from their peers or identify themselves as lesbian, gay, or bisexual.

Some gay/lesbian individuals may have subconsciously accepted a negative view of homosexuals as abnormal and even deviant and thus experience self-loathing and lack of self-acceptance; this is termed **internalized homophobia**. It is often manifested as low self-esteem and self-loathing resulting in high-risk activities such as substance abuse and high-risk sexual activity.

Heterosexism, on the other hand, refers to viewing the world through the lens of heterosexuality as the norm and a lack of realization or acknowledgement that alternatives to this exist. This is acted out constantly in everyday society by the assumption that everyone is heterosexual and that anything else is not "normal." Examples of heterosexism in health care systems abound. Asking clients about their marital status is itself a heterosexist assumption, as most gays or lesbians cannot be or are not married. This situation is changing in Canada; however, with legislation protecting the rights of same-sex couples to marry having been enacted in the recent past. The usual choices for partner status include married, separated/divorced, widowed, or single. How does a lesbian woman who is in a long-term relationship answer this question? Heterosexism serves to alienate gays and lesbians, and while it is not as overtly threatening as homophobia, the social and psychological effects are far reaching and are known to delay entry into the health care system. In contrast, individuals who are gay-positive recognize the diversity of human sexual and emotional attraction and are open to gay, lesbian, and bisexual individuals and couples.

Many health care providers describe themselves as being neutral in their practice related to the sexual orientation of their clients. This is based on the belief that health care should be accessible to all and not based on the particular needs of any one group or population (Brotman et al., 2002). This may result in health care providers not asking about sexual orientation when meeting a new client or ignoring disclosure in an attempt to appear accepting. It is more appropriate to acknowledge this disclosure and reflect acceptance and caring, which will further encourage the client to share sensitive information that may influence care (Williams-Barnard et al., 2001). Acting in neutral manner may in fact be seen as a negative response (Boehmer & Case, 2004).

HEALTH CARE RISKS RELATED TO HOMOSEXUALITY

Because of the invisibility of sexual minorities in our society, the reality of their health care needs and health risks are not readily apparent. Up until the mid-1970s, homosexuality was classified as a mental illness, and much attention was focused on "curing" homosexuals (Brotman et al., 2002). This usually involved intensive psychiatric therapy, including classical aversion therapy by using electric shocks. In the 1980s the HIV/AIDS epidemic appeared and attention was primarily focused on gay men as vectors and victims of this disease. Lesbians in the health care system are often even more invisible and unless they identify as such may be regarded as single women. Because many lesbians do not have children, they are at increased risk of cancers such as breast and ovarian cancer, which are both associated with childlessness. Smoking and other substance abuse rates are also higher among lesbians than the general population, and this may be related to the stress of living as a sexual minority, internalized homophobia, or social factors such as peer group acceptance of these behaviours (Lehmann, Lehmann, & Kelly, 1998).

Many health care providers equate sexual orientation with sexual behaviour and focus exclusively on the apparent link between the two. They thus see gays and lesbians only in the context of their sexual activities and perceived risks associated with these and ignore other health care risks that are not associated with gender. Health care providers frequently make assumptions about both the health care status and risks for disease of their gay/lesbian/bisexual clients, and these assumptions are often erroneous (Bonvicini & Perlin, 2003). Examples of these assumptions include the belief that all gay men have anal intercourse and are at high risk for HIV and other STIs, and that lesbians never have penetrative sex. While gay men have been disproportionately affected by the HIV/AIDS epidemic since the 1980s, many gay men do not have anal intercourse, preferring other acts of sexual expression that do not place them at higher risk for HIV infection, and some lesbians do have penetrative sex with men occasionally and yet continue to identify as lesbian. Even participating in anal sex can be safe if condoms are used consistently.

Homosexual youth are often assumed to be HIV infected regardless of their risk activities (Ginsburg, Winn, Rudy, Crawford, Zhao, & Schwarz, 2002).

The most significant health risk for gays and lesbians is thought to be the avoidance of routine health care due to a variety of concerns (Harrison & Silenzio, 1996); many of these concerns are related to the actual or perceived reactions of the health care providers to the client's homosexuality. Lesbians do not have mammograms and Pap tests as often as heterosexual women, and gay men are less likely to seek out preventive health care for themselves. Mental health issues such as depression are also major concerns for this population; however, how this is viewed is vitally important. As lesbians and gay men age, these issues persist and may be compounded by lack of social support, difficulties finding assisted housing where the individual or couple may feel comfortable, and lack of knowledge about financial planning (McMahon, 2003).

Homosexuality is not a mental health problem, but society's traditional view of homosexuality as deviant has contributed to gay and lesbian people having conflicting feelings about their sexual orientation. This results in high levels of depression in this population and an increased risk of suicidal ideation and attempts (Igartua, Gill, & Montoro, 2003). Internalized homophobia is seen to be central to this phenomenon; if individuals find it difficult to accept who they are because of negative societal messages that have been absorbed, this causes a significant amount of self-doubt and self-loathing, resulting in destructive behaviours and high-risk activities. The stresses that many in this population are exposed to have been termed "minority stress," referring to the negative effects on mental health of stigma, prejudice, and discrimination (Meyer, 2003). Encompassed in this concept is the expectation of rejection, the need to hide and conceal, internalized homophobia, and coping mechanisms used to adapt to the hostile environment that is created.

Gay youth are more likely to be targets of hate crimes and violence in schools and may experience abuse in their intimate partner relationships, often associated with substance and alcohol abuse (Bonvicini & Perlin, 2003). The consequences of bullying are far reaching and may continue into adulthood, where the occurrence of post-traumatic stress disorder has been associated with bullying at school (Rivers, 2004). Gay youth are also more likely to become homeless; they are either evicted from their family home due to conflict about their sexual orientation or flee for their safety when emotional, sexual, and/or physical abuse becomes untenable (Rew, Whittaker, Taylor-Seehafer, & Smith, 2005). (See Chapter 27.)

Gay men, lesbians, and bisexuals of colour and/or with visible or invisible disabilities face additional challenges, both within larger society and within the gay/lesbian community (Parks, Hughes, & Matthews, 2004). They have to confront the norms of both the majority and minority communities and cultures in which they live. Aboriginal or First Nations people who are gay or lesbian face additional challenges based on historical and familial patterns of abuse and trauma with high levels of psychological distress and increased use of mental health services (Balsam, Huang, Fieland, Simoni, & Walters, 2004).

DISCLOSURE OF SAME-SEX ATTRACTION OR RELATIONSHIP

Coming Out

Disclosure of sexual orientation is recognized as being difficult no matter when it occurs in the lifespan. The amount of difficulty relates to the nature of the relationship (telling a parent), the age of the individual (adolescent versus adult), and the value placed on the relationship (friend or relative versus stranger). Hiding one's sexual orientation is thought to lead to poor health outcomes (Cole, Kemeny, Taylor, & Visscher, 1996) as well as risk-taking behaviour such as smoking and alcohol and substance abuse (Case et al., 2004). Gay/lesbian adolescents are at increased risk for suicide, and as many as 30% to 40% of homosexual teens have attempted or seriously contemplated harming themselves. Risk of suicide has been noted to be highest around the time when disclosure to parents is being planned or has occurred (Igartua et al., 2003). Youth who are in the process of coming out experience health risks dependent on where in the process they are. Those who do not have connections in the gay and lesbian community appear to suffer significant psychological distress as they struggle to accept their sexual orientation. Later in the process, when they are connected to a social group, their risk for alcohol and substance abuse increases, as does high-risk sexual activity. This may reflect the reality of where young gay and lesbian people meet their peers; interactions frequently occur at bars and other places where this population is able to meet and may centre around activities that are not always healthy (Wright & Perry, 2006).

Transgender youth are especially vulnerable as society is particularly blind to the existence of individuals who do not fit into the traditional male or female mold. Gender-atypical behaviour is less acceptable in boys than in girls, and these youth experience significant adversity in school and the family. They often run away, become involved in street activities, and suffer the consequences of survival sex (exchanging sex for food, shelter, or money) and all that this entails (Grossman & D'Augelli, 2006). These youth often dress as the sex they feel like and are open to ridicule, harassment, and sometimes violence. Fear of the consequences of disclosing their transgender status is a major factor in mental health and contributes to fear of personal safety in many social as well as family situations.

Disclosing to Health Care Providers

Communication is seen to be a central part of the problems that gays and lesbians face in their health care interactions. Coming out or disclosing sexual orientation is an essential element of good health for gays, lesbians, and two-spirited people; however, in the health care arena, it is a constant process, as with each new care provider encountered the process must be repeated and the same fears and concerns about the reaction are experienced over and over again (Brotman et al., 2002). Not disclosing (being "closeted") is associated with

shame and hiding, and leads to ill health, both physically and mentally. Lesbians have been noted to find it more difficult to disclose to health care providers (Klitzman & Greenberg, 2002), which may reflect the lack of power many women experience in society and in the health care system. However, other evidence suggests that women are more likely than men to disclose to their health care providers (Neville & Henrickson, 2006). The difference may lie in the gender of the health care provider, as many women prefer a female care provider and may feel more comfortable disclosing than a male homosexual to a male health care provider.

Canadian Research Box 23.1

Brotman, S., Ryan, B., & Cormier, R. (2003). The health and social service needs of gay and lesbian elders and their families in Canada. *The Gerontologist, 43*(2), 192–202.

This qualitative study explored the experiences of elderly gay and lesbian individuals and their families in accessing a range of health and social services. The researchers also explored how the agencies providing health and social support deliver services to this population. Results portray an overwhelming experience of marginalization in both social and political spheres. Five key themes emerged: (1) historical experiences of discrimination, (2) homophobia in everyday life, (3) profound invisibility, (4) their ability to access long term care services in spite of the invisibility, homophobia, and discrimination, and (5) gay and lesbian support networks that do not adequately address their needs.

Discussion Questions:

1. What differences might there be for young gay men and women of today when they grow older compared with the experiences of these older individuals?

2. What determinants of health could influence the health of gays and lesbians?

SOCIAL INCLUSION

So what can nurses do to be inclusive with gay/lesbian/bisexual clients? The first step is to address our own assumptions, beliefs, and attitudes about homosexuality. (See the *Gay Affirmative Practice Scale,* Appendix 23A.) These are likely to be reflective of the attitudes we absorbed growing up in our own families. Many of us may not ever have explored our attitudes to homosexuality and may not be aware of how heterosexist we are. Think about what you believe about homosexuality and where those beliefs came from. Have they changed over the years, or are they the same as they were when you were growing up? Do you know anyone who is lesbian, gay, bisexual, or transgender? Can you recall caring for a self-identified homosexual client and what that was like? What did you have to do to overcome assumptions or attitudes that got in the way of providing nonjudgmental care? Perhaps this has never presented a challenge to you, or perhaps you cannot remember taking care of a gay/lesbian client. This may be because you have never asked the right questions or have appeared to be non-accepting and so a gay/lesbian client has never disclosed to you. It is highly unlikely that you have *never* come across a gay/lesbian client; you just did not know at the time that the client was gay or lesbian!

Reflect whether you regularly use inclusive language when taking a history from a new client. Do you ask if the client has a partner and if that partner is a man or woman? Most heterosexual clients will readily tell you that their partner is a man (or woman), and even if gay/lesbian clients do not disclose to you at that point, or state that they are not partnered at the present time, you have indicated by your choice of language that you are aware something other than heterosexual relationships exist. This may allow the gay/lesbian client to be more open at this or a future appointment. If the client does identify as being gay/lesbian or bisexual, do not ignore the comment but rather acknowledge this fact and inform the client that openness will allow for a better therapeutic relationship. Another way of asking this question is to ask whether the client is sexually active, and if so, whether sex is with men, women, or both. This removes the assumption that sex is only something that happens in the context of a relationship and may allow disclosure of bisexuality that occurs outside of an established relationship. Directly asking if the client is gay or lesbian can itself raise a barrier, as the client may not self-identify as such but may in fact be having sexual relations with someone of the same or the opposite sex.

Consider the forms that we ask clients to complete. Is the language contained in these forms inclusive or exclusive? Think about advocating for a change in the section usually marked as "marital status." This can be changed to "relationship or partner status" and include the option of same-sex relationship (gay, lesbian, or bisexual) along with the usual single, married, separated/divorced, or widowed. However, for clients who are in same-sex marriages, the term "married" does apply and should be used.

It is also important to be truthful about the level of confidentiality that is possible related to the clients and their health history. Many gay/lesbian/bisexual clients, especially teens, are very concerned about this (Ginsburg et al., 2002). Though complete confidentiality is a goal to aim toward, it is not always possible, and the clients need to know what information about them may be accessible to others and to tailor their disclosure and health-related information accordingly.

Think about the educational material that is given to clients and look to see if there are any images of same-sex couples used as illustration. The same goes for posters that are displayed on the walls of clinics and hospitals. These seemingly minor details can speak volumes to the gay/lesbian clients who attend the clinic/hospital about their safety in disclosing sexual orientation. Familiarize yourself with resources in the community that are gay/lesbian friendly; know the names and contact information for gay-positive or gay-identified counsellors and other health care providers. Have information on hand to give out to clients, including websites and other resources that target gay/lesbian/bisexual individuals.

ROLE OF THE COMMUNITY HEALTH NURSE

Community health nurses have a vital role to play in both modelling and encouraging respect and tolerance in all aspects of daily life and especially in the various arenas where they work with members of the community. Nurses who work in schools have a particularly important role to play in affecting the health and physical and mental safety of gay, lesbian, bisexual, or transgender youth. It is vitally important that the needs of this vulnerable and invisible population are identified and addressed both on an individual and school-based level. There is much work to be done in sensitizing teachers, coaches, aides, and other youth to the challenges facing these youth every day in our schools and playgrounds. This needs to occur within the context of the client's cultural and religious affiliations; communities where homosexuality is strictly forbidden present a challenge for the individual who wants to come out but also wants to maintain ties with family and members of the community.

Case Study

You are a community health nurse in an inner-city clinic and you are contacted by the guidance counsellor at a local high school. She wants you to take part in some educational sessions she is organizing at the high school for World AIDS Day. She tells you that she is concerned that the gay students in the school are not practising safe sex, and wants you to make sure they know about condoms.

Discussion Questions

1. What additional questions would you need to ask this counsellor before agreeing to participate in any activity at the school?

2. How do you identify gay students in a high school and specifically target them for education?

3. How would you approach this topic in a high school population?

Community health nurses can also advocate for social inclusion and equity in health in our diverse nation by influencing the attitudes and knowledge of community members. This may start at the level of the family, where nurses can help a young gay person come out to their family and support the family in accepting this. This work can then extend to the school, the community centre, and perhaps even to the level of civic and provincial politics. As advocates for our clients and communities, we can both support their best interests and encourage change when inequity and disparity are identified. Creating a society based on tolerance and respect is the responsibility of each of us as citizens, and nurses, by virtue of the trust granted us by the people we work with, are ideally suited to encourage this.

Though it is important to consider our own attitudes, beliefs, and practices, it is also important to challenge these same attitudes and actions among fellow students, co-workers, and colleagues. While you may be gay-positive, other people you encounter in class and in clinics and hospitals may not be, and they will have equal opportunities to interact with gay/lesbian/bisexual clients and potentially cause harm through their words and actions. Including fellow students in an exploration of attitudes, knowledge, and beliefs will give you a good idea of how easy or difficult it may be to change homophobic or heterosexist attitudes and practices.

Summary

This chapter has described some of the challenges that lesbians, gay men, bisexuals, and transgenders face in our society as a whole and our health care systems in particular. It has also presented strategies for nurses to confront their own attitudes to gay, lesbian, bisexual, and transgender clients and to help in the development of greater accessibility for this population to our health care system.

KEY TERMS

homosexuality
homosexual
lesbians
gay
bisexual
transgenders
coming out
homophobia
internalized homophobia
heterosexism

INDIVIDUAL CRITICAL THINKING EXERCISES

1. What is your theory about homosexuality? Do you think it is genetic or learned (i.e., nature or nurture)? What in your life may have influenced your thinking?

2. A client comes to you and discloses that she is a lesbian. Do you enter this into her chart or tell other members of the health team about this? Why or why not?

3. How would you address a transgender client who has male genitalia but dresses as a woman?

GROUP CRITICAL THINKING EXERCISES

1. Identify homophobic or heterosexist attitudes that you have witnessed as a student at the university and during clinical experiences. How did you deal with these?

2. Do you think that a gay nurse should be "out" in the workplace? Why or why not?

3. Would you be comfortable working with another nurse who is gay, lesbian, or bisexual? What if any concerns do you have and why?

REFERENCES

Balsam, K., Huang, B., Fieland, K., Simoni, J., & Walters, K. (2004). Culture, trauma, and wellness: A comparison of heterosexual and lesbian, gay, bisexual, and two-spirit native Americans. *Cultural Diversity and Ethnic Minority Psychology, 10*(3), 287–301.

Blank, T. O. (2005). Gay men and prostate cancer: Invisible diversity. *J. Clin. Oncol, 23*(12), 2593–2596.

Boehmer, U., & Case, P. (2004). Physicians don't ask, sometimes patients tell: Disclosure of sexual orientation among women with breast carcinoma. *Cancer, 101*(8), 1882–1889.

Bonvicini, K., & Perlin, M. (2003). The same but different: Clinician–patient communication with gay and lesbian patients. *Patient Education and Counseling, 51,* 115–122.

Brotman, S., Ryan, B., Jalbert, Y., & Rowe, B. (2002). The impact of coming out on health and health care access: The experiences of gay, lesbian, bisexual and two-spirit people. *Journal of Health and Social Policy, 15*(1), 1–29.

Case, P., Austin, S. B., Hunter, D. J., Manson, J. E., Malspeis, S., Willett, W. C., et al. (2004). Sexual orientation, health risk factors, and physical functioning in the Nurses' Health Study II. *Journal of Women's Health (Larchmt.), 13*(9), 1033–1047.

Cole, S. W., Kemeny, M. E., Taylor, S. E., & Visscher, B. R. (1996). Elevated physical health risk among gay men who conceal their homosexual identity. *Health Psychology, 15*(4), 243–251.

Ginsburg, K., Winn, R., Rudy, B., Crawford, J., Zhao, H., & Schwarz, D. (2002). How to reach sexual minority youth in the health care setting: The teens offer guidance. *Journal of Adolescent Health, 31,* 407–416.

Grossman, A., & D'Augelli, A. (2006). Transgender youth: Invisible and vulnerable. *Journal of Homosexuality, 51*(1), 111–128.

Harrison, A., & Silenzio, V. (1996). Comprehensive care of lesbian and gay patients and families. *Primary Care, 23*(1), 31–47.

Igartua, K., Gill, K., & Montoro, R. (2003). Internalized homophobia: A factor in depression, anxiety, and suicide in the gay and lesbian population. *Canadian Journal of Community Mental Health, 22*(2), 15–30.

Klitzman, R., & Greenberg, J. (2002). Patterns of communication between gay and lesbian patients and their health care providers. *Journal of Homosexuality, 42*(4), 65–75.

Lehmann, J., Lehmann, C., & Kelly, P. (1998). Development and health care needs of lesbians. *Journal of Women's Health, 7*(3), 379–387.

McMahon, E. (2003). The older homosexual: Current concepts of lesbian, gay, bisexual, and transgender older Americans. *Clinics in Geriatric Medicine, 19,* 587–593.

Meyer, I. (2003). Prejudice, social stress, and mental health in lesbian, gay, and bisexual populations: Conceptual issues and research evidence. *Psychological Bulletin, 129*(5), 674–697.

Neville, S., & Henrickson, M. (2006). Perceptions of lesbian, gay and bisexual people of primary healthcare services. *Journal of Advanced Nursing, 55*(4), 407–415.

Parks, C., Hughes, T., & Matthews, A. (2004). Race/ethnicity and sexual orientation: Intersecting identities. *Cultural*

Diversity and Ethnic Minority Psychology, 10(3), 241–254.

Rew, L., Whittaker, T., Taylor-Seehafer, M., & Smith, L. (2005). Sexual health risks and protective resources in gay, lesbian, bisexual and heterosexual homeless youth. *JSPN, 10*(1), 11–19.

Rivers, I. (2004). Recollections of bullying at school and their long-term implications for lesbians, gay men, and bisexuals. *Crisis, 25*(4), 169–175.

Williams-Barnard, C., Mendoza, D., & Shippee-Rice, R. (2001). The lived experience of college student lesbians' encounters with health care providers. *Journal of Holistic Nursing, 19*(2), 127–142.

Wright, E., & Perry, B. (2006). Sexual identity distress, social support, and the health of gay, lesbian, and bisexual youth. *Journal of Homosexuality, 51*(1), 81–110.

ADDITIONAL RESOURCES

Websites

Alberta Teachers' Association—List of Resources (books, videos, etc.)

www.teachers.ab.ca/Issues+In+Education/ Diversity+and+Human+Rights/Sexual+Orientation/ Resources+for+Teachers/selected+readings.htm

Egale Canada, a national organization that advances equality and justice for lesbian, gay, bisexual, and trans-identified people and their families across Canada

www.egale.ca

PFLAG Canada, a registered charitable organization that provides support, education, and resources to parents, families, and individuals who have questions or concerns about sexual orientation or gender identity

www.pflagcanada.ca

About the Author

Anne Katz, RN, PhD, was born and raised in South Africa. She emigrated to Canada after completing her basic nursing training with a specialty in midwifery. Her nursing experience in Winnipeg includes caring for HIV/AIDS-infected individuals at the Village Clinic, a centre of excellence for the care of individuals with HIV/AIDS. She is an adjunct professor at the University of Manitoba and is currently the clinical nurse specialist and sexuality counsellor at the Manitoba Prostate Centre.

Appendix 23A
Gay Affirmative Practice Scale

This questionnaire is designed to measure clinicians' beliefs about treatment with gay and lesbian clients and their behaviours in clinical settings with these clients. There are no right or wrong answers. Please answer every question as honestly as possible.

Please rate how strongly with you agree or disagree with each statement about treatment with gay and lesbian clients on the basis of the following scale:

> SA = Strongly agree
> A = Agree
> N = Neither agree nor disagree
> D = Disagree
> SD = Strongly disagree

1. In their practice with gay/lesbian clients, practitioners should support the diverse makeup of their families. _____
2. Practitioners should verbalize respect for the lifestyles of gay/lesbian clients. _____
3. Practitioners should make an effort to learn about diversity within the gay/lesbian community. _____
4. Practitioners should be knowledgeable about gay/lesbian resources. _____
5. Practitioners should educate themselves about gay/lesbian lifestyles. _____
6. Practitioners should help gay/lesbian clients develop positive identities as gay/lesbian individuals. _____
7. Practitioners should challenge misinformation about gay/lesbian clients. _____
8. Practitioners should use professional development opportunities to improve their practice with gay/lesbian clients. _____
9. Practitioners should encourage gay/lesbian clients to create networks that support them as gay/lesbian individuals. _____
10. Practitioners should be knowledgeable about issues unique to gay/lesbian couples. _____
11. Practitioners should acquire knowledge necessary for effective practice with gay/lesbian clients. _____
12. Practitioners should work to develop skills necessary for effective practice with gay/lesbian clients. _____
13. Practitioners should work to develop attitudes necessary for effective practice with gay/lesbian clients. _____
14. Practitioners should help clients reduce shame about homosexual feelings. _____
15. Discrimination creates problems that gay/lesbian clients may need to address in treatment. _____

Please rate how frequently you engage in each of the behaviours with gay and lesbian clients on the basis of the following scale:

> A = Always
> U = Usually
> S = Sometimes
> R = Rarely
> N = Never

16. I help clients reduce shame about homosexual feelings. _____
17. I help gay/lesbian clients address problems created by societal prejudice. _____
18. I inform clients about gay affirmative resources in the community. _____
19. I acknowledge to clients the impact of living in a homophobic society. _____
20. I respond to a client's sexual orientation when it is relevant to treatment. _____
21. I help gay/lesbian clients overcome religious oppression they have experienced based on their sexual orientation. _____
22. I provide interventions that facilitate the safety of gay/lesbian clients. _____
23. I verbalize that a gay/lesbian orientation is as healthy as a heterosexual orientation. _____
24. I demonstrate comfort about gay/lesbian issues to gay/lesbian clients. _____
25. I help clients identify their internalized homophobia. _____
26. I educate myself about gay/lesbian concerns. _____
27. I am open-minded when tailoring treatment for gay/lesbian clients. _____
28. I create a climate that allows for voluntary self-identification by gay/lesbian clients. _____
29. I discuss sexual orientation in a non-threatening manner with clients. _____
30. I facilitate appropriate expression of anger by gay/lesbian clients about oppression they have experienced. _____

Scoring, Reliability, and Validity Information

Scoring instructions: Using the chart below, please give each answer the indicated number of points. After all questions have been answered, add up the total number points. Higher scores reflect more affirmative practice with gay and lesbian clients.

Items 1–15	Items 16–30	Points
Strongly agree	Always	5
Agree	Usually	4
Neither agree nor disagree	Sometimes	3
Disagree	Rarely	2
Strongly disagree	Never	1

Source: Copyright © 2002, Catherine Lau Crisp, PhD. Illegal to photocopy or otherwise reproduce without expressed permission of author. In addition, please do not change any of the wording on the version at http://ccrisp.googlepages.com/GAP.doc.

Reliability information: Initial evidence for reliability is provided in the following table.

	Cronbach's Alpha	Standard Error of Measurement
Items 1–15	.9307	1.91
Items 16–30	.9375	2.71

Validity information: Initial evidence for validity is provided in the following table.

	Pearson's R	Instrument
Items 1–15	.624 ($p_1 = .000$)[1]	HATH[1]
Items 16–30	−.466 ($p_2 = .000$)[2]	ATLG[2]
Items 1–30	.021 ($p_3 = .691$)[3]	SDS (M − C 1[10])[3]
Factorial validity	All items load on their intended domain ≥ .60	

1. Heterosexuals' Attitudes Toward Homosexuals (HATH).
   Source: Larsen, K., Reed, M., & Hoffman, S. (1980). Attitudes of heterosexuals toward homosexuality: A Likert-type scale and construct validity. *Journal of Sex Research, 16*(3), 245–257.
   Correlation was significant and in the expected direction.

2. Attitudes Toward Lesbians and Gay Men (ATLG).
   Source: Herek, G. (1988). Heterosexuals' attitudes toward lesbians and gay men: Correlates and gender differences. *Journal of Sex Research, 25*(4), 451–477.
   Correlation was significant and in the expected direction.

3. Marlowe-Crowne Social Desirability Scale (short version) (SDS M-C 1[10]).
   Source: Strahn, R., & Gerbasi, K. C. (1972). Short, homogeneous versions of the Marlowe-Crowne Social Desirability Scale. *Journal of Clinical Psychology, 28*, 191–193.
   Correlation was non-significant, suggesting that the GAP does not measure social desirability.

Disaster Nursing and Emergency Preparedness

Mary Anne Simpson and Lucia Yiu

OBJECTIVES

After studying this chapter, you should be able to:

1. Define the various types of disasters and their consequences.

2. Discuss the role of the National Incident Management System and the Incident Command System in disaster management.

3. Understand the roles and responsibilities of the Public Health Agency of Canada in emergency preparedness.

4. Identify the key functions of community health nurses during and following a disaster.

5. Discuss the skill set that will prepare a community health nurse to respond effectively to emergencies.

INTRODUCTION

Each disaster is unique. The way in which a disaster will impact a community depends upon the individual community's social, cultural, economic, and health makeup. In order to respond effectively in a disaster situation across different communities, special expertise in emergency management is required. Ongoing threats of harm have become a major issue in today's world, bringing with them enormous social and economic consequences affecting large numbers of people. The consequences of different types of disasters vary in severity, each with its own degree of death, mass injury, illness, and loss. As part of a public health workforce, community health nurses (CHNs) must be well prepared to react and provide essential services in caring for people affected by disasters.

Disaster nursing is an emerging specialty. This chapter provides an overview of the role of CHNs in providing care to people affected by a disaster situation. It highlights different types of disasters, and how the National Incident Management System (NIMS) and the Incident Command System (ICS) function as a comprehensive model to manage major incidents. The Jennings Disaster Nursing Management Model will be introduced to guide nurses in understanding disaster nursing.

DISASTERS IN CANADA

According to the Canadian Disaster Database (Public Safety and Emergency Preparedness Canada, 2005), chemical and fuel spills, floods, snowstorms, and forest fires were the most common disasters recorded in Canada in the last decade. (See Table 24.1.)

WHAT IS A DISASTER?

Disastrous events typically occur suddenly and can be caused by nature, human error, biological hazards, or diseases. They include earthquakes, floods, fires, hurricanes, cyclones, major storms, volcanic eruptions, spills, air crashes, droughts, epidemics, food shortages, and civil strife (Landesman, 2005). Disasters often are perceived as random killers. When disasters strike, they affect everyone in the community in which they occur. Individuals at greatest risk include vulnerable groups such as women, children, the elderly, the poor, and people with mental and physical disabilities (Cohen, 2000). Life-threatening conditions brought on by disasters and the adverse health effects borne of these conditions often result in increased mortality and morbidity.

Types of Disasters

Natural Disasters **Natural disasters** are unpredictable; they can happen very quickly or slowly. However, with advance warning such as weather reports, the impacts can sometimes be mitigated. Some examples of natural disasters include droughts, heat waves, blizzards, cold waves, heavy snowfalls, earthquakes, cyclones, tsunamis, tornadoes, flood or thunderstorms, volcanoes, and wildfires. On December 24, 2004, the world was shocked when a strong earthquake triggered a massive tsunami that hit Southeast Asia in Indonesia, Sri Lanka, southern India, Thailand, Malaysia, the Maldives, Bangladesh, Burma, Mauritius, Somalia, Kenya, Seychelles, and Tanzania, leaving 280 931 dead.

Man-made Disasters **Man-made disasters** may result—and have resulted—in mass numbers of civilian injuries and deaths, leaving the communities they touch with long-term adverse effects. Bioterrorism, bombings, and technical disasters, such as nuclear disasters, are all examples of man-made disasters. Some man-made disasters, such as those caused by a bioterrorist attack, are brought about intentionally. **Bioterrorism** is "the use of a microorganism with the deliberate intent of causing infection in order to achieve certain goals" (Public Health Agency of Canada [PHAC], 2001). The release of a biological agent, such as smallpox or anthrax, with the intent to infect humans is an example of a bioterrorist attack. Ideological or politically inspired bombings, civil and political disorder as seen in countries at war, riots, and economic emergencies resulting in social instability are also examples of man-made disasters.

TABLE 24.1
Selected Canadian Disasters

Date and Location	Disaster	Human Consequences
1900—Ottawa & Hull	Fire	15 000 evacuated 7 died
1910—British Columbia (Rogers Pass)	Snow avalanche	62 railway workers died
1918 to 1925—Canada	Spanish flu	2 million people ill > 50 000 died
1927—Newfoundland	Hurricane	56 died
1994—Alberta (Lethbridge)	Chemical release/derailment	200 evacuated
1996—Quebec (Saguenay)	Flood	10 died 15 825 people evacuated
1998—Nova Scotia (Peggy's Cove)	Aircraft accident	229 died
2000—Ontario (Walkerton)	Drinking water contamination	7 died 2300 people injured
2003—Ontario (Toronto)	SARS epidemic	44 died (of 438 cases)
2003—Southeastern B.C. and Southwestern Alberta	Forest fires (started by lightning, careless fire use)	~50 000 residents evacuated
2005—Saskatchewan (Cumberland House, Cree First Nation)	Flood	~2000 residents evacuated
2005—Alberta (14 communities)	Floods	2 dead 7028 residents evacuated ~4000 homes damaged

Source: Public Safety and Emergency Preparedness Canada. (2005). Canadian Disaster Database. Retrieved October 3, 2007, from http://ww5.ps-sp.gc.ca/res/em/cdd/search-en.asp.

The terrorist attacks on the World Trade Center in New York and the Pentagon in Washington on September 11, 2001, represent one of the most recent and well watched examples of a man-made disaster of this type (Rodriguez & Long, 2006). Twenty-four Canadians were counted among the 2823 killed when terrorists flew commercial airliners into the World Trade Center towers in New York City. This attack, combined with the anthrax exposures that followed, prompted an increased awareness of the need for bioterrorism preparedness. The threat of bioterrorism remains even more real and pressing today when we consider that more than 30 diseases previously unknown have emerged as viruses or bacteria, including for example Ebola virus, Legionnaire's disease, E-coli O157:H7 associated with hemolytic uremic syndrome, HIV/AIDS, hepatitis C, and H5N1 Influenza A or avian influenza (Naylor, 2003).

Technological malfunctions resulting from man-made disaster most often occur in communities with industrial sites and can be triggered by a natural disaster. Contamination of the water or food supply, the unintentional release of deadly

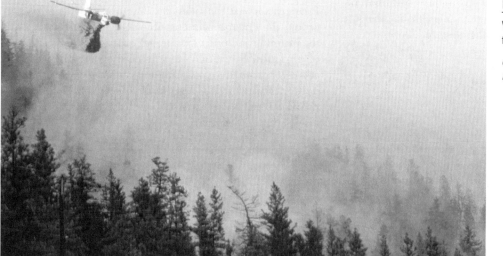

Photo 24.1

Water bomber extinguishing a forest fire in British Columbia.

Credit: © Gunter Marx Photography/CORBIS

airborne substances such as anthrax, fires, explosions, and exposure to hazardous materials are all conduits for technological disasters. Building or bridge collapses, transportation crashes, dam or levee failures, nuclear reactor accidents, and breaks in water, gas, or sewer lines may also result in a disaster of this type (Landesman, 2005). Both man-made and natural disasters leave people injured, put emergency responders at risk, and have a lasting impact on the health of the communities they affect.

Epidemics Another type of disaster is that brought about by way of disease epidemic. An **epidemic** can occur when an infectious disease enters a community and spreads rapidly. Transmission of an infectious disease that is easily transmitted or highly contagious can quickly result in an emergency situation if the right conditions exist. Such conditions as a densely populated area, lack/loss of proper sanitation and hygiene practices, and lack of or disrupted public health services may provide a breeding ground for an epidemic. Even if these conditions are not present, the nature of the disease itself may still result in a disaster situation if the disease is sufficiently serious that there will be high levels of morbidity and mortality. This is particularly so if social and economic disruption occurs once the disease is present, if there is a lack of trained professional personnel with experience available to manage the epidemic, and if there is a lack of equipment and supplies. Epidemics are further complicated if the disease is or may become susceptible to international transmission.

PUBLIC SAFETY AND EMERGENCY PREPAREDNESS IN CANADA

Disaster preparedness and response at a national and provincial/territorial level ensures support for public health authorities and other officials who are responsible for managing the health of their community before, during, and after a disaster occurs. Public health officials attend to prevention of infectious disease and injury. They routinely conduct surveillance for infectious disease and they work in collaboration with other agencies within the health sector. They have governmental jurisdiction to oversee the public's health, and they use triage skills in disaster situations (Landesman, 2005).

Government Authority and Legislative Framework

Federal legislation with respect to emergencies and emergency preparedness is found in two complementary acts, the Emergencies Act and the Emergency Preparedness Act. Both pieces of legislation were enacted in 1988, at which time the Emergencies Act replaced the War Measures Act as the source of the federal government's authority to act in the event of a national emergency.

The Emergencies Act The **Emergencies Act** (Department of Justice Canada, 2007a) allows the federal government to grant the use of special powers to ensure the safety and security of Canadians during a national emergency. The Emergencies Act defines a national emergency as "an urgent and critical situation of a temporary nature that seriously endangers the lives, health or safety of Canadians and is of such proportions or nature as to exceed the capacity or authority of a province to deal with it, or seriously threatens the ability of the Government of Canada to preserve the sovereignty, security and territorial integrity of Canada, and cannot be effectively dealt with under any other law of Canada" (p. 1). The federal government intervention is restricted to only the most serious of emergency situations, while respecting the authority of the provinces and territories to govern accordingly within their own geographical jurisdictions.

There are four categories of "national emergency":

1. public welfare emergencies, such as a major natural disaster or accident, which are beyond the authority of the province or territory in which the disaster occurs to address;

2. public order emergencies, wherein there is a serious security threat to the nation;

3. international emergencies arising from acts of coercion or intimidation or the serious use of force or violence, which threaten the sovereignty, security, or territorial integrity of Canada or its allies; and

4. a state of war, either active or imminent, involving Canada or its allies.

The Emergencies Act contains further safeguards designed to ensure a measured response in the event that a situation falls within one of the categories described above. It is important to note that the extraordinary powers extended by the federal government must be tailored to the specific disaster event, and may not exceed what is necessary to deal with the particulars of the situation at hand. The Emergencies Act is not designed to justify the arbitrary or excessive use of power on the part of the federal government.

The Emergency Preparedness Act The **Emergency Preparedness Act** (Department of Justice Canada, 2007b) functions as companion legislation to the Emergencies Act. Where the Emergencies Act provides the authority for government action, the Emergency Preparedness Act provides a basis for the planning and programming necessary to address disasters of all kinds. Specifically, the Emergency Preparedness Act addresses the need for cooperation between the provinces and territories at the federal level to establish responsibilities and the need for public awareness, as well as providing a structure for training and education.

Emergency Management

Emergency management is an essential discipline involving a diverse group of skilled professionals, with the ultimate responsibility resting with the government to assess and deal with risk in an effort to protect the health and safety of the public (Haddow & Bullock, 2006). The four areas of emergency management in the life-cycle process of a disaster include (Veenema, 2003):

1. mitigating or preventing the effects of an emergency;
2. preparing for emergencies or disasters;
3. responding to an emergency or disaster to reduce the impact on public loss; and
4. recovering from an emergency or disaster by assisting communities to return to normal.

ORGANIZATIONAL STRUCTURE AND CHAIN OF COMMAND

National Incident Management System

An international system known as the **National Incident Management System (NIMS)** was developed by the Department of Homeland Security in the United States and released in March 2004. The NIMS was quickly adopted by the Government of Canada and now provides the framework for all levels of government in Canada to develop emergency response plans. The NIMS supports an effective management system for disaster preparedness regardless of the nature of the incident or its level of complexity (Qureshi, Gebbie, & Gebbie, 2006).

Incident Command System

The **Incident Command System (ICS)** is a standardized, on-scene incident management concept designed specifically to allow public health officials to respond efficiently in an emergency situation by implementing an organized and integrated response across jurisdictional boundaries, irrespective of the nature of the emergency (Qureshi et al., 2004; Weiner & Irwin, 2003). The ICS was crafted in the early 1970s in California to assist firefighters in responding to any size or type of wildfire emergency. The ICS is part of the NIMS and improves communication using a structured chain of command and control, with key management positions, action plans, and sections to meet the requirements of the situation.

CRISES IN PUBLIC HEALTH: THE WALKERTON E-COLI EXPERIENCE AND SARS

The face of emergency preparedness in Canada has also been shaped by two recent events that highlighted the gaps and weaknesses in the Canadian public health system and infection control capacity. In the year 2000, improper execution of safe water practices in Walkerton, Ontario, led to the contamination of the town's water supply by way of E-coli O157:H7 and *Campylobacter jejuni* bacteria. One year later,

the same strain of E-coli contaminated the drinking water in North Battleford, Saskatchewan. The *Walkerton Commission of Inquiry Reports* (O'Connor, 2002) called for 93 recommendations that would ensure the quality of drinking water to reduce the risk of infection and death. A similar inquiry was called on account of the breakdown in the town water filtration plant in North Battleford. In 2003, Canadians again faced the need for emergency response following the outbreak of sudden acute respiratory syndrome (SARS). SARS emerged from China in 2002 and spread quickly across the globe to Toronto (Naylor, 2003).

Since these events, four comprehensive reports have been released, each of which calls for a renewal in the national public health system. Both *The Health of Canadians—The Federal Role* (Kirby & LeBreton, 2002) and *Reforming Health Protection and Promotion in Canada: Time to Act* (Kirby, 2003) called for the federal government to provide funding support and to take a stronger leadership role to strengthen the public health infrastructure and health promotion efforts in Canada.

Learning from SARS: Renewal of Public Health in Canada: A report of the National Advisory Committee on SARS and Public Health, known as the Naylor Report (2003), addressed a lack of capacity in the clinical and public health systems and epidemiological investigation of the outbreak; dysfunctional relationships between various orders of governments; absence of protocols for data- or information-sharing among different government levels; and inadequate business processes between and across jurisdictions for outbreak management and emergency response. The report recommends the need for a Canadian Agency for Public Health, with a chief Public Health Officer of Canada heading the agency and reporting to the Minister of Health; development of a National Health Strategy with specific health targets and benchmarks; public health partnership programs to build capacity in public health at the local/municipal level; and a national strategy to renew and sustain public health human resources (including public health nurses, public health physicians, infection control practitioners, and microbiologists). The report draws specific attention to the role of CHNs in emergency preparedness. Naylor notes that public health nurses (PHNs), making up one-third of the public health workforce, will face a shortage of 7000 registered nurses by 2011. He notes that the essential contributions by public health nurses during the SARS outbreak have received little public attention.

For the Public's Health: A Plan of Action, or the Walker Report (2004), targeted all sectors of Ontario's health care system involved in planning for, funding, and delivering public health programs and services in Ontario. The recommendations directly impacted local public health and emergency medical services to build a public health model, establish infection control networks and standards, improve emergency preparedness, develop a communications infrastructure in the event of an emergency, enhance surveillance, and increase enrolment in key public health professions.

Canadian Research Box 24.1

Campbell, A. (2006, December). *The SARS Commission—Spring of fear: Final report*. Ontario Ministry of Health and Long-Term Care. Retrieved January 22, 2007, from http://www.health.gov.on.ca/english/public/pub/ministry_reports/campbell06/online_rep/index.html.

This retrospective qualitative study was based on public hearings, government and hospital documents, and interviews of more than 600 people involved with the SARS outbreak in 2003 in Ontario. The report aims to address the system failure in the public health infrastructure and its deficiencies in health protection and emergency response laws in Ontario.

SARS killed 44 people, and almost 375 fell ill over 5 months in 2003. In a heath care setting, 72% were infected; of this group, 45% were health workers, mostly nurses working closely with sick patients. Thematic problems emerged in all hospital and government agencies in (1) communication; (2) preparation/planning; (3) accountability; (4) worker safety; (5) infection control and surveillance; (6) infrastructure and resources; and (7) precautionary principle and action in risk reduction. In contrast, the spread of SARS in a British Columbia hospital was rapidly brought under control because of the government's commitments to worker safety and intervention with safety and compliance inspections in the early stages of the outbreak.

The final report recommends (a) increased funding to strengthen the public health infrastructure; (b) changes to hospital practices, disease surveillance, and provincial public health and emergency legislation; (c) embracing precautionary principles to safeguard the front-line workers; and (d) using lessons learned from SARS to better prepare for potential threats such as the H5N1 pandemic flu or unexpected health crises.

Discussion Questions:

1. Relate what CHNs must do in the event of a disaster.
2. Discuss key lessons learned from the SARS crisis for emergency preparedness planning.

THE PUBLIC HEALTH AGENCY OF CANADA

On September 24, 2004, the Government of Canada established the Public Health Agency of Canada (PHAC) and appointed the first Chief Public Health Officer (CPHO) of Canada. On December 16, 2006, the Public Health Agency of Canada Act (PHAC, 2006) was given Royal Assent, recognizing the Agency with enabling legislation and establishing the dual role of the CPHO as head of the PHAC and lead public health professional in Canada. Several branches, centres, and directorates report to the Chief Public Health Officer, including the Centre for Emergency Preparedness and Response (CEPR), the National Microbiology Laboratory, the Laboratory for Foodborne Zoonoses, the Pandemic Preparedness Secretariat, the Infectious Disease and Emergency Preparedness (IDEP) Centre, and the Office of Public Health Safety. The agency shares Canadian expertise and works with global partners including the World Health Organization, the United States Centers for Disease Control and Prevention, and the new European Centre for Disease Prevention and Control.

PUBLIC HEALTH RESPONSE IN A DISASTER

Federal, provincial/territorial, and local public health professionals are responsible for the health of their communities in both preparing for a disaster and responding once a disaster has occurred. The seven phases of a functional disaster response model for public health activities in preparing and responding to a disaster include (Landesman, 2005):

1. Planning—apply basic concepts of local public health to disaster management;
2. Prevention—control/prevent outbreaks, organize services and treatment, manage injuries, and provide long-term counselling and mental health interventions;
3. Assessment—determine the incidence of disease and causal factors;
4. Response—communicate plans and needs;
5. Surveillance—establish syndromic surveillance information systems;
6. Recovery—mobilize resources; and
7. Evaluation—determine whether emergency plans and disaster response are effective and efficient.

Each phase is linked with specific responsibilities and skill sets possessed by a network of public health professionals for disaster planning and relief.

ROLE OF COMMUNITY HEALTH NURSING ORGANIZATIONS IN DISASTERS

International Council of Nurses

The International Council of Nurses (ICN) represents more than 124 national nurses' associations worldwide. It works to establish sound policies that condemn violations of human rights commonly seen during and after a disaster (ICN, 2006). The ICN provides assistance to countries in disaster planning by influencing banks and international financial institutions and ensuring that countries at increased risk for disasters have quick access to other care services. It urges countries to include disaster planning in their assistance programs, and promotes and facilitates disaster information, training, and technology while encouraging international networks. The ICN states that "nurses with their technical skills and knowledge of epidemiology, physiology, pharmacology, cultural-familial structures, and psychosocial issues can assist in disaster preparedness programs, as well as during disasters. [They] can play a strategic role cooperating with health and social disciplines, government bodies, community groups, and non-governmental agencies, including humanitarian organizations" (p. 2).

Canadian Nurses Association

The Canadian Nurses Association (CNA) provides information related to global nursing issues including disasters. CNA has partnered with PHAC's Centre for Emergency Preparedness and Response to provide expertise and consultation in developing the role of nurses in a national emergency plan. As members of the ICN, the CNA responded to SARS in 2003, the tsunami disaster in South and Southeast Asia in 2004, and hurricane Katrina in 2005.

EMERGENCY PREPAREDNESS: PLANNING AND PREPARING FOR A DISASTER

Core Competencies

Before CHNs can effectively contribute during a disaster, they must be competent to respond in an emergency. Jennings-Sanders (2004) described **disaster nursing** as "the systematic and flexible utilization of knowledge and skills specific to disaster-related nursing, and the promotion of a wide range of activities to minimize the health hazards and life threatening damage caused by disasters in collaboration with other specialized fields" (p. 69). A set of core competencies to educate nursing students related to mass casualty incidents with examples should be incorporated into the nursing curriculum (Jennings-Sanders, Frisch, & Wing, 2005). (See the box "Core Competencies Related to Mass Casualty Incidents.")

Core Competencies Related to Mass Casualty Incidents

1. Critical thinking: Uses an approved ethical framework to support decision making and prioritizing needed in disaster situations.
2. Assessment: Assesses the safety issues for self, the response team, and victims in any given response situation in collaboration with the incident response.
3. Technical skills: Demonstrates safe administration of immunizations, including smallpox vaccination.
4. Communication: Describes the local chain of command and management system for emergency response during a mass casualty incident.

The Jennings Disaster Nursing Management Model

The literature has a limited number of disaster planning models to guide nurses to respond to a disaster. The *Jennings Disaster Nursing Management Model*, originally introduced to teach disaster nursing to nursing students, focuses on assisting community health nurses in planning for and managing disasters at their work site (Jennings-Sanders, 2004). There are four phases of the Jennings Disaster Nursing Management model:

Phase I (Pre-disaster) This phase involves assessing resources, risks, and planning to achieve primary prevention such as providing information to help the public at large prepare for a disaster. During this phase the nurse must be able to respond effectively by identifying and allocating human resources and material resources such as shelters, planning cooperative agreements with other community agencies, defining the roles of everyone involved, assisting special needs groups to develop plans, and developing or activating the disaster plan.

Phase II (Disaster Occurs) In this phase the nurse assumes multiple roles providing care, education, and case management to disaster victims, by using a holistic approach that considers emotional, physical, psychosocial, and cultural aspects of care to improve the overall health of disaster victims. The impact of a disaster varies in time and severity. Children, older adults, and people with mental illness are among the highest-risk groups for serious mental health morbidity and mortality. CHNs must recognize symptoms of serious mental illness and depression, and must make every effort to reduce devastating outcomes (Landesman, 2005). Their own family safety, pet care, and personal safety at work, as well as food, water, sleep, shelter, and rest periods while at work, are also of concern among nurses responding in the event of an emergency (Jennings-Sanders, 2004).

CHNs may find themselves working in different roles, such as operating a walk-in clinic, working in a shelter or evacuation centre, and triaging people at mass clinics while providing prophylactic medication or administering vaccine. The nurse as case manager may need to liaise between the victim and a community agency or clinic. Nurses must recognize problems through diagnosis and, through secondary prevention, provide immediate treatment, including making referrals to an emergency room or community site where a clinic has been organized.

Phase III (Post-disaster) During this phase the nurse performs tertiary prevention through assessment, planning, and implementation. Nurses ensure that victims in the disaster are receiving treatment, and they decrease disabilities through tertiary preventive interventions such as rehabilitation. Nurses will also assess the emergency disaster plan and evaluate the severity of the disaster on the community. They will coordinate recovery operations to help local residents of the community reduce their exposure to risk and disease. They will apply epidemiological principles to ensure that the community does not become infected with disease, and they will implement infection control measures.

Phase IV (Positive Client/Population Outcomes) In this phase, nurses must measure the overall impact of the disaster to organize the coordination of community services to help residents in their recovery, reduce mortality rates, and reduce health care costs while improving the health status of the client/population. Positive outcomes include increased community relations, improved knowledge of disasters, improved disaster nursing plans, and decreased costs related to the disaster. (See Canadian Research Box 24.1 on p. 354.)

HIGH-RISK SITUATIONS: CORE COMPETENCIES FOR PUBLIC HEALTH NURSES

According to Berkowitz (2002) and Pattillo (2003), public health nursing skills and competencies are critical to bioterrorism preparedness and a public health nurse response. Eight domains of core competencies and skills were developed by a council of major public health and health care organizations to provide essential public health services to respond during an emergency. These skills were cross-referenced with ten essential services. (See Table 24.2 and the Case Study below.)

Case Study

In February 2007, the Public Health Agency of Canada is notified by the World Health Organization (WHO) that a pandemic influenza emergency has been declared in the world. The WHO confirms that the avian influenza (H5N1) virus has killed 1 million people in Asia as a result of human-to-human transmission. The virus is spreading across Europe. It is estimated that in three months the strain will arrive in North America from Asia and Europe. The Public Health Agency of Canada has informed provincial and territorial governments that they need to implement their pandemic plans at the provincial/territorial and community levels. Local public health units are taking the lead in each community to implement pandemic plans.

Discussion Questions

1. Determine the type of disaster in an avian influenza pandemic.

2. Describe the steps you would take to prepare for this pandemic situation.

3. Referring to Table 24.2, briefly outline the needed core competencies and skills and public health services required for the pandemic planning.

TABLE 24.2
Core Competencies and Skills and Essential Public Health Services

Eight Domains of Core Competencies and Skills	Ten Essential Public Health Services
■ Analytic assessment skill ■ Policy development/program planning ■ Communication ■ Cultural competency ■ Community dimensions of practice ■ Basic public health sciences ■ Financial planning and management ■ Leadership and systems thinking	■ Monitor health status to identify community health problems ■ Diagnose and investigate health problems and health hazards in the community ■ Educate and empower people about health issues ■ Mobilize community partnerships to identify and solve health problems ■ Develop policies and plans that support individual and community health efforts ■ Enforce laws and regulations that protect health and ensure safety ■ Link people to needed personal health service and ensure the provision of health care when otherwise unavailable ■ Ensure a competent public health and personal health care work force ■ Evaluate effectiveness, accessibility, and quality of personal and population-based health services ■ Research for new insights and innovative solutions to health problems

SAFETY OF VULNERABLE POPULATIONS

Nursing organizations and home health nurses must know the types of disasters and biological agents that could occur or be released in their community to provide medical management for their clients while ensuring their own personal protection when responding to an emergency (Sawyer, 2003). Sawyer states that management must provide education and training of home health nurses (HHNs) to understand the agency emergency preparedness plan, document skill sets of each staff member, know how to answer questions, and establish a clear communication plan in an emergency response.

Clients receiving home care may be ventilator dependent, threatening their life if an electrical failure should occur. Many clients may be hearing impaired, unable to access a telephone due to physical limitations, and have no close support from their family members who may live out of town. The "Hazard Vulnerability Analysis" assessment tool can be used by HHNs to determine the level of risk to their caseload of clients by focusing on *preparation* and *prevention* (Rodriguez & Long, 2006). In the event of an emergency, HHNs are in an excellent position to provide increased surveillance of those patients who make up their caseload After assessing the client's home environment, family and social support networks, and community partners, the HHN can develop a plan to ensure communication, protect the client from death, and reduce the impact of a disaster on those most susceptible. As participants in a community emergency, HHNs can also report any suspected evidence of a biological agent, monitor and support those individuals who are quarantined in their homes, and offer skills in health screening and administer vaccines at community sites.

In order to ensure that vulnerable populations are protected in the event of an emergency or disaster, long term care facilities and community-based support services must be integrated into local and regional disaster planning to provide for clear communication and appropriate response plans. These organizations often deal with low staffing ratios and are not well coordinated with hospitals, yet share common resources during a disaster and make unique contributions (Saliba, Buchanan, & Kington, 2004).

Summary

This chapter has outlined the types of disasters and challenges to which the nursing profession must learn to competently respond during a community disaster. An explanation for the renewed infrastructure of public health in Canada provides knowledge about the PHAC, leadership from the chief public health officer, and established emergency procedures, legislation, regulations, and processes that continue to build the current framework and legislation essential to health care delivery during any emergency.

Canadian nurses must develop an agenda to strengthen education in disaster nursing. An understanding of disaster training combined with community health, public health nursing experience, and technological knowledge strengthens the role of public health nurses in bioterrorism emergency preparedness and response. This can happen only when nursing research is applied to emergency response practice, education, and health policy. CHNs play a vital role in emergency preparedness. A strong, effective public health workforce of community health nurses must be established to meet the challenges of unpredictable threats on the community.

KEY TERMS

natural disasters
man-made disasters
bioterrorism
epidemic
Emergencies Act
Emergency Preparedness Act
emergency management
National Incident Management System (NIMS)
Incident Command System (ICS)
disaster nursing

INDIVIDUAL CRITICAL THINKING EXERCISES

1. What competencies do beginning nurses require to be able to respond to mass casualty incidents?

2. What technical skills do nurses require to respond during an emergency?

GROUP CRITICAL THINKING EXERCISES

A tornado has left many families without homes. Local politicians and emergency response planners have declared a disaster in the area and ordered citizens to evacuate to a shelter.

1. Discuss what essential public health services are needed in this situation.

2. How could nursing students assist in this emergency response?

REFERENCES

Berkowitz, B. (2002). One year later: The impact and aftermath of September 11: Public health nursing practice: Aftermath of September 11, 2001. *Online Journal of Issues in Nursing,7*(3), Manuscript 4. Retrieved January 6, 2007, from http://www.nursingworld.org/ojin/topic19/tpc19_4.htm.

Cohen, R. E. (2000). *Mental health services in disasters: Instructor's guide.* Washington, D.C.: PAHO Publications.

Department of Justice Canada. (2007a). *Emergencies Act, R.S., 1985*, c. 22 (4th Supp.). Retrieved January 9, 2007, from http://laws.justice.gc.ca/en/showtdm/cs/E-4.5.

Department of Justice Canada. (2007b). *Emergency Preparedness Act, R.S., 1985, c. 6 (4th Supp.).* Retrieved January 9, 2007, from http://laws.justice.gc.ca/en/showtdm/cs/E-4.6.

Haddow, G. D., & Bullock, J. A. (2006). *Introduction to emergency management* (2nd ed.). Burlington, MA: Elsevier Butterworth-Heinemann.

International Council of Nurses. (2006, revised). *ICN position statement: Nurses and disaster preparedness.* Retrieved January 9, 2007, from http://www.icn.ch/psdisasterprep01.htm.

Jennings-Sanders, A. (2004). Teaching disaster nursing by utilizing the Jennings Disaster Nursing Management Model. *Nurse Education in Practice, 4,* 69–76.

Jennings-Sanders, A., Frisch, N., & Wing, S. (2005). Nursing students' perception about disaster nursing. *Disaster Management and Response, 3,* 80–85.

Kirby, M., & LeBreton, M. (2002, October). *The health of Canadians—the federal role final report.* Vol. 6: Recommendations for Reform. The Standing Senate Committee on Social Affairs, Science and Technology.

Retrieved January 9, 2007, from http://www.parl.gc.ca/37/2/parlbus/commbus/senate/com-e/soci-e/rep-e/repoct02vol6-e.htm.

Kirby, M. (2003, November). *Reforming health protection and promotion in Canada: Time to act.* The Standing Senate Committee on Social Affairs, Science and Technology. Retrieved September 17, 2006, from http://www.parl.gc.ca/37/2/paribus/commbus/senate/Com-e/SOCI-E/rep-e/repfinnov-3-e.htm.

Landesman, L. Y. (2005). *Public health management of disasters: The practice guide* (2nd ed.). Washington, D.C.: American Public Health Association.

Naylor, D. (2003). *Learning from SARS: Renewal of public health in Canada: A report of the National Advisory Committee on SARS and Public Health.* Ottawa: Health Canada.

O'Connor, D. R. (2002). *Walkerton Commission of Inquiry reports: A strategy for safe drinking water* (ISBN: 0-7794-2621-5). Toronto: Ontario Ministry of the Attorney General. Retrieved January 9, 2007, from http://www.attorneygeneral.jus.gov.on.ca/english/about/pubs/walkerton/.

Patillo, M. M. (2003). Mass casualty disaster nursing course. *Nurse Educator, 28*(6), 271–275.

Public Safety and Emergency Preparedness Canada. (2005). *Canadian disaster database.* Retrieved January 9, 2007, from http://www.psepc-sppcc.gc.ca/res/em/cdd/search-en.asp.

Public Health Agency of Canada (PHAC). (2001). Bioterrorism and public health. *Canada Communicable Disease Report, 27*(4). Retrieved January 9, 2007, from http://www.phac-aspc.gc.ca/publicat/ccdr-rmtc/01vol27/dr2704ea.html.

Public Health Agency of Canada (PHAC). (2006). *Act to establish public health agency comes into force,* Retrieved January 9, 2007, from http://www.phac-aspc.gc.ca/media/nr-rp/2006/2006_11_e.html.

Qureshi, K. A., Gershon, R. M., Merrill, J. A., Calero-Breckheimer, A., Murrman, M., Gebbie, K. M., Moskin, L. C., May, L., Morse, S. S., & Sherman, M. (2004). Effectiveness of an emergency preparedness training program for public health nurses in New York City. *Family Community Health, 27*(3), 242–249.

Qureshi, K., Gebbie, K. M., & Gebbie, E. N. (2006, Oct. 27). *Public Health Incident Command System: A guide for the management of emergencies or other unusual incidents within public health agencies.* New York: U of Albany.

Rodriguez, D., & Long, C. O. (2006). Preparedness for the home healthcare nurse. *Home Healthcare Nurse, 24*(1), 21–27.

Saliba, D., Buchanan, J., & Kington, R. S. (2004). Function and response of nursing facilities during community disaster. *American Journal of Public Health, 94*(8), 1436–1441.

Sawyer, P. P. (2003). Bioterrorism: Are we prepared? *Home Healthcare Nurse, 21*(4), 220–223.

Veenema, T. G. (Ed.). (2003). *Disaster nursing and emergency preparedness for chemical, biological, and radiological terrorism and other hazards,* New York, Springer Publishing Co. Inc.

Walker, D. (2004, April). Final report of the Ontario expert panel on SARS and infectious disease control. *For the public's health: A plan of action.* Toronto: SARS Expert Panel Secretariat, Ontario, Ministry of Health and Long-Term Care.

Weiner, B., & Irwin, M. (2003). Current initiatives for emergency preparedness response: Commentary on "New challenges for public health care: Biological and chemical weapons awareness, surveillance, and response." *Biological Research for Nursing, 4*(4), 255–257.

ADDITIONAL RESOURCES

Websites

CDC Bioterrorism Preparedness & Response
  www.bt.cdc.gov/
  www.bt.cdc.gov/Documents/Planning/PlanningGuidance.PDF

Center for Research on the Epidemiology of Disasters (CRED)
  www.cred.be/

International Federation of the Red Cross (IFRC)
  www.ifrc.org

Pan American Health Organization (PAHO)
  www.paho.org

Public Health Agency of Canada's Centre for Emergency Preparedness and Response
  www.phac-aspc.gc.ca/cepr-cmiu/index.html

Readings

Rowitz, L. (2006). *Public health for the 21st century: The prepared leader.* Toronto: Jones and Bartlett Publishers.

Wynd, C. (2006, Sept. 30). A proposed model for military disaster nursing. *OJIN: The Online Journal of Issues in Nursing, 11*(3). Retrieved from http://www.nursingworld.org/ojin/topic31/tpc31_4.htm.

About the Authors

Mary Anne Simpson, RN (Victoria Hospital, London), BScN, MSc (Windsor), is Manager of Vaccine Preventable Diseases in the Communicable Disease and Sexual Health Services at the Middlesex-London Health Unit (London, Ontario). She is a member of the Association of Public Health Nursing Management in Ontario (AND-SOOHA), the Registered Nurses' Association of Ontario (RNAO), the Canadian Public Health Association (CPHA), and the Community and Hospital Infection Control Association (CHICA). She has been involved in several emergency response situations including meningococcal immunization and hepatitis A immunization campaigns in Middlesex–London. She was deployed to the Ministry of Health and Long-Term Care in 2003 during SARS, and was involved in the rubella outbreak in Oxford County, Ontario, in 2005.

Lucia Yiu, RN, BScN, BA (Windsor), BSc (Toronto), MScN (Western Ontario), is an Associate Professor in the Faculty of Nursing, University of Windsor, and an Educational and Training Consultant in community nursing. Her practice and research include multicultural health, international health, experiential learning, community development, breast health, and program planning and evaluation.

Adolescent Sexual Health and Pregnancy

Cynthia Mannion

chapter 25

OBJECTIVES

After studying this chapter, you should be able to:

1. Examine adolescent sexuality issues in the context of the determinants of health.

2. Recognize the developmental aspects of adolescents with the potential to influence the outcomes of sexual behaviour.

3. Discuss issues/factors linked to sexual awareness and adolescent sexual activity within the current context.

4. Examine tensions and the occurrence of violence in the teenage relationship.

5. Discuss the roles of the community health nurses can play in supporting pregnant adolescents and adolescents who are at risk for pregnancy.

INTRODUCTION

This chapter will discuss sexual awareness, sexual activity in teenagers, and teenage pregnancy. Throughout, evidence from three recent Canadian surveys will be reported: (1) the 2003 *Canadian Youth, Sexual Health and HIV/AIDS Study* (CYSHHAS) (Council of Ministers of Education, 2003); (2) the 2002 *Canadian Contraception Study Part 2* (CCS) (Fisher, Boroditsky, & Morris, 2004); and (3) the 2003 *Canadian Community Health Survey* (CCHS) (Statistics Canada, 2005). The 2003 CYSHHAS included 11 074 students ranging from 12 to 16 years old from all provinces and territories except Nunavut. The 2002 CCS examined sexual-health–related knowledge and contraceptive practices of 249 adolescents aged 15 to 18 years. The 2003 CCHS is based on a sample of 18 048, weighted to be representative of Canadian households including adolescents aged 15 to 24 years. Although these reports cannot be representative of all teens, they provide insight into contraceptive and sexual health practices of adolescents and those behaviours that may precede pregnancy.

The determinants of health outlined by the Public Health Agency of Canada (PHAC) (2003) help us understand the multidimensional nature of health and factors that affect health status, teen sexuality, and sexual practices. They include:

1. income and social status,

2. social support networks,

3. education and literacy,

4. employment and working conditions,

5. social environments,

6. physical environments,

7. personal health practices and coping skills,

8. healthy child development,

9. biology and genetic endowment,

10. health services,

11. gender, and

12. culture.

BASIC CONCEPTS OF SEX, SEXUALITY, AND SEXUAL HEALTH

It is useful to consider globally held concepts of sex, sexuality, and sexual health, as described in Table 25.1. The terms in Table 25.1 do not represent an official WHO position or definition, as they are still under revision by world experts.

TEEN PREGNANCY

Worldwide, there has been a trend toward lower adolescent pregnancy and birth rates. The decline in teen pregnancy rates can be interpreted in a number of ways. Premarital sexual activity is more acceptable today than 20 years ago; and the stigma of unwed pregnancy has decreased. There is also a wider acceptance of goals other than motherhood for women and therefore a delay of marriage and childbearing years.

The **teen pregnancy rate** is a composite of the number of live births, still births, and abortions. In 2000, the number of pregnancies among 15- to 19-year-old women was 38 600, a decline from 61 242 in 1974 (McKay, 2004). The abortion rate has remained fairly steady, at 20.2 per 1000 between 1974 and 2000.

TABLE 25.1
Basic Concepts of Sex, Sexuality, and Sexual
Health

Sex	Refers to the biological characteristics that define humans as female or male.
Sexuality	Refers to a core dimension of being human that includes sex, gender, sexual and gender identity, sexual orientation, eroticism, emotional attachment/love, and reproduction. It is experienced or expressed in thoughts, fantasies, desires, beliefs, attitudes, values, activities, roles, and relationships. Sexuality is a result of the interplay of biological, psychological, socioeconomic, cultural, ethical, and religious/spiritual factors. While sexuality can include all these aspects, not all of these dimensions need to be experienced or expressed. However, in sum, our sexuality is experienced and expressed in all that we are, what we feel, think and do.
Sexual health	The experience of the ongoing process of physical, psychological, and socio-cultural well-being related to sexuality.

Sources: Pan American Health Organization & World Health Organization. (2000). Promotion of sexual health: Recommendations for action. *Proceedings from the Regional consultation Antigua Guatemala, pp. 26–29. Retrieved April 27, 2007, from http://www.who.int/reproductive-health/gender/ sexualhealth.html.*

Canadian Research Box 25.1

McKay, A. (2006). Trends in teen pregnancy in Canada with comparisons to U.S.A. and England/Wales. *The Canadian Journal of Human Sexuality, 15*(3–4), 157–61.

Trends in teen pregnancy can be viewed as an indicator of teenagers' control over their sexual and reproductive health. In the countries examined, teenagers from the United States and England/Wales share similar attributes. The teen pregnancy rate, independent from the abortion rate, has been declining over the past 10 years, and more so among younger teens (15–17 years of age). In Canada, the prairie provinces and the territories have higher teenage pregnancy rates than the national average, perhaps reflecting ethno-cultural differences. The findings in this study indicate that greater sexual information and access to contraception have increased women's choices regarding sexual behaviour and reproduction. Culture and religion continue to influence many.

Discussion Questions:

1. Speculate as to why teenagers living in rural communities may have a higher pregnancy rate than the national average. What ethno-cultural factors may influence this?

2. What social issues may have influenced the change in the teenage pregnancy rate?

CONTRACEPTION

Oral contraceptives (OCs) and condoms are the most commonly used contraceptive methods among teenagers, although use is inconsistent (Fisher et al., 2004). Condoms are favoured because they offer birth control and prevention of sexually transmitted infection (STI). Sixty-six percent reported using OCs and 44% used condoms, but overall the 2002 CCS reported a lack of consistent adherence to any method of contraception among teens in the study. This finding is mirrored by the two other Canadian surveys. Although 85% of 15- and 18-year-olds and 91% of 16- and 17-year-olds used contraception having intercourse the first time, 25% of 15-year-olds and 17 % of 16-year-olds responded that they only "usually" used contraception.

According to the 2003 CYSHHAS (Council of Ministers of Education, 2003), teens were also familiar with the morning-after pill but less aware of other methods of contraception. None of the sexually active teens surveyed used spermicidal methods or IUDs. In 1997, Canada approved depot medroxy-progesterone acetate (DMPA), a long-acting injectable birth control method (Boonstra, 2002). The 2002 CCS reported that 6% of sexually active teens aged 15 to 18 used DMPA. The effect of this contraceptive measure on teen pregnancy rate in Canada has yet to be determined (Fisher et al., 2004).

RISKS OF PREGNANCY

Adolescents who engage in sexual activity are at risk for pregnancy due to non-compliance with contraception, failure of birth control, and lack of pregnancy prevention knowledge. Adolescent pregnancies are complicated by the lack of early and consistent prenatal care. The lack of prenatal monitoring of weight gain, blood pressure, and fetal growth places both the young mother and the fetus at risk for pre-eclampsia, cephalopelvic disproportion, preterm birth, and low birth weight. Untreated sexually transmitted infections hold specific and often chronic disease risks for the fetus, including blindness, congenital syphilis, and exposure to herpes virus.

The pregnant adolescent must meet her own nutritional needs in addition to the needs of the growing fetus. Both are at risk for nutritional insufficiencies of calcium, folic acid, and protein, and particularly iron deficiency anemia. The lack of cessation of smoking and recreational drug and alcohol use increases the risk for low birth weight infants, congenital anomalies, the whole range of fetal alcohol spectrum disorders (FASD) and sudden infant death. Pregnant teens need support, information, and prompt, consistent prenatal care to support a healthy pregnancy outcome.

CONSEQUENCES OF PREGNANCY

Teen pregnancy interrupts the developmental tasks of adolescence and forces redirection of personal goals and social processes. Teenaged mothers and fathers face enormous social and financial challenges, particularly if estranged from their family of origin. The low literacy skills that accompany limited education increase the risk of unemployment and herald a decline in income and social status. Poverty is associated with poorer health practices, higher morbidity, and earlier death, but this is also borne preferentially by women (Spitzer, 2005). The young mother is likely to have limited knowledge of healthy child development, limited access to healthy physical environments, and less ability to prepare her children for school. She may be unfamiliar with appropriate health services and lack access to them.

Generally, most teens are not developmentally prepared to parent and often do so within adverse social and economic conditions. The adolescent relationship is ill equipped to cope with a pregnancy and often fails without strong family support. This is not to say that all adolescent relationships lack depth and meaning, but the emotional maturity required for parenting may be lacking. Marriage does not alleviate these pressures, and many teen marriages end in divorce, leaving many young women the head of single-parent families with poor economic resources. A young father facing financial insecurity is most likely to be uninterested in childrearing and become increasingly uninvolved (Rhein et al., 1997). The resulting family instability tends to translate into higher rates of child abuse and neglect (MacMillan, 2000).

NEEDS OF TEENAGE MOTHERS

Nurse researchers have invited adolescent mothers to participate in qualitative research to better understand the adolescent mother's experience. Peterson, Sword, Charles, & DiCenso (2007) found nursing care qualities in the postpartum period that contributed to satisfactory experiences of adolescent mothers: foremost was the state of being calm, followed by demonstrations of confidence in the young mother and the anticipation of unstated needs. Overwhelmingly, adolescent mothers wanted to be treated the same way older mothers were treated.

Teenage Mothers

- Adolescent mothers need anticipatory guidance for parenting tasks.
- Adolescents need access to accurate, factual information about human sexuality, STIs, and contraception when they are contemplating sexual activity.
- Adolescents may not view oral sex, anal sex, or mutual masturbation as "sex," but the risk of STIs remains.

Recent studies (Herrman, 2006; Rentschler, 2003; Stiles, 2005) have documented teen experiences in motherhood and child rearing. Although these studies are not generalizable to

all teens, they provide insight into the successes and difficulties that teen mothers experience and provide some guidance for CHNs. The studies identified that development of peer support groups specifically designed for pregnant adolescents and adolescent parents have been successful strategies to support young mothers and mothers-to-be.

In a naturalistic study, teen mothers identified their needs as support and knowledge (Stiles, 2005). Their goals were happiness, independence, and a career, and to attain these they visualized using such strategies as support groups, life skills education, and completion of formal education and employment (Stiles). An ethnographic study explored the experience of 16 young mothers with respect to their current life context, their relationships, their vocations, and their personal characteristics and parenting. Their perceptions reflected costs and rewards and a desire to seek a better life (Herrman, 2006).

SEXUAL HEALTH OF TEENS

The 2003 CYSHHAS addressed that the health determinants that have been linked to the sexuality and sexual activity of teens include parental income and occupation, educational achievement, degree of religiosity, gender identity, and disability. Interpersonal determinants such as coping ability and self-esteem also help determine healthy sexuality and encourage responsible decision making.

Characteristics of sexually healthy teens include an appreciation and understanding of their body and the bodily functions associated with puberty, the reproductive cycle, and the psychosocial aspects of sexuality. This knowledge can help teens to understand the consequences of their actions. Teens who identify their own values within their self-identity can make decisions as to what is right for them in the face of media messages and peer pressure. The 2003 CYSHHAS reports that girls with lower self-esteem ratings are at risk for high-risk sexual behaviours.

Issues in sexual health include STIs, unintended pregnancy, sexual well being, intimate partner violence (IPV), and safe sexual practices. Both the sexually active teen and the sexually naïve teen are vulnerable, as they may not have access to factual and accurate information or to services providing care in sexuality and fertility, and may be at risk for sexual coercion and abuse from older and sexually experienced acquaintances or strangers.

Given an unplanned pregnancy, teens are no less deserving of accessible and timely medical care and genetic counselling than the married young adult residing in a seemingly more stable and socially acceptable situation. However, for teens, access to health care and particularly prenatal care may be hampered by fear of disclosure and unfamiliarity with reproductive health care services. If adolescents are expected to make mature and responsible decisions regarding sexual behaviour, they need information, education, and other access to supportive health care services.

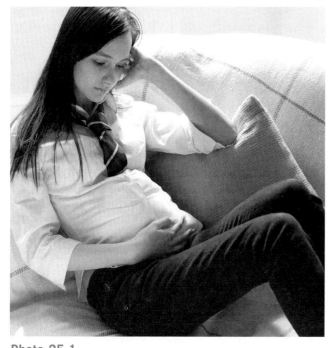

Photo 25.1

A pregnant teen.

Credit: Chris Rout/Alamy

ASSOCIATED RISK BEHAVIOURS

High risk behaviours such as alcohol and drug use are associated with early initiation of sexual experiences and unplanned pregnancy. Adolescents who use substances prior to engaging in sexual intercourse are less likely to use birth control or STI protection (Boyce, Doherty, Fortin, & MacKinnon, 2003). The 2003 CYSHHAS polled students about alcohol, drug, and tobacco use. Having had too much alcohol or drugs was listed as the third reason why condoms were not used the last time Grade 11 males and females had sexual intercourse (Boyce et al., 2006). Alcohol use increased as adolescents progressed from Grades 9 to 11, but adolescents also reported using other addictive substances such as solvents, LSD/acid, ecstasy, cocaine/crack, magic mushrooms, and chewing tobacco. Hashish and marijuana use was most prevalent, and 27% of Grade 11 students reported using these at least once per month.

TOO YOUNG FOR SEXUAL ACTIVITIES?

In Canada, the age for sexual consent—renamed "the age of protection"—was changed in 2007 to 16 years from 14 years. This change has important social, legal, and political implications. Age of initiation of sexual intercourse for teens participating in the 2002 CCS was 13 years (5%), and by 19+ years 98% of respondents reported having had intercourse. The median age of initiation of sexual intercourse was approximately 16.5 years. Of concern is that youths less than 16 years old will be less likely to seek health care information or services regarding sexual issues.

HEALTHY CHILD DEVELOPMENT

The development of sexuality begins early in human development with the establishment of trust and love within the primary relationship between a parent/caregiver and infant. Adolescence is generally considered to occur between the ages of 12 and 19 years and is marked by enormous psychological and physical changes. Accompanying adolescent physical development are psychosocial tasks that include developing a sense of identity and self-esteem, autonomy, and independence; seeking psychological and physical intimacy; and developing sexual identity. Sexual interest and sexual behaviours increase as adolescents enter puberty and achieve physiological sexual maturity. As this period spans a broad passage of development from teen to adulthood, sexual health recommendations for early adolescents may not be applicable for those in mid or late adolescence.

The family can have a profound effect on the sexual and emotional health of adolescents (Boyce, 1999). Parents who encourage psychological autonomy increase the likelihood that their teen will make their own decision regarding initiation of sexual behaviours rather than succumb to social pressures. In the 2003 CYSHHAS, 72% of students reported living with parents, 13% with mother alone, and 3% with father alone. More than 71% of boys and girls all ages reported "I have a happy home life," which is an important determinant for emotional and physical health. In a large American survey of almost 10 000 Grade 6 to Grade 12 students, Fulkerson, Story, Mellin, Leffert, Neumark-Sztainer, & French (2006) found that regular family rituals such as family dinners served as a protective factor reducing high-risk behaviours including sexual behaviours among adolescents.

Some families present teens with greater obstacles to overcome in completing the psychosocial tasks of adolescence than others. Families where physical, emotional, or sexual abuse occurs are at high risk for low self-esteem and make easy victims for coercive or controlling behaviour. This places the teen at risk for peer/date violence and potentially abusive sexual relationships (Renker, 2002). The 2003 CYSHHAS found a gender difference among boys and girls responding to self-esteem measures. Fewer Grade 9 to 11 girls than boys stated that they possessed confidence. Boys were also more likely to report that they liked themselves than girls did across the grades.

Boyce (1999) reported that some parental behaviours relate to sexual risk-taking of adolescents. Parental monitoring of daily activities is strongly associated with low-risk sexual behaviour among sexually active teens. In an American study of approximately 2000 boys and girls examining when and where sexual activity occurred, a strong, positive independent association was found between the amount of unsupervised time teens had and sexual behaviours. More than one-half of students reported being home alone for more than four hours per day. Of those who had intercourse, 91% said it occurred after school in someone's home or their own (Cohen , Farley, Taylor, & Martin, 2002). In a small U.S. study, adolescents who reported that their parents knew where they were and what activities outside the home they were involved in expressed thoughts less favourable toward initiating intercourse than did those with more unrestricted time (Sieverding, Adler, Witt, & Ellen, 2005).

SOCIAL AND PHYSICAL ENVIRONMENTS

Peers form an important social network for teens. Teens are connected with their peer group through school and by cell phone, telephone, and internet. In 2003, 64% of Canadian households reported regularly using the internet (Statistics Canada, 2006). It was estimated that the number of Canadian households that have access to the internet was growing by 5% per year, implying that by now the majority of households are "on the net." For teens, friend networking sites increase the number of relationships formed and feedback on posted profiles can enhance or decrease self-esteem (Valkenburg, Peter, & Schouten, 2006). Health and sexual information is transmitted and shared this way.

The physical environment, a determinant of health, influences teen decision making. Television, radio, film, and advertising are inundated with sexual innuendo and herald overt sexual behaviour far more socially acceptable than it was in the past. The internet allows unsupervised access to sexual images and information that may exceed the viewer's understanding and ethic, placing the broad gamut of human sexuality out of the context of mutually caring and age-appropriate relationships. The public face of overt sexuality is one-sided as it lacks sexual responsibility and the consequences of sexual activity are rarely addressed. These include sexually transmitted infections that can result in chronic disease and infertility, unplanned/unwanted pregnancies, and the devastating impact of teen pregnancy on family coupled with the interrupted social development of the teen.

Peer pressure exerts a strong influence on adolescent decisions to engage in sexual activity. Initiation of sexual behaviours is strongly bound to social pressure (Sant'Anna, Catunda, Carvalho, & Coates, 2007), and peers create a sense of normalcy surrounding sexual behaviours. The risk of early sexual initiation increases as the age difference increases between boyfriends and girlfriends (Vanoss Marin, Coyle, Gomez, Carvajal, & Kirby, 2000). The longer the exposure to sexual intercourse and the more sexual partners a teen has, the higher the risk for sexually transmitted infections and unintended pregnancy.

SEXUAL ACTIVITIES OF TEENS

Teens may engage in a variety of sexual activities, including oral and anal sex or mutual masturbation. There is some evidence that they do not consider these activities as "sex" and reserve that term for sexual intercourse (Randall & Byers, 2003). A recent study reported that oral sex is viewed as less risky and more acceptable, and that more adolescents intend to engage in it rather than vaginal sex (Halpern-Felsher, Cornel, Kropp, & Tschann, 2005). Only 25% of students considered oral sex and only 2% to 14% considered touching or masturbatory behaviours—in the presence of another or on the telephone or computer—to be having sex (Randall & Byers). These other sexual activities were favoured because they avoided the risk of pregnancy and retained virginity. One-third of students in Grade 9 and one-half of students in Grade 11 reported having had oral sex at least once (Council of Ministers of Education, 2003). Multiple partners were reported by 40% of sexually active 18-year-olds: 20% had two partners in the past two years, 10% had three partners, 5% had four partners, and 5% had five or more partners (Fisher et al., 2004).

VIOLENCE

During the past decade, public awareness regarding intimate partner violence has been growing steadily, but violence within adolescent relationships has escaped careful examination. In a prospective qualitative study of pregnant adolescents aged 18 to 20 years, Renker (2002) found that teens experienced abuse from a variety of individuals, including intimate partners, former partners, and family members. Intimate violence in adolescent relationships is likely underreported for many reasons, but also because adolescents have legitimate concerns about their safety following disclosure to authorities. They may fear retaliation from the perpetrator or fail to have the personal stamina and coping resources to break away from the pattern of violence that is mixed within the status and security of being in a relationship.

Peer approval in a sexual relationship may foster tolerance to violence. This is reinforced if the victim's family uses abuse to deal with conflict, fails to recognize or support the adolescent who is experiencing intimate violence, or responds with rejection. Personality characteristics in the adolescent victim can contribute to continuing violence. The perpetrator may have poor social skills, have limited problem solving abilities, or be heavily involved in substance abuse. Violent or controlling behaviour may be misinterpreted as an indication of love and commitment by adolescent girls (Seimer, 2004).

Intimate partner violence that began prior to pregnancy is likely to continue during pregnancy and into the postpartum period. Raphael (2006) reports on domestic violence and birth control sabotage from a survey of teen mothers aged 15 to 17 years. Younger mothers experienced more domestic violence than older teenaged mothers. Four hundred and seventy-four American girls accepting welfare responded to a written survey in health clinics; more than half of the respondents reported some level of domestic violence in the previous 12 months; 41% reported severe levels (kicking, beating, or being threatened with a weapon). Girls with older boyfriends were more likely to have experienced domestic violence that was more severe than those with younger boyfriends (Raphael).

Partners play a role in the choice and use of birth control. Fifty-one percent of teens reported experiencing a form of birth control sabotage from their partner either verbally or by the destruction of birth control measures. Some teens did not use OCs but used injections (DMPA) as they were easier to conceal from their partners. Domestic violence and birth control sabotage are correlated: 66% of those teens reporting domestic violence also experienced birth control sabotage (Raphael, 2006).

WORKPLACE CONSTRAINTS

Access to sexual and reproductive health is the right of teens, but there is no designated health care professional or institutional body directly responsible for this. Although strategically placed, the CHN's role is complicated, given workplace constraints. Existing policies in some school boards (religious/private) stipulate what content matter can be included in health promotion activities. The CHN may not be free to target sexual-health services to teens in a school setting.

COMMUNITY HEALTH NURSES AND TEEN PREGNANCY

Some evidence suggests that the way community health care is delivered can impact on the health of the teenage family. Early-intervention programs offering intense home visitation by public health nurses were associated with infants of teenage mothers who had fewer days of hospitalization and increased immunization rates during the first year of life compared with those who received traditional public health nursing care (Koniak-Griffin, Anderson, Brecht, & Verzemnieks, 2002). Secco et al. (2007) suggest that interventions to improve peer support such as involving adolescent friends in prenatal support and education may enhance the adolescent mother's coping abilities with respect to infant care. Offering knowledge and exploring the pregnant adolescent's expectations around infant care and motherhood can help the new mother to successfully and appropriately respond to her infant.

The way in which care is given is important. It is important for the CHN to take her lead for assessment and intervention from the teen, to listen sensitively and carefully as the teen tries to make sense of the pregnancy, of childbearing and childrearing and attempts to develop responsive skills. Some of these behaviours should be reinforced and others managed to gently suggest rather than admonish. Becoming a mother is yet another identity the teen must find within her own emerging self-identity. The imposition of societal norms may increase maternal anxiety and cause the teen to turn from a resource if she feels it is judgmental and imposing.

Emerging evidence indicates that CHNs should make an effort to acknowledge and involve the fathers of the children (Rhein et al., 1997; Spear, 2004). Too often, the biological father is displaced; many teen fathers wish to be involved but require information about childbearing and childrearing. Continuous paternal involvement should be encouraged if possible, in prenatal classes, prenatal visits, and in the provision of information as to the health and progression of the pregnancy. Confusion about child care can translate into paternal lack of interest and predict uninvolvement (Rhein).

ROLES OF THE COMMUNITY HEALTH NURSE

Community health nurses (CHNs) are in a unique position to reach teens contemplating or engaging in sexual activity. They may also be the first health care professionals available to a pregnant teen. Schools also provide an ideal setting for CHNs to provide factual information about human sexuality, low-risk sexual activities, and current information on contraception and STI prevention and treatment. (See Chapter 16.)

CHNs should be suspicious if an adolescent presents with vague complaints or symptoms that do not appear to have an organic cause, as this may be indicative of abuse or sexual exploitation (Seimer, 2004). Should a teen present with pregnancy, the nurse can provide a prompt referral to the medical service that supports the teen's decision, be that sensitive prenatal care or other therapeutic services. Younger adolescents should be asked directly about involvement in sexual activity, STI prevention, and contraceptive use. A respectful and non-judgmental approach is favoured. Because the teen may not consider some activities to be "sex," the nurse must be specific in addressing a particular sexual behaviour such as oral sex or anal sex. Options and STI prevention information should be offered. Adherence to consistent use of contraception and condoms should be reinforced along with a reminder that OCS use does not confer STI protection.

Case Study

Liza is 16 years old and the eldest daughter of a traditional Italian family. Liza has had a steady relationship for 18 months with a 19-year-old young man whom her family approve of. They have been having unprotected sexual relations for 6 months. Liza presents with morning nausea, fatigue, and amenorrhea. The test for pregnancy is positive. Liza's mother, suspicious about the symptoms, demands the result and an immediate abortion referral if the test is positive.

Discussion Questions

1. Who should be invited to take part in the conversations you will have about Liza's future?

2. What is the responsibility and role of the young man?

3. Liza has asked you to intervene with her mother. What will you say to her mother?

Summary

Teenagers begin sexual activity in early adolescence, inconsistently use contraception, and have multiple partners over time. Prevention of STIs and adherence to reversible contraceptive methods are major individual and public health challenges. CHNs must continually educate themselves using the most accurate and current information and be familiar with the guidelines regarding sexual health to reduce the inconsistencies the population faces across the country. Prevention of unintended pregnancy has far-reaching implications. Healthy child development is powerfully influenced by prenatal and early childhood experiences, and teenage parents may be disadvantaged to provide it optimally. Among other things, birth weight—an indicator of fetal health—is affected by maternal nutrition patterns, drug and alcohol intake, and maternal weight gain. Child physical health is a result of genetic endowment, access to nutritious foods, healthy social and physical environments, and access to medical care.

Although the rate of teenage pregnancy is declining, the effect of the rise in age of consent may reduce access to information and services. It is imperative that CHNs understand the trends in adolescent sexual behaviour, refine communication skills unique to this population, and provide the best information and care within the constraints of the environment within which they work. Given an adolescent pregnancy, the CHN will find the strengths in the young woman and man, support and guide where possible, and assist to strengthen the capabilities inherent in the adolescent parent and provide resources where weaknesses emerge.

KEY TERMS

teenage pregnancy rate
sex
sexuality
sexual health

INDIVIDUAL CRITICAL THINKING EXERCISES

1. What are the factors that will help sexually active adolescents make responsible sexual choices?

2. How do we understand the differences between teens who demonstrate low-risk sexual behaviours and those who do not?

GROUP CRITICAL THINKING EXERCISES

1. Can you think of a way of presenting information to teens to dispel myths such as (a) a woman cannot become pregnant the first time she has sex, (b) a girl cannot become pregnant if she has not yet had her first menstrual period, and (c) having sex standing up prevents pregnancy.

2. On Friday May 4, 2007, the House of Commons passed a bill to raise Canada's age of sexual consent from 14 years to 16 years, as it is in the UK, Australia, and much of the U.S. The legislation renamed the age of consent the "age of protection." Behind the change is the belief that this will offer teens protection from exploitive sexual activity such as pornography or prostitution, including activities that may occur over the internet. Consenting teens who engage in sexual activity cannot be criminally charged if their sexual partner is less than five years different in age and not in a position of authority over them. This "close in age" clause does not apply to those under age 14.

The legislation has been criticized for challenging the sexual autonomy of youths and increasing the difficulty of access to information on safe sexual practices, STI protection contraception, and the prevention of unintended pregnancy. Consider the following sites to prepare your arguments opposing or supporting the bill.

- The Canadian Federation for Sexual Health (CFSH): www.ppfc.ca/ppfc/content.asp?articleid=86

- The Department of Justice Canada: www.justice.gc.ca/en/dept/clp/faq.html

- Library of Parliament—Canada's Legal Age of Consent to Sexual Activity: www.parl.gc.ca/information/library/PRBpubs/prb993-e.htm

REFERENCES

Boonstra, H. (2002). Teen pregnancy: Trends and lessons learned. *The Guttamacher Report, 5*(1), 10–13.

Boyce, R. K. (1999). Parenting processes related to sexual risk-taking behaviours of adolescent males and females. *Journal of Marriage and the Family, 61,* 99–109

Boyce, W., Doherty, M., Fortin, C., & MacKinnon, D. (2003). *Canadian youth, sexual health, and HIV/AIDS study: Factors influencing knowledge, attitudes and behaviours.* Toronto: *Council of Ministers of Education.*

Boyce, W., Doherty-Poirier, M., MacKinnon, D., Fortin, C., Saab, H., King, M., & Gallupe, O. (2006). Sexual health of Canadian youth: Findings from the Canadian youth, sexual health and HIV/AIDS study. *The Canadian Journal of Human Sexuality, 15*(2), 59–68.

Council of Ministers of Education. (2003). *Canadian youth, sexual health and HIV/AIDS Study: Factors influencing knowledge, attitudes and behaviours.* Toronto: Author.

Cohen, D. A., Farley, T. A., Taylor, S. N., & Martin, D. H. (2002). When and where do youths have sex? The potential role of adult supervision. *Pediatrics, 12:110*(6), 66.

Fisher, W., Boroditsky, R., & Morris, B. (2004). The 2002 Canadian contraception study: Part 2. *J Obstet Gynaecol Can. I, 26*(7), 646–656.

Fulkerson, J. A., Story, M., Mellin, A., Leffert, N., Neumark-Sztainer, D., & French, S. (2006). Family dinner meal frequency and adolescent development: Relationships with developmental assets and high-risk behaviours. *Journal of Adolescent Health, 39*(3), 337–345.

Halpern-Felsher, B. L., Cornel, J. L., Kropp, R. Y., & Tschann, J. M. (2005). Oral vs. vaginal sex among adolescents: Perceptions, attitudes and behaviour. *Pediatrics, 115*(4), 845–851.

Herrman, J. W. (2006). The voices of teen mothers: The experience of repeat pregnancy. *MCN American Journal Maternal Child Nursing, 31*(4), 243–249.

Koniak-Griffin, D., Anderson, N. L., Brecht, M. L., & Verzemnieks, I. (2002). *J Adolescent Health, 1*(30), 44–54.

McKay, A. (2004). Adolescent sexual and reproductive health in Canada: A report card in 2004. The Sex Information and Education Council of Canada. *The Canadian Journal of Human Sexuality, 13*(2), 67–81.

MacMillan, H. L. (2000). Preventive health care, 2000 update: Prevention of child maltreatment. Canadian Task Force on Preventive Health Care. *CMAJ 163*(11), 1451–1458.

Peterson, W. E., Sword, W., Charles, C., & DiCenso, A. (2007). Adolescents' perceptions of inpatient postpartum nursing care. *Qual Health Res 17*(2), 201–212.

Public Health Agency of Canada. (2003). *What determines health?* Retrieved on April 21, 2007, from http://www.phac-aspc.gc.ca/phsp/phdd/determinants/index.html#determinants.

Randall, H. E., & Byers, E. S. (2003). What is sex? Students' definitions of having sex, sexual partner, and unfaithful sexual behaviour. *The Canadian Journal of Human Sexuality, 12*(2), 87–96.

Raphael, J. (2006). Teens having babies: The unexplored role of domestic violence. *School Nurse News, 23*(3), 38–24.

Renker, P. R. (2002). Keep a blank face. I need to tell you what has been happening to me. *MCN American Journal Maternal Child Nursing, 27*(2), 109–116.

Rentschler, D. D. (2003). Pregnant adolescents' perspectives of pregnancy. *MCN Am J Maternal Child Nursing, 28*(6), 377–383.

Rhein, L. M., Ginsburg, K. R., Schwarz, D. F., Pinto-Martin, J. A., Zhao, H., Morgan, A. P., et al. (1997). Teen father participation in child rearing: Family perspectives. *J Adolesc Health. 21*(4), 244–252.

Sant'Anna, M. J., Catunda, J. K., Carvalho, K. A., & Coates, V. (2007). Pregnant teenager involvement in sexual activity and the social context. *Scientific World Journal, 25*(6), 998–1007.

Secco, M. L., Profit, S., Kennedy E., Walsh, A., Letourneau, N., & Stewart, M. (2007). Factors affecting postpartum depressive symptoms of adolescent mothers. *J Obstet Gynecol Neonatal Nurs, 36*(1), 47–54.

Seimer, B. S. (2004). Intimate violence in adolescent relationships: Recognizing and intervening. *MCN, 29*(2), 117–121.

Sieverding, J. A., Adler, N., Witt, S., & Ellen, J. (2005). The influence of parental monitoring on adolescent sexual initiation. *Archives of Pediatrics and Adolescent Medicine, 159*(8), 1–10.

Spear, H. J. (2004). A follow-up case study on teenage pregnancy: "Havin' a baby isn't a nightmare, but it's really hard." *Pediatr Nursing, 30*(2), 120–125.

Spitzer, D. L. (2005). Engendering health disparities. *Can J Public Health. 96*(2), S78–96.

Statistics Canada. (2005, December 20). *Canadian Community Health Survey*. Retrieved May 14, 2007, from http://www.statcan.ca/cgi-bin/imdb/p2SV.pl?Function=getSurvey&SDDS=3226&lang=en&db=IMDB&dbg=f&adm=8&dis=2.

Statistics Canada. (2006). *Canada Year Book 2006—Internet use in Canada*. 56F0003XIE, 0-660-19563-1, Ottawa: Author.

Stiles, A. S. (2005). Parenting needs, goals, & strategies of adolescent mothers. *MCN AMJ Maternal Child Nursing, 30*(5), 327–333.

Vanoss Marin, B., Coyle, K. K., Gomez, C.A., Carvajal, S. C., & Kirby, D. B. (2000). Older boyfriends and girlfriends increase risk of sexual initiation in young adolescents. *Journal of Adolescent Health, 27*(6), 409–418.

Valkenburg, P. M., Peter, J., & Schouten, A. P. (2006). Friend networking sites and their relationship to adolescents' well-being and self-esteem. *Cyberpsychol Behav, 9*(5), 584–590.

ADDITIONAL RESOURCES

Website

Teenage Pregnancy Trends in Canada
www.statcan.ca/english/kits/preg1.htm

Readings

Barrett, A. (2004). Oral sex and teenagers: A sexual health educator's perspective. *SIECCAN Newsletter, 39*(1–2), 197–200.

Hampton, M. R., Jeffery, B., McWatters, B., & Smith, P. (2005). Influence of teens' perceptions of parental disapproval and peer behaviour on their initiation of sexual intercourse. *The Canadian Journal of Human Sexuality, 14,* 105–121.

McKay, A. (2004). Sexual health education in the schools: Questions and answers. *The Canadian Journal of Human Sexuality, 13*(3–4), 129–141.

Steenbeek A., Tyndall M., Rothenberg R., & Sheps, S. (2006). Determinants of sexually transmitted infections among Canadian Inuit adolescent populations. *Public Health Nursing, 23,* 531–534.

About the Author

Cynthia Mannion, RN, MSc (A) (McGill University School of Nursing, 1985), PhD (Dietetics and Human Nutrition, McGill University, 2004), is an Assistant Professor in the Faculty of Nursing at the University of Calgary. She practised nursing in Montreal in acute care settings and had a community private practice providing prenatal classes, labour support, and breastfeeding consultation. In 1997 she relocated to Calgary and was employed by the University of Calgary in 2002. Her research interests involve dietary behaviour, nutritional assessment, and dietary intake and outcomes in maternal/child health.

Violence in Families

Margaret M. Malone

OBJECTIVES

After studying this chapter, you should be able to:

1. Analyze critically the concept of "family violence."

2. Connect family violence to health implications for women, children, and seniors.

3. Examine the impact of gender, race, age, class, sexuality, and culture on family violence.

4. Investigate how community health nurses can work to eliminate family violence.

5. Explore critical theories and approaches that inform community health nurses' strategies to raise community awareness about family violence and its health impacts.

6. Develop health-promoting interventions to address family violence in communities.

INTRODUCTION

Family violence is a major social and public health problem of epidemic proportion in Canada with devastating effects for women, children, seniors, and families. The direct and indirect health and "financial costs of such violence are staggering as are the social and human costs that cause untold damage to the economic and social fabric of communities" (World Health Organization [WHO], 2004, p. vii). To date, societal responses have focused primarily on identification, crisis intervention, and services to individuals and families.

Nurses frequently are the first members of the health care team to interface with family members experiencing violence and abuse. Moreover, community health nurses (CHNs) are strategically located within communities where assessment, intervention, and health promoting initiatives can be developed, researched, implemented, and evaluated. In this chapter, we describe theoretical frameworks rooted in social justice—that is, critical social theory and an analysis that studies the intersections of gender, race, class, ethnicity, sexuality, age, ability, and culture. We illustrate how these frameworks can inform strategies for earlier identification of violence occurring in families, raise critical awareness of its health impacts, and guide nurses' prevention, health promoting, and empowering strategies to eliminate violence in society.

A CRITICAL ANALYSIS OF FAMILY VIOLENCE AND HEALTH IMPLICATIONS

Many cling to a family ideal that includes love between members, shared norms and values, happiness, caring and nurturing relationships, and, above all, *safety*. Moreover, we often assume that violent acts occur between strangers, but violence to newborn infants, children, adolescents, women, pregnant women, Aboriginal women, immigrant and refugee women, disabled people, same-sex partners, or seniors does not happen to strangers. It happens in our families, and among our neighbours, friends, co-workers, and clients.

Violence is located within social, historical, cultural, economic, environmental, and political contexts and cuts across gender, social class, race, ability, education level, sexuality, age, ethnicity, culture, religion, and nationality. For example, while sexual assault against men and boys is a significant problem, often underreported and largely neglected in research (WHO, 2002), women are "more likely than men to be the victims of the most severe forms of spousal assault, as well as spousal homicide, sexual assault, and criminal harassment (stalking)" (Statistics Canada, 2006, p. 13). Spousal violence rates for Aboriginal women are more than three times higher than for non-Aboriginal women or men, as are the severity and impacts (Statistics Canada).

The World Health Organization (2004) argues for "prevention of interpersonal violence as a whole rather than focusing on individual sub-types" (p. 3). When developing prevention and health promotion strategies, it is equally important to attend to at-risk populations while focusing on common underlying and cross-cutting risk factors. In the following, we draw attention to at-risk populations and combine individual and community-based assessment, prevention, and health promotion strategies in the work needed to eliminate violence.

Women, Family Violence, and Health

Violence against women includes "any act of gender-based violence that results in, or is likely to result in, physical, sexual, and psychological harm or suffering to a woman, including threats of such acts, coercion, or arbitrary deprivation of liberty, whether occurring in public or private life" (Statistics Canada, 2006, p. 8). It encompasses dowry-related violence;

honour killing; rape, including marital rape; and trafficking. The most common type of violence against women worldwide is *domestic violence*—that is, the physical, emotional, and/or sexual abuse of women by their intimate partners or ex-partners (WHO, 2001, p. 5).

The National Violence Against Women Survey (Statistics Canada, 1994) reported that of the 12 300 women surveyed, 25% of women 16 years of age and older reported they had been abused by an intimate partner and 10% had been assaulted at least once during the previous 12 months. According to Statistics Canada (2004), data from 94 reporting police agencies across Canada indicate that females were the victims in 85% of reported cases of spousal violence. Half of all family homicides involved spouses, with 62% of female homicides committed by male spouses, either current or estranged. This figure is three times the number of men killed by their spouses. The rate of spousal homicide for Aboriginal women was eight times the rate for non-Aboriginal women (Statistics Canada, 2006).

Health Canada (1999a) states, "Ignoring violence as a factor in women's health and well-being not only leads to misdiagnosis and inadequate treatment, it also disregards the full extent of the personal and social consequences of violence" (p. 2). In 1995, it was estimated that violence against women may cost $4.2 billion annually (Statistics Canada, 2006).

Children, Youth, Family Violence, and Health

Child maltreatment refers to "the harm, or risk of harm, that a child or youth may experience while in the care of a person they trust or depend on, including a parent, sibling, other relative, teacher, caregiver or guardian" (National Clearinghouse on Family Violence, 2006, p. 1). Harm may occur through direct actions or neglecting to provide basic human needs: "human nurturance, food, clothing, shelter, necessary health care, and provisions for safety and medical care" (McAllister, 2000, ¶ 8).

Due to underreporting and definitional problems, we still do not know how many children and youth experience abuse and neglect. However, Trocme et al.'s (2005) research reveals the extent of "reported" child abuse and neglect by Canadian child welfare services, excluding Quebec, for children under 16. Of the 103 297 primary "substantiated" child maltreatments in Canada in 2003, neglect was the most common form of child abuse (30%), followed by exposure to domestic violence (28%), physical abuse (24%), emotional maltreatment (15%), and sexual abuse (3%). Girls were often victims of sexual abuse (63%) and emotional maltreatment (54%), and boys were often victims of physical abuse (54%). Furthermore, Onyskiw (2002) notes that "exposure to family violence has an adverse effect on children's health and use of health services" (p. 416) and that "these children generally fared less favourably on several measures of health than children of non-violent families" (p. 419). In 2003, the estimated cost of child abuse to child victims and adults was $15 billion (Statistics Canada, 2006).

Older Adults, Family Violence, and Health

Elder abuse is "the mistreatment of older people by those in a position of trust, power, or responsibility for their care" (Health Canada, 1999b, p. 1). **Elder neglect** involves "the failure of a caregiver to meet the needs of an older adult who is unable to meet those needs alone" (p. 2). Such behaviours as denial of food, water, medication, medical treatment, therapy, nursing services, health aids, clothing, and visitors are included. Caution has been expressed about subsuming elder abuse under "family violence" in case we miss the importance of elder abuse and neglect for the elder population (MacLean & Williams, 1995).

Only a small proportion of elder abuse comes to the attention of the health, social service, and justice systems. Abuse and maltreatment of older adults are least likely to be reported (14 times lower than the rate for 18- to 24-year-olds) because of emotional, physical, or financial dependence on the abuser, because of embarrassment (especially if the abuser is an adult child), or because they fear institutionalization (Statistics Canada, 1998, 2003). The health and social costs of elder abuse have yet to be fully determined.

Aboriginal Peoples, Family Violence, and Health

In 2004, "RCMP detachments in Nunavut reported 498 domestic assaults against women and 58 against men, likely a small percentage of those that occurred. In many communities, violent crime is increasing rather than decreasing" (Pauktuutit Inuit Women of Canada, 2006, p. 2). Women and children are often the victims of violence. Moreover, eight out of every ten Aboriginal women and four out of every ten children have been abused or assaulted (Hare, 1991). Family violence and its effects on Aboriginal peoples has led to disproportionately high health disparities and inequities directly and indirectly associated with or related to social, economic, cultural, and political inequities (Adelson, 2005).

Attitudinal change is vital in removing the barriers faced by First Nations women and children experiencing family violence. The emotional, psychological, physical, and mental health of Aboriginal women, children, and men must be addressed in a culturally safe (McMurray, 2007) and appropriate way. While patriarchal attitudes and gender relations are important considerations, Aboriginal women's experience of violence must also be understood through "the important prisms of racism, colonialism, and classism" (Mandell & Duffy, 2000, p. 308).

Immigrants, Family Violence, and Health

Canada is one of the most culturally diverse countries in the world, yet there is a dearth of specific data addressing differential experiences of family violence by race, ethnicity, class, and culture. Fong's (2000) research with Chinese Canadian women showed that immigrant women "experienced a great deal of pain and hardship due to their isolation, burden of childcare responsibilities, lack of English skills, unfamiliarity with the new environment and new culture, lack of an adequately paid job, and/or financial dependence on their husbands" (p. iv), in addition to an abusive relationship. Yet these same women "employed a wide range of strategies to resist the abuse and protect themselves from different dangerous situations" (p. iv). Drawing on case studies, reports, and interviews, Agnew (1998) captured similar experiences for immigrant women from Asia, Africa, and the Caribbean who have suffered wife abuse.

Immigration and resettlement experiences exert enormous influence on the health of immigrants and refugees (Beiser, 2005; Guruge & Khanlou, 2004) and can be factors related to and/or compounded by experiences of family violence. Consideration of the unique needs of diverse immigration populations while taking into account cultural, linguistic, and systemic barriers to health and healthy behaviours must be taken into account when developing prevention and health promotion strategies related to violence occurring in immigrant and refugee families.

Lesbians and Gays, Family Violence, and Health

Prevalence rates of family violence among lesbian and gay couples (with or without children) have been more difficult to assess; however, "experts estimate rates comparable to heterosexual couples" (Seelau & Seelau, 2005, p. 363). Mandell and Duffy (2000) argue that these occurrences push "feminists to focus on power and control perspectives rather than the interplay of genders" (p. 309). The Society of Obstetricians and Gynecologists of Canada issued an alert to health care workers regarding the need to assess for partner abuse in lesbian relationships while being sensitive to the difficulties in disclosing sexual orientation compounded by revealing experiences of partner abuse (Davis, 2000).

Canadian Research Box 26.1

Jiwani, Y. (2005). Walking a tightrope: The many faces of violence in the lives of racialized immigrant girls and young women. *Violence against Women, 11*(7), 846–875.

In this participatory research, Jiwani reveals a paucity of Canadian studies examining the realities and experiences of girls from immigrant and refugee families who are racialized. Through interviews and/or focus groups, participants who were young women of colour identified racism as the dominant and most pervasive form of violence they encountered in their daily lives. The analysis revealed gendered racism, gendered violence, sexualization, violence between girls of different racial backgrounds, and parental conflict. Racism, as a form of systemic violence, influences and shapes the lives of young women and girls from racialized immigrant communities. Stigmatization of these communities can result in further isolation and marginalization. Fear can become a part of this process, inhibiting women in these communities from disclosing violence.

Discussion Questions:

1. Given that schools are locations where girls and young women spend time, how would you develop a health promotion program to recognize and reduce the impact of racism as a major form of violence? Whom would you involve and how? When and where in the process would you involve them? What issues would you address? What strategies would you use to address them? How would you implement and evaluate these strategies?

2. What safety and ethical issues should be considered in your program?

3. Analyze the relevance of these issues to preventing violence in families and communities.

The health risks, interpersonal stresses, and psychological challenges faced by lesbian and gay youth, especially when compounded by family violence and social discrimination, are outlined by Gochros and Bidwell (1996). They challenge health care workers to develop innovative early intervention programs for lesbian and gay youth while acknowledging the formidable barriers to providing these services.

STRATEGIES TO ELIMINATE FAMILY VIOLENCE

Brown (1991) asserted that "violence in any society persists because there is a role for it, because it serves a purpose. Violence persists . . . because people opposed to it have been addressing its manifestations rather than its root causes" (p. 104). Most researchers, critical theorists, and people working with individuals and populations agree that violence is a social act rooted in issues of power and control. Moreover, woman, child, and elder abuse "occurs within familial relationships because these are sites of power, and locations that permit it to happen" (Neysmith, 1995, p. 48). Definitional problems about what constitutes violence and abuse persist, but this does not preclude acting now to prevent violence and promote health.

THEORETICAL FRAMEWORKS AND APPROACHES

Critical Social Theories

Critical social theories include liberation work against poverty and illiteracy; feminist scholarship on the oppression of women; lesbian and gay liberation studies; and critical perspectives on race and ethnic relations, gender inequalities, and health promotion (Stevens & Hall, 1992). Included are theories of violence against women, children, youth, elders, older lesbians, and men. In defining a violent society, critical theorists analyze the social, economic, and political ways individuals and groups are harmed by social institutions and the state. Research methods that raise critical questions, while examining lived experiences, are integrated with a view toward social justice and social change.

Inclusive Race, Class, and Gender Analytical Frameworks

Understanding the intersections of race, ethnicity, class, gender, abilities, sexualities, culture, age, and religious beliefs expands our capacity to work effectively against violence in families and communities. As CHNs, we must understand the concerns of the marginalized groups and provide culturally safe and sensitive services to those who have experienced violence within their communities. Similarly, when developing health promotion programs related to violence for immigrant women, CHNs must be respectful of the need to maintain culture and tradition while at the same time working for change (Choudhry et al., 2002). Changing our thinking requires not only assessing data, but also examining our own biases, beliefs, and feelings about these issues. The capacity to reflect on our own experiences is a major principle in CHN practice (Community Health Nurses Association of Canada, 2003).

Empowerment and Community Participation Approaches

Empowerment is a dynamic, action-oriented process that focuses on power relations and intervention strategies in creating relationships with greater equity in resources, status, authority, and health. The process of community empowerment can begin at any point along a continuum that includes personal, small group, community organization, partnerships, and social and political action (Laverack, 2004). CHNs can engage community participants in problem identification, planning, development, implementation, and evaluation processes using community-based participatory research. In this process, "power over" becomes "power with" in the personal and collective work to eliminate violence and its associated health disparities in families.

ROLE AND FUNCTION OF THE COMMUNITY HEALTH NURSE

Assessment at the individual level can facilitate critical awareness of the extent of family violence in the community. The process includes addressing the safety of the person in addition to being critically aware of family violence, indicators of abuse and neglect, the importance of asking about abuse, how to ask about abuse, individual risk factors, routine universal comprehensive screening, community resources, prevention

and health promoting strategies, and connecting individual harm with the social, political, economic, and cultural context in which it occurs to make political action possible.

First, *safety of the person* is key. Poorly designed and implemented assessment strategies put women, children, and elders in violent, abusive, or neglectful relationships at substantial risk. The environment must *be safe* and individuals must *feel safe* before they can discuss their experiences. A short-form ABCD-ER Mnemonic Tool may be used as a guide in this process. (See the text box "Short-Form ABCD-ER Mnemonic Tool: Guiding Principles for Screening".)

Short-Form ABCD-ER Mnemonic Tool: Guiding Principles for Screening

A: *Attitude* and *Approachability* of health care professionals

B: *Belief* in the woman's account of her own experience of abuse

C: *Confidentiality* is essential for disclosure

D: *Documentation* that is consistent and legible

E: *Education* about the serious health effects of abuse

R: *Respect* for the integrity and authority of each woman's life choices and *Recognition* that the process of dealing with the identified abuse must be done at her pace, directed by her decisions.

Source: Reproduced with permission from the Middlesex-London Health Unit, London, Ontario, Canada. (2000). Task force on the health effects of women abuse: Final report (p. 34). London, ON: Author. While the information contained in the materials is believed to be accurate and true, no responsibility is assumed by MLHU for its use.

Second, CHNs must become more *critically aware* of family violence and abuse, understanding that it cuts across all ages, races, genders, sexualities, cultures, religions, abilities, classes, and other socially organized structures. The London Battered Women's Advocacy Centre developed a Power and Control Wheel (Figure 26.1) that outlines some of the tactics used by the abuser in woman abuse situations.

Third, CHNs need to know *indicators* of emotional abuse and neglect for children, adults, and elders. Some indicators manifest themselves in health effects. Indicators for both children and adults include depression, withdrawal, low self-esteem, severe anxiety, fearfulness, being overly passive or compliant, sleep disturbances, suicide attempts, and other forms of physical abuse, present or suspected. For children, indicators include failure to thrive in infancy, emotional instability, physical complaints with no medical basis, over- or underachievement, and inability to trust. For adults, indicators also include feelings of shame and guilt, substance abuse, discomfort or nervousness around caregivers or relatives, and social isolation (Health Canada, 1996).

FIGURE 26.1 Battering in Intimate Relationships: "The Power and Control Wheel"

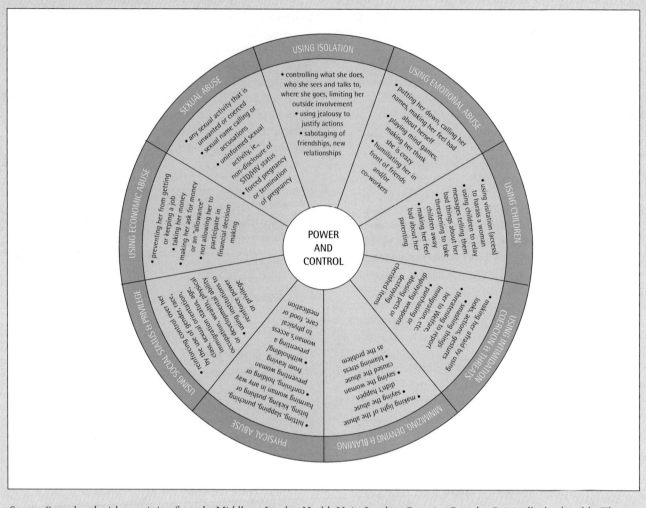

Source: Reproduced with permission from the Middlesex-London Health Unit, London, Ontario, Canada. Originally developed by The Domestic Abuse Intervention Project, Duluth, USA. Further adapted by The London Battered Women's Advocacy Centre.

Fourth, CHNs must understand the importance of *asking about abuse*. Asking increases the chances of preventing further abuse and is an important signal of support. It lets a woman know she is believed, respected, supported, and heard. Moreover, naming the problem raises awareness and makes it public and political. Cultural safety, sensitivity, and linguistic considerations must be built into CHNs' strategies and practice.

Fifth, CHNs need to learn *how* to ask about abuse. Privacy is key. Direct and specific questions are best and should be non-threatening, non-blaming, open-ended, and always preceded by genuinely supportive statements of concern. (See the text box "Screening for Woman Abuse: Developing a Personal Style".)

Sixth, CHNs need to understand *individual risk factors* to intervene in the cycle of violence. The social determinants of health, which include income and social status, employment and working conditions, personal health, coping skills, gender, race, ethnicity, age, sexuality, religion, culture, and social environment, should be considered when assessing risk factors.

Seventh, through *routine universal comprehensive screening*, CHNs can demonstrate connections between individual harm and social context. "Screening means imbedding questions about abuse in a health history or incorporating validated screening instruments into the history and assessment process" (Registered Nurses' Association of Ontario, 2005, p. 15).

- **Universal screening** refers to the characteristics of the group to be screened and occurs when nurses ask every woman over a specified age about her experience of abuse.
- **Routine screening** refers to the frequency with which screening is carried out. Routine screening is performed on a regular basis regardless of whether or not signs of abuse are present.
- **Indicator-based screening** refers to screening whereby nurses observe one or more indicators that suggest a woman may have been abused and subsequently question her about the indicator(s) (RNAO, 2005).

Screening for Woman Abuse: Developing a Personal Style

A screening protocol should be flexible so that it can be altered to fit the context of the particular situation. The process may vary depending on the health care or community setting, the relationship of the CHN to the woman, the presenting problem, the woman's history, and the role of the particular CHN in meeting the woman's health needs.

A few suggestions:

- Ask simple, direct questions.

- Maintain a matter-of-fact tone of voice and relaxed demeanour.

- Be sure your body language, facial expressions, and words all convey the same thing: that you are willing to hear what the woman has to say and are willing to help.

- Emphasize that all women are screened routinely for abuse as part of health care interactions.

- Use the screening process as an opportunity to educate the woman about the prevalence, dynamics, and health effects of abuse.

- Use neutral terms in asking about abuse. (Someone of the same sex may have abused the woman.)

Ways to Ask about Abuse: Some Sample Questions

- We know that abuse and violence in the home affect many women and directly affect their health. I wonder if you ever experience abuse or violence at home?

- Have you ever felt unsafe or threatened in your own home?

Physical Abuse

- The injuries you have suggest to me that someone may have hit you. Did anyone hit you?

Emotional Abuse

- Does anyone close to you call you names, criticize your friends or family, or try to control what you do?

Sexual Abuse

- Have you ever been forced to have sex with your partner when you did not want to?

Sources: Adapted from Health Canada. (1999). A handbook for health and social services professionals responding to abuse during pregnancy (p. 24). Ottawa, ON: Health Canada, Health Promotion and Services Branch. (Cat. No. H72-21/165-1998E); and Middlesex-London Health Unit. (2000). Task force on the health effects of women abuse: Final report (pp. 33–34). London, ON: Author.

The most comprehensive approach is one that combines routine and universal screening for all females 12 years of age and older (RNAO, 2005, p. 23).

Eighth, CHNs must *make appropriate referrals* in their communities to assist abused women, children, seniors, and men. Support services could include:

police; shelters; victim assistance and services (police based, court based, other); sexual assault support; women's centres; child advocacy centres; children's aid services; crisis telephone lines (e.g., kids-help lines, distress lines); medical services and health care centres; counseling services for women, children, Aboriginals, immigrants, and seniors; legal assistance (legal aid, lawyer referral services, other); Aboriginal services; immigrant and refugee services; ethnocultural organizations that address abuse issues; child welfare authorities; programs for men that abuse women and for men that have been abused; self-help clearinghouses and networks; community resources centres; and other related services (Health Canada, 1999c, p. 41).

Ninth, CHNs must work collaboratively to *develop broad-based, comprehensive health promoting strategies* in their communities that include primary, secondary, and tertiary prevention approaches to family violence. These should include ethical, research, and evaluative components. CHNs should also address the diversity of their community by attending to gender, race, class, age, ethnicity, ability, sexuality, language, literacy, and culture.

Tenth, when CHNs *connect individual harm with the social, economic, cultural, and political context*, it makes violence public and political. Here, CHNs can initiate political actions supported by critical theoretical frameworks (Stevens & Hall, 1992). This means:

- *Taking a stand.* CHNs have a responsibility to diverse communities that are vulnerable to the oppressive, health-damaging conditions of violence.

- *Asking critical questions* to demystify oppressive situations. For example, why has a unified effort to eradicate violence in its many forms not occurred? Whose interests are served by violence?

- *Working with communities* to solve health problems. Targeting problems people identify, such as violence and abuse, situates CHNs' efforts in communities' struggles.

- *Acting collectively.* Forming alliances with community members and groups concerned with violence in families creates solidarity and uses collective strength to work for healthy social change. Sustaining these alliances requires an ongoing commitment supported by sufficient funding.

Learning how to do this work takes time, commitment, and a caring presence. To assist in this endeavour, we have listed references, resources, and websites at the end of this chapter. Other resources may be obtained at women's centres, clinics, shelters, and health and social service agencies.

Case Study

Serena, a 30-year-old Mexican Canadian woman, recently gave birth to her first child, a small, healthy baby girl. During her short hospital stay, Serena attended the post-natal classes, including one on breastfeeding. She appeared to be confident in her care of the baby. However, in the presence of her husband during the discharge planning, the nurse noted Serena appeared quite nervous.

You do a follow-up home visit as part of the "Healthy Mother, Healthy Baby" program co-sponsored by the Community Health Department and the hospital. You are welcomed by Serena, who informs you that her husband is out buying groceries. You assess the health of mother and baby and offer support and advice about breastfeeding. You invite Serena to the local "Mothers and Babies Group," but Serena, who seems quite interested, does not think her husband will let her go. She mentions that when the baby cried for a while last evening her husband became angry, telling her to keep the baby quiet because he needed his sleep. Serena appears anxious about her husband's impending return.

Discussion Questions

1. Given her concerns about her husband, what is your first response to Serena?

2. How do you initiate an assessment of her situation?

3. What are your priorities?

Summary

Violence is a social act that involves a serious abuse of power and control. Violence is endemic in our families and our communities, cutting across class, race, age, ethnicity, sexualities, abilities, religions, and national boundaries. Violence is located within historical, economic, cultural, social, environmental, and political contexts. There are connections between what happens in our families and in our society, and between what happens in our society and in our families. In our work to address and eradicate violence, CHNs and our allies must make these connections. Simultaneously, CHNs can work collaboratively to facilitate social changes at the level of individual, family, group, community, and population.

CHNs who guide their practice with critical theories and intersectional frameworks while working with people where they live affirm those who are dealing with experiences of violence in families as active, engaged subjects in their own struggle. Participatory empowering strategies can facilitate this process. "Empowerment influences people's ability to act through collective participation by strengthening their personal and organizational capacities, challenging power inequities, and achieving outcomes on many reciprocal levels in different domains" (Wallerstein, 2006, p. 19), while working collaboratively to eliminate violence in families and communities.

KEY TERMS

family violence
violence against women
child maltreatment
elder abuse
elder neglect
critical social theories
empowerment
universal screening
routine screening
indicator-based screening

INDIVIDUAL CRITICAL THINKING EXERCISES

1. Consider your experiences with people in your practice placements or your community who have experienced violence or abuse. Examine critically your own perspectives, assumptions, and biases, including thinking about where, when, from whom, and/or how you developed these ideas.

2. How is family violence represented in the media? Give two examples. Drawing on the material in this chapter, provide a comparative critical analysis of your examples, addressing the strengths and limitations of each. Include a critical analysis of the implications these media representations have for the community's understanding of family violence, for health and health care, and for CHN theory and practice.

GROUP CRITICAL THINKING EXERCISE

1. You are a nurse in an urban community health centre serving a mixed-income, ethnically/racially diverse community. A number of women have recently disclosed that they have been victims of "family violence." After reading on this topic and talking with other health care providers, you realize that family violence is much more pervasive than you had imagined. You decide to address this issue within the community.

2. You and your colleagues begin to think about strategies to stop family violence. Using critical theories and other CHN frameworks and approaches, develop a health promotion program to address this problem.

REFERENCES

Adelson, N. (2005). The embodiment of inequity: Health disparities in Aboriginal Canada. *Canadian Journal of Public Health, 96*(S2), S45–S61.

Agnew, V. (1998). *In search of a safe place: Abused women and culturally sensitive services.* Toronto: University of Toronto Press.

Beiser, M. (2005). The health of immigrants and refugees in Canada. *Canadian Journal of Public Health, 96*(S2), S30–S44.

Brown, R. (1991). Attack violence at its roots. *Canadian Woman Studies/Les Cahiers de la Femme, 12*(1), 12–15.

Choudhry, U. K., Jandu, S., Mahal, J., Singh, R., Sohi-Pabla, H., & Mutta, B. (2002). Health promotion and participatory action research with South Asian women. *Journal of Nursing Scholarship, 34*(1), 75–81.

Community Health Nurses Association of Canada. (2003). *Canadian community health nursing standards of practice.* Retrieved September 27, 2007, from http://www.communityhealthnursescanada.org.

Davis, V. (2000). Lesbian health guidelines. SOGC clinical practice guidelines. *Journal of the Society of Obstetricians and Gynecologists of Canada, 2*(3), 202–205.

Fong, J. S. (2000). *Silent no more: How women experienced wife abuse in the local Chinese community.* Unpublished doctoral dissertation, York University, Toronto.

Gochros, H., & Bidwell, R. (1996). Lesbian and gay youth in a straight world: Implications for health care workers. *Journal of Gay and Lesbian Social Services, 5*(1), 1–17.

Guruge, S., & Khanlou, N. (2004). Intersectionalities of influence: Researching the health of immigrant and refugee women. *Canadian Journal of Nursing Research, 36*(3), 32–47.

Hare, S. (1991). Breaking free: A proposal for change to Aboriginal family violence. *Canadian Woman Studies/Les Cahiers de la Femme, 11*(4), 79–80.

Health Canada. (1996). *Emotional abuse.* Information from the National Clearinghouse on Family Violence. (Cat. No. 72-22/18-1996E). Retrieved December 21, 2006, from http://www.phac-aspc.gc.ca/ncfv-cnivf/familyviolence/.

Health Canada. (1999a). *Violence against women* (last updated March 28, 2006). Retrieved February 5, 2007 from www.hc-sc.gc.ca/english/women/ facts_issues/ facts_violence.htm

Health Canada. (1999b). *Abuse and neglect of older adults: Information from the National Clearinghouse on Family Violence.* Ottawa: Public Health Agency of Canada. (Cat. No. H72-22/6-1998E).

Health Canada. (1999c). *A handbook for health and social services professional responding to abuse during pregnancy.* Ottawa: Health Canada, The National Clearinghouse on Family Violence. (Cat. No. H72-21/165-1998E).

Laverack, G. (2004). *Health promotion practice: Power & empowerment.* Thousand Oaks, CA: SAGE Publications.

MacLean, M. J., & Williams, R. M. (1995). Introduction. In M. J. MacLean (Ed.), *Abuse & neglect of older Canadians: Strategies for change* (pp. ix–xii). Toronto: Thompson Educational.

Mandell, N., & Duffy, A. (2000). *Canadian families: Diversity, conflict, and change.* Toronto: Harcourt Brace Canada.

McAllister, M. (2000). Domestic violence: A life-span approach to assessment and intervention [Electronic version]. *Lippincott's Primary Care Practice, 4*(2), 174–189.

McMurray, A. (2007). *Community health and wellness: A socio-ecological approach* (3rd ed.). Marrickville, AU: Elsevier Australia.

National Clearinghouse on Family Violence. (2006). *Child maltreatment in Canada: Overview paper.* Prepared by S. Jack et al. Ottawa: Public Health Agency of Canada.

Neysmith, S. M. (1995). Power in relationships of trust: A feminist analysis of elder abuse. In M. J. MacLean (Ed.), *Abuse and neglect of older Canadians: Strategies for change* (pp. 43–54). Toronto: Thompson Educational.

Onyskiw, J. E. (2002). Health and the use of health services of children exposed to violence in their families. *Canadian Journal of Public Health, 93*(6), 416–420.

Pauktuutit Inuit Women of Canada. (2006). *National strategy to prevent abuse in Inuit communities and sharing knowledge, sharing wisdom: A guide to the national strategy.* Ottawa: Author.

Registered Nurses' Association of Ontario. (2005). *Woman abuse: Screening, identification and initial response.* Toronto: Author.

Seelau, S. M., & Seelau, E. P. (2005). Gender-role stereotypes and perceptions of heterosexual, gay and lesbian domestic violence. *Journal of Family Violence, 20*(6), 363–371.

Statistics Canada. (1994). *Violence against women survey.* Ottawa: Author. (Cat. No. 11-001E).

Statistics Canada. (1998). *Family violence in Canada: A statistical profile, 1998.* Ottawa: Author. (Cat. No. 85-224-XPB).

Statistics Canada. (2003). *Family violence in Canada: A statistical profile, 2003.* Ottawa: Author. (Cat. No. 85-224-XIE).

Statistics Canada. (2004). *Family violence in Canada: A statistical profile, 2004.* Ottawa: Canadian Centre for Justice Statistics.

Statistics Canada. (2006). Measuring violence against women: Statistical trends 2006. Ottawa: Author. (Cat. No. 85-570-X1E).

Stevens, P., & Hall, J. (1992). Applying critical theories to nursing in communities. *Public Health Nursing, 9*(1), 2–9.

Trocme, N., Fallon, B., MacLaurin, B., Daciuk, J. Felstiner, C., Black, T., et al. (2005). *Canadian incidence study of reported child abuse and neglect—2003: Major findings.* Ottawa: Minister of Public Works and Government Services Canada. Cat. No. HP5-1/2005E.

Wallerstein, N. (2006). *What is the evidence of empowerment to improve health?* Copenhagen: WHO Regional Office for Europe (Health Evidence Network Report). Retrieved September 5, 2006, from http://www.who.dk/Document/E88086.pdf.

World Health Organization. (2001). *Putting women first: Ethical and safety recommendations for research on domestic violence against women.* Geneva, Switzerland: WHO, Department of Gender and Women's Health, Family and Community Health.

World Health Organization. (2002). *World report on violence and health.* Geneva: Switzerland: Author.

World Health Organization. (2004). *Preventing violence: A guide to implementing the recommendation of the world report on violence and health.* Geneva, Switzerland: Author.

ADDITIONAL RESOURCES

Websites

Assaulted Women's Help Line
  www.awhl.org
Boost–Child Abuse Prevention & Intervention
  www.boostforkids.org

Metropolitan Action Committee on Violence against Women and Children (METRAC)

www.metrac.org

National Clearinghouse on Family Violence

www.phac-aspc.gc.ca/ncfv-cnivf/familyviolence/

World Health Organization—Prevention of Violence

www.who.int/violence_injury_prevention/violence/en/

www.who.int/violence_injury_prevention/violence/ global_campaign/en/index.html

www.who.int/violence_injury_prevention/violence/ activities/child_maltreatment/en/index.html

Readings

Davila, Y. R. (2005). Teaching nursing students to assess and intervene for domestic violence. *International Journal of Nursing Education Scholarship, 2*(1), 1–11.

Jaffe, P. G., Baker, L. L., & Cunningham, A. J. (Eds.). (2004). *Protecting children from domestic violence: Strategies for community intervention.* New York: The Guilford Press.

Sev'er, A. (2002). *Fleeing the house of horrors: Women who have left abusive partners.* Toronto: University of Toronto Press.

World Health Organization and the International Society for the Prevention of Child Abuse and Neglect. (2006). *Preventing child maltreatment: A guide to taking action and generating evidence.* Geneva, Switzerland: WHO. (Available at http://whqlibdoc.who.int/publications/2006/ 9241594365_eng.pdf).

About the Author

Margaret M. Malone, RN, PhD, is an Associate Professor, School of Nursing, Ryerson University. A nurse sociologist, Margaret has taught sociology and women's studies at the University of Toronto, Trent University, and Wilfrid Laurier University. Currently, she teaches community, population, and global health, with an emphasis on diversity and health promotion, in the post-diploma undergraduate and graduate programs. Her research addresses health promotion, community development, violence against women and children, marital separation, divorce, and an emerging social theory of gender, emotions, and knowledge. Academic awards include a Ruth Wynn Woodward Postdoctoral Fellowship in Women's Studies, Simon Fraser University, and a Donner/Bajnok Merit Award. As Co–Principal Investigator, in 2006 she was awarded a grant to develop a Nursing Centre for Research and Education on Violence against Women and Children.

Poverty, Hunger, and Homelessness

Cathy Crowe

OBJECTIVES

After studying this chapter, you should be able to:

1. Describe the context and social policy origins of poverty, hunger, and homelessness in Canada.

2. Analyze and discuss the issues and impact of poverty, hunger, and homelessness on the health of individuals, families, and communities.

3. Describe the role of the nurse and nursing organizations in anti-poverty from a social justice perspective.

INTRODUCTION

Poverty is entrenched in every Canadian community and it is now widely accepted that low income leads to poor health, reduced ability to sustain health, and an earlier death. *Hunger,* perhaps the most vicious outcome of poverty, leaves children without the energy to focus in school or even play, and adults to succumb to numerous ailments, frustration, and despair. *Homelessness,* a direct result of government policies that have dehoused people, has now been declared a national disaster by hundreds of organizations, including the Big City Mayors' Caucus of the Federation of Canadian Municipalities (National Housing and Homelessness Network [NHHN], 2004). This chapter will discuss the issues of poverty, hunger, and homelessness and provide practical means to involve community health nurses in solutions, both at an individual and systemic or policy level.

POVERTY

Poverty is a human rights violation. It is not exclusive to developing countries; in fact, poverty may be the most pressing social justice issue that impacts negatively on the health of people in Canada, whether it is a First Nations community without access to safe drinking water and proper housing; a senior living alone on a pension with $80 left per month after rent, "surviving" on canned salmon and toast; a mother unable to afford to send her child on a school trip; or a new immigrant working the night shift and feeding his family of five on minimum wage. **Poverty** can be defined as the lack of food, clothing, and shelter plus other necessities "required to maintain long-term physical well being" (Sarlo, 1996, p. 25). Poverty is often at the root of poor health, a higher incidence of disease, a shortened life expectancy, extreme isolation, and social exclusion. Poverty is both a cause and product of social exclusion, affecting Aboriginal people, immigrants and refugees, racial-

ized groups, people with disabilities, single parents, children and youth in disadvantaged circumstances, lesbians, gays, bisexuals, and transgendered people. **Social exclusion** refers to the various types of structures and practices—legal, economic, social—that through their processes and results support inequality, barriers, and stigma (Galabuzi, 2004).

The United Nations' *International Covenant on Economic, Social and Cultural Rights* states that every person has the right to an adequate standard of living, including the right to be free from hunger, to have a job, be paid fair wages, and to get an education (Office of the United Nations High Commissioner for Human Rights, 1966). Every five years, governments are required to report on how they are implementing the Covenant to the Committee on Economic, Social and Cultural Rights (CESCR), which has been set up by the United Nations to monitor how governments are meeting their international commitments. Although Canada is a party to the Covenant, which requires countries to turn these rights into realities, the United Nations Committee's reviews of Canada have repeatedly demonstrated systematic government policy decisions and policy omissions that have led to a worsening poverty rate, racialization of poverty, hunger, and homelessness. The Committee's 1998 report (CESCR, 1998) addressed the variety of ways that Canada's economic and social safety net has been dismantled. (See the text box "CESCR 1998 Review of Canada: Selected Articles".) The 2006 report (CESCR, 2006) is even clearer, noting that almost none of their 1993 or 1998 recommendations were implemented. They noted the absence of a Canadian official poverty line; insufficient minimum wages and social assistance rates to ensure an adequate standard of living; high poverty rates among disadvantaged and marginalized individuals and groups such as African Canadians and persons with disabilities; and ongoing homelessness and food insecurity. They made numerous specific recommendations such as the need to include domestic violence as a specific offence in the Criminal Code.

CESCR 1998 Review of Canada: Selected Articles

17. The Committee is greatly concerned at the gross disparity between Aboriginal people and the majority of Canadians with respect to the enjoyment of Covenant rights. . . . In particular, the Committee is deeply concerned at the shortage of adequate housing, the endemic mass unemployment and the high rate of suicide, especially among youth in the

→

Aboriginal communities ... (and) the failure to provide safe and adequate drinking water to Aboriginal communities on reserves.

24. The Committee is gravely concerned that such a wealthy country as Canada has allowed the problem of homelessness and inadequate housing to grow to such proportions that the mayors of Canada's ten largest cities have now declared homelessness a national disaster.

27. The Committee expresses its grave concern at learning that the Government of Ontario proceeded with its announced 21.6% cuts to social assistance in spite of claims that it would force large numbers of people from their homes.

28. The Committee is concerned that the significant reductions in provincial social assistance programs, the unavailability of affordable and appropriate housing and widespread discrimination with respect to housing create obstacles to women escaping domestic violence.

30. The Committee notes with concern that at least six provinces in Canada (including Quebec and Ontario) have adopted "workfare" programs that either submit the right to social assistance to compulsory employment schemes or reduce the benefit of social assistance when recipients, who are usually young, assert their right to choose freely what type of work they wish to do. In many cases, these programs constitute work without the protection of fundamental labour rights and labour standards legislation.

33. The Committee is perturbed to hear that the number of food banks has almost doubled between 1989 and 1997 in Canada and are able to meet only a fraction of the increased needs of the poor.

35. The Committee is concerned at the crisis level of homelessness among youth and young families. According to information received from the National Council of Welfare, over 90% of single mothers under 25 live in poverty. Unemployment and underemployment rates are also significantly higher among youth than among the general population.

36. The Committee is also concerned about significant cuts to services on which people with disabilities rely, such as cuts to home care, attendant care, special needs transportation systems and tightened eligibility rules for people with disabilities. Programs for people who have been discharged from psychiatric institutions appear to be entirely inadequate, (and) . . . a large number of those patients end up on the street, while others suffer from inadequate housing with insufficient support services.

Source: Office of the High Commissioner for Human Rights.

In addition, the United Nations' (1948) Declaration of Universal Human Rights, Article 25, signed by Canada in 1948 states:

> Everyone has the right to a standard of living adequate for the health and well-being of himself [*sic*]) and of his [*sic*] family, including food, clothing, housing, and medical care and necessary social services, and the right to security in the event of unemployment, sickness, disability, widowhood, old age or other lack of livelihood in circumstances beyond his [*sic*] control. (p. 7)

Many of Canada's social programs and labour practices had their origins after the Depression and World Wars I and II, where large numbers of people collectively organized and campaigned for improved public policies. For example, workers involved in the Winnipeg General Strike in 1919 organized for an eight-hour day and a living wage, the mothers' pension movement that sought a guaranteed income for widows after the war, unemployment benefits, and pensions that were introduced after WWII (Swanson, 2001). Medicare, the Canada Assistance Plan, the Employment Insurance Act, and the Canada Pension, have all been popular programs introduced in the latter half of the twentieth century.

Yet the past three decades have seen both an erosion and demolition of these valuable social programs, and poverty, hunger, and homelessness are widely seen to be a direct result of these actions. It is evident that when a movement or campaign for social programs becomes part of our cultural and popular history, people are more likely to embrace it and fight to keep it. For example, most Canadians are familiar with the origins of our national health care program and believe it should not be allowed to be diminished or privatized. Less widely known are the origins of Canada's national housing program, which resulted from World War II veterans and their families who, facing a housing shortage, protested in cities such as Ottawa, Montreal, and Vancouver by literally taking over empty army barracks to demand housing. This led to the National Housing Act and the Canada Mortgage and Housing Corporation. This lapse in our collective history may explain the almost virtual silence across the country when the national housing program was cancelled by the federal government in 1993.

The economic recessions in the 1980s and 1990s coincided with cuts to social spending by federal, provincial, and territorial governments. Not only did governments cut transfers to provinces for social programs, but they also cut taxes, benefiting high income earners the most.

In 1996, the federal government eliminated the Canada Assistance Plan and drastically reduced the unemployment insurance program. This led to an overall decline in government income-support programs such as welfare.

The combination of reduced government spending and increased tax cuts has led to a growing income gap between rich and poor (Yalnizyan, 2000). For example, the poorest 10% of young families earned less than $11 567 in 1989, but by 1997 the number earning less than $11 567 swelled to 14% of the population of households raising children, and the poorest 10% earned less than $6591 in 1997. Not only are there more families in the lowest income category, they are poorer. Meanwhile, the richest 10% of families had an average income of $144 699 in 1989. The National Council of Welfare (2006a, 2006b) released Welfare Incomes 2005 and Poverty Profile 2002 and 2003. They reported 4.8 million Canadians living below the poverty line, with poverty rates growing among children (17.6%), senior women (19.1%), and female lone parents (48.9%), and high poverty rates for recent immigrants, visible minorities, Aboriginal peoples, and peoples with disabilities. (See the text box "Poverty Facts.")

Poverty Facts

- Number of people living in poverty in Canada: 4.9 million
- Family type with highest poverty rate: Single-parent mothers (48.9%)
- Number of children living in poverty: 1.2 million, or 17.6%
- One in ten people using a food bank reported that their primary source of income is paid employment
- Seniors living in poverty received about 90% of their incomes from government programs such as Canada and Quebec Pension Plans, Old Age Security, and the Guaranteed Income Supplement
- Increase in after-tax incomes since 1980: By the richest 20% of family units +14.4%; by the poorest 20% of family units +4.3%
- Canada's gross domestic product in 2003: $1.2 trillion

Source: National Council of Welfare. (2006a). Adapted from Poverty Facts 2003. *Retrieved October 2, 2007, from* http://www.ncwcnbes.net/documents/researchpublications/Research Projects/PovertyProfile/2002-03Report_Summer2006/Fact Sheets/PovertyFacts2003.pdf.

Other factors, including the influences of free trade, have meant that the current economy for workers includes an increase in precarious forms of employment, with more temporary jobs and more part-time, contract, and seasonal employment. This means fewer workers are able to obtain jobs that provide enough hours, pay, and benefits to make ends meet. A federal government withdrawal from social programs, a shift to privatization, and government budgets that emphasize tax cuts have all led to public policy choices that have contributed to the worsening state of poverty in the country.

In 1989, the House of Commons pledged to eliminate child poverty by the year 2000. Hundreds of studies have now demonstrated that the material and social deprivation associated with poverty is a primary cause of poor health in Canadians. For children, that means higher infant mortality, an increase in low birth weights, poor functional health (such as vision, hearing, and mobility), a higher incidence of asthma and chronic disease such as type II diabetes, more deaths from injury, cognitive impairment, and learning disabilities (Raphael, 2007).

Despite widespread public awareness and sympathy for child poverty and the particular vulnerabilities of small bodies and minds to poverty, poverty reduction has not been a primary goal of senior levels of government in Canada. Child poverty remains inextricably linked to women's poverty and poverty overall (Figure 27.1).

HUNGER

Hunger is the symptom of food insecurity. **Food insecurity** has been broadly defined in academic circles as the limited, inadequate, or insecure access of individuals and households to sufficient, safe, nutritious, personally acceptable food to meet their dietary requirements for a healthy and productive life (Tarasuk, 2003). Hunger or food insecurity is probably one of the most obvious and immediate results of poverty. The causes of poverty are the same as the causes of hunger. Although the most widely used measures of poverty are Statistics Canada's *low-income cut-offs,* or LICOS (an income threshold formula used to define poverty), there is not one province or territory with minimum wage rates or welfare rates above the LICO (Canadian Association of Food Banks [CAFB], 2005). For example, the income of a single mother with two children who is working 40 hours a week at minimum wage is at less than 50% of Statistics Canada's low-income cut-off. In real dollars she earns $15 000 a year but requires $31 000 to meet the basic needs of her family and to be above the poverty line (CAFB 2005, p. 20).

Food Banks originated in the early 1980s in Canada and are now institutions across the country. The statistics are staggering. According to a survey by the CAF Banks, HungerCount 2005, 823 856 people used a food bank in one month in 2005. Food bank use has become one marker of food insecurity. Other markers include the growing number of people who rely on drop-in centres, food programs such as "soup kitchens," and even panhandling for access to food.

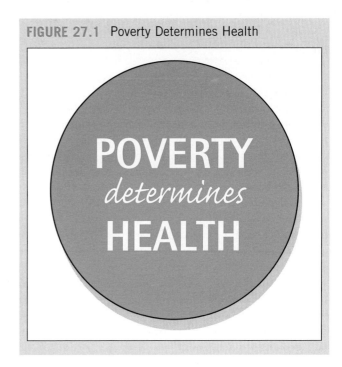

FIGURE 27.1   Poverty Determines Health

Historically, child poverty and child hunger have been the focus of campaigns to end hunger. However, they have tended to ignore that if children are hungry, so too are the families they are part of. Researchers have now demonstrated that low-income single mothers compromise their own food intake to provide their children with adequate nutrition. The women failed to meet caloric and many essential nutrient intake requirements, such as folate, vitamin C, vitamin A, iron, zinc, and calcium (McIntyre et al., 2003). In addition, homeless adults and people living on inadequate incomes experience hunger. In the late 1990s, street nurses began to notice signs of malnutrition, weight loss, and the prevalence of hunger in their clients, issues that had not been prevalent before. They also began to speak out. During that period, food assistance programs in community centres or drop-in centres began to face funding challenges and cuts, exacerbating food shortages.

In Ontario, where social assistance rates were cut by 21.6% in 1995, a province-wide campaign to raise the social assistance rates by 40% and the minimum wage to $10 per hour highlights the obvious—increased rates means money for food on the table and the ability to pay rent. Toronto nurse Kathy Hardill believes that one of the most useful things she can do as a nurse is to assist someone who is homeless to obtain a higher income level so they can afford to eat and find a place to live (K. Hardill, personal communication, July 5, 2005). In Ontario, that means assisting someone with the complicated assessment and forms required to obtain Ontario Disability Support if he or she can qualify. Working with a local anti-poverty group, the Ontario Coalition Against Poverty, Hardill helped to organize a group of like-minded professionals called Health Care Providers Against Poverty. They proceeded to operate "special diet clinics" to assist low-income people who were on social assistance to receive a not widely known special diet benefit of up to $250 per month per person. This project successfully put millions of dollars into the hands of poor Ontarians who could then put food on the table for their families. In October 2005, 1000 people were assisted in a special diet clinic held on the grounds of the Ontario legislature building.

HOMELESSNESS

The word homelessness has many definitions, meanings, and stereotypes attached to it. In Canada, **homelessness** is widely recognized to include those who are living outdoors—for example, on sidewalks, on grates, in parks, in ravines—and in emergency hostels or Violence Against Women shelters. However, *homelessness* also encompasses people who are precariously housed—for example, families who are doubled up with other families, sharing crowded living space, and people who are living in inadequate housing, such as without access to potable water or full bathroom facilities, or housing that is in severe state of disrepair. It also includes those in "core housing need," i.e., people who are paying more than 30% of their income on rent. Historically, the absence of a comprehensive definition of homelessness has led to avoidance of the necessary solutions (Layton, 2000).

Canadian Research Box 27.1

Kerr, M., Frost, D., & Bignell, D. (2004). *Don't we count as people?* Saskatchewan Social Welfare Policy and Women's Health. Saskatchewan: Prairie Women's Health Centre of Excellence.

This participatory action research project examined social assistance policies in Manitoba and Saskatchewan and their impact on women's health. In 2003, seven focus groups were held with women from urban, rural, and Aboriginal communities. The participating women were all living on social assistance. The qualitative research provided a voice for women who described the daily reality of their lives and the impact of social assistance policies on their physical and emotional health. They reported health problems that were made worse by inadequate nourishment, cold and damp suites, and the many stresses of living in poverty. The women described how the low level of welfare benefits prevented them from meeting their fundamental needs, including food/special diet, safe and affordable housing, transportation, health care, and medications. One woman had to put her ill son back into foster care because she did not have enough money for food; women routinely diverted food money for rent payments; women were forced to live in cheap housing where mice and rat infestations were the norm; mothers were unable to afford the costs of personal hygiene supplies for their daughters; and they felt the shame of having to rely on charity. School disruptions due to frequent moves as a result of eviction, family breakdown, and addictions are some of the stress-producing situations they often encountered. The report concluded with recommendations for the provincial Minister Responsible for Welfare Policies in Saskatchewan, such as the notion that decision makers be challenged to live on a welfare income in order to fully understand the implication of existing policies.

Discussion Questions:

You are asked to replicate this study to examine the impact of provincial social assistance policies on women in your community.

1. How would you go about planning the research, and who would you involve as key partners?

2. How would you include the voices of low-income women?

3. How would you disseminate your report?

Homelessness, more visible in Canada during the 1980s, reached new and dangerous levels in the mid 1990s. This social phenomenon is widely seen as a direct result of the federal government's cancellation of its national housing program in 1993 and by a similar pattern of cuts by most provinces to their housing programs. As a result, in large cities like Toronto, Vancouver, and Calgary, homelessness grew out of control. Not only were shelters and drop-in centres overflowing, but also visible numbers of people were now evident on the street and eventually in outdoor encampments and squats such as the famous Tent City in Toronto. Around this time, a new specialty was emerging called *street nursing*, the term having been coined by a homeless man at the corner of Sherbourne and Dundas streets in downtown Toronto.

It was initially these nurses, along with workers in drop-ins and shelters, who began to see the following: worsening physical and mental health, hunger, the return of tuberculosis, infections that quickly spread through crowded sleeping places such as shelters and church basements, and large numbers of people at threat of heat injury requiring rehydration efforts in the summer or winter injuries such as frostbite or steam burns from sleeping on hot air grates. They also observed that there were numerous funerals of homeless people in the community and eventually clusters of deaths began to occur—one of the most famous being the three 1996 "freezing deaths" in Toronto that led to an inquest and national media coverage on homelessness.

One of the earliest pieces of research on homelessness in Canada, the 1992 *Street Health Report,* was praised by the World Health Organization as sound, community-based nursing research. The report identified the poor health status of homeless people, the barriers to health, and the policy solutions (Ambrosio, Baker, Crowe, & Hardill, 1992). In 2005, Street Health produced an updated *Research Bulletin* that once again demonstrated the poor health and systemic barriers. The research highlighted that more than half of homeless people have a serious health condition such as cardiovascular or respiratory disease, hepatitis, diabetes, anemia, epilepsy, cancer, or HIV/AIDS; 33% of these people did not have a usual source of health care or used an emergency department as their usual source of care; and 49% of people in the study with serious health conditions did not receive any kind of government income benefits (Street Health, 2005).

These observations by frontline workers and nurses (including this author) ultimately led to the formation of the Toronto Disaster Relief Committee in 1998 and the declaration that homelessness qualified as a social welfare disaster (Toronto Disaster Relief Committee, 1998).

Homelessness, once prominent only in large cities, is now an emergency in almost every Canadian community, both urban and rural. Most communities report the same problem: a growing number of homeless families, a shortage of shelter space, concern about disease outbreaks and an increasing death rate among the homeless, and long waiting lists ranging from 2 to 12 years for affordable housing. In fact, the National Housing and Homelessness Network reports that 1.7 million Canadians are suffering from the nation-wide affordable housing crisis and homeless disaster across the country (NHHN, 2005). At least 250 000 people are estimated to be homeless during the year, 60 000 of whom are youth and 10 000 are children (Gulliver & Driemeyer, 2006). Housing advocacy groups across the country continue to work to convince the federal government to reintroduce a national housing program by calling for the "One Percent Solution." In the early 1990s, federal, provincial, and territorial and municipal governments spent about 1% of their overall budgets on housing, prior to cancelling any new spending on affordable housing. The One Percent Solution would require the federal government to spend an additional $2 billion annually. Provinces and territories would be required to match that amount (Shapcott, 2004).

WORKING WITH THE POOR

Historically, nurses have both cared for those living in poverty "downstream" and attempted to alleviate the causes of the poverty "upstream." (See Chapter 6.) In medieval times, members of religious and secular nursing orders cared for those who were shunned or discriminated against: lepers, orphaned children, and the poor. Today, poverty may be less obvious, but it is just as persistent. Nurses, no matter where they are working, cannot assume the people they are caring for have adequate shelter, enough food, a well-paying job, or benefits. They may not have the financial means to carry on health care treatments at home, to buy required medications, to follow the ideal diabetic diet, or to return to clinic by public transportation for their next appointment. Nurses can ensure that program and funding commitments take into account the special needs of impoverished populations.

Canadian nursing history is rich with examples of nurses working in and against horrific conditions of poverty. Public health nurses working in inner-city and rural communities, Victorian Order of Nurses and St. Elizabeth nurses providing home visiting, district nurses relying on horses to get to rural communities in the West, outpost nurses working in northern First Nations communities, nurses specializing in tuberculosis, and the most recent nursing specialty of street nursing—nurses providing health care for people who are homeless and under-housed through outreach to drop-ins, shelters, and the street.

In many situations, advocacy is inherent in the work of nurses working in the community. In the 1960s, Peggy Ann Walpole was a young nurse working in the emergency department of Toronto's St. Michael's Hospital when she asked herself where all the homeless women spent their time after they left the ER. She knew these were women with addictions, women who had been abused, had mental health problems, or were in trouble with the law. She rented an unused beverage room in an old hotel in the downtown core, eventually relocating it to a larger space on Yonge Street and then to its current location on Pembroke. It's called Street Haven, and it is a model that includes a continuum of care: an outreach program, a drop-in, a short-term hostel, and supportive housing. Walpole was widely known and respected in the early years of the expansion of homeless services in Toronto (Street Haven, n.d.).

A more recent example is the work of street nurses who have continued to point out that homelessness in Canada constitutes a national disaster and insist that the single and foremost solution—rather than their nursing interventions—is the reintroduction of Canada's national housing program, which was cancelled in 1993. Yet, despite strong grassroots nursing involvement in the issues of poverty, hunger, and homelessness, professional nursing associations have begun to address the issue more systematically only recently. The

Association of Registered Nurses of Alberta, in its 2005 Position Statement on Vulnerability, refers to the Canadian Nurses Association Code of Ethics for Registered Nurses: "Nurses should be aware of broader health concerns such as environmental pollution, violations of human rights, world hunger, homelessness, violence, etc. and are encouraged to the extent possible in their personal circumstances to work individually as citizens or collectively for policies and procedures to bring about social change, keeping in mind the needs of future generations" (College & Association of Registered Nurses of Alberta, 2005, p. 6).

The specific issues of poverty, homelessness, and hunger are now fully integrated into the work of the Registered Nurses' Association of Ontario (RNAO). They are incorporated into all aspects of political advocacy through the speeches and actions of the RNAO leadership, through involvement of members in regular "action alerts," and through hands-on support of grassroots initiatives such as the special diet campaign work of Ontario's street nurses. Most promising is the initiative of the Canadian Nursing Student Association, which has highlighted the need to respond to the crisis of homelessness and the lack of affordable housing both in its national conferences and through position papers (Canadian Nursing Students' Association, 2006).

SOCIAL ACTION

Social action refers to organized activities that seek to improve human welfare and deepen community involvement in social change. In a healthy community, social action promotes the values of social justice and human rights and ensures that no one is left behind, living in poverty, facing hunger, living homeless. *Individual and systemic advocacy* are the tools and the means for social action. They are the upstream efforts that can make the long-term difference. Nurses both as individuals and as part of organized movements can be part of social change.

Christine's Story

Christine Cherniski is an activist in Thunder Bay. The following is an excerpt from a speech she gave to a housing conference in May 2006.

I've been asked to talk about not having enough to get by. I always wonder how to express what it's like to go without most of the key components that make life life. I've imagined having the things our family needed, cutting vegetables in the bright afternoon sun; my daughter doing homework; not complaining of a hunger headache; with the tools, education, resources, support, and nutrition to meet what is meant for her to do. No one's ambition is an empty cupboard, but this is where many hungry kids end up. The need for food assistance is happening at a rate not seen since the Great Depression.

I think of low wage workers barely getting by for every bit as hard a day's work, countless women abused and raped to keep their kids from cold Canadian winters...and the time I've spent there myself. I think of children kept home because there is no lunch to send to school when Health Canada says poverty is worse for them than *smoking*. If our children are hungry their parents are even more so. It is not acceptable for part of our population to suffer.

Poverty is a lack of access to our world, culture, resources and fun. It means isolation and doing without most of what we need to exist. It means complete instability and causes developmental risks to health, behaviour, socialization and learning. It causes sleep disturbance, mental illness, exacerbated health conditions, obesity, a shorter life and more; and all costing hateful tax payers increasing animosity toward me.

Always being without is degrading and demoralizing. How many people are without their honoured place in our world? The Declaration of Human Rights says we are all entitled—*every one*—to food, shelter, clothing and dignity. Martin Luther King Jr. said that a time comes when silence is betrayal; that we are called to speak for the weak, voiceless...of our nation. These are basic human needs, and they should not be able to be taken away.

There is never-ending cash for social workers, services providers, and high-paid legal and medical professionals pacifying poverty and political salaries to entrench it. What we need are better social assistance rates and a minimum wage adequate to support well-being and honest, respectful delivery of service. I think if many caring service providers have a chance to help, they do. We have to untie their hands so they can act with us against these abuses.

We need to facilitate low-income people to speak out and show them their opinions make a difference, even if spoken haltingly or between work and childrearing, and they need to be protected when they do. There is room for everyone to be prosperous, and the money in government is there to make it happen. We can eradicate homelessness and wipe out poverty in our country. We just need your help to do it. Margaret Mead said, "Never doubt that a small group of thoughtful citizens can change the world. Indeed, it's the only thing that ever has."

Source: Christine Cherniski, Activist

Case Study

You are doing a postnatal visit to a family that is new to Canada. They are living in a dark, illegal basement apartment and sharing the space with an adult relative. Dad was an engineer in his home country but the family is currently on social assistance, and he is forced to look for work. Only he speaks English. Mom is breastfeeding, but you notice cans of formula on the kitchen counter. Their phone has recently been disconnected. Their biggest concern today is that they have had to throw out their mattress because of bedbugs. Baby girl is two weeks old.

Discussion Questions

1. How would you assess this family's needs and in what priority?

2. How would you support this family in the next few weeks?

Summary

This chapter has addressed the issues and impact of poverty, hunger, and homelessness on the health of individuals, families, and communities. The idea that it is wrong to discriminate against someone based on the colour of their skin is now common sense, but it was a fight that took well over 300 years and that fight continues. The idea that it is wrong to discriminate against women is also common sense, but that fight took well over 100 years and that fight continues. The processes of social and economic exclusion in Canada, which leave hundreds of thousands of people relegated to poverty, hunger, and homelessness, are equally discriminatory and wrong. Nurses are trusted and well positioned in the community to be part of the strategies to build a healthier community that has less poverty, hunger, and homelessness.

KEY TERMS

poverty
social exclusion
hunger
food insecurity
homelessness
social action

INDIVIDUAL CRITICAL THINKING EXERCISES

1. Discuss the impact of homelessness on health.

2. As a CHN, discuss some of the ways you would approach helping someone with a health problem who is sleeping in a shelter or outdoors.

3. Consider some of the systemic and attitudinal barriers that homeless people face within the health care system. Taking into account the principles of primary health care and human rights, what are some of the changes that could take place to improve access and health care for homeless people? How could nurses make those changes happen?

GROUP CRITICAL THINKING EXERCISES

1. Recent extreme heat waves in the summer have led to growing public health concern regarding the elderly, people with chronic and debilitating health conditions, and people living in poverty and in inadequate housing

such as rooming houses. Existing public health measures seem to rely on public service announcements that encourage the public to drink lots of fluid and go to air-conditioned spaces such as libraries. Provide a critique of these measures and consider possible solutions and advocacy measures.

2. October 17 is the day the United Nations identifies as the International Year to Eradicate Poverty. You have been asked to lead a delegation on a tour of the poverty "hotspots" in your community. Whom would you pick to be in your delegation? Where would you take them? What information would you provide? And how would you present it at each stop on the tour?

REFERENCES

Ambrosio, A., Baker, D., Crowe, C., & Hardill, K. (1992). *The Street Health report. A study of the health status and barriers to health care of homeless women and men in the City of Toronto.* Toronto: Street Health. Retrieved September 30, 2007, from http://tdrc.net/index.php?page=resources.

Canadian Association of Food Banks. (2005). *Time for action. Hunger count 2005.* Retrieved August 10, 2006, from http://www.cafb-acba.ca.

Canadian Nursing Students Association. (2006). *Position statement: Health and homelessness.* Retrieved August 8, 2006, from http://www.cnsa.ca/publications/archives/2006-01Position Statements.pdf.

College & Association of Registered Nurses of Alberta. (2005). *Position statement on vulnerability.* (2005). Retrieved August 10, 2006, from http://www.nurses.ab.ca/pdf/Vulnerability.pdf.

Committee on Economic, Social and Cultural Rights. (1998, December). *Concluding observations of the committee on economic, social and cultural rights: Canada* (10/12/98. E/C.12/1/Add.31.). Retrieved November 3, 2006, from http://www.unhchr.ch/tbs/doc.nsf/(Symbol)/E.C.12.1.Add.31.En?OpenDocument.

Committee on Economic, Social and Cultural Rights. (2006, May). *Consideration of reports submitted by state parties under articles 16 and 17 of the covenant. Concluding observations of the Committee on Economic, Social and Cultural Rights: Canada* (22/05/06. E/C.12/CAN/CO/4, E/C.12/CAN/CO5). Retrieved November 4, 2006, from http://www.equalityrights.org/NWG/resources/nwg/UN/CESCR-06Observations-e.pdf.

Galabuzi, G. (2004). Social exclusion. In D. Raphael (Ed.), *Social determinants of health: Canadian perspectives* (pp. 235–251). Toronto: Canadian Scholars' Press.

Gulliver, T., & Driemeyer, R. (2006). *Toronto Disaster Relief Committee pre-budget submission. Standing Committee on Finance.* Retrieved September 30, 2007, from http://tdrc.net/resources/public/financecommittee2006.doc.

Layton, J. (2000). *Homelessness. The making and unmaking of a crisis.* Toronto: Penguin/McGill Institute. [A new edition is anticipated in spring 2008. Working title: Still Homeless!]

McIntyre, L., Glanville, N. T., Raine, K. D., Dayle, J. B., Anderson, B., & Battaglia, N. (2003). Do low-income lone mothers compromise their nutrition to feed their children? *Canadian Medical Association Journal, 168*(6), 686–691.

National Council of Welfare. (2006a). *Poverty facts 2003*. Retrieved October 2, 2007, from http://www.ncwcnbes. net/documents/researchpublications/ResearchProjects/ PovertyProfile/2002-03Report_Summer2006/FactSheets/ PovertyFacts2003.pdf.

National Council of Welfare. (2006b). *Welfare incomes 2005*. Retrieved October 22, 2007, from http://www.ncwcnbes. net/documents/researchpublications/ResearchProjects/Welf areIncomes/2005Report_Summer2006/ReportENG.pdf.

National Housing and Homelessness Network. (2004). Ending homelessness: The one percent solution. In D. Hulchanski & M. Shapcott (Eds.), *Finding room: Policy options for a Canadian rental housing strategy* (pp. 381–388). Toronto: University of Toronto Press.

National Housing and Homelessness Network. (2005). *Promises made, promises betrayed: National report card grades federal housing efforts as failure.* Retrieved September 30, 2007, from http://tdrc.net/resources/public/05-NHHN- Housing%20Report%20Card.pdf.

Office of the United Nations High Commissioner for Human Rights. (1966). Poverty: Human rights dimension of poverty. Retrieved November 16, 2006, from http://www. ohchr.org/english/issues/poverty/index.htm.

Raphael, D. (2007). *Poverty and policy in Canada: Implications for health and quality of life.* Toronto: Canadian Scholars' Press.

Sarlo, C. (1996). *Poverty in Canada* (2nd ed.). Vancouver, B.C.: Fraser Institute.

Shapcott, M. (2004). Where are we going? Recent federal and provincial housing policy. In D. Hulchanski & M. Shapcott (Eds.), *Finding room: Policy options for a Canadian rental housing strategy* (pp. 195–212). Toronto: University of Toronto Press.

Street Haven. (n.d). *Peggy Ann's gift of hope.* Retrieved November 3, 2006, from http://www.streethaven.com/ pages/PeggyAnn.html.

Street Health. (2005). *Street Health research bulletin. Fall 2005.* Retrieved November 4, 2006, from http://www. streethealth.ca/Downloads/ResearchBulletin1005.pdf.

Swanson, J. (2001). *Poor bashing.* Toronto: Between the Lines Press.

Tarasuk, V. (2003). Low income, welfare and nutritional vul- nerability. *Canadian Medical Association Journal, 168*(6), 709–710.

Toronto Disaster Relief Committee. (1998). *State of emergency declaration: An urgent call for emergency humanitarian relief and prevention measures.* Retrieved September 30, 2007, from http://tdrc.net/resources/public/Report-98-TDRC.htm.

United Nations. (1948). *Universal declaration of human rights.* Retrieved November 3, 2006, from http://www.un.org/ Overview/rights.html.

Yalnizyan, A. (2000). *Canada's great divide: The politics of the growing gap between rich and poor in the 1990s* [Electronic version]. Toronto: Centre for Social Justice. Retrieved November 2, 2006, from http://www.socialjustice.org/ pdfs/canadasgreatdivide.pdf.

ADDITIONAL RESOURCES

Websites

Canadian Nursing Students' Association
www.cnsa.ca

Campaign 2000
www.campaign2000.ca

National Anti-Poverty Organization
www.napo-onap.ca

Toronto Disaster Relief Committee/National Housing and Homelessness Network
www.tdrc.net

Films

Cavalier, N., & Schofield, L. (Director). (2006). *Raise the rates.* [Documentary]. Canada: uncorp.pro. 27 minutes (Available from www.ocap.ca).

Connolly, M. (Director). (2003). *Shelter from the Storm.* [Documentary]. Canada: Brink Inc. 59 minutes (Available from www.tdrc.net).

Saywell, S. (Writer/ Director). (2002). *Street Nurse.* [Documentary]. Canada: Shelley Saywell. 45 minutes (Available from www.tdrc.net).

Books

Bates, C., Dodd, D., & Rousseau, N. (Eds.). (2005). *On all frontiers: Four centuries of Canadian nursing.* Ottawa: University of Ottawa Press.

Crowe, C. (2007). *Dying for a home: Homeless activists speak- out.* Toronto: Between the Lines.

Raphael, D. (Ed.). (2004). *Social determinants of health: Canadian perspectives.* Toronto: Canadian Scholars' Press.

About the Author

Cathy Crowe, RN (Toronto General Hospital), BAAN in Nursing (Ryerson), MEd in Sociology (Ontario Institute for Studies in Education), has worked in the area of home- lessness for more than 19 years. Cathy follows the pulse of health issues affecting homeless people, including access to health care, overall deteriorating health, the return of tuberculosis, deplorable shelter conditions, and an escalat- ing death rate. In 1998 Cathy co-founded the Toronto Disaster Relief Committee (TDRC), which declared homelessness a national disaster. Its signature "One Percent" slogan refers to the demand that all levels of gov- ernment commit an additional 1% of their budgets to an affordable social housing program. A 2002 documentary film on Cathy's work, *Street Nurse,* was directed by Emmy and Gemini award winner Shelley Saywell.

CHAPTER
28

Substance Abuse

Hélène Philbin Wilkinson

OBJECTIVES

After studying this chapter, you should be able to:

1. Understand and discuss the reasons why people use psychoactive substances.
2. Identify the differences between substance use and abuse, and understand the concept of dependency.
3. Describe the scope of substance use and abuse in Canada.
4. Discuss socio-demographic factors that are commonly associated with substance abuse patterns.
5. Explain the harms associated with substance abuse.
6. Articulate the components of effective substance abuse strategies.
7. Understand and begin to apply the concepts of health promotion, harm reduction, and resiliency theory.
8. Articulate your own values and attitudes toward substance abuse.

INTRODUCTION

Substance abuse is a complex public health issue that can have severe and permanent consequences for individuals, families, and communities. The overall cost of substance abuse (including alcohol, tobacco, and illicit drugs) was estimated to cost Canadians $39.8 billion in 2002 (Rehm et al., 2006). It is also associated with high rates of diseases and other lifestyle-related causes of death and injury. For example, in 2002 in Canada, substance abuse accounted for 21% of all deaths (through cancer, cardiac and pulmonary disease, as well as overdoses, motor vehicle accidents, and death by fire), 25% of years of potential life lost, and 19.4% of hospitalizations (Rehm et al., 2006).

Considerable non-monetary costs to Canadian society also exist, such as the pain, suffering, and bereavement experienced by families, friends, and victims, which can have profound and lasting effects that cannot be measured in dollars.

Just as substance abuse causes poor health, poor health and other socioeconomic disadvantages can contribute to substance abuse (Single, 1999). This socio-environmental perspective has guided the development of holistic substance abuse strategies that recognize the interrelationships among the person, the substance, and the environment. This chapter is intended to introduce the community health nurse (CHN) to the practice of developing comprehensive community-based responses to substance abuse. It is also intended to stim-

ulate further discussion and research about a multifaceted public health issue that you will undoubtedly encounter at some point in your career.

WHY DO PEOPLE USE DRUGS?

People use different drugs for different reasons, and the reasons vary from drug to drug, from person to person, and from circumstance to circumstance. While certain psychoactive drugs may be prescribed to relieve anxiety, tension, stress, or insomnia, some people may self-medicate to improve performance or to resolve physical or emotional discomfort. The mere availability of a drug may cause individuals to be curious enough to experiment. The danger, however, is that experimental use may lead to other reasons for using, which may in turn result in abuse and/or dependence.

Other people may take drugs to boost their self-confidence or to forget about or cope with traumatic life events or situations. Immediate gratification from drugs may make people feel good and/or can quickly reduce or eliminate uncomfortable emotions, albeit temporarily. Social pressures to use drugs can be very strong for both young people and adults. However, children are especially vulnerable as they may imitate and interpret their parents' use as a necessary part of having fun or relaxing. Young people may use drugs to rebel against unhappy situations or because they feel alienated, have an identity crisis, or need to be accepted by their peers. The media are also considered a powerful source of influence. Ads often promote drinking or smoking as a social activity or as a factor in the achievement of success.

TERMINOLOGY

The term **drug** refers to a **psychoactive substance** that affects a person's physiological or psychological state or behaviour. In this chapter, *drugs* will be referred to as substances consumed for medicinal and non-medicinal purposes, legally or illegally, and the term will be used interchangeably with the term *psychoactive substances*.

Most people don't think of **alcohol** as a drug, but it is. Ethyl alcohol is present in beer, wine, spirits, and liqueurs, and methyl alcohol is found in solvents, paint removers, antifreeze, and other household and industrial products. At low doses, alcohol acts as a central nervous system depressant, producing relaxation and a release of inhibitions. At higher doses, it can produce intoxication, impaired judgment and coordination, even coma and death.

Tobacco leaves, which are shredded and dried, can be smoked in cigarettes, cigars, or pipes, or be chewed or inhaled. More than 4000 chemicals are found in tobacco, including nicotine, the main psychoactive component that stimulates the central nervous system.

Illicit drugs (illegal drugs) include cannabis (marijuana and hashish), phencyclidines (PCP, ketamine), hallucinogens (LSD, mescaline, psilocybin, MDA), stimulants other than caffeine and nicotine (amphetamines, cocaine, crack), depressants (barbiturates, methaqualone, benzodiazepine), and opiates (heroin, morphine, methadone, codeine). **Inhalants**, also known as volatile solvents, are depressant drugs that produce feelings of euphoria, exhilaration, and vivid fantasies. Their use can cause brain damage, asphyxiation, and death. Using inhalants such as gasoline or certain illicit drugs such as PCP can cause immediate and serious problems regardless of how or when they are taken.

Licit drugs (legal drugs) that are used for medicinal purposes are legally available by prescription or sold over the counter and include drugs to relieve pain, control anxiety, or combat insomnia. Licit drugs used for non-medicinal purposes include alcohol and tobacco, either of which can be legally purchased and used by those who are of legal age.

Substance use refers to any consumption of psychoactive drugs, which can result in benefits or harm. **Substance abuse** or misuse refers to drug use that leads to adverse physical or psychological consequences, which may or may not involve **dependence**. Drug dependency is progressive in nature and affects the physiological, cognitive, behavioural, and psychological dimensions of a person's health. It is manifested by continuous use despite the presence of problems that are caused by the pattern of repeated self-administration that results in tolerance, withdrawal, and compulsive substance-taking behaviour (American Psychiatric Association, 1994). Dependence can be physical and/or psychological. **Physical dependence** occurs when an individual's body reacts to the absence of a drug, and **psychological dependence** occurs when drug use becomes central to a person's thoughts and emotions. You may wish to consult your psychiatric nursing text to further explore this topic.

THE SCOPE OF SUBSTANCE USE AND ABUSE IN CANADA

Canadian researchers have found that approximately 20 million people in Canada consume psychoactive substances. Despite the fact that overall rates of use have decreased among Canada's general population, the abuse of tobacco and alcohol continue to be leading causes of preventable death and illness (Federal, Provincial, and Territorial Advisory Committee on Population Health [FPTACPH], 1999).

Prevalence patterns of substance use and abuse are influenced by both individual and socio-demographic factors such as age, gender, education, changes in lifestyle, attitudes, and beliefs. For example, researchers have found that men are more likely than women to report alcohol and other drug use, and that use tends to decline with increasing age (Adlaf &

Ialomiteanu, 2002). The additional resources at the end of this chapter provide further details about the differences in consumption patterns across Canada and the individual, social, geographical, and historical factors that can influence the use and abuse of substances.

Tobacco

Smoking is the single most serious public health problem in our country, killing more Canadians than alcohol, car accidents, suicides, and murders combined (Health Canada, 2001). Smoking rates continue to be highest among males and young people, but the gender gap is narrowing as young adolescent females are now more likely to smoke than their male peers. Smoking also appears to be strongly related to employment, income, and education: the higher the education and income levels, the lower the percentage of smoking (FPTACPH, 1999).

Alcohol

Approximately 12.7 million Canadians are regular drinkers. Overall, men tend to drink twice as much as women, and high rates of consumption appear more prevalent among youth 18 to 24 years of age, single persons, and persons with less formal education (Demers & Poulin, 2005).

Significant social problems caused by the misuse of alcohol in our country include driving under the influence of alcohol and domestic and interpersonal violence. Although impaired driving rates have dropped over the last couple of decades, the largest number of alcohol-related deaths stem from impaired driving accidents, many of which involve young people (Single, Rehm, Robson, & Van Truong, 2000).

Canadian Research Box 28.1

Heaman, M. I., & Chalmers, K. (2005). Prevalence and correlates of smoking during pregnancy: A comparison of Aboriginal and non-Aboriginal women in Manitoba. *Birth, 32*(4): 299–305.

The research literature confirms that the prevalence of smoking among Aboriginal people in Canada is higher than in the general population; however, little is known about the smoking rates among Aboriginal women who are pregnant or the characteristics of Aboriginal women who are more likely to smoke during pregnancy. The researchers in this study examined the prevalence of smoking during pregnancy among Aboriginal and non-Aboriginal women who were giving birth in the province of Manitoba.

Interviews were conducted with 684 postpartum women who delivered a live single infant in two tertiary care hospitals in Manitoba. A stratified analysis was used to describe effect–measure modification for correlates of smoking among both Aboriginal and non-Aboriginal groups. A multivariable logistic regression was conducted for the total sample.

The researchers found that a significantly higher proportion of Aboriginal women (61.2%) than non-Aboriginal women (26.2%) smoked while pregnant. Although no specific correlates of smoking were observed among Aboriginal women, several maternal characteristics were associated with smoking and pregnancy for the total sample. These included inadequate prenatal care, low support from others, single marital status, illicit drug use, Aboriginal race/ethnicity, and non-completion of high school among non-Aboriginal women. The findings confirm a high prevalence of smoking during pregnancy, particularly among Aboriginal women. As such the researchers recommend greater coordination of efforts aimed at prevention and cessation.

Discussion Questions:

1. How did you respond to the findings of this study? Were you surprised by the higher prevalence of smoking among Aboriginal women who are pregnant? How do these findings support or refute what you have observed in your own community or province?

2. The findings in this study illustrate how substance use/abuse can be influenced by the complex interactions between individual characteristics, culture/ethnicity, social and economic factors, and physical environments. Discuss how marital status, social support networks, education. and personal health practices influence pregnant Aboriginal and non-Aboriginal women in your area.

Illicit Drugs

Cannabis is the most widely used illicit drug in Canada. Other commonly used illicit drugs include hallucinogens, LSD, speed, heroin, and cocaine. Although the overall consumption of illicit drugs is relatively low compared with that of alcohol and tobacco, research reports indicate that the use of illicit drugs other than cannabis has risen during the past decade (Adlaf & Ialomiteanu, 2005). Illicit drug use is more common among males and young people, especially among street youth (FPTACPH, 1999).

Tragically, suicides account for almost half of illicit drug–related deaths. Although mortality resulting from illicit drug use is lower than from alcohol and tobacco, illicit drug–related deaths tend to involve younger people (Single, Robson, Rehm, & Xie, 1999).

Approximately 7% of Canadians use at least one **injectable drug** (cocaine/crack, LSD, amphetamines, heroin, or steroids), and two out of five of these individuals share needles, a known risk for the transmission of HIV, hepatitis B, and other blood borne pathogens (FPTACPH, 1999). AIDS acquired through the use of illicit drugs accounts for approximately 8% of deaths related to the use of illicit drugs.

As for inhalants, approximately 1% of Canadians use solvents or glue, but children and youth are the highest users (MacNeil & Webster, 1997). For example, some studies involving inmates of detention centres reveal that inhalants were the first drugs ever used by this group. Other studies also indicate that street youth, inner-city youth, and First Nations and Inuit youth living in rural and remote areas have higher rates of solvent abuse. Of note is that heavy solvent use is often a response to poor life conditions.

Licit Drugs

Nearly 5 million Canadians use, appropriately and inappropriately, one or more licit drugs, including over-the-counter and prescription pain pills, sleeping pills, tranquilizers, antidepressants, and diet pills. Of the prescription drugs, narcotic pain relievers (e.g., codeine, Demerol, morphine) are the group most commonly used by Canadians, particularly women and young people (Riley, 1998). Females also use more tranquilizers, antidepressants, and sleeping pills, and the elderly have the highest use of sleeping pills and antidepressants (MacNeil & Webster, 1997). Of particular concern is the use of medications among older persons since the aging process is frequently accompanied by an increase in chronic or acute illness and an increase in the total number of prescribed drugs.

HARMFUL CONSEQUENCES OF SUBSTANCE ABUSE

All drugs have adverse and undesirable effects. For example, the long-term use of tobacco can cause lung damage; alcohol abuse can cause liver damage; sniffing cocaine can damage nasal passages; people who inject drugs intravenously can become infected with blood borne diseases such as HIV or hepatitis B; and exposure to second-hand smoke among neonates, infants, children, and adults is associated with an increased risk of a number of acute and chronic conditions.

People who use drugs that have been obtained illegally can never really know what they are taking. For example ecstasy and crystal meth, both of which belong to the amphetamine family, can be easily manufactured in unregulated illegal labs. As a result, the chemicals and processes vary affecting the strength, purity, and effect of the final product. The consequences can be devastating, including severe dependency and drug reactions, and fatal overdoses. Other associated harms can include an increase in crime and violent acts; strained relationships; workplace and school absenteeism; and health problems such as ulcers, liver and kidney damage, pancreatic diseases, heart disease, cancer, sexual and reproductive issues, and pre- and postnatal complications.

As little as one drink of alcohol every other day can help adults gain some protection against heart disease; however, heavy drinking does raise blood pressure and can also increase the risk of stroke and heart failure.

The consumption of alcohol during pregnancy can result in **fetal alcohol spectrum disorder** (FASD), which is manifested by developmental, neurological, and behavioural delays in infants and young children. Though the major cause of these conditions is the frequency and volume of an expectant mother's alcohol intake, other contributing factors to consider include genetic predisposition, poor nutrition, age, the lack of prenatal care, and the use of other drugs. Since a safe level of alcohol consumption during pregnancy or while breastfeeding has not been established, public health professionals advise expectant and breastfeeding mothers not to drink alcohol, even in moderation. Consult your maternity and pediatric nursing texts for additional information about the incidence and clinical symptoms of FASD.

The Response to Substance Abuse

Given the wide range of individual, social, and cultural factors that can influence patterns of drug use, strategies have shifted from the view that substance abuse is not merely caused by individual psychological or moral factors. This shift in perspective has stimulated the development of public health models that combine elements of primary, secondary, and tertiary prevention, which have been described and referred to in previous chapters.

The Risk Continuum The **risk continuum**, initially developed by the Ontario Ministry of Health (1988), is a conceptual framework that has been widely used to design community-based strategies that correspond to the different risks associated with the use and abuse of different substances. Composed of risk categories (see Figure 28.1), the continuum is based on the principle that the degree of risk associated with drug use is related to the amount of the substance being consumed and the conditions under which it is consumed, thus reflecting socio-behavioural and environmental approaches. Strategies are based on this premise but also reflect the nature of the substance. For example, the "low risk" category is not applicable to the use of illicit drugs and inhalants as they are considered harmful even at low doses. Similarly, the concept of "no risk" is not consistent with the use of prescription drugs because there is always some risk of side effects when taking any medication.

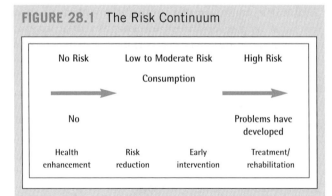

FIGURE 28.1 The Risk Continuum

Source: Ontario, Ministry of Health. A Framework for the Response to Alcohol and Drug Problems in Ontario. 1988. ISBN 0772947889, p. 8. Adapted with permission.

The risk continuum illustrates that a comprehensive community-based substance abuse strategy combines activities that are related to both health promotion and health recovery. For example, more and more communities are introducing strategies that combine treatment, prevention, law enforcement, and harm reduction. Depending on the level of risk, activities may include health enhancement, risk avoidance, risk reduction, early identification and intervention, and treatment and rehabilitation, all of which draw from the concepts of primary, secondary, and tertiary prevention.

Planning any of these strategies in the community typically consists of four fundamental steps:

- identify priority population groups;
- establish intermediate and ultimate objectives for each target population group;
- determine existing programs, services, and policies that can address these objectives; and
- identify and involve appropriate groups, agencies, and organizations.

Substance abuse is a multifaceted issue and therefore requires the collaboration of several sectors, including home, schools, workplaces, health care settings, recreational settings, enforcement and justice systems, and so on. Examples of activities that can be implemented in a few of these sectors are provided in Table 28.1.

Health Promotion

Health promotion consists of activities related to health enhancement, risk avoidance, and risk reduction. **Health enhancement** is a strategy involving activities that are designed to increase resilience. The main focus in this strategy is to develop or enhance health rather than reduce substance use or abuse. It combines both behavioural and socio-environmental approaches. For example, abstaining from the consumption of drugs is often promoted and integrated with other healthy lifestyle choices and supported by healthy environments.

Risk avoidance, another socio-environmental approach, reinforces the adoption of low-risk consumption. It is intended to increase the likelihood that drinking (for example) will take place at a level and in a context that has a low association with health and social problems. This approach is intended to reduce drug consumption before health and social problems develop, particularly among people who find themselves in the "moderate risk" category of the continuum.

An effective substance abuse strategy combines education, policy change, and environmental support, as they are mutually complementary and strengthen the impact of other prevention activities. Education helps people make healthy decisions and participate in health activities by increasing knowledge and motivation, changing attitudes, and increasing the skills that are required to avoid or reduce risk. These activities can consist of programs and services that impart knowledge about substances and help develop refusal skills. Policy changes are intended to create an environment that is conducive to healthy practices by making it easier to adopt

TABLE 28.1
Examples of Substance Abuse Prevention Activities by Sector, Stakeholders, and Target Group

Sector	Stakeholders	Target Group	Activities
Home	Parents, children, local media, mass media, public health, community organizations and groups, health agencies	• Children • Youth • Parents	• Discuss substance use/abuse issues with children and youth. • Provide skill development programs for parents. • Promote educational materials. • Encourage the development of a home drinking policy. • Encourage alternative healthy activities/behaviours.
Elementary and secondary schools	School administration, public health, students, parents, teachers, guidance counsellors, physical education and health consultants, parent teacher group, community alcohol and drug consultants	• Students (K–12) • Staff • Parents • Teachers • Peer leaders	• Develop school policies on alcohol and drugs. • Encourage an integrated drug education curriculum that spans the school years. • Provide ongoing training for those delivering the drug education curriculum. • Hold special events to supplement drug education curriculum. • Organize student interest groups (e.g., students against drunk driving). • Provide early identification and intervention programs in the schools.

Source: Ontario, Ministry of Health, Health Promotion Branch. Community Mobilization Manual [vol. 4] Ideas for Action on Alcohol. 1991. ISBN 0772968616, p. 9. Adapted with permission.

healthy behaviours and more difficult to adopt unhealthy practices. Such policies as tobacco by-laws or alcohol legislation can create healthy social and physical environments. **Environmental support** helps to ensure healthy conditions, practices, and policies that make it easier for people to achieve and maintain their health. For example, the presence of recreational activities and self-help groups can provide important environmental supports for a community (Ontario Ministry of Health, Health Promotion Branch, 1991).

Health Recovery Early identification and intervention programs and treatment and rehabilitation programs are strategies designed for people who have started to experience problems related to their substance abuse. The emphasis is on the early identification of signs and symptoms in order to intervene and reduce consumption levels and effectively manage the problems that have developed. Treatment and rehabilitation (health recovery) is intended to assist people with substance abuse problems as their consumption is considered to be "high risk." These individuals should be provided with comprehensive assessments in order to match their recovery needs and their personal circumstances with the appropriate treatment services. Overall, the purpose in health recovery is to prevent further deterioration and reduce the harms that have resulted from a problematic drug-consumption pattern.

Treatment and rehabilitation services in Canada typically include detoxification services, assessment and referral, inpatient and outpatient treatment programs, and aftercare and follow-up. Additionally, special programs have been designed to address the unique needs of certain population groups such as women, youth, Aboriginal people, impaired driving offenders, and inmates of correctional institutions.

Harm Reduction and Resiliency Theory **Harm reduction** and resiliency theory can be powerful tools to minimize the harms associated with substance abuse. They also offer a wide spectrum of opportunities for the CHN to help strengthen the capacity of individuals and communities experiencing the adverse effects of substance abuse.

Harm reduction is a public health philosophy that has gained popularity in the last two decades; however, some claim that it is a new name for an old concept. It is described as a program or policy designed to reduce drug-related harm without requiring the cessation of drug use (Centre for Addiction and Mental Health, 2002). Examples include alcohol server training programs and impaired driving countermeasures. In the treatment field, the most pre-eminent harm reduction strategies are needle exchanges and methadone maintenance programs, both of which allow the individual to live with a certain level of dependency while minimizing risks and other disruptive effects to the person and the community. For example, in addition to clean needles and syringes, needle exchange programs provide condoms and sexual health counselling as a means of reducing the risk of spreading HIV by sexual activity (Laurie & Green, 2000). Some may argue that harm reduction cannot be applied to tobacco since even small quantities of tobacco can be harmful. But consider the recent harm reduction measures that have been put in place that have created protection for non-smokers in restaurants in various provinces across Canada. It is often said that harm reduction is not what's nice, it's what works. The focus is therefore not on the use or the extent of use, but on the harms that are associated with the use. While becoming drug free may be the ultimate goal, it is not required from the outset. The goal is to reduce more immediate and tangible harms.

A harm reduction message to the public is somewhat different from other types of prevention messages, for example *avoid problems when you drink* vs. *drinking less is better* (Single, 2000). As you work through the case study in this chapter, you will learn that many policies, such as the promotion of low-alcohol beverages, are based on harm reduction principles. Consequently, harm reduction stands in contrast to other models and philosophies such as abstinence-based health promotion initiatives and population-based measures like alcohol tax policies and restrictions on availability making it more difficult to get. Although these are necessary to control underage drinking and the excessive promotion of alcohol, they do not target individuals who are most at risk for alcohol problems. Harm reduction focuses on lowering the risk and severity of adverse consequences without necessarily reducing consumption. Although different, they are complementary and both have an important role in addressing substance abuse problems in our communities.

When harm reduction emerged as a public health strategy, it initially involved socially marginal populations such as injection drug users and correctional inmates. It may therefore provoke debate and controversy as an appropriate strategy for some communities or organizations. Consider the progress that has been made, however, since the introduction of clean needle and syringe exchange programs. Strong community stakeholder endorsement is key with this approach in order to prevent a public outcry on its appropriateness, which would inadvertently shift the focus from its intended purpose to a debate about other peripheral social issues. On the other hand, such a dialogue may be crucial given its potential to produce a shift in knowledge, attitudes, and values.

The theory of **resiliency** consists of two fundamental concepts—risk and protective factors—both of which contribute to one's sense of resiliency. Resiliency is described as the capability of individuals, families, groups, and communities to cope successfully in the face of significant adversity or risk (Mangham, McGrath, Reid, & Stewart, 1995). **Risk factors** are considered stresses that challenge individuals, including their own personal and environmental characteristics. When stresses such as substance abuse are greater than one's protective factors, even those who have been resilient in the past may become overwhelmed. **Protective factors** are skills, personality factors, and environmental supports that act as buffers when people are faced with stressful events. Individual protective factors may include literacy and interpersonal skills. Community-based protective factors may consist of shared values and strong volunteer participation.

The application of resiliency in the development of substance abuse strategies is particularly valuable as both risk and protective factors must be examined and analyzed in order to recognize the aspects of an individual's or community's health that can be enhanced or reduced. Using the framework helps to identify predominant risk factors and ensure that responses are anchored in resiliency for a specific situation, as opposed to lifetime resiliency. For example, analyzing such factors as age or social isolation, which may lead to compulsive patterns of drug use, can help generate knowledge and understanding about why some individuals and communities respond differently to this kind of adversity. As illustrated in Figure 28.2, protective factors can influence outcomes, thus making it critical to capitalize on the individual's or community's strengths. The framework is especially useful because it supports the integration of other determinants of health, such as employment, and considers the linkages with a person's or a community's socio-cultural and economic environment.

Case Study

A local Junior A hockey team plays in your community's municipally owned arena. Team officials have been selling beer during home games as a means of generating revenue for the team. There have been recent and well-publicized complaints about people becoming intoxicated and creating disturbances during and after games. Community officials and private entrepreneurs are looking for the support of the local police department and your public health unit in order to effectively address this issue and prevent further disturbances. The well-attended hockey games represent the main source of entertainment for many families during the long winter season. Your public health board has requested a substance abuse program to explore this issue and develop an appropriate strategy to reduce these emerging alcohol-related problems.

Discussion Questions

1. Discuss the health, social, and legal risks that are commonly associated with the practice of serving alcohol during sports events in municipally owned facilities.

2. Explore various prevention and enforcement strategies that can be adopted to minimize the risks that are associated with the service of alcohol.

3. Identify the various groups of stakeholders that should be targeted as part of these strategies.

Summary

In this chapter, we have explored the impact that substance abuse can have on the health of individuals and communities. Three types of drug consumption, including the use and abuse of drugs, and the concept of dependency were briefly presented. The reasons why people use and abuse drugs were discussed, as well as how a maladaptive pattern of substance abuse progresses toward physical and psychological dependence.

The scope of alcohol, tobacco, and illicit and licit drug use and abuse was discussed. Socio-demographic characteristics commonly associated with certain prevalence patterns

FIGURE 28.2   Framework of Community Resilience

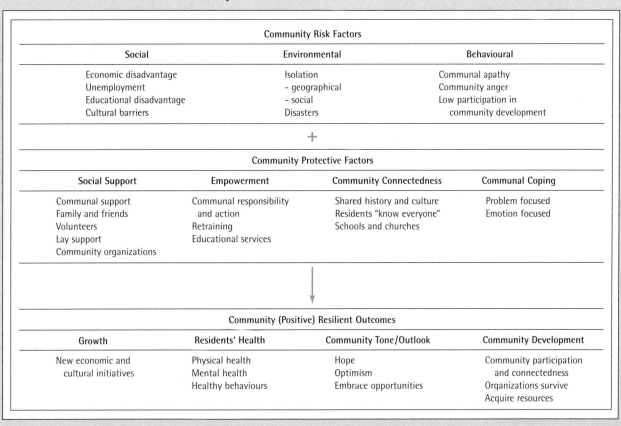

Community Risk Factors		
Social	**Environmental**	**Behavioural**
Economic disadvantage	Isolation	Communal apathy
Unemployment	– geographical	Community anger
Educational disadvantage	– social	Low participation in
Cultural barriers	Disasters	community development

+

Community Protective Factors			
Social Support	**Empowerment**	**Community Connectedness**	**Communal Coping**
Communal support	Communal responsibility	Shared history and culture	Problem focused
Family and friends	and action	Residents "know everyone"	Emotion focused
Volunteers	Retraining	Schools and churches	
Lay support	Educational services		
Community organizations			

Community (Positive) Resilient Outcomes			
Growth	**Residents' Health**	**Community Tone/Outlook**	**Community Development**
New economic and	Physical health	Hope	Community participation
cultural initiatives	Mental health	Optimism	and connectedness
	Healthy behaviours	Embrace opportunities	Organizations survive
			Acquire resources

Source: Statistical Report on the Health of Canadians, Health Canada (1999). Reproduced with the permission of the Minister of Public Works and Government Services Canada, 2007.

were examined because it is essential to understand that substance abuse can cause poor health, just as poor health and other social, health, and economic disadvantages can contribute to substance abuse. Although substance abuse affects many Canadians, some populations are particularly vulnerable to its effects, including women, infants and children, adolescents, street youth, and the Aboriginal population. Harms commonly associated with substance abuse were identified, including fetal alcohol syndrome, impaired driving, suicides, and interpersonal violence.

Responding to substance abuse problems in the community requires sound data, a plan grounded in theory, and strong intersectoral collaboration. The public health and substance abuse strategies presented in this chapter reflect both behavioural and socio-environmental frameworks, including health promotion, harm reduction, and the resiliency theory, all of which draw from the models of primary, secondary, and tertiary prevention. The risk continuum is an effective tool to determine strategies that appropriately correspond to the different risks associated with various levels of drug consumption. A community's substance abuse strategy should combine health promotion and health recovery activities, including education, policy, and environmental support. No single activity can be effec-

tive on its own; they are mutually complementary and strengthen the overall strategy. The theories of harm reduction and resiliency were presented, both of which can support and enhance other approaches. The application of the conceptual frameworks presented in this chapter can serve to guide the CHN in the development of comprehensive substance abuse strategies linking the individual, the drug, and the environment.

KEY TERMS

drug
psychoactive substance
alcohol
tobacco
illicit drugs
inhalants
licit drugs
substance use
substance abuse
dependence
physical dependence
psychological dependence
injectable drug

fetal alcohol spectrum disorder
risk continuum
health promotion
health enhancement
risk avoidance
environmental support
harm reduction
resiliency
risk factors
protective factors

INDIVIDUAL CRITICAL THINKING EXERCISES

1. Privately explore the first thing that comes to mind when you read each of the following expressions. Then, explore your reactions to each expression. Do they differ from each other? If so, consider the reasons why. Did any of your reactions surprise you? If yes, think about how your personal values could influence your professional practice.

- A homeless alcoholic
- Needle exchange program
- Abstinence-based treatment
- Problem drinker
- Methadone treatment
- Parent with hangover
- IV drug user
- Crack dealer
- Professor smoking marijuana

- Pregnant speed addict
- Crystal meth addict
- Chain (tobacco) smoker
- Female cocaine user
- Drunk driver
- Twenty-year-old buying booze for underage sibling
- Person with HIV
- Gas sniffer
- Underage drunk
- Coffee drinker

2. Read your local newspaper or a magazine, or watch the news, a television program, or a movie. Pay attention to the images and messages about the consumption of alcohol, tobacco, and illicit or licit drugs. Who are these messages aimed at? What are they portraying? Consider the degree of influence that these images have on drug consumption patterns in society.

GROUP CRITICAL THINKING EXERCISES

1. Select a particular issue or harm that is associated with substance abuse in your community (e.g., impaired driving, FASD). What sources of information (local, regional, provincial, and national) can be used to help your group accurately define the problem?

2. For the issue identified in question 1, have your group map your community's current capacity in terms of substance abuse prevention and treatment (health promotion and health recovery) services and programs. You may use the telephone directory or contact local health and social service agencies. For example, you should highlight how peo-

ple access general information about the issue and, if appropriate, where people access treatment services. Make note of any gaps your group observes.

3. Using the results of the mapping exercise in question 2, discuss as a group the risk factors that you believe have contributed to the development of the issue or harm identified in question 1. Additionally, your group should explore the protective factors that have acted as buffers or that will have the capacity to create positive outcomes for your target population or for the community.

REFERENCES

Adlaf, E. M., & Ialomiteanu, A. (2002). *CAMH monitor e-report: Addiction and mental health indicators among Ontario adults in 2001, and changes since 1997.* CAMH Research Doc. Series No. 12. Toronto: Centre for Addiction and Mental Health. Retrieved October 15, 2006, from http://www.ocat.org/pdf/CAMH_report_prevalence.pdf.

Adlaf, E. M., & Ialomiteanu, A. (2005). Other drug use and problems. In *Canadian addiction survey [CAS]: A national survey of Canadians' use of alcohol and other drugs.* Ottawa: Health Canada.

American Psychiatric Association. (1994). *Diagnostic and statistical manual of mental disorders* (4th ed.). Washington, D.C.: Author.

Centre for Addiction and Mental Health. (2002). *CAMH position on harm reduction: A background paper on its meaning and applications for substance use issues.* Toronto: Author.

Demers, A., & Poulin, C. (2005). Alcohol use. In *Canadian addiction survey [CAS]: A national survey of Canadians' use of alcohol and other drugs.* Ottawa: Health Canada.

Federal, Provincial, and Territorial Advisory Committee on Population Health. (1999). *Statistical report on the health of Canadians.* Ottawa: Health Canada.

Health Canada. (2001). The federal tobacco control strategy—A framework for action. Ottawa: Health Canada.

Laurie, M. L., & Green, K. L. (2000). Health risk and opportunities for harm reduction among injection-drug-using clients of Saskatoon's needle exchange program . *Canadian Journal of Public Health, (91)*5, 350.

MacNeil, P., & Webster, I. (1997). *Canada's alcohol and other drugs survey, 1994: A discussion of findings.* Ottawa: Health Canada.

Mangham, C., McGrath, P., Reid, G., & Stewart, M. (1995). *Resiliency: Relevance to health promotion: Discussion paper.* Ottawa: Health Canada.

Ontario Ministry of Health. (1988). *A framework for the response to alcohol and drug problems in Ontario.* Toronto: Author.

Ontario Ministry of Health, Health Promotion Branch. (1991). *A guide for community health promotion planning.* Toronto: Author.

Rehm, J., Ballunas, D., Brochu, S., Fischer, B., Gnam, W., Patra, J., Popovas, S., Sarnocinska-Hart, A., & Taylor, B. (2006). *The costs of substance abuse in Canada, 2002 highlights.* Retrieved October 13, 2007, from http://www.ccsa.ca/NR/rdonlyres/18F3415E-2CAC-4D21-86E2-CEE549EC47A9/0/ccsa0113322006.pdf.

Riley, D. (1998). Drugs and drug policy in Canada: A brief review and commentary. Canadian Foundation for Drug Policy. Retrieved October 15, 2006, from http://www.cfdp.ca/sen1841.htm.

Single, E. (1999). *Substance abuse and population health: Workshop on addiction and population health. Edmonton, Alberta, June, 1999.* Ottawa: Canadian Centre on Substance Abuse. Retrieved October 15, 2006, from http://www.ccsa.ca/NR/rdonlyres/5CC1D7F6-4C32-49A3-8C7E-2F5E53690105/0/ccsa0003891999.pdf.

Single, E. (2000). *The effectiveness of harm reduction and its role in a new framework for drug policy in British Columbia.* Presentation to the National Federal/Provincial/Territorial Meeting on Injection Drug Use, Vancouver. Retrieved October 15, 2006, from http://www.ccsa.ca/pdf/ccsa-003201-2000.pdf.

Single, E., Rehm, J., Robson, L., & Van Truong, M. (2000). The relative risks and etiologic fractions of different causes of death and disease attributable to alcohol, tobacco and illicit drug use in Canada. *Canadian Medical Association Journal, 162*(12), 1669–1675.

Single, E., Robson, L., Rehm, J., & Xie, X. (1999). Morbidity and mortality attributable to substance abuse in Canada. *American Journal of Public Health, 89*(3), 385–390.

ADDITIONAL RESOURCES

Websites

Canada's Drug Strategy
www.hc-sc.gc.ca/ahc-asc/activit/strateg/drugs-drogues/index_e.html

Canadian Centre for Ethics in Sport
www.cces.ca

Canadian Centre on Substance Abuse (CCSA)
www.ccsa.ca

Canadian Centre on Substance Abuse Addictions Database
www.ccsa.ca/CCSA/EN/Addiction_Databases/AddictionsOrgsForm.htm

Canadian Community Epidemiology Network on Drug Use
www.ccsa.ca/CCSA/EN/Partnerships/CCENDU

Canadian Foundation for Drug Policy
www.cfdp.ca

Canadian Health Network, Substance Use/Addictions
www.canadian-health-network.ca/servlet/ContentServer?cid=1048003176982&pagename=CHN-RCS%2FPage%2FGTPageTemplate&c=Page&lang=En

Health Canada, First Nations and Inuit Health, Treatment Centre Directory
www.hc-sc.gc.ca/fnih-spni/substan/ads/nnadap-pnlaada_dir-rep_e.html

MADD Canada Mothers Against Drunk Driving
www.madd.ca

National Database of FASD and Substance Use During Pregnancy Resources
www.ccsa.ca/fas/

National Native Alcohol and Drug Abuse Program (NNADAP)
www.hc-sc.gc.ca/fnih-spni/substan/ads/nnadap-pnlaada_e.html

Alberta Alcohol and Drug Abuse Commission (AADAC)
www.aadac.com

British Columbia Ministry of Health, Mental Health and Addictions
www.health.gov.bc.ca/mhd/

Addictions Foundation of Manitoba
www.afm.mb.ca

New Brunswick Department of Health and Wellness, Addiction and Mental Health Services
www.gnb.ca/0051/0055/index-e.asp

Newfoundland and Labrador Department of Health and Community Services, Addictions Services
www.health.gov.nl.ca/health/commhlth_old/factlist/drugdepts.htm

Government of the Northwest Territories, Department of Health and Social Services
www.hlthss.gov.nt.ca

Nova Scotia Department of Health, Addictions Resources
www.gov.ns.ca/heal/policywatch/add.html

Ontario Centre for Addiction and Mental Health
www.camh.net

Prince Edward Island Addiction Services
www.gov.pe.ca/hss/addiction/

Québec Ministère de la Santé et des Services Sociaux
http://dependances.gouv.qc.ca/index.php?accueil

Saskatchewan Health, Alcohol and Drug Services
www.health.gov.sk.ca/ps_alcohol_and_drugs.html

Yukon Health and Social Services, Alcohol and Drug Services
www.hss.gov.yk.ca/programs/alcohol_drugs

International Resources

Alcoholics Anonymous World Services
www.alcoholics-anonymous.org

Drug Policy Alliance
www.drugpolicy.org

National Council on Alcoholism and Drug Dependence (U.S.)
www.ncadd.org

University of Washington, Alcohol and Drug Abuse Institute
http://depts.washington.edu/adai

About the Author

Hélène Philbin Wilkinson, RN, BScN (Laurentian University), MN (Athabasca University), is the program manager of the forensic mental health program at the Northeast Mental Health Centre (NEMHC) in North Bay, Ontario. Prior to joining the NEMHC, Hélène was a senior health planner with the Northern Shores District Health Council, where she oversaw the planning portfolios of addiction, mental health, and French-language health services. After spending the early part of her career in hospital she turned to the community, where she worked as a public health nurse then as a senior program consultant with the Centre for Addiction and Mental Health, where she provided leadership in several research and program evaluation projects that focused on alcohol and drug policy. She was instrumental in designing "Setting a New Direction: A Resource Guide for Alcohol, Tobacco and Other Drug Policies for Summer Camps," which was distributed to residential summer camps across Canada. Hélène has also developed curriculum in the areas of social marketing and program evaluation, and worked as a part-time instructor and mentor in nursing and health promotion certificate and degree programs. She dedicates her chapter to her godmother Ella, one of the first public health nurses in Northeastern Ontario.

Sexually Transmitted Infections and Blood Borne Pathogens

Wendi Lokanc-Diluzio, Alison Nelson, Janet L. Wayne, and Janet B. Hettler

OBJECTIVES

After studying this chapter, you should be able to:

1. Understand the different types of sexually transmitted infections and blood borne pathogens and the issues surrounding their transmission, testing, treatment, and prevention.

2. Recognize the potential physical, psychological, and financial implications of sexually transmitted infections and blood borne pathogens through analysis of Canadian statistical trends and issues raised in the literature.

3. Identify population-specific issues related to sexually transmitted infections and blood borne pathogens.

4. Identify various applications of the population health promotion model when developing health promotion and prevention strategies for sexually transmitted infections and blood borne pathogens.

5. Describe innovative interventions involving community health nurses that address sexually transmitted infections and blood borne pathogens in different regions of Canada.

INTRODUCTION

Sexually transmitted infections (STIs) and **blood borne pathogens (BBPs)** such as **human immunodeficiency virus (HIV)** are significant public health issues in Canada. Historically and currently, those affected by STIs and HIV have encountered stigmatization and discrimination as STIs and HIV often elicit emotional reactions such as anxiety, fear, and shame. The continued stigma of STIs and HIV may impede people from protecting themselves, as well as from seeking testing and treatment. Societal reactions of intolerance toward people at risk for STIs and HIV, as well as those living with HIV and acquired immune deficiency syndrome (AIDS), may further marginalize specific populations who already experience inequities in health status.

In this chapter, community health nurses (CHNs) are challenged to promote health, build capacity, and facilitate access and equity through innovative community strategies to address STIs and BBPs. Historical and current challenges regarding STI and BBP prevention and healthy public policies are discussed. Additionally, an overview of the main categories of STI and their incidence and/or prevalence in Canada is presented along with a review of selected BBPs, their trans-

mission, and current rates. Implications for CHNs working with marginalized populations related to STI and BBP prevention and risk reduction are discussed. Examples of how CHNs address STIs and BBPs through innovative prevention strategies are presented.

HISTORY OF STIS AND BBPS AND THEIR EFFECTS ON HEALTHY PUBLIC POLICY

Over the years, STIs have been labelled in different ways including *venereal disease* (VD), which referred to Venus, the Roman goddess of love. In the 1970s, the term VD was viewed as inaccurate and replaced by sexually transmitted disease (STD), because "love often plays little or no role in the transmission of such diseases" (Shriver, Byer, Shainberg, & Galliano, 2002, p. 136). Recently in Canada, the term STI has become preferred, as STI is viewed as an encompassing term that includes infections that may be asymptomatic (Shriver et al., 2002).

Healthy public policies and guidelines need to be constantly revisited and updated based on research to assist in protecting the public from the consequences of STI and BBP. Currently, researchers are investigating the complex relationship between STI and HIV. To date, what is known about STI and HIV co-infection is that STI and HIV infections often coexist. In other words, having an STI likely increases the susceptibility to HIV infection (Public Health Agency of Canada [PHAC], 2006a). Community health nursing interventions that support people to take precautions to prevent STI may also reduce the risk of HIV infection.

Prior to the discovery of antibiotics, STIs were not treatable, and serious illness was common. Healthy public policies were implemented to test men and women for syphilis prior to marriage and to test women during pregnancy to prevent neonatal infection. With the advent of antibiotic treatment, new policies were developed. For example, for more than 100 years silver nitrate eye drops, or more recently other antibiotics such as erythromycin, were recommended by the Canadian Pediatric Society (CPS) for all newborns to prevent blindness from gonorrhea (CPS, 2006). As well, the CPS advises that all pregnant women be screened for gonorrhea and chlamydia and treated as needed (CPS, 2006).

Currently, all Canadian provinces and territories have developed recommendations and/or guidelines for prenatal HIV testing to promote informed decision making related to neonatal HIV prevention (PHAC, 2005). Antiretroviral medications are an effective way to reduce the risk of HIV transmission to newborns and young children when given to HIV-positive women during pregnancy and/or before birth (PHAC, 2005).

Healthy public policies have also been developed in response to community action. For example, the infection of people with HIV through blood transfusions prompted a national reaction to implement strict blood bank surveillance guidelines. Since 1985, all blood donors are screened for HIV. The risk of HIV transmission via blood transfusion has decreased considerably from 1985 to 2003 from roughly 1 in 16 000 to 1 in greater than a million (PHAC, 2003).

SEXUALLY TRANSMITTED INFECTIONS AND BLOOD BORNE PATHOGENS

STIs can be categorized as bacterial, viral, or ectoparasitic infections. Some viral diseases such as HIV and hepatitis B are found in the blood and are spread through unprotected (condomless) sexual contact as well as contact with infected blood. The following is a brief summary of the most common STIs and BBPs in Canada.

Bacterial STIs

The most common **bacterial STIs** are chlamydia, gonorrhea, and syphilis. *Chlamydia* and *gonorrhea* are primarily transmitted through unprotected vaginal and anal intercourse, and less often through unprotected oral intercourse. The infections can also pass from mother to newborn baby during delivery (PHAC, 2006a). Symptoms in females may include abnormal vaginal discharge or bleeding, lower abdominal pain, or burning during urination (PHAC, 2006a). Symptoms in males may include unusual penile discharge, burning while urinating, or pain or swelling of the testes. Additionally, rectal pain and discharge may indicate infection through anal intercourse. Most often, however, individuals do not experience any symptoms, resulting in the ongoing spread of infection and/or serious complications (PHAC, 2006a). In women, untreated chlamydia and/or gonorrhea infections may lead to pelvic inflammatory disease (PID), which is an inflammation of the upper female genital tract (PHAC, 2006a). Complications of PID may include chronic pelvic pain, infertility, and ectopic pregnancy (PHAC, 2006a).

Many people avoid having STI testing because of their fear of pain and embarrassment. Within a supportive and non-judgmental environment, however, those fears can be alleviated. Chlamydial and gonorrheal infections are detected via urine testing and/or cervical/penile/anal/throat swabbing (Sexuality Information and Education Council of the United States [SIECUS], 2003). Both infections are relatively easy to treat with antibiotics if detected early (PHAC, 2006a).

In Canada, chlamydia is the most prevalent reportable STI. From 1997 to 2004, the chlamydia rate increased by 70% from 113.9 to 197.1 per 100 000 population (PHAC, 2006b). A disproportionate number of women and youth are affected with chlamydia (PHAC, 2006b). Gonorrhea is the

second most prevalent reportable STI in Canada. From 1997 to 2004, the reported rate nearly doubled, from 14.9 to 28.9 per 100 000 population (PHAC, 2006b). Males accounted for greater than 60% of all gonorrhea cases (PHAC, 2006b).

Syphilis is primarily transmitted via unprotected vaginal, oral, or anal sexual contact (PHAC, 2006a). The signs and symptoms of syphilis are often overlooked because in the early stages it manifests as painless sores (chancres) with flu-like symptoms. Diagnosis is often delayed until later stages, when there is already extensive damage to the central nervous or cardiovascular system, resulting in complications such as paralysis or mental illness (PHAC, 2006a). Syphilis is diagnosed through blood tests, swabs with dark-field microscopy, and clinical symptoms (e.g., chancres and rash) (PHAC, 2006a). Syphilis infections are easily treated with antibiotics, and long-term outcomes are reduced with early diagnosis (PHAC, 2006a).

In Canada, syphilis is the least common of the reportable STIs. However, from 1996 to 2004 the rate of infectious syphilis slowly increased from 0.4 to 3.5 per 100 000 population (PHAC, 2006b). In 2004, males accounted for nearly 90% of all syphilis cases (PHAC, 2006b). Recently, there have been several outbreaks in Canada linked to the sex-trade worker and men who have sex with men populations (PHAC, 2006a).

Viral STIs

Genital herpes and *human papillomavirus (HPV)* are highly prevalent **viral STIs** among sexually active people. These viruses are easy to spread, difficult to prevent and detect, and non-reportable. Herpes and HPV are transmitted through vaginal, oral, and/or anal sexual intercourse but mostly through skin-to-skin sexual contact (PHAC, 2006a). Herpes can also be spread from mother to baby through childbirth and can cause serious complications (PHAC, 2006a).

Genital herpes often appears as one or a group of painful, itchy, fluid-filled blisters in or around the genitals, buttocks, and/or thighs. People may experience burning during urination, fever, flu-like symptoms, and swollen glands. After becoming infected with genital herpes, some people experience only one herpes outbreak while others can have an outbreak every month or so. It is important to note that 60% of infections are asymptomatic (PHAC, 2006a).

Herpes is diagnosed through clinical examination or a culture of the fluid drawn from a sore (PHAC, 2006a). There are two types of herpes: type 1 (most commonly found on the mouth) and type 2 (most commonly found on the genitals) (PHAC, 2006a). Both types 1 and 2 are found on the genitals and/or mouth due to the increased occurrence of oral sex. There is no cure for herpes; however, outbreaks can be managed through intensive and/or preventive doses of antiviral medication (PHAC, 2006a).

Many people infected with HPV have no symptoms. There are more than 140 strains of HPV (PHAC, 2006a). Some cause genital warts; others cause abnormal cell growth on the cervix, which may lead to cervical cancer if left untreated. Abnormal cervical changes resulting from HPV are detected only through a Pap test (PHAC, 2006a). Abnormal cervical changes may be monitored by repeat Pap tests, or through referral for colposcopy for more intensive diagnostic testing and treatment. Genital warts appear as groups of cauliflower-like growths in the genital area. HPV is diagnosed through clinical examination and special testing to visualize the genital warts. Freezing, burning, or laser therapies are used to treat genital warts. Because HPV is non-reportable, its incidence is unknown. It is estimated that approximately 70% of adults will experience at least one type of HPV infection in their lifetime (PHAC, 2006a).

Ectoparasites

Ectoparasites include pubic lice (crabs) and scabies, both of which can be transmitted through sexual or non-sexual (e.g., contact with infected towels or bed linens) contact. *Pubic lice* are most commonly found in genital and surrounding hair; however, they can also be found in chest, armpit, or facial hair (PHAC, 2006a). The adult louse lays nits (eggs) in the hair, and within 5 to 10 days the nits hatch. Symptoms of lice include itching and skin irritation.

Scabies are parasites that burrow under the skin, leaving red bumps that cause symptoms of irritation and itchiness (PHAC, 2006a). Scabies can be found on any part of the body; however, they prefer warm moist places such as the genital area. Both conditions can be diagnosed through careful examination of infected areas and are treated with over-the-counter products (e.g., Nix) containing insecticides such as permethrin (PHAC, 2006a).

Vaginal Infections

Vaginal infections include bacterial vaginosis, candidiasis (yeast), and trichomoniasis. Not all these infections are transmitted sexually, but they are often included in the category of STIs. For more information on these conditions, please refer to the *Canadian Guidelines on Sexually Transmitted Infections*, 2006 Edition (PHAC, 2006a).

Blood Borne Pathogens

BBP such as HIV and hepatitis B need special consideration as they are not solely transmitted by sexual activity. Transmission can also occur by reusing drug, tattooing, or piercing equipment that has residual traces of infected blood and from mother to neonate during pregnancy or birth. Additionally, HIV can be transmitted through breast milk, and hepatitis B can be transmitted by sharing razors or toothbrushes with an infected person (Canadian AIDS Society, 2004; PHAC, 2006a).

Many people live with HIV for several years without feeling seriously ill. Even with treatment, however, HIV will eventually progress into AIDS. It is estimated that up to 90% of those infected experience primary or acute HIV symptoms, which occur two to four weeks after infection (PHAC, 2006a). Symptoms are generally mild and include flu-like symptoms such as sore throat, fatigue, fever, and nausea (PHAC, 2006a). The chronic symptomatic phase occurs when the HIV weakens the immune system and the body exhibits long-term symptoms such as swollen lymph nodes, skin lesions, fever, and diarrhea. AIDS is diagnosed when multiple opportunistic infections occur, such as pneumonia, lymphomas, and fungal infections (PHAC, 2006a).

HIV is diagnosed through a special blood test that became available in Canada in 1985. There is a window period of three to six months during which HIV antibodies may remain undetectable, requiring an individual to return for follow-up testing (PHAC, 2006a). Pre- and post-test counselling by CHNs is important because they can engage clients, prepare them for the potential impact of test results, and raise awareness of risk-reduction practices such as condom use. Some provinces regrettably forgo pre- and post-test counselling as it is assumed to be time-consuming and costly. Unfortunately, there is no cure for HIV infection, but there is treatment. A variety of antiretroviral drugs are now available that delay the progression of HIV infection to AIDS (PHAC, 2006a).

From 1985 to 2005, approximately 60 160 positive HIV tests were reported in Canada (PHAC, 2006c). In 2005, 43.5% of all positive HIV tests were among the men who have sex with men (MSM) population, 30.9% were among the heterosexual population, and 19.5% were among injection drug users (PHAC, 2006c). Though Aboriginal people compose only 3.3% of Canada's population, in 2005, 22.4% of all new HIV infections were among Aboriginal people (PHAC, 2006d). In Canada, males are five times more likely to be HIV-positive than are women (PHAC, 2006c).

Many people are infected with hepatitis B without knowing it because they often do not experience any symptoms. Approximately 30% to 50% of adults infected with hepatitis B will show nonspecific symptoms including fatigue, nausea, vomiting, jaundice (yellowing of the skin or whites of the eyes), decreased appetite, and joint swelling or pain (PHAC, 2006a, 2006e). Most people infected with hepatitis B recover; however, some people become chronic carriers. Most carriers have no symptoms but can infect others. Carriers may eventually develop liver cancer or cirrhosis (PHAC, 2006a; PHAC, 2006e). Hepatitis B is diagnosed through blood testing. Combination antiviral drugs are available for those with chronic active hepatitis B (PHAC, 2006e).

It is estimated that fewer than 5% of Canadians have markers of past hepatitis B infection, and fewer than 1% are carriers of hepatitis B (PHAC, 2006e). Certain sub-populations tend to be at greater risk for the virus, including those who were born in endemic areas, men who have sex with men, sex-trade workers, and injection drug users (PHAC, 2006e). The widespread availability of hepatitis B vaccine has assisted in prevention of the infection. Publicly funded vaccination programs are offered in all Canadian provinces and territories. Hepatitis B vaccine is routinely offered to all Canadian children/adolescents. If parents are hepatitis B carriers and/or they were born in endemic areas, the vaccination is offered to children during the first year of life (PHAC, 2006e).

IMPLICATIONS OF STI AND BBP

All STIs and BBPs are underreported, as many Canadians do not go for testing or do not know they are infected. CHNs are aware of the large number of people living with incurable, non-reportable STIs such as herpes and HPV. Rates of reportable STIs (e.g., chlamydia) and BBPs (e.g., HIV) provide CHNs with some understanding regarding the scope of the problem. If STIs and BBPs remain inadequately addressed and treated, they can lead to ongoing spread of the infection, infertility, neonatal complications, pelvic inflammatory disease, or even death (PHAC, 2006b). STIs can negatively impact a person's relationships, self-esteem, mental health, coping abilities, and work productivity. Additionally, there are societal economic implications due to the medical costs associated with diagnosis and treatment, especially if there are complications such as infertility and neonatal infection.

CHNs must attempt to address not only medical issues such as treatment, but also the social and economic issues. For example, CHNs can raise awareness in the workplace and community to increase the funding for HIV medication, research, and alternative employment during times of intense treatment. Some CHNs work with groups that support people living with HIV or herpes who wish to pursue loving, sexual relationships with an understanding partner.

STI and BBP Prevention and Risk Reduction

Accurate and consistent use of latex or polyurethane **male condoms** or polyurethane **female condoms** is important to decrease the transmission of STIs. However, condoms may not be 100% effective in protecting against herpes or HPV (e.g., genital warts on the testicles or labia). Abstinence from all types of sexual activity is the only 100% effective method of preventing STI. Infection by BBPs, such as HIV and hepatitis B, are prevented by condom use and by using clean needles and equipment for tattooing, piercing, and injecting drugs. Condoms and/or dental dams should always be used for oral sex (PHAC, 2006b).

Community health nurses are challenged with the issue of "safer sex fatigue," which is a term used to describe an individual's tiredness regarding complying with and hearing about safer sex messages, resulting in an increase in risky behaviour (Canadian AIDS Society, 2004). Interventions such as sexual health education are important, but to have an impact they must be timely and relevant to the target population. It is vital to find innovative ways to promote the use of male and female condoms and dental dams. CHNs must "think upstream" and use health promotion approaches that address the issues of their target population. CHNs can reach individuals through street outreach, counselling, and peer mentoring programs. Furthermore, CHNs can explore innovative ways to make these risk reduction measures appealing to groups or communities through poster and social marketing campaigns. CHNs can work with other sectors and multidisciplinary groups to develop healthy public policy to address STI and BBP issues.

Offering chlamydia urine testing in outreach vans and putting condom machines in schools are examples of health promotion activities resulting from healthy public policies.

Special Populations

The following is not an exhaustive discussion of all the hard-to-reach or marginalized populations in Canada. However, it is meant to raise awareness of some special groups and their risk for acquiring or transmitting STIs and BBPs.

Men Who Have Sex with Men In Canada, the MSM population has the highest proportion of HIV and AIDS when compared to other subpopulations (PHAC, 2006c). A survey of Ontario self-identified gay and bisexual MSM determined 35% to 40% of respondents had participated in unprotected anal intercourse within the last year; approximately 17% had unprotected anal intercourse with a partner whose HIV status was unknown; and 4% had unprotected anal intercourse with a partner who tested positive for HIV (Myers et al., 2004).

Although health education messages addressing condom use are constantly being reinforced, it is clear from this study that certain cohorts of MSM are still not being reached with current prevention strategies. It is important for CHNs to *work with* the MSM population to develop messaging that is innovative and relevant. Additionally, it is important for CHNs to deliver messaging at venues frequented by the MSM population. For example, Myers et al. (2004) noted that MSM search for sexual relations in a number of different sites including gay bars (60.3%), the internet (35.3%), and bath houses (31.4%). These sites can therefore serve as venues for prevention messaging.

Sex-Trade Workers Sex-trade workers are at increased risk for contracting and spreading STIs and BBPs for several reasons, including their high numbers of sexual partners; limited ability to access social, health, and legal services; lifestyle risks such as substance use; and limited economic resources (PHAC, 2006a). Condom use varies among sex-trade workers and the choice to use condoms is frequently controlled by the customer (Rekart, 2005). Customers often refuse to use condoms or offer additional pay for "condomless" sex (Rekart, 2005).

CHNs working with this group can promote a variety of risk-reduction strategies (e.g., correct use of male or female condoms) to prevent this population from acquiring and/or spreading STI and BBP. Since access to and the cost of condoms may deter sex-trade workers from using them, it is paramount that condoms are available for free. Peer education strategies have proven promising in terms of increasing knowledge related to STI and HIV and safer sex practices (Rekart, 2005). CHNs can work with sex-trade workers to educate their peers regarding risk-reduction strategies such as condom negotiation. Overall, it is important that the services developed for sex-trade workers (e.g., peer education, hepatitis B vaccinations, STI testing and/or treatment) are delivered innovatively (e.g., from a mobile van, hotel room, community centre) and with the workers' input (Rekart, 2005).

Street Youth It is estimated that approximately 150 000 youth in Canada live on the streets on any given day (PHAC, 2006f). This population is extremely vulnerable because, for many, addressing the basic necessities of life is of greater priority than preventing or addressing potential health risks (PHAC, 2006g). As a result, youth involved in street culture often do not take effective action in preventing STIs and BBPs (PHAC, 2006g).

In a 2003 Canadian-based study of street youth, it was determined that street youth had a chlamydia rate that was approximately 10 times more, and a gonorrhea rate that was 20 to 30 times more, than that of mainstream youth, and that approximately 25% of street youth were involved in the sex trade at some point (PHAC, 2006g). Resources must be allocated for both sufficient outreach with this population and comprehensive programming that entails prevention, screening, and treatment services (PHAC, 2006g).

Injection Drug Users Injection drug users represent a growing concern for CHNs, as the craving for "another hit" overrides the importance of using a clean needle to prevent the transmission of HIV or hepatitis B (PHAC, 2006d). Some injection drug users may take years to rehabilitate. Offering better access to condoms and clean needles/drug equipment via needle exchange programs and safer injection facilities may help these populations lower their risk of contracting HIV while they search for effective treatment. Needle exchange programs and safer injection facilities are discussed further below.

New Immigrants In 2005, more than 260 000 immigrants arrived in Canada (Citizenship and Immigration Canada, 2006). Language, cultural, socioeconomic, and educational barriers may deter this population from seeking health services. This includes STI and HIV testing, education, and counselling (PHAC, 2006a). New immigrants are overwhelmed with adapting to new cultural and health care practices. Many come from countries where HIV, hepatitis, and other STIs are more prevalent and treatment is inaccessible (PHAC, 2006a). Cultural beliefs may also influence a person's motivation to access health services. Some may try a variety of herbs or culturally accepted medications before seeking medical treatment for an STI or HIV. Many Canadian provinces lack services and resources that are translated, culturally sensitive, and accessible to newcomers (PHAC, 2006a). It is important that CHNs be attentive to the stressful and complex issues faced by immigrants as they integrate into Canadian culture (PHAC, 2006a).

Unwilling or Unable Population Researchers have identified that some HIV-positive individuals are "unwilling or unable" (e.g., refuse to disclose HIV-positive status to sexual partners) to prevent the spread of HIV. The research has determined these individuals often present with one or more of the following issues: psychiatric issues (e.g., depression, fetal alcohol syndrome); addictions; social deficits (e.g., lack of support and housing, involvement in the sex trade); and health deficits (e.g., lack of HIV knowledge) (Calgary Coalition on HIV/

AIDS, 2004). Researchers believe these variables contribute to higher-risk activities (e.g., having sex without a condom) and can impede a person's efficacy at implementing risk-reduction practices. Health authorities across Canada are addressing this issue in different ways, ranging from implementing comprehensive referral systems to providing housing and treatment.

Innovative STI and BBP Prevention Interventions in Canada

The PHPM (Hamilton & Bhatti, 1996) provides a comprehensive tool for CHNs to utilize when planning STI and BBP prevention interventions with individuals, groups, and populations. (Refer to Chapter 6 for more information on the PHPM.) Novel and innovative strategies are being implemented across Canada in an attempt to lower the prevalence of STIs and BBPs.

Needle Exchange Programs and Safer Injection Facilities Injection drug use is a mounting public health concern in Canada. Individuals who participate in high-risk drug injection behaviours (e.g., sharing needles) pose a number of potential health risks to themselves and others, such as transmission of HIV and hepatitis B and C (Elliott, Malkin, & Gold, 2002). Some Canadian communities have addressed the issue of needle sharing with harm-reduction strategies such as needle exchange programs and safer injection facilities. The harm-reduction model acknowledges that abstinence from all drugs is not realistic for all people and therefore, although drug use is not condoned, it is seen as essential to implement risk-reduction strategies to reduce harmful outcomes related to drug use (Elliott et al., 2002).

Case Study

A fictitious community called Realville has a large population of immigrant women living with HIV. Several CHNs work in a lower-income sector of the city with this population. The women's literacy levels are low and their cultural beliefs influence them to have large families. The CHNs understand, through a literature review and talking with their clients, that appropriate accessible services are lacking for immigrant women with HIV.

Using the PHPM, the CHNs focus on addressing access to health services that consider the women's cultural beliefs and practices. They collaborate with a group of representatives from health, social services, and business sectors to discuss the lack of services for this group. The group conducts an assessment to determine if there are any gaps in health services for immigrant women in the city. They work together to apply for and secure sustained funding to develop adequate support groups,

→

outreach services, and appropriate treatment services staffed by professionals and peer mentors who are aware of the cultural issues. Culturally appropriate HIV teaching is conducted with these groups to address cultural barriers to accessing and using condoms.

Discussion Questions

1. What determinants of health will the CHNs need to be aware of when working with the immigrant women of Realville?

2. What health promotion strategies can the CHNs and community agencies implement to address the issues of these clients?

3. How can the CHNs involve the women and community agencies who work with immigrant women in the development of these strategies?

Canadian Research Box 29.1

Flicker, S., Skinner, H., Read, S., Veinot, T., McClelland, A., Saulnier, P., et al. (2005). Falling through the cracks of the big cities: Who is meeting the needs of HIV-positive youth? *Canadian Journal of Public Health, 96*(4), 308–312.

The purpose of the research was to investigate, from a Canadian perspective, the manner in which professionals can better support youth (ages 12 to 24) living with HIV. The researchers utilized a qualitative, community-based participatory research approach for their investigation. Youth participants were recruited via flyers, personal invitations, community-based agencies, and hospital clinics. Youth interested in participating contacted the research team directly. In-depth, semi-structured interviews and a short demographic survey were completed with 34 Ontario-based youth.

The researchers collaborated with HIV-infected youth and the professionals working with them to analyze the data. Thematic analysis determined there were three major areas in the lives of youth where support was needed:

(a) *Personal feelings regarding HIV.* Youth indicated they experience an array of emotional responses to their HIV infection status. Feelings of hopelessness, isolation, and loneliness were predominant.

(b) *Obstacles to societal participation.* Various social (e.g., stigma surrounding HIV and a lack of family support) and structural (e.g., poverty and homophobia) obstacles hinder youth from fully participating in society.

(c) *Types of supports needed.* Youth experience difficulty accessing HIV support services and expressed mixed feelings toward existing services.

The researchers stated that better supporting the needs of youth infected with HIV not only will positively impact this population but also may limit the spread of HIV to oth-

ers. They concluded by stating that as the number of HIV-infected youth increases, it is timely to re-evaluate present tertiary prevention interventions targeting this population.

Discussion Questions:

1. How can CHNs involve youth living with HIV in developing HIV-prevention strategies?

2. What determinants of health can be targeted to improve the health of youth living with HIV?

Needle exchange programs (NEPs) provide injection drug users with free, sterile injecting equipment to reduce their risk of contracting and/or spreading infection (Elliott et al., 2002). Evaluation research conducted on a Vancouver-based NEP demonstrated a reduction in needle sharing (Wood et al., 2002). Although NEPs are controversial, they are widely accepted as a method for minimizing the spread of blood borne diseases (Elliott et al., 2002; Wood et al., 2002).

Safer injection facilities (SIFs) provide a safe location for drug users to inject their own drugs with clean equipment under the supervision of medically trained professionals. The main objectives of SIFs are to decrease the spread of infectious disease, improve contact between the health care system and injection drug users, decrease the use of drugs in public places, decrease fatal and non-fatal drug overdoses, and increase recruitment of injection drug users into addiction treatment and rehabilitation programs (Wood et al., 2004a). Although SIFs are an innovative public health intervention, they are extremely controversial in various countries, including Canada.

In 2003, health care providers in Vancouver piloted the first medically supervised SIF in North America (Kerr, Tyndall, Montaner, & Wood, 2005). Evaluation research of this program indicated several positive outcomes including decreased syringe sharing (Kerr et al., 2005), decreased injection-related litter, decreased numbers of individuals injecting in public, and decreased numbers of syringes discarded in public (Wood et al., 2004b).

Social Marketing Campaigns *Social marketing* can be defined as "a program-planning process that applies commercial marketing concepts and techniques to promote voluntary behavior change" (Grier & Bryant, 2005, p. 319). In Canada, these types of campaigns are becoming more innovative as they provide blatant and, at times, provocative messages to different segments of the population. Unfortunately, many of these campaigns are not properly evaluated for their short- or long-term impact on the target population.

One campaign that did have evaluation results was launched in 2001 by the AIDS Committee of Toronto. The "Welcome to Condom Country" campaign targeted Toronto-based MSM (SHEA & Company, 2002). The primary objectives of the campaign were to raise awareness regarding the increasing incidence of HIV infection among MSM, and to promote the adoption of safer sex practices. A variety of promotional materials (e.g., television and newspaper advertisements, posters, brochures, post cards) were produced. The

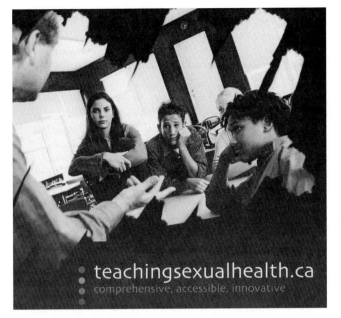

Photo 29.1

Website That Promotes Sexual Health.

Credit: teachingsexualhealth.ca

controversy generated by the campaign also contributed to the success of the project as it received significant media coverage locally, provincially, nationally, and internationally, which prompted more opportunities for discussion about the key campaign messages. Nearly 2500 men from Toronto participated in the evaluation questionnaire. Approximately 81% of the respondents remembered seeing campaign promotional materials and almost 43% indicated they were more likely to participate in safer sex practices as a result of the campaign. Additionally, 75% felt that the campaign was effective in reaching the MSM population (SHEA & Company, 2002).

Telehealth and Web-Based Resources   *Telehealth* and *web-based resources* have become important in terms of health education and prevention of STIs and BBPs, as well as support for those living with HIV (Kalichman, Benotsch, Weinhardt, Austin, Luke, & Cherry, 2003; White & Dorman, 2001). Telehealth is the utilization of advanced telecommunications technology in order to exchange health-related information and administer health services that transcend cultural, time, social, and geographical barriers (Care, Gregory, Whittaker, & Chernomas, 2003). Electronic mail and the internet are means of providing telehealth services to those seeking information (Care et al., 2003) about STIs and BBPs. Individuals may experience increased comfort utilizing email as a form of communicating, especially if their questions or concerns are personal or sensitive in nature (Care et al., 2003).

Although telehealth is promising for sexual health promotion, it is important for CHNs to acknowledge its downfalls. First, "liability for care practices and potential misdiagnosis . . . provided through the medium of distance or electronic technologies are issues warranting careful exploration" (Care et al., 2003, p. 249). Second, this technology may be inaccessible to those who cannot afford computers.

Finally, when communication is conducted electronically, the contextualization of the client's situation may be lost.

Websites can also be used to disseminate STI and BBP prevention information. For example, www.teachingsexual health.ca (see Photo 29.1) was developed to provide accurate, relevant, and timely resources for Alberta-based sexual health educators, parents, and students. The website provides educators with teaching strategies while considering diversity issues such as ethnicity, differing abilities, and gender in the learning setting.

HPV Vaccination   In July 2006, Health Canada approved a vaccine that protects against the various strains of HPV that cause the majority of cervical cancer and genital warts. The vaccine is considered a medical milestone in terms of cancer prevention. It is anticipated that the long-term implications of the vaccine will result in a reduction of cervical cancer cases, although the need for women to have regular Pap tests will continue. The National Advisory Council on Immunization (NACI) released a *Statement on Human Papillomavirus Immunization* in 2007 to inform Canadian health care providers regarding appropriate use of the vaccine (NACI, 2007). The Society of Obstetricians and Gynecologists of Canada (SOGC) has developed an innovative website, (www. hpvinfo.ca) to provide information to teens, adults, parents, teachers, and health professionals (SOGC, 2006).

Summary

This chapter discusses the complex issues surrounding STIs and BBPs in Canada. The history of STIs and how healthy public policy addresses STI and BBP prevention are briefly outlined. A review of STI and BBP statistical trends and epidemiology are presented. The special needs of marginalized populations who may present unique challenges to CHNs related to STI and BBP are illustrated. Suggestions on how CHNs can use the PHP model to plan innovative prevention strategies are made. In conclusion, the PHP model provides a strong guide for CHNs when planning future STI and BBP promotion and prevention programs within communities.

KEY TERMS

sexually transmitted infections (STIs)
blood borne pathogens (BBPs)
human immunodeficiency virus (HIV)
bacterial STIs
viral STIs
male condoms
female condoms
needle exchange programs (NEPs)
safer injection facilities (SIFs)

INDIVIDUAL CRITICAL THINKING EXERCISES

1. The rate of HIV infection in pregnant women is rising in Canada. More than half of pregnant women being diagnosed with HIV are from a country where HIV is endemic. Transmission from mother to neonate can be

reduced to almost zero through prenatal HIV testing and the use of chemoprophylaxis treatment during pregnancy, labour, and birth and for the neonate (O'Connor & MacDonald, 2002). How can CHNs work with pregnant immigrant/refugee women to use health promotion strategies to reduce HIV transmission during pregnancy?

2. STI rates are increasing in males 15–24 years old. The Public Health Agency of Canada (2006a) states that testing and education are important to prevent STIs. Unfortunately, many youth at risk for STIs leave school early and become street involved, thus missing the benefit of sexual health education opportunities. What determinants of health could be addressed by CHNs related to the issues of street youth and STI?

GROUP CRITICAL THINKING EXERCISES

1. Gay youth often face rejection from significant support systems such as family and friends when they come out. Some youth quit school and leave home to live on the street. Some rely on panhandling and prostitution to support themselves and pay for drugs that help them cope. High-risk activities and a lack of resources increase gay youths' risk for STIs and HIV. How can a CHN use the *Canadian Community Health Nursing Standards of Practice (CCHNSP)* (see Appendix A) to plan care for gay youth within a sexual health clinic?

2. To address the complications associated with STI and HIV, healthy public policy has been initiated and developed by policy-makers and health professionals, but often with little input from the public. How can CHNs use primary health care's principle of public participation (CNA, 2000) to inform the development of healthy public policy related to STI and HIV?

REFERENCES

Calgary Coalition on HIV/AIDS. (2004). *Phase two: Guidelines for working with U2 clients.* Calgary: Author.

Canadian AIDS Society. (2004). *HIV transmission: Guidelines for assessing risk* (5th ed.). Retrieved August 7, 2006, from http://www.cdnaids.ca/web/repguide.nsf/pages/cas-rep-0307.

Canadian Pediatric Society (CPS). (2006). *Position Statement: Recommendations for the prevention of neonatal ophthalmia.* Retrieved September 5, 2006, from http://www.cps.ca/English/statements/ID/ID02-03.htm.

Care, W.D., Gregory, D., Whittaker, C., & Chernomas, W. (2003). Nursing, technology, and informatics: An easy or uneasy alliance? In M. McIntyre, & E. Thomlinson (Eds.), *Realities of Canadian nursing: Professional, practice and power issues* (pp. 243–261). Philadelphia: Lippincott Williams & Wilkins.

Citizenship and Immigration Canada. (2006). *Facts and figures 2005: Immigration overview.* Retrieved August 25, 2006, from http://www.cic.gc.ca/english/pub/facts2005/index.html.

Elliott, R., Malkin, I., & Gold, J. (2002). *Establishing safe injection facilities in Canada: Legal and ethical issues.* Ottawa: Canadian HIV/AIDS Legal Network.

Flicker, S., Skinner, H., Read, S., Veinot, T., McClelland, A., Saulnier, P., et al. (2005). Falling through the cracks of the big cities: Who is meeting the needs of HIV-positive youth? *Canadian Journal of Public Health, 96*(4), 308–312.

Grier, S., & Bryant, C. A. (2005). Social marketing in public health. *Annual Review of Public Health, 26,* 319–339.

Hamilton, N., & Bhatti, T. (1996). *Population health promotion: An integrated model of population health and health promotion.* Ottawa: Public Health Agency of Canada, Health Promotion Development Division. Retrieved August 31, 2006, from http://www.phac-aspc.gc.ca/ph-sp/phdd/php/php.htm.

Kalichman, S. C., Benotsch, E. G., Weinhardt, L., Austin, J., Luke, W., & Cherry, C. (2003). Health-related internet use, coping, social support, and health indicators in people living with HIV/AIDS: Preliminary results from a community survey. (2003). *Health Psychology, 22*(1), 111–116.

Kerr, T., Tyndall, M., Montaner, J., & Wood, E. (2005). Safer injection facility use and syringe sharing in injection drug users. *Lancet, 366,* 316–318.

Myers, T., Allman, D., Calzavara, L., Maxwell, J., Remia, R., Swantee, C., et al. (2004). *Ontario's men survey final report.* Retrieved August 25, 2006, from http://cbr.cbrc.net/modules.php?name=News&file=article&sid=275.

National Advisory Council on Immunization (NACI). (2007). Statement on human papillomavirus vaccine. *Canadian Communicable Disease Report, 33*(ACS-2), 1–32. Retrieved April 29, 2007, from http://www.phac-aspc.gc.ca/publicat/ccdr-rmtc/07pdf/acs33-02.pdf.

O'Connor, K. S., & MacDonald, S. E. (2002). Aiming for zero: Preventing mother-to-child transmission of HIV. *Canadian Medical Association Journal, 166*(7), 909–910.

Public Health Agency of Canada (PHAC). (2003). *Transfusion transmitted injuries section: Transfusion transmitted diseases/infections.* Retrieved August 31, 2006, from http://www.phac-aspc.gc.ca/hcai-iamss/tti-it/ttdi_e.html.

Public Health Agency of Canada (PHAC). (2005). *HIV/AIDS epi update May 2005: Perinatal transmission of HIV.* Retrieved August 31, 2006, from http://www.phac-aspc.gc.ca/publicat/epiu-aepi/epi-05/pdf/epi_05_e.pdf.

Public Health Agency of Canada (PHAC). (2006a). *Canadian guidelines on sexually transmitted infections 2006 edition.* Retrieved August 1, 2006, from http://www.phac-aspc.gc.ca/std-mts/sti_2006/sti_intro2006_e.html.

Public Health Agency of Canada (PHAC). (2006b). *Canadian sexually transmitted infections surveillance report, 2004: Pre-release.* Retrieved August 1, 2006, from http://www.phac-aspc.gc.ca/std-mts/stddata_pre06_04/index.html.

Public Health Agency of Canada (PHAC). (2006c). *HIV and AIDS in Canada: Surveillance report to December 31, 2005.* Retrieved August 10, 2006, from http://www.phac-aspc.gc.ca/publicat/aids-sida/haic-vsac1205/index.html.

Public Health Agency of Canada (PHAC). (2006d). *Focusing on populations at risk.* Retrieved September 28, 2006, from http://www.phac-aspc.gc.ca/aids-sida/populations_e.html.

Public Health Agency of Canada (PHAC). (2006e). *Canadian immunization guide* (7th ed.). Retrieved April 29, 2007, from http://www.phac-aspc.gc.ca/publicat/cig-gci/index.html.

Public Health Agency of Canada (PHAC). (2006f). *Street youth in Canada: Findings from enhanced surveillance of Canadian street youth, 1999–2003.* Retrieved July 15,

2006, from http://www.phac-aspc.gc.ca/std-mts/reports_06/youth_e.html.

Public Health Agency of Canada (PHAC). (2006g). *Sexually transmitted infection in Canadian s treet youth: Findings from enhanced surveillance of Canadian street youth, 1999–2003.* Retrieved July 15, 2006, from http://www.phac-aspc.gc.ca/std-mts/reports_06/sti-youth_e.html.

Rekart, M. L. (2005). Sex work harm reduction. *Lancet, 366,* 2123–2134.

SHEA & Company. (2002). *Welcome to condom country campaign final evaluation report.* Retrieved August 10, 2006, from http://www.actoronto.org/website/research.nsf/pages/condomcountryreportfinal.

Shriver, S. P., Byer, C. O., Shainberg, L. W., & Galliano, G. (2002). *Dimensions of human sexuality* (6th ed.). Boston: McGraw-Hill.

Sexuality Information and Education Council of the United States (SIECUS). (2003). *Fact sheet: The truth about STI.* Retrieved April 29, 2007, from http://www.siecus.org/pubs/fact/fact0019.html.

Society of Obstetricians and Gynaecologists of Canada (SOGC). (2006). *SOGC media advisory: Interim statements on HPV immunization.* Retrieved April 29, 2007, from http://www.sogc.org/media/advisories%2D20061019%5Fe.asp.

White, M., & Dorman, S. M. (2001). Receiving social support online: Implications for health education. *Health Education Research: Theory & Practice, 16*(6), 693–707.

Wood, E., Tyndall, M. W., Spittal, P. M., Li, K., Hogg, R. S., Montancr, J. S., et al. (2002). Factors associated with persistent high-risk syringe sharing in the presence of an established needle exchange programme. *AIDS, 16*(6), 941–3.

Wood, E., Kerr, T., Montaner, J. S., Strathdee, S. A., Wodak, A., Hankins, C. A., et al. (2004a). Rationale for evaluating North America's first medically supervised safer-injecting facility. *The Lancet Infectious Diseases, 4*(5), 301–6.

Wood, E., Kerr, T., Small, W., Li, K., Marsh, D. C., Montaner, J. S. G., et al. (2004b). Changes in public order after the opening of a medically supervised safer injecting facility for illicit injection drug users. *Canadian Medical Association Journal, 171*(7), 731–734.

ADDITIONAL RESOURCES

Websites

Canadian AIDS Society
   www.cdnaids.ca

Canadian Federation for Sexual Health
   www.cfsh.ca

Canadian HIV/AIDS Legal Network
   www.aidslaw.ca

Public Health Agency of Canada: *Canadian Guidelines on Sexually Transmitted Infections* 2006 Edition
   www.phac-aspc.gc.ca/std-mts/sti_2006/sti_intro2006_e. html

Public Health Agency of Canada, Sexual Health and Sexually Transmitted Infections
   www.phac-aspc.gc.ca/std-mts

Sex Information and Education Council of Canada
   www.sieccan.org

Society of Obstetricians and Gynaecologists of Canada
   www.sexualityandu.ca

Teaching Sexual Health
   www.teachingsexualhealth.ca

About the Authors

Wendi Lokanc-Diluzio, RN, BN (University of Calgary), MN (University of Calgary), has worked in public health since 1997. Since 2002, she has worked as a Sexual Health Specialist for the Calgary Health Region, where she provides leadership in the area of sexual health promotion and has had the opportunity to develop, implement, and evaluate many health promotion projects. In 2006, Wendi codeveloped and cotaught a blended learning school health promotion course to an inter-professional group of students attending the University of Calgary.

Alison Nelson, RN, BScN (University of Alberta), MN (University of Calgary), has worked as a public/community health nurse in rural and urban Alberta and B.C. since 1991. She was an Instructor with the Faculty of Nursing, University of Calgary from 2001 to 2006 and taught in the areas of community health nursing and sexual health promotion. Alison was Co-Director of the Faculty's Community Health Nursing Unit, where she was involved in several projects focusing on building capacity and/or creating continuing education opportunities for Community Health Nurses (see www.chnalberta.org). Currently, Alison is co-chair of the Alberta Society for the Promotion of Sexual Health (www.aspsh.ca). She is the former Manager of Sexual & Reproductive Health in the Calgary Health Region. Presently, she is the Decision Support and Evaluation Manager, Screening Programs, Population Health and Information, Alberta Cancer Board.

Janet L. Wayne, RN, BScN (University of Alberta), MN (University of Calgary), is currently a Quality Improvement Consultant for the Calgary Health Region. Janet has worked in the area of sexual and reproductive health and communicable disease for more than a decade. She has spearheaded and managed a number of large, innovative health promotion and telehealth projects involving community and cross-ministry partners such as

→

teachingsexualhealth.ca. Janet has presented these sexual health projects at various conferences across Canada and to university classes in Calgary.

Janet B. Hettler, RN, DipN (Kelsey Institute of Applied Arts and Sciences, Saskatoon), BScN (University of Saskatchewan), MN (University of Calgary), is currently the Manager of the Crisis Nursery at Calgary Children's Cottage Society. Janet has worked in public health since 1981, initially as a public health nurse in rural Alberta. In 1988, she began working in the area of sexual and reproductive health, first in a rural health unit outside Calgary then with the Calgary Health Region as a Sexual and Reproductive Health Clinical Nurse Specialist. During her time in sexual and reproductive health she oversaw a number of sexual health promotion projects.

Future Directions

Lynnette Leeseberg Stamler and Lucia Yiu

In Villeneuve and MacDonald's report *Towards 2020: Visions for Nursing* (2006), we find scenarios of nursing in a future that looks quite different from what the majority of your teachers were taught, as well as what you will see as you graduate in the near future from basic nursing programs. In describing the health care system, Rosemary Goodyear (as cited in Villeneuve & MacDonald, 2006) suggests that "communities are moving away from doctors as primary care provider and are more open to alternative providers like NPs and RNs" (p. 94). *Primary health care* is the way to achieve health all for all. (See Chapter 7.) The *Towards 2020* report identifies self-care as the "largest contributor to the creation and maintenance of health" (Villeneuve & MacDonald, 2006, p. 95). Self-care is described as taking place "in the socio-environmental-political-cultural context of the individual and is influenced by resources available" (p. 95). The second-largest contributor is identified as "all the community health and social resources in place to support health and keep people well" (p. 95). In other words, nurses play a key role in providing a supportive environment for people to attain good health in their own communities—where they live, work, learn, and play.

According to the Canadian Institute for Health Information (2007), two-thirds of nurses currently work in institutional settings. Villeneuve and MacDonald (2006) suggest that by 2020 the percentages will have reversed, with two-thirds working in community-based care. Further, they identify that nurses will "develop and implement broad programs of health promotion and illness prevention in schools, workplaces and communities, and [be] a strong, visible presence" (p. 99). Finally, they identify that nursing research will "place less emphasis on nurses and nursing processes than was the case 20 years ago, focusing instead on health, the needs of patients and communities, and providing sound evidence to guide policy and practice" (p. 99).

Other futuristic documents support this new picture and offer additional details (Porter-O'Grady, 2001a, 2001b). It is clear that if the futuristic picture is an accurate one, the changes in the next few years will be profound. There are implications for nursing education as well as nursing practice.

How are we preparing for such changes? First, let's look at changes in nursing practice, specifically community nursing practice. We know that the demographics of the Canadian population are changing, as seen in the age stratifications, the cultural mix, and the increase in Aboriginal people. Strategies to improve population health will need to be targeted to specific groups. The "one-size" approach will no longer fit all. As the Canadian population becomes increasingly diverse, nurses must be mindful to move beyond cultural sensitization and awareness and direct their care to promoting cultural harmony and acceptance of individual cultural differences. By doing so, nurses will move one step closer to promoting equality and social justice in the communities we care for.

With longer life expectancy, we encounter various illnesses such as cancer, diabetes, heart conditions, or Alzheimer's disease during our life course. New advances in genetics and other treatments will radically change how we adapt and age. The need for emergency preparedness will not diminish, but will be always present, albeit with a variety of concerns, from HIV/AIDS to avian flu. Nurses face new health challenges in helping individuals and populations through chronic disease management, reducing dependence on hospital services, and supporting people at home. We need to work interprofessionally and intraprofessionally to create a seamless health system. This system is expected to provide timely access to appropriate services and care to the clients. Health promotion and illness prevention will be key to reducing health care costs and to promoting our communities in the healthiest state possible.

What will not change is the importance of using frameworks such as the determinants of health to assist CHNs in proactively planning for the future and positioning ourselves as co-creators of change in practice. We must be politically savvy and go beyond local and national needs. CHNs must make every effort to be well informed of how socioeconomic and political trends and environmental changes such as global warming may impact the health of various communities.

Some steps have already been taken at the national level. In response to many factors, including public inquiries into specific disease outbreaks, investments have been made into areas of public health at the national level. These investments have included the creation of the Public Health Agency of Canada (PHAC), the creation of the position of Chief Public Health Officer, and also the identification of a federal cabinet minister for public health. The PHAC has been working with practitioners to develop a set of core competencies for all workers in public health, as well as specific competencies for individual professions, in collaboration with the Community Health Nurses Association of Canada (CHNAC) Standards of Practice (both reprinted in this book's Appendices). The standards and competencies are complementary documents, describing the desired practice of a nurse with two years of experience in community health. CHNAC has also partnered with the Canadian Nurses Association (CNA) to create a nursing certification in community health nursing. Nursing graduates have the opportunity to achieve initial and continuing certification through examination and continuing education.

Concerns about nursing shortages are not limited to acute-care facilities. At this time there are difficulties providing sufficient numbers of practitioners to fulfill current needs, much less a new future. One way to accomplish this task is to increase the number of nursing students in basic programs. However, this capacity building is not limited to increasing the numbers of nursing students but also to increasing the number of faculty members (and, in some cases, enhancing their skills) to produce the numbers of community nurses required to influence the health of Canadians. Further, increased globalization has forced our profession to consider such things as ethical hiring practices for international nurses, and global standards for basic nursing education.

As well, there are changes in community nursing education. Community nursing has always been part of a baccalaureate nursing curriculum, with a broad-based approach and the individual, family, group, aggregate, and population identified as clients. Public health nursing is identified as having a stronger focus on population health. However, there are both challenges and new opportunities peeking over the horizon. The Canadian Association of Schools of Nursing created a task force that has since become a permanent sub-committee specifically related to public health education. Members of the sub-committee are working with nurse educators, employers, and other stakeholders to examine the competencies and standards as they apply to new graduates, and how that might change basic nursing curricula. The Canadian Nurse Practitioner Initiative (CNPI) from the CNA has worked with provincial organizations and schools of nursing to create curricula for primary health care nurse practitioner programs. Individual groups, such as the Professional Education Working Group, are looking at specific areas of specialty (e.g., vaccine providers) and ascertaining the education and skills required for competent practice. All of these continue to inform basic and continuing education in nursing.

Graduate opportunities are also increasing in number, scope, and variety. Specific to community nursing, graduate nursing students have opportunities to tailor master's in nursing degrees to a community specialty or consider one of the new interdisciplinary Master's in Public Health programs that are springing up across the country. In addition, schools of public health are proposed in several universities—representing additional opportunities for advanced interdisciplinary work and research in community health with a strong nursing contribution.

Research in community nursing is also increasing; a recent project funded by the Canadian Health Services Research Fund examines Canadian community and public health nursing capacity to ascertain exactly what is being done and what needs to be done in the future (Underwood, 2006). It is such research as this that assists nursing to be proactive in building capacity and in translating knowledge to practice to advance our nursing profession. This translation is one of community nursing's strengths. We add to the national picture through the knowledge and data of our local communities, and then, when national priorities and strategies have been formulated, we tailor them to our local communities to enhance success. We are the health profession that clearly contributes to both arenas. At the end, the concerted efforts played by all community nursing educators, researchers, and practitioners will benefit the communities for whom we care.

So, what of the future? As each of us gazes into our cloudy crystal ball, a few things are discernable. One is that nurses, including CHNs, have the skills and knowledge to be a political force for the health of Canadians, if we so choose. By supporting our professional organizations, by being proactive in the political process, and by using our knowledge to affect and change healthy public policy, we can contribute significantly to influencing the movement and direction of health care in Canada.

In addition, CHNs now nurse a global community. Though it will be up to us to make a concerted effort to ensure that our voices are heard and that we stand together to protect the health of Canadians, we must, at the same time, position ourselves and partner with nurses in other countries to influence and support health care on a global scale. The challenges of preparing practitioners in community health nursing and producing the evidence on which our practice is based will continue to arise. And at the heart of it all will be our nurse–client relationships, with a focus to promote and protect the health of the community. What an exciting future to behold!

REFERENCES

Canadian Institute for Health Information. (2007). *Percentage distribution of RNs employed in nursing by place of work and territorial/provincial location, Canada, 2005.* Retrieved April 20, 2007, from http://secure.cihi.ca/cihiweb/en/statistics_RNDB_2005_employment_fig18_e.html.

Porter-O'Grady, T. (2001a). Profound change: 21st century nursing. *Nursing Outlook, 49,* 182–6.

Porter-O'Grady, T. (2001b). Into the new age: The call for a new construct for nursing. *Geriatric Nursing, 22*(1), 12–15.

Underwood, J. (Principal Investigator). (2006). *Building Community & Public Health Nursing Capacity.* Proposal to Canadian Health Services Research Foundation REISS Competition.

Villeneuve, M., & MacDonald, J. (2006). *Towards 2020: Visions for nursing.* Ottawa: Canadian Nurses Association.

About the Authors

Lynnette Leeseberg Stamler, RN, PhD, is Professor and Graduate Chair at the College of Nursing, University of Saskatchewan. She completed her BSN at St. Olaf College, Minnesota; her MEd at the University of Manitoba; and her PhD at the University of Cincinnati. Her research interests include patient/health education, breast health, diabetes education, quality of nursing care, and nursing education. She was a VON nurse for four years prior to her teaching career, and is a researcher with NCE—Auto 21. She is active in national and international nursing organizations, and is President Elect of the Canadian Association of Schools of Nursing.

Lucia Yiu, RN, BScN, BA (Windsor), BSc (Toronto), MScN (University of Western Ontario), is an Associate Professor in the Faculty of Nursing, University of Windsor, and an Educational and Training Consultant in community nursing. Her practice and research include multicultural health, international health, experiential learning, community development, breast health, and program planning and evaluation.

Appendix A

THE CANADIAN COMMUNITY HEALTH NURSING STANDARDS OF PRACTICE*

The model in the figure below illustrates the dynamic nature of community health nursing practice, embracing the present and projecting into the future. The values and beliefs (shaded) ground practice in the present yet guide the evolution of community health nursing practice over time. The community health nursing process (unshaded) provides the vehicle through which community health nurses work with people, and supports practice that exemplifies the standards of community health nursing. The standards of practice revolve around both the values and beliefs and the nursing process with the energies of community health nursing always being focussed on improving the health of people in the community and facilitating change in systems or society in support of health. Community health nursing practice does not occur in isolation but rather within an environmental context, such as policies within their workplace and the legislative framework applicable to their work.

THE STANDARDS OF PRACTICE

Knowledge of, and adherence to, the following standards is an expectation of every community health nurse working in any of the domains of practice, education, administration or research. These standards serve as a benchmark for novice community health nurses and become basic practice expectations after two years of experience. The practice of expert community health nurses will extend beyond these standards. While each standard is relevant to the practice of both home health nurses and public health nurses, the emphasis in practice on elements of specific standards will vary according to the practice focus.

Standard 1: Promoting Health

Community health nurses view health as a dynamic process of physical, mental, spiritual and social well-being. They believe that individuals and/or communities realize aspirations and satisfy needs within their cultural, social, economical and physical environments. Community health nurses consider health as a resource for everyday life that is influenced by circumstances,

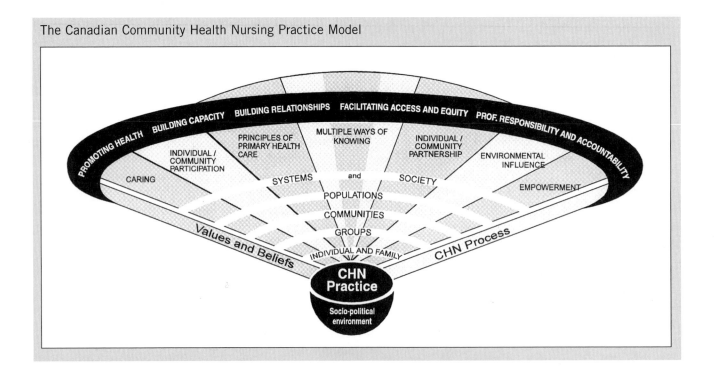

The Canadian Community Health Nursing Practice Model

Reprinted by permission of the Community Health Nurses Association of Canada www.communityhealthnurses.org

beliefs and the determinants of health including social, economic and environmental health determinants: a) income and social status, b) social support networks, c) education, d) employment and working conditions, e) social environments, f) physical environments, g) biology and genetic endowment, h) personal health practices and coping skills, i) healthy child development, j) health services, k) gender, and l) culture (Health Canada, 2000). It includes self-determination and a sense of connectedness to the community.

Community health nurses promote health using the following strategies: a) health promotion, b) illness and injury prevention and health protection, and c) health maintenance, restoration, and palliation. It is recognized that it may be relevant to use these strategies in concert with each other when providing care and services. This standard incorporates these strategies by drawing upon the frameworks of primary health care (WHO, 1978), the Ottawa Charter for Health Promotion (WHO, 1986), and the Population Health Promotion Model (Health Canada, 2000).

A) HEALTH PROMOTION Community health nurses focus on health promotion and the health of populations. Health promotion is a mediating strategy between people and their environments—a positive, dynamic, empowering, and unifying concept that is based in the socio-environmental approach to health. This broad concept is envisioned as bringing together people who recognize that basic resources and prerequisite conditions for health are critical for achieving health. The population's health is closely linked with the health of its constituent members and is often reflected first in individual and family experiences from birth to death. Healthy communities and systems support increased options for well-being in society. Community health nurses consider socio-political issues that may be underlying individual/community problems.

The community health nurse:

1. Collaborates with individual/community and other stakeholders in conducting a holistic assessment of assets and needs of the individual/community.
2. Uses a variety of information sources to access data and research findings related to health at the national, provincial/territorial, regional, and local levels.
3. Identifies and seeks to address root causes of illness and disease.
4. Facilitates planned change with the individual/community/ population through the application of the Population Health Promotion Model.
   - Identifies the level of intervention necessary to promote health
   - Identifies which determinants of health require action/change to promote health
   - Utilizes a comprehensive range of strategies to address health-related issues.
5. Demonstrates knowledge of and effectively implements health promotion strategies based on the Ottawa Charter for Health Promotion.
   - Incorporates multiple strategies addressing: a) healthy public policy; b) strengthening community action; c) creating supportive environments; d) developing personal skills; and e) re-orienting the health system
   - Identifies strategies for change that will make it easier for people to make a healthier choice.
6. Collaborates with the individual/community to assist them in taking responsibility for maintaining or improving their health by increasing their knowledge, influence and control over the determinants of health.
7. Understands and uses social marketing and media advocacy strategies to raise consciousness of health issues, place issues on the public agenda, shift social norms, and change behaviours if other enabling factors are present.
8. Assists the individual/community to identify their strengths and available resources and take action to address their needs.
9. Recognizes the broad impact of specific issues such as political climate and will, values and culture, individual/ community readiness, and social and systemic structure on health promotion.
10. Evaluates and modifies population health promotion programs in partnership with the individual/community and other stakeholders.

B) PREVENTION AND HEALTH PROTECTION The community health nurse adopts the principles of prevention and protection and applies a repertoire of activities to minimize the occurrence of diseases or injuries and their consequences to individuals/communities. Health protection strategies often become mandated programs and laws by governments for the larger geo-political entity.

The community health nurse:

1. Recognizes the differences between the levels of prevention (primary, secondary, tertiary).
2. Selects the appropriate level of preventative intervention.
3. Helps individuals/communities make informed choices about protective and preventative health measures such as immunization, birth control, breastfeeding, and palliative care.
4. Assists individuals, groups, families, and communities to identify potential risks to health.
5. Utilizes harm reduction principles to identify, reduce or remove risk factors in a variety of contexts including home, neighbourhood, workplace, school and street.
6. Applies epidemiological principles in using strategies such as screening, surveillance, immunization, communicable disease response and outbreak management and education.
7. Engages collaborative, interdisciplinary and intersectoral partnerships to address risks to the individual, family, community, or population health and to address prevention and protection issues such as communicable disease, injury and chronic disease.

8. Collaborates in developing and using follow-up systems within the practice setting to ensure that the individual/community receives appropriate and effective service.

9. Practices in accordance with legislation relevant to community health practice (e.g. public health legislation, child protection).

10. Evaluates collaborative practice (personal, team, and/or intersectoral) in achieving individual/community outcomes such as reductions in communicable disease, injury and chronic disease or reducing the impacts of a disease process.

C) HEALTH MAINTENANCE, RESTORATION AND PALLIATION Community health nurses provide clinical nursing care, health teaching and counselling in health centres, homes, schools and other community based settings to individuals, families, groups, and populations whether they are seeking to maintain their health or dealing with acute, chronic or terminal illness. The community health nurse links people to community resources and co-ordinates/facilitates other care needs and supports. The activities of the community health nurse may range from health screening and care planning at an individual level to the forming of intersectoral collaborations and resource development at the community and population level.

The community health nurse:
1. Assesses the individual/family/population's health status and functional competence within the context of their environmental and social supports.

2. Develops a mutually agreed upon plan and priorities for care with the individual/family.

3. Identifies a range of interventions including health promotion, disease prevention and direct clinical care strategies (including those related to palliation), along with short and long term goals and outcomes.

4. Maximizes the ability of an individual/family/community to take responsibility for and manage their health needs according to resources and personal skills available.

5. Supports informed choice and respects the individual/family/community's specific requests while acknowledging diversity, unique characteristics and abilities.

6. Adapts community health nursing techniques, approaches and procedures as appropriate to the challenges inherent to the particular community situation/setting.

7. Uses knowledge of the community to link with, refer to or develop appropriate community resources.

8. Recognizes patterns and trends in epidemiological data and service delivery and initiates improvement strategies.

9. Facilitates maintenance of health and the healing process for individuals/families/ communities in response to significant health emergencies or other diverse community situations that negatively impact upon health.

10. Evaluates individual/family/community outcomes systematically and continuously in collaboration with the individuals/families, significant others, other health practitioners and community partners.

Standard 2: Building Individual/Community Capacity

Building capacity is the process of actively involving individuals, groups, organizations and communities in all phases of planned change for the purpose of increasing their skills, knowledge and willingness to take action on their own in the future. The community health nurse works collaboratively both with the individual/community affected by health compromising situations and the people and organizations who control resources. Community health nurses start where the individual/community is at to identify relevant issues and assess resources and strengths. They determine the individual's or community's stage of readiness for change and priorities for action. They take collaborative action by building on identified strengths and facilitate the involvement of key stakeholders: individuals, organizations, community leaders and opinion leaders. They work with people to improve the determinants of health and "make it easier to make the healthier choice". Community health nurses use supportive and empowering strategies to move individuals and communities toward maximum autonomy.

The community health nurse:
1. Works collaboratively with the individual/community, other professionals, agencies and sectors to identify needs, strengths and available resources.

2. Facilitates action in support of the five priorities of the Jakarta Declaration to:
   - Promote social responsibility for health
   - Increase investments for health development
   - Expand partnerships for health promotion
   - Increase individual and community capacity
   - Secure an infrastructure for health promotion.

3. Uses community development principles:
   - Engages the individual/community in a consultative process
   - Recognizes and builds on the group/community readiness for participation
   - Uses empowering strategies such as mutual goal setting, visioning and facilitation
   - Understands group dynamics and effectively uses facilitation skills to support group development
   - Enables the individual/community to participate in the resolution of their issues
   - Assists the group/community to marshal available resources to support taking action on their health issues.

4. Utilizes a comprehensive mix of community/population based strategies such as coalition building, intersectoral partnerships and networking to address issues of concern to groups or populations.

5. Supports the individual/family/community/population in developing skills for self-advocacy.

6. Applies principles of social justice and engages in advocacy in support of those who are as yet unable to take action for themselves.

7. Uses a comprehensive mix of interventions and strategies to customize actions to address unique needs and build individual/community capacity.

8. Supports community action to influence policy change in support of health.

9. Actively works to build capacity for health promotion with health professionals and community partners.

10. Evaluates the impact of change on individual/community control and health outcomes.

Standard 3: Building Relationships

Building relationships within community health nursing is based upon the principles of connecting and caring. Connecting is the establishment and nurturing of a caring relationship and a supportive environment that promotes the maximum participation of the individual/community, and their own self-determination. Caring involves the development of empowering relationships, which preserve, protect, and enhance human dignity. Community health nurses build caring relationships based on mutual respect and on an understanding of the power inherent in their position and its potential impact on relationships and practice.

The community health nurse's most unique challenge is building a network of relationships and partnerships with a variety of relevant groups, communities, and organizations. These relationships occur within a complex, changing, undefined and often ambiguous environment that may present conflicting and unpredictable circumstances.

The community health nurse:

1. Recognizes her/his personal attitudes, beliefs, assumptions, feelings and values about health and their potential effect on interventions with individuals/communities.

2. Identifies the individual/community beliefs, attitudes, feelings and values about health and their potential effect on the relationship and intervention.

3. Is aware of and utilizes culturally relevant communication in building relationships. Communication may be verbal or non-verbal, written or pictorial. It may involve face-to-face, telephone, group facilitation, print or electronic means.

4. Respects and trusts the family's/community's ability to know the issue they are addressing and solve their own problems.

5. Involves the individual/community as an active partner in identifying relevant needs, perspectives and expectations.

6. Establishes connections and collaborative relationships with health professionals, community organizations, businesses, faith communities, volunteer service organizations, and other sectors to address health related issues.

7. Maintains awareness of community resources, values and characteristics.

8. Promotes and facilitates linkages with appropriate community resources when the individual/community is ready to receive them (e.g. hospice/palliative care, parenting groups).

9. Maintains professional boundaries within an often long-term relationship in the home or other community setting where professional and social relationships may become blurred.

10. Negotiates an end to the relationship when appropriate, e.g. when the client assumes self-care, or when the goals for the relationship have been achieved.

Standard 4: Facilitating Access and Equity

Community health nurses embrace the philosophy of primary health care and collaboratively identify and facilitate universal and equitable access to available services. Community health nurses engage in advocacy by analyzing the full range of possibilities for action, acting on affected determinants of health, and influencing other sectors to ensure their policies and programs have a positive impact on health. Community health nurses collaborate with colleagues and with other members of the health care team to promote effective working relationships that contribute to comprehensive client care and the achievement of optimal client care outcomes. Community health nurses use advocacy as a key strategy to meet identified needs and enhance individual and/or community capacity for self-advocacy. They are keenly aware of the impact of the determinants of health on individuals, families, groups, communities and populations. The practice of community health nursing occurs with consideration for the financial resources, geography and culture of the individual/community.

The community health nurse:

1. Assesses and understands individual and community capacities including norms, values, beliefs, knowledge, resources and power structure.

2. Provides culturally sensitive care in diverse communities and settings.

3. Supports individuals/communities in their choice to access alternate health care options.

4. Advocates for appropriate resource allocation for individuals, groups and populations to facilitate access to conditions for health and health services.

5. Refers, co-ordinates or facilitates access to service within health and other sectors.

6. Adapts practice in response to the changing health needs of the individual/community.

7. Collaborates with individuals and communities to identify and provide programs and delivery methods that are acceptable to them and responsive to their needs across the life span and in different circumstances.

8. Uses strategies such as home visits, outreach and case finding to ensure access to services and health-supporting conditions for potentially vulnerable populations (e.g. persons who are ill, elderly, young, poor, immigrants, isolated, or have communication barriers).

9. Assesses the impact of the determinants of health on the opportunity for health for individuals/families/communities/populations.

10. Advocates for healthy public policy by participating in legislative and policymaking activities that influence health determinants and access to services.

11. Takes action with and for individuals/communities at the organizational, municipal, provincial/territorial and federal levels to address service gaps and accessibility issues.

12. Monitors and evaluates changes/progress in access to the determinants of health and appropriate community services.

Standard 5: Demonstrating Professional Responsibility and Accountability

Community health nurses work with a high degree of autonomy in providing programs and services. They are accountable to strive for excellence, to ensure that their knowledge is evidence-based, current and maintains competence, and for the overall quality of their own practice. Community health nurses are accountable to initiate strategies that will help address the determinants of health and generate a positive impact on people and systems.

Within a complex environment, community health nurses are accountable to a variety of authorities and stakeholders as well as to the individual/community they serve. This places them in a variety of situations with unique ethical dilemmas. These include whether responsibility for an issue lies with the individual/family/community/population, or with the nurse or the nurse's employer, the priority of one individual's rights over another's, individual or societal good, allocation of scarce resources and dealing with issues related to quality versus quantity of life.

The community health nurse:

1. Takes preventive and/or corrective action individually or in partnership with others to protect individuals/communities from unsafe or unethical circumstances.

2. Advocates for societal change in support of health for all.

3. Utilizes nursing informatics (information and communication technology) to generate, manage and process relevant data to support nursing practice.

4. Identifies and takes action on factors which impinge on autonomy of practice and quality of care.

5. Participates in the advancement of community health nursing by mentoring students and novice practitioners.

6. Participates in research and professional activities.

7. Makes decisions using ethical standards/principles, taking into consideration the tension between individual versus societal good and the responsibility to uphold the greater good of all people or the population as a whole.

8. Seeks assistance with problem solving as needed to determine the best course of action in response to ethical dilemmas and risks to human rights and freedoms, new situations, and new knowledge.

9. Identifies and works proactively to address nursing issues that will affect the population through personal advocacy and participation in relevant professional associations.

10. Contributes proactively to the quality of the work environment by identifying needs/issues and solutions, mobilizing colleagues, and actively participating in team and organizational structures and mechanisms.

11. Provides constructive feedback to peers as appropriate to enhance community health nursing practice.

12. Documents community health nursing activities in a timely and thorough manner, including telephone advice and work with communities and groups.

13. Advocates for effective and efficient use of community health nurse resources.

14. Utilizes reflective practice as a means of continually assessing and seeking to improve personal community health nursing practice.

15. Seeks professional development experiences that are consistent with current community health nursing practice, new and emerging issues, the changing needs of the population, the evolving impact of the determinants of health and emerging research.

16. Acts upon legal obligations to report to appropriate authorities situations of unsafe or unethical care provided by family, friends or other individuals to children or vulnerable adults.

17. Uses available resources to systematically evaluate the availability, acceptability, quality, efficiency and effectiveness of community health nursing practice.

Appendix B

CORE COMPETENCIES FOR PUBLIC HEALTH IN CANADA

What Are Core Competencies?

Core competencies are the essential knowledge, skills and attitudes necessary for the practice of public health. They transcend the boundaries of specific disciplines and are independent of program and topic. They provide the building blocks for effective public health practice, and the use of an overall public health approach. Generic core competencies provide a baseline for what is required to fulfill public health system core functions. These include population health assessment, surveillance, disease and injury prevention, health promotion and health protection.[1]

WHY DO WE NEED CORE COMPETENCIES?

Core competencies may improve the health of the public by:

- contributing to a more effective workforce
- encouraging service delivery that is evidence-based, population-focused, ethical, equitable, standardized and client-centred
- helping to create a more unified workforce by providing a shared understanding of key concepts and practices
- helping to explain the nature of public health and health goals.

Core competencies will benefit the people who work in public health by:

- providing guidelines for the basic knowledge, skills and attitudes required by individual practitioners in public health
- supporting the recruitment, development and retention of public health practitioners
- providing a rational basis for developing curricula, training and professional development tools
- improving consistency in job descriptions and performance assessment
- supporting the development of discipline- and program-specific sets of competencies.

Core competencies can help public health organizations to:

- identify the knowledge, skills and attitudes required across an organization or program to fulfill public health functions
- help identify the appropriate numbers and mix of public health workers in a given setting
- identify staff development and training needs
- provide a rationale for securing funds to support workforce development
- develop job descriptions, interview questions, and frameworks for evaluation and quality assurance
- facilitate collaboration, shared goals and interdisciplinary work.

1.0 Public Health Sciences

Competency Statements	Practice Examples
1.1 Demonstrate knowledge about the following concepts: the health status of populations, inequities in health, the determinants of health and illness, strategies for health promotion, disease and injuring prevention and health protection, as well as the factors that influence the delivery and use of health services.	*Front line provider:* Discuss the need for a prenatal nutrition program in an Aboriginal community as well as contributing factors such as income, education, culture and traditional foods.
1.2 Demonstrate knowledge about the history, structure and interaction of public health and health care services at local, provincial/territorial, national, and international levels.	*Front line provider:* Recall public health events such as the implementation of universal immunization programs in order to explain to parents the importance of this measure for maintaining public health.
1.3 Apply the public health sciences to practice.	*Front line provider:* Apply the epidemiology triangle (host, environment and agent) to the issue of West Nile virus. *Consultant/Specialist:* Integrate Geographic Information System (GIS) software for mapping cases of West Nile Virus to account for seasonal trends.
1.4 Use evidence and research to inform health policies and programs.	*Front line provider:* Discuss how evidence from a recent research study can be utilized in practice. *Consultant/Specialist:* Summarize key findings from a contact tracing report to support policy changes in communicable disease services.
1.5 Demonstrate the ability to pursue lifelong learning opportunities in the field of public health.	*Front line provider:* Register for a Skills Online module with the Skills Enhancement for Public Health Program.

---

1. Advisory Committee on Population Health. *Survey of Public Health Capacity in Canada. Highlights Report to the Federal, Provincial, Territorial Deputy Ministers of Health.* Ottawa: Health Canada, 2001.

2.0 Assessment and Analysis

Competency Statements	Practice Examples
2.1 Recognize that a health concern or issue exists.	*Front line provider:* Describe a situation in a school community recognizing that the lack of healthy food choices in the school cafeteria is an issue.
2.2 Identify relevant and appropriate sources of information, including community assets and resources.	*Front line provider:* Identify key informants such as student leaders and service providers.
2.3 Collect, store, retrieve and use accurate and appropriate information on public health issues.	*Front line provider:* Use data collection tools (e.g., IPHIS) to document practice. *Consultant/Specialist:* Design data collection tool on Fetal Alcohol Spectrum Disorder (FASD) and obtain relevant provincial/territorial statistics on the prevalence of FASD.
2.4 Analyze information to determine appropriate implications, uses, gaps and limitations.	*Front line provider:* Identify the limitations of information resulting from a telephone survey in a diverse community.
2.5 Determine the meaning of information, considering the current ethical, political, scientific, socio-cultural and economic contexts.	*Front line provider:* Identify how smoking affects men and women differently and how reasons for smoking differ between genders, and among socioeconomic groups and different cultures.
2.6 Recommend specific actions based on the analysis of information.	*Consultant/Specialist:* Make recommendations for health policies regulating artificial tanning salons due to the increasing incidence of skin cancers.

3.0 Policy and Program Planning, Implementation and Evaluation

Competency Statements	Practice Examples
3.1 Describe selected policy and program options to address a specific public health issue.	*Front line provider:* Identify potential school intervention programs and activities to address increasing rates of sexually transmitted infections among youth.
3.2 Describe the implications of each option, especially as they apply to the determinants of health and recommend or decide on a course of action.	*Front line provider:* Explore the social and economic implications of a folic acid education program directed at adolescents and decide whether or not to proceed.
3.3 Develop a plan to implement a course of action taking into account relevant evidence, legislation, emergency planning procedures, regulations and policies.	*Consultant/Specialist:* Prioritize the components of a restaurant inspection logic model including appropriate rationale and develop the implementation plan for each component.
3.4 Implement a policy or program and/or take appropriate action to address a specific public health issue.	*Consultant/Specialist:* Act according to the organization's emergency response plan in the event of an outbreak or emergency.
3.5 Demonstrate the ability to implement effective practice guidelines.	*Front line provider:* Use universal infection control measures appropriately.
3.6 Evaluate an action, program or policy.	*Front line provider:* Develop and implement an evaluation plan for a smoke-free workplace program in collaboration with stakeholders.
3.7 Demonstrate an ability to set and follow priorities, and to maximize outcomes based on available resources.	*Front line provider:* Set priorities for action on safer crack use in a local harm reduction program based on existing resources.
3.8 Demonstrate the ability to fulfill functional roles in response to a public health emergency.	*Front line provider:* Be familiar with the organization's emergency management manual. *Manager/Supervisor:* Arrange a debriefing session after a public health incident to identify lessons learned and assess the need for recovery intervention for team members involved.

4.0 Partnerships, Collaboration and Advocacy

Competency Statements	Practice Examples
4.1 Identify and collaborate with partners in addressing public health issues.	*Front line provider:* Explain the roles of the provincial government, local recreation department, school boards, boards of health and the Boys and Girls Club in addressing childhood obesity to a parent group.
4.2 Use skills such as team building, negotiation, conflict management and group facilitation to build partnerships.	*Front line provider:* Assist the school in developing a school health team. *Consultant/Specialist:* Facilitate the development of the terms of reference for a partnership between school boards and public health.

4.3	Mediate between differing interests in the pursuit of health and well-being, and facilitate the allocation of resources.	*Front line provider:* Interview key community members to determine the range of opinions on the implementation of a local tobacco by-law. *Consultant/Specialist:* Synthesize input from individuals and organizations in order to prepare a report on the readiness of a community to offer a needle exchange clinic.
4.4	Advocate for healthy public policies and services that promote and protect the health and well-being of individuals and communities.	*Consultant/Specialist:* Using information from the Canadian Community Health Survey and feedback from principals, make a presentation to the Board of Health to advocate for a provincial school nutrition policy.

5.0 Diversity and Inclusiveness

Competency Statements	**Practice Examples**
5.1 Recognize how the determinants of health (biological, social, cultural, economic and physical) influence the health and well-being of specific population groups.	*Consultant/Specialist:* Develop a funding proposal in collaboration with key stakeholders for a community kitchen project in a disadvantaged area with a culturally diverse population.
5.2 Address population diversity when planning, implementing, adapting and evaluating public health programs and policies.	*Front line provider:* Provide access to vaccines for people of all cultural groups and populations (e.g., drive-through vaccine clinics for disabled population groups).
5.3 Apply culturally relevant and appropriate approaches with people from diverse cultural, socioeconomic, and educational backgrounds, and persons of all ages, genders, health status, sexual orientations and abilities.	*Front line provider:* Collaborate with members of an Afghanistan community to develop a tuberculosis screening program in their neighbourhood. *Manager/Supervisor:* Negotiate with primary care team to provide cancer screening clinics staffed with female practitioners for Muslim women.

6.0 Communication

Competency Statements	**Practice Examples**
6.1 Communicate effectively with individuals, families, groups, communities and colleagues.	*Front line provider:* Revise oral presentations to meet the needs of various audiences.
6.2 Interpret information for professional, non-professional and community audiences.	*Front line provider:* Develop immunization schedule fact sheets for people with low literacy levels. *Consultant/Specialist:* Discuss population health information about health status and demographics with front line providers.
6.3 Mobilize individuals and communities by using appropriate media, community resources and social marketing techniques.	*Front line provider:* Use multiple strategies to effectively communicate health messages appropriate to audiences (e.g., community newspapers, local television, radio, billboards, face-to-face events). *Manager/Supervisor:* Use community networks to receive and provide information about issues affecting the health of citizens.
6.4 Use current technology to communicate effectively.	*Consultant/Specialist:* Forward workplace health information from a health promotion listserv to staff members on a workplace health committee.

7.0 Leadership

Competency Statements	**Practice Examples**
7.1 Describe the mission and priorities of the public health organization where one works, and apply them in practice.	*Front line provider:* Illustrate how a program logic model incorporates the organization's mission into program specific goals and outcomes. *Manager/Supervisor:* Apply the priorities of the organization to the work plan of an interdisciplinary team.
7.2 Contribute to developing key values and a shared vision in planning and implementing public health programs and policies in the community.	*Front line provider:* Involve parents, teachers, and students in developing a vision and health goals for the school community.
7.3 Utilize public health ethics to manage self, others, information and resources.	*Consultant/Specialist:* Develop a research protocol that protects the privacy of participants from a local women's shelter. *Manager/Supervisor:* Facilitate a lunch and learn session for the interdisciplinary team with a local ethicist to discuss vaccine security.

→

7.4	Contribute to team and organizational learning in order to advance public health goals.	*Front line provider:* Participate on a staff committee whose purpose is to facilitate the incorporation of best practice guidelines into policies and practice.
		Consultant/Specialist: Participate in a mentoring program with other employees.
7.5	Contribute to maintaining organizational performance standards.	*Front line provider:* Assist in the collection of data for inclusion in the organization's annual performance report.
		Manager/Supervisor: Develop a plan to form an accreditation team to review and use the Public Health Standards of the Canadian Council on Health Services Accreditation.
7.6	Demonstrate an ability to build community capacity by sharing knowledge, tools, expertise and experience.	*Front line provider:* Facilitate discussion with a community group that is developing an active living program, to identify factors that could impact on program delivery such as resources, space and previous community experience.
		Manager/Supervisor: Sponsor and participate in a continuing education session for an interdisciplinary team on working effectively with community groups to achieve public health goals.

Source: Public Health Agency of Canada. Core Competencies for Public Health in Canada, Release 1.0. (2007). Retrieved October, 30, 2007, from http://www.phac.aspc.gc.ca/ccph-cesp/pdfs/cc-manual-eng-090407.pdf.

Answers to Study Questions

Chapter 1

1. The two forms of community health nursing that evolved in Canada in the early twentieth century were public health nursing and visiting/district nursing. PHNs were employed by civic, provincial, or federal health departments to carry out preventive programs in the community. In the later part of the twentieth century, PHNs took on new roles in health promotion and community development. Visiting/district nurses offered bedside nursing services in the home. They were most frequently employed by charitable organizations. Visiting nursing is now more commonly referred to as home care nursing.

2. The social gospel movement was one important impetus for the development of community-based social services. It was an ecumenical and evangelical stream within the Protestant churches that had as its goal the establishment of God's kingdom on earth.

   Another important social movement was maternal feminism. Maternal feminists had a particular interest in the health and welfare of women and children. The social gospel movement and maternal feminism created an important strategic alliance after World War I and their efforts are theorized to have had an important influence on the rise of the Canadian welfare state.

   The last important social movement was the public health movement. Sanitarianism, bacteriology, and health education were all important paradigms within the early public health movement. All contributed to the overarching belief that the application of scientific knowledge would create a healthy nation.

3. Early community health nursing programs focused on women, children, the poor, the working class, and immigrants. There were several interrelated reasons for this emphasis. All these groups were vulnerable within a society where political and economic power was held by elite and middle-class males. Their vulnerability was clearly demonstrated by the higher mortality rates these groups experienced. Another reason for the focus on these groups was the need to create a strong and healthy pool of future citizens to establish Canada's pre-eminence in the twentieth century. Immigrants were an important target group because elite and middle-class reformers believed that they needed to adopt Canadian beliefs and practices rather than retain those of their countries of origin.

4. The earliest public health programs that employed nurses were TB control, school health, and infant welfare. TB was a leading cause of death in early-twentieth-century Canada and a particular problem among the urban poor. Early efforts to control TB were based on the belief that a reduction in the incidence of this disease would, as well as alleviating suffering, reduce the costs of public welfare and health care programs.

   School-health programs were established to identify health problems among school-age children. As working-class children entered the public school system, it became apparent that they suffered from many preventable health problems that detracted from their capacity to learn.

   Infant welfare programs were established to reduce infant mortality rates. In the early twentieth century, immigration, industrialization, and urbanization created unprecedented urban squalor.

5. The British North America Act reflected nineteenth-century beliefs about the role of the state. In keeping with the philosophy of laissez faire, the state had no role to play in the provision of health care and social welfare for its citizens. These were private matters, which were the responsibility of individuals and families. Those who could not provide for their families were compelled to obtain charitable assistance from local governments or, more likely, voluntary philanthropic agencies. The BNA Act left responsibility for health care in the hands of the provinces, which also took only a limited interest in this area. Enabling legislation for the establishment of health departments was passed by several provinces prior to the end of the nineteenth century, but permanent health departments were not established in most Canadian cities and provinces until the twentieth century. Prior to the end of World War II, local and provincial health departments received no assistance from the federal government. Their capacity to respond to the health needs of the communities for which they were responsible was constrained by their ability to fund programs from local tax revenues.

6. The Canadian welfare state had its origins in the early twentieth century as provincial and municipal departments of health began to provide publicly funded public health programs at the local level. Some provinces, cities, and municipalities, particularly those in Western Canada, were virtually bankrupted by their attempts to respond to widespread unemployment and poverty. They put pressure on the federal government to assist them. However, other provinces, more concerned about maintaining strict divisions between provincial and federal powers, opposed any initiatives that would enable the federal government to intervene into what had previously been

provincial responsibilities. Several attempts by the federal government to take a greater role in health and welfare programs were stopped by the Supreme Court, which used the BNA Act as the basis of its decisions. In 1940, the Royal Commission on Dominion-Provincial Relations recommended that the federal government undertake responsibility for old-age pensions and unemployment insurance, but leave responsibility for health with the provinces.

In the 1940s, 1950s, and 1960s, a series of cost-sharing arrangements enabled the federal government to establish a national health care system by creating incentives for the provinces to spend more money in this area and to extend those services to all citizens regardless of ability to pay. The National Health Grants Program (1948), the National Hospital Insurance and Diagnostic Services Act (1957), and the Medical Care Insurance Act (1968) were key elements in the increased federal role in the provision of health care.

7. First, they often pioneered community health nursing programs, thus demonstrating both the need for and the effectiveness of these programs. Second, they provided community health programs in communities where local governments were either unable or unwilling to do so. Third, they created educational programs to prepare nurses to practise in this area. Fourth, they provided funding to support local initiatives to create community health nursing programs.

Chapter 2

1. North America's first universal health insurance program was initially implemented in 1947 at a provincial level in Saskatchewan. It was not until 1957, a full decade later, that similar legislation, the Hospital Insurance and Diagnostic Services Act (HIDS), was passed by the federal government. The HIDS provided financial incentives for the provinces to establish hospital insurance plans.

In 1962, Saskatchewan led the country again with legislation providing universal, publicly funded, medical insurance. In 1966, the federal government followed suit with the passage of the National Medical Care Insurance Act (Medicare). This Act was implemented in 1968, and by 1971 all provinces were fully participating.

As a result of the strain on the federal budgets caused by the blanket 50/50 cost-sharing between the federal and provincial/territorial governments, in 1977 the federal government passed the Established Programs Financing Act (EPF), which changed the federal share of health costs to per capita block grants assigned to provinces and tied to economic performance.

In 1984, the Canada Health Act, which banned extra-billing and user fees by physicians, was passed.

2. The Canadian Nurses Association intensely lobbied for the Bill's passage into law. In addition, they were successful in amending it. As it was introduced into Parliament in 1983, Bill C-3 identified only physicians as providers of insurable services. The CNA amendment changed the language to include other health care workers as potential providers of insurable services, opening the door for the public to have direct access to nursing care through insured services.

3. Although the 1867 Constitution Act did not explicitly assign responsibility for health policy to either the federal or provincial governments, historically both levels of government have been involved in ensuring the availability of health services for Canadians, and in funding those services. Responsibility for hospitals is assigned by the Act exclusively to provinces and, as a result, health care in Canada has sometimes been erroneously interpreted to fall under provincial jurisdiction. The federal government assumes responsibility for delivering a few direct health services, e.g., Aboriginal populations, veterans, and military personnel. Provincial governments are responsible for the delivery of the remainder of health care services, including public health.

Funding for health care is another matter, however. The federal government's involvement in funding health care relates both to its mandate to equalize services among provinces and its responsibilities to ensure provinces are in compliance with the Canada Health Act.

4. *Public health* in Canada is funded by a combination of provincial and/or municipal tax dollars, although federal grants may be available for specific initiatives. Without a national public health program, however, provinces are free to make changes in funding mechanisms that can further destabilize the system and deepen disparities among and within provinces.

In all 12 provinces/territories, the ministries or departments of health and/or social/community services maintain control over home care budgets and funding levels. However, contrary to other forms of health care provided in Canada, home care has retained a significant private-sector component. So while all provincial governments finance home care services to some extent, often user fees or co-payments are required.

5. With respect to stopping the practices of extra-billing and charging user fees, the CHA fulfilled its purpose. However, the issue of provincial/territorial non-compliance with the five criteria of the Act remains to be adequately addressed.

- The intent of the Act was to relate federal cash contributions not only to insured health services but also to extended health care services. In that respect the CHA has not been effective.
- The Act endorsed health promotion but limited its focus to medically necessary hospital and physicians' services. Health promotion services, largely provided by provincial public health, were left unprotected by federal legislation. The resulting variability of health promotion and disease prevention services within and among jurisdictions violates the Act's principle of portability.

- Canadians enjoy relatively good health when compared with other countries. Canada also spends less per capita and less of its gross domestic product on health than some other countries, including the United States. However, there is room for improvement, particularly in respect to outcomes such as infant mortality rates, which are still higher than in a number of other developed countries.

6. The Health Council of Canada was created as part of the 2003 First Ministers' Accord on Health Care Renewal to monitor and report on renewal of the health system and to ensure transparency and accountability. In 2004 those responsibilities were expanded to include reporting annually on health status and health outcomes.

    - The Health Council of Canada consists of 26 Councillors, 12 to represent their respective jurisdictional governments and 14 non-government representatives. The Council accomplishes its work through the work of the Councillors and the support of a highly skilled Secretariat.
    - In meeting its mandate, the Health Council of Canada consults with Canadians and monitors the status of health care system activities, particularly in the areas that have been identified as priorities. It publishes its findings and makes them available to Canadians on its website.

Chapter 3

1. - Public health nurses work in client homes, schools, workplaces, community centres, clinics, mobile street clinics, within the community on coalitions, and with other partner agencies.
   - Home health nurses provide direct care to clients in homes and schools.
   - Community health centre or outreach nurses provide primary health care in clinics settings or may be involved in mobile clinics.
   - Outpost nurses may work out of clinics or in clients' homes or schools.
   - Parish nurses work with members of a congregation in the parish place of worship or homes of parishioners.
   - Occupational health nurses work primarily in the workplace, which could range from the manufacturing industry shop floor and corporate office settings to the hospitality industry's casino setting.

2. - Teacher to individuals and groups
   - Direct care provider to individuals requiring nursing care and interventions in the form of treatment, supportive therapy, or hygiene care
   - Policy advocate for supportive healthy environments
   - Counsellor to supplement the holistic aspect of client care

3. - Through population-based health promotion
   - Public policy support (i.e., smoke-free public places, sidewalk by-laws to encourage active living, alcohol policy for safe serving, safe playgrounds to prevent injuries)
   - Public education through marketing and use of mass media
   - Target multiple targets and sites with health education messages
   - Community mobilization to empower communities to gain control over life
   - Skill development and education and counselling with individual

4. - Implement holistic strategies that involve the client in their plan of care
   - Encourage as much independence as possible
   - Use collective decision-making in nursing care planning
   - Nursing care is enabling and holistic and as non-invasive as possible

5. - Process for professional development
   - Support for leadership development
   - Control over practice and scheduling
   - A safe work environment
   - Reasonable remuneration and benefits to enhance staff morale and support nurses in delivering quality nursing services

6.

	HHN	PHN	PHCNP	SANE	FCN	Entrepreneur
1. Promoting health	Health education in the home	Community-wide campaign	Lifestyle counselling	Holistic health assessments	Community health education	Education re prevention
2. Building individual or community capacity	Referrals to support agencies	Healthy public policy advocacy	Advocacy for client services	Referrals for long-term support for victims	Uses community development principles	Counselling

	HHN	PHN	PHCNP	SANE	FCN	Entrepreneur
3. Building relationships	Family consultations	Coalition work	Collaboration with HC team	Team meetings for collaboration	Group work	Marketing of service
4. Facilitating access and equity	Advocacy for policy to support care access	Advocacy for multicultural resources	Flexibility in practice	24/7 on call availability for the service	Promote social justice	Pro bono work as required to clients in need
5. Demonstration of professional responsibility and accountability	Professional development Mentorship Professional Associations Participates in research	(As in HHN)	(As in HHN)	(As in HHN)	(As in HHN)	(As in HHN)

Chapter 4

1. See Table 4.1.
2. See Table 4.2.
3.
   i. Promoting health: CHNs promote health through a) health promotion; b) prevention and health protection; and c) health maintenance, restoration, and palliation.

   ii. Building individual/community capacity: CHNs begin where individuals and communities are, helping them to identify relevant health issues and to assess their strengths and resources. CHNs use strategies that involve advocacy and empowerment.

   iii. Building relationships: CHNs establish and nurture caring relationships with individuals and communities that promote maximum participation and self-determination.

   iv. Facilitating access and equity: CHNs collaboratively identify and facilitate universal and equitable access to available health care services and the socioeconomic, social, and physical environmental determinants of health.

   v. Demonstrating professional responsibility and accountability: CHNs must adhere to federal and provincial professional standards, laws, and codes of ethics and must use resources effectively and efficiently. They have a responsibility to be knowledgeable, competent, and current, and must also help others around them, such as colleagues and students, to develop and maintain competence.

4. The first, the harm principle, requires that power be exercised over individuals against their will only to prevent harm to others. Restricting the liberty of mentally competent people to protect their own well-being is not a sufficient justification.

   The second principle, least restrictive or coercive means, stipulates that the full force of governmental authority and power should not be used, unless less coercive method are unavailable or have failed. Education,

negotiation, and discussion should come before regulation and incarceration (Upshur, 2002).

   The third, the reciprocity principle, indicates that if a public action is warranted, social entities, such as a public health department, are obligated to assist individuals in meeting their ethical responsibilities. In addition, because complying with the requests of the public health department may impose burdens on individuals, such as time and money, the reciprocity principle demands that compensation be given (Upshur, 2002).

   The fourth, the transparency principle, refers to the way in which decisions are made. All relevant stakeholders should participate in decision-making in an accountable and equitable fashion that is free of political interference or coercion (Upshur, 2002).

5. In order for CHNs to assist clients in making informed choices, at least two elements must be considered: the exchange of information between the client and CHN and respect for the client's autonomy. The process of consent includes CHNs disclosing, unasked, whatever a reasonable person would want to know if they were in the position of the client. The nurse must provide the information that the average prudent person in the client's particular position would want to know. CHNs must provide information about the nature of the treatment/procedures they are providing, including benefits and risks, alternative treatments, and consequences if the treatment is not given. The presentation of this information must consider the client's education, language, age, values, culture, disease state, and mental capacity. When clients provide their consent it must be done voluntarily (i.e., without being coerced) and they must have the capacity (i.e., mental competence) to do so. The only exceptions to not needing consent for treatment are in emergency situations and as required by law.

6. There are four key elements that must be proven to make a finding of negligence: (a) that there was a relationship between the person bringing the claim (i.e., plaintiff, e.g., client, family) and the person being sued (i.e., defendant, e.g. nurse), (b) that the defendant breached the standard

of care, (c) that the plaintiff suffered a harm, and (d) that the harm suffered was caused by the defendant's breach of the standard of care.

Chapter 5

1. A discourse is a patterned system of texts, messages, talk, dialogue, or conversations that can be identified in communications and located in social structures. Key ideas are patterned expressions that can be located within social structures.

2. Primary health care is a balanced combination of medical care, health promotion and prevention, consumer protection, effective health care systems, appropriate technology, and inter-sectoral cooperation organized to ensure effective action on the determinants of health and to shape environments in support of healthful living and healthy lifestyles.

    A Primary Health Care Model suggests a balanced combination of medical care, health promotion and prevention, consumer protection, effective health care systems, appropriate technology, and inter-sectoral cooperation (Green & Ottoson, 1999; RNABC, 2002).

3. The difference between these two views originates in how each perspective conceptualizes health. Traditionally, the medical model defines health as the absence of disease, whereas the systems view envisions health as shaped by myriad physical, social, environmental, and organizational factors.

4. The challenge to nurses is to be aware of the view of health that dominates in their practice environment and to begin practice from the client's perspectives on health, working collaboratively within this view in the interest of the client.

5. The Lalonde Report shifted perspectives on health from illness care to health care by suggesting that health is embedded in a web of factors including physical, social, and environmental factors.

6. In the ecological perspective, health is viewed as a consequence of the interdependence between the individual and the family, community, culture, and physical and social environments.

7. In a relational nursing practice, the nurse builds trusting relationships, collaborates with clients to identify and address their health-related issues, fosters clients' strengths, promotes and protects clients' rights, practises in an inter-sectoral manner to address the determinants of health, and strives for a respectful, integrated, and accessible system of health care delivery.

8. Through the development of a series of charters and frameworks that flesh out the elements of systems views of health, Canada has played a leading role in shaping discourses of health toward a systems view. These works, in combination with the scholarly and advocacy efforts of an army of academics and health advocates, have been fundamental in arguing to maintain a single-payer system for health care in Canada—a system consistent in its philosophy with a systems view of health rather than a bio-medical model view of health. Canada's charters and framework of health promotion, population health, and primary health care, along with the related health care system, are models in the international arena for a health care system that advances a systems view of health.

9. The authors invite students to offer their views on the metaphors of nursing practice provided in this chapter by e-mail communication to the first author, Lynne Young, at leyoung@uvic.ca. The author will model a relational process while facilitating the discussion by ensuring that all voices are heard and all opinions are respected. The facilitator will share her observations and reactions and summarize the discussion.

Chapter 6

1. Answers can be found in Table 6.1.
2.
   - an umbrella term referring to any activity designed to foster health
   - a synonym for health education
   - the marketing or selling of health
   - a strategy concerned with lifestyle behaviour change
   - health education plus environmental and legislative measures designed to facilitate the achievement of health and prevention of disease
   - an approach that encompasses a set of values that include concepts of empowerment, equity, and collaboration

    The first four interpretations (but especially the second, third, and fourth) reflect the behavioural approach to health promotion, whereas the latter two reflect the socio-environmental approach.

3.
   - The first time a national government had made an official statement regarding the importance of health promotion as a key strategy for improving population health
   - Concept of "health" expanded to include the notion of increased functional ability and wellness
   - Challenged the dominant thinking of the time that access to health services was the key to population health
   - Weakness was the assumption that the main determinant of health was individual behaviour or lifestyle
   - Weakness is underlying belief that health professionals should use any means possible to encourage or coerce individuals to change to healthier behaviours
   - Can lead to victim blaming—you chose the behaviour—you have the health challenge

4. The description of each behavioural strategy is found in Table 6.2. Regulatory measures coincide with healthy public policies used in the socio-environmental approach.

5. Approaches that focus solely on individual behaviour change and individual responsibility for health can lead to victim-blaming, whereby individuals end up being implicitly blamed for being sick because they have "chosen" unhealthy lifestyles or they have unhealthy coping

styles when, in fact, their social and economic circumstances have often left them with limited options.

6. ■ Ideological responses to the behavioural approach: influence of social movements, concern with "social justice," the "common good," social change, and social responsibility for health.

   ■ Theoretical developments: ecological perspective, which suggested that health is a product of the interdependence between the individual and subsystems of the ecosystem, and belief that the environment sets limits on individual behaviour but also that behaviour influences environments.

   ■ Limitations of population-level disease prevention initiatives in changing individual behaviours, and failure to address inequalities in health.

   ■ Epidemiological evidence that the distribution of disease in any given society is the result of the economic, political, and social relationship between individuals and groups in society, not the result of individual behaviours.

7. Empowerment is the central concept. It refers to the process or outcome of individuals, communities, and populations gaining power, knowledge, skills, and/or other resources that allow them to achieve positive change, including increased self-efficacy. Empowerment relates directly to the concept of health promotion as a process of enabling individuals, communities, and populations to increase control over the determinants of health.

8. Health promotion:

   ■ involves the population as a whole and the context of their everyday lives, rather than focusing on people at risk for specific diseases;

   ■ is directed toward action on the determinants or causes of health;

   ■ combines diverse, but complementary, methods or approaches;

   ■ aims particularly at effective and concrete public participation; and

   ■ recognizes that health professionals, particularly those in primary health care, have an important role in nurturing and enabling health promotion.

9. ■ By working on their individual practices (e.g., including SDOH in client assessments and treatment and follow-up plans)

   ■ By helping to reorient the health care system (e.g., ensuring that health promotion programs go beyond lifestyle and behaviour to include SDOH)

   ■ By advocating for healthy public policies (e.g., using stories from patients to help advocate for policies that address SDOH or by making decision-makers aware of the research on the links between socioeconomic factors and health)

10. ■ Focus on health and building capacity for health.
    ■ Think "upstream."
    ■ Look for partnership opportunities.
    ■ Be patient.

Chapter 7

1. ■ *Primary health care* refers to a range of comprehensive (from primary to tertiary) care, essential health care services that are practical and scientifically sound, based on acceptable methods and technology, universally accessible to individuals and families in the community, and at a cost that is affordable to help members of the community to attain self-reliance and self-determination.

   ■ *Primary care* refers to health services that are provided at the first entry point to the health care system. Usually, the care is based in the community and acute or rehabilitative care in nature.

2. Health promotion is a common theme in all three terms.

   ■ *Primary health care* is an approach to health promotion. It uses five principles to guide the planning and delivery of essential health services to communities: health promotion, inter-sectoral cooperation, appropriate technology, accessibility, and public participation. Primary health care is often the focus of international development efforts to reduce such inequalities.

   ■ *Population health* is an approach that focuses on the interrelated connections and factors that influences the health of the population over the life course.

   ■ *Health promotion* is the process of enabling people to increase their control over and improve their health and to achieve a higher level of health functioning.

3. Refer to the text box on PHC principles in the chapter (p. 112) on CNA's definitions for health promotion, inter-sectoral cooperation, appropriate technology, accessibility, and public participation.

4. ■ Review health data related to the homeless population to understand the issue at hand.

   ■ Make a list of the community stakeholders that could advocate for the needs of the homeless population and investigate how to engage and mobilize the community partners.

   ■ Many ways of increasing the access of homeless persons to the essential elements of primary health care exist. A multiple intervention approach will be required. Many of the stakeholder people and organizations identified in the suggested approach could be involved (e.g., municipalities, health and social service organizations, non-governmental social planning organizations, and public health, housing, and social assistance departments and staff).

   ■ The following table suggests intervention strategies to achieve each of the elements (described in PHC):

	Political Action	Community Organization	Coalition Building and Advocacy	Small Group Development	Personal Care
Education concerning prevailing health problems and the methods of preventing and controlling them			■	■	■
Promotion of food supply and proper nutrition	■	■			
Maternal and child health care, including family planning		■		■	■
An adequate supply of safe water and basic sanitation	■	■	■		
Immunization against the major infectious diseases		■			■
Prevention and control of locally endemic diseases		■	■		
Appropriate treatment of common diseases and injuries					■
Provision of essential drugs	■	■			■

5. ■ *International health* is concerned with development, strengthening of health care systems, and efforts to improve health conditions in developing countries. It can address health crises and public health emergencies frequently arising in developing countries, such as the tsunami that killed several hundred thousand South East Asians in December 2004 or refugees living in occupied land.

   ■ *Global health* refers to health challenges that span national borders and present global health challenges. An example is the severe acute respiratory syndrome (SARS) or the avian influenza. Global health issues are increasing in prominence as a result of changing demographics, evolving migration patterns, increasing cultural interactions, and ease of travel.

Chapter 8

1. Any five of:
   ■ consistency: the same events happen over and over again under the same conditions
   ■ strength: the greater the exposure, the more likely the problem or event will result
   ■ specificity: the cause is linked to a specific problem
   ■ time relationship: there is logic between the time of the stressor and the event problem—the problem does not come before the stressor
   ■ congruence: the comparable logic between what is already known (e.g., natural history of the disease) and what is being examined
   ■ sensitivity: is this factor the distinct cause, or could other factors be responsible for the disease/problem?
   ■ biological/medical: the strength of the causal factor combined with the receptiveness/risk of the host
   ■ plausibility: new information may contradict previously held beliefs, but may be credible
   ■ experiments and research: new or existing information based on rigorous scientific research will add to credibility of causality
   ■ analogy factors: refers to transfer of knowledge from a known to an unknown situation

2. Mortality statistics look at the deaths due to specific diseases/conditions; morbidity looks at people who become ill with specific diseases/conditions. Morbidity informs epidemiologists how frequently the illness occurs and mortality tells them how likely the person is to die from the illness. Both types of data assist in planning future foci for health professionals and health promotion, as well as evaluating the usefulness of interventions.

3. ■ Cohort: a study in which the researcher examines the individual characteristics of a group of people who manifest a particular disease or health challenge, to find out what common factors they share and what differences can be discerned. Example research questions: 1)

What factors are common or different in a group of teens who are involved in front-end automobile collisions? 2) What are the dietary habits and hygiene practices of 10-year-olds with no dental caries?

- Case-control: the individuals in the cohort with a disease or health choice are matched to individuals who are similar in some characteristics (for example, age, gender, time, geographic residence) but who have not manifested the disease or health choice in question. The health histories or characteristics of the individuals in both groups are then obtained. These data are compared and any common and different factors are identified between the two populations. Example research questions: 1) What are the similarities and differences in maternal age, presence of family support system, education, and level of anxiety between teen mothers who choose to breastfeed and those who do not? 2) What are the differences and similarities between women in province X who have multiple sclerosis and those who do not?

- Cross-sectional: snapshots of the present that are used to suggest relationships that can be tested in future research. Example research questions: 1) What coping behaviours do nursing students use to manage community clinical practice and what are their anxiety levels? 2) How do stress scores differ between people who exercise regularly three or more times a week and those who do not?

4. ■ Environment: the context in which the event occurs. Examples of environments are physical, economic, and psychological.
   ■ Agent: the contagious or noncontagious force that begins or continues a health challenge.
   ■ Host: the human being in which the event occurs.

5. *Incidence* is a measure of the new cases of a particular disease/health condition in a given space of time (usually one year); *prevalence* is the number of persons in a given population who have a given condition/disease at the current time. If prevalence and incidence are different, the disease may be chronic in nature, with death or recovery frequently experienced a long time after diagnosis, e.g., rheumatoid arthritis. If prevalence and incidence are similar, the disease is probably short lived, with recovery or death a short time after diagnosis, e.g., the flu or Ebola virus.

6. *Prospective* is a study in which individuals are followed for a period of time to see if they acquire the disease in question or to find out what happens to them. Example research questions: 1) What illnesses/injuries are experienced by women working in an automobile-manufacturing plant compared with women working in a food-processing plant over a ten-year period? 2) Is the use of health professionals different over time between women who are in professional university programs and those who are not?

Retrospective is a study in which individuals are grouped in the present relative to a particular issue or disease and then examined for past events or situations that

may or may not have influenced their susceptibility to the present issue or disease. Example research questions: 1) What are the common factors in the histories of a group of women who required hysterectomies for nonmalignant causes in their third decade? 2) What are common wellness strategies that a group of octogenarians have used over their lifetimes?

Chapter 9

1. Communicable diseases are illness caused by a specific agent that arises from direct or indirect transmission of that from an infected host through an intermediate environment. The control and management of communicable diseases is based on a sound understanding of epidemiological investigation and the interplay of the host–agent–environment factors.

2. There are two modes of transmission: direct and indirect contact with infected hosts or with their excretions. Most disease are transmitted, or spread, through contact or close proximity because the causative bacteria or virus is airborne.

3. Contact tracing begins with interviewing this student (initial case definition) to gather data to confirm the exhibiting signs and symptoms and place and time of exposure to the TB. Usually the investigation is done by PHNs at the local health unit. A list of contacts will be gathered to identify the *index case* or first case. The follow-up will include investigation and surveillance of each of these contacts for the needed screening, diagnosis, and treatment as deemed necessary.

4. The first step would be to validate that the meningitis is a confirmed medical diagnosis. If the diagnosis is confirmed, report to the health unit, and work with the health unit staff to ensure that investigation and follow-up will be carried out in a timely manner. Advise the day care staff to remove the child until the infectious period is passed. Provide information on meningitis re mode of transmission, incubation period, signs and symptoms, period of communicability and control measures. (See Table 9.1.) Educate the staff and parents in the control and management of the disease. This will alleviate much unneeded anxiety and will gain cooperation.

5. ■ First review the principles of communicable diseases and epidemiology and evidence from the latest research studies to ensure that you will have a sound theoretical base to guide your practice.
   ■ Understand your role by reviewing the agency guidelines and protocol in communicable disease control and management, including the latest directives from the Public Health Agency of Canada for communicable disease control measures.
   ■ Conduct your own community assessment to better understand the health and risks of residents in your community. Assess the agent, host, and environment factors by conducting a community scan and by examining local health data. Assess the relationship

of your community to the larger communities for mortality and morbidity data to see how healthy your community is and why your community is at risk for hepatitis. Validate and conclude your assessment of the hepatitis situation in your community by discussing your findings and questions with your team to formulate a community plan of action with a focus on hepatitis A prevention.

6. You would need full disclosure of all the contacts and the nature of the contacts in a timely manner. This will enable you to identify whether these contacts are at risk through confidential case contact tracing. Health education on the disease and its mode of transmission can be carried out at the same time to avoid further spread of the infection and to encourage early treatment.

Chapter 10

1. ■ Balancing work and family life
   ■ Finances (more than one million Canadian children live in low-income families, and low income is most prevalent in lone-parent families headed by women)
   ■ Lack of time with family members
   ■ Boomerang kids: children living at home until older, returning home between jobs and school
   ■ Caring for elderly parents (For more and updated information visit the websites for Statistics Canada and the Vanier Institute of the Family as cited at the end of Chapter 10.)

2. ■ Stay at home longer to save money while attending postsecondary institution
   ■ Move home between jobs to save money
   ■ Move home between school terms to save money
   ■ Move home between marriages or relationships
   ■ Difficulty in finding full-time employment that pays an adequate wage

3. ■ Provider of direct care
   ■ Health promoter/educator
   ■ Partner/collaborator
   ■ Advocate
   ■ Case manager
   ■ Researcher
   ■ Leader
   ■ Administrator/manager

4. ■ A relationship with mutual respect between the nurse and the family for each other's roles, expertise, and responsibilities
   ■ A relationship in which joint decision making exists
   ■ A relationship that encourages cooperation for shared goals

5. ■ The family can be defined as "being unique and whomever the person defines as being family. They can include, but are not limited to parents, children, siblings, neighbours, and significant people in the community"

■ A pet may even be considered a family member

6. ■ The whole family is the focus of assessment, diagnosis, planning, and intervention.
   ■ The structure, function, development, and interactions of the family would be assessed. Individual members are in the background.
   ■ Strengths, resources, and limitations of the family as a unit are identified.
   ■ The nurse needs to be familiar with family nursing theories and their conceptual sources.
   ■ The nurse needs to be aware of the impact of the social determinants of health on families and communities.

Chapter 11

1. ■ CHNs work in many settings: homes, schools, health clinics, community centres, physicians' offices, family health teams, and health units.
   ■ Most CHNs work as home health nurses (HHNs) and public health nurses (PHNs). HHNs care for individuals and families and PHNs care for the community or population at large. Both groups of nurses apply nursing process with a focus to promote the health of residents living in their community. See Chapter 3 for the roles and functions of other CHNs such as nurse practitioners, occupational health nurses, and nurses working in the faith community or correctional setting.
   ■ Home health nurses may be employed by VONs, St. Elizabeth, ParaMed, or ComCare. They mainly provide direct care from managing acute or post surgical problems to rehabilitative or palliative care.
   ■ Some other CHNs work in public health for official health agencies such as health units. They carry out services as set by the Health Protection and Promotion Act and the focus of care is population-focused care.
   ■ Depending on the settings and the nature of the work, CHNs carry out various functions in consultation, counselling, health teaching, case management, referral and follow-up, screening, outreach, disease surveillance, policy development and enforcement, social marketing, advocacy, community organizing, coalition building, and collaboration.

2. Healthy communities are those with competent community dynamics that foster public participation, mutual support, and community action to promote optimal community growth. Characteristics of healthy communities are:
   ■ Affordable and adequate access to food, water, housing, recreation, and transportation
   ■ Clean and safe physical environment
   ■ Conservation of natural environment and resources
   ■ Accessible and quality health and social services
   ■ Opportunities for education and skill development

- Robust economy with high employment rate
- Peace and low crime rates
- Supportive family and work life
- Strong sense of community belonging
- Strong culture, heritage, and spiritual beliefs
- Equity, social justice, and diversity
- Citizen participation in decision-making
- Committed leadership
- Healthy public policy

3. To promote the health of the community, CHNs must understand the characteristics and needs of their populations and the community. They need to possess strong community assessment skills to get a realistic profile of the community dynamics and to critically analyze and explore the roots of the community strengths or problems, and assess the effects of various social determinants of health on the health of the population.

   CHNs need to develop a community plan to mobilize resources to help the community to attain optimal health. These population-focused health promotion strategies include but are not limited to advocacy for healthy public policy, strengthening of community action, and the creation of supportive environments. The ability to work in partnership with the stakeholders and engage them at the grassroots level is critical throughout the nursing process.

   Overall, CHNs must possess a sound knowledge base of community health promotion strategies to guide their practice. Strong research and critical thinking skills are essential for CHNs to analyze the problems and strengths and help translate knowledge to practice from their evidence-based practice.

4. CHNs systematically assess all components that will affect the health of the population and the community dynamics and functions. These components are outlined in Figure 11.1 and Table 11.4 as follows: population, physical environments, socioeconomic environments, education and healthy child development, culture and religion, health and social services, transportation, law and safety, government and politics, and communication.

5. *Population health* aims to maintain and improve the health status of 1) the entire population (i.e., community-focused), 2) a specific target population (i.e., systems-focused), or 3) the individuals (i.e., individual-focused) within the community (Minnesota Department of Health, 2001). It strives to reduce inequities in health status between population groups by addressing what determines their health.

   Community engagement is a process involving citizens at various levels of participation based on interpersonal communication and trust and a common understanding and purpose.

   Community governance is a method of community engagement that ensures effective involvement and empowerment of local community representatives in the planning, direction setting, and monitoring of health

organizations to meet the health needs and priorities of the populations within local neighbourhood communities.

   Community development is the process of involving a community in the identification and reinforcement of those aspects of everyday life, culture, and political activity that are conducive to health. This might include support for political action to modify the total environment and strengthen resources for healthy living, as well as reinforcing social networks and social support within a community and developing the material resources and economic base available to the community.

   Capacity building is a process that strengthens the ability of an individual, organization, community, or health system to develop and implement health promotion initiatives and sustain positive health outcomes over time. It involves organizational development, human resource development, leadership, partnership, resource allocation, and policy formulation.

6. Community dialogue encourages a two-way communication among community members to share and discuss their experiences, lessons learned, problems, needs, visions, and goals. Members engage in the discussions, they exchange information, and become an open learning community and a support for one another.

   When working with a population that the CHNs are not familiar with or when there is a need to introduce new information or resolve old community issues, community dialogue is an effective way for both parties to learn about each other's cultures, needs, values, expectations, and reasons why differences exist. Once a common understanding is reached, mutual goals can be developed and community partnership for actions can be built.

Chapter 12

1. The components of an effective occupational health and safety program are:

   - management commitment;
   - worker involvement;
   - assessing and controlling the work environment;
   - addressing injuries, illnesses, and incidents; and
   - administration of health and safety in the workplace.

   Each of these components includes specific elements that make up an effective program.

2. The occupational health and safety team includes the OHN, occupational physician, occupational hygienist, safety professional, and ergonomist. Other team members can include a counsellor, physiotherapist, or other health safety professionals.

3. The role of occupational physicians is to diagnose and treat occupational injuries and illnesses. Their focus is on workers and worker health. These professionals consider the effects of the work environment on worker health.

   The focus of occupational hygienists and safety professionals is on worker health and safety as well; however, they focus more directly on the work environment. Occupational hygienists look for, measure, and control hazards.

Safety professionals also look for hazards using a loss-control perspective. They also conduct investigations of incidents so that controls can be recommended to minimize future human and economic losses.

4. ■ Safety: exit doorway that is blocked with supplies
   ■ Physical: noise
   ■ Chemical: cold sterilizing solution
   ■ Biological: hepatitis B
   ■ Ergonomic: computer workstation not properly set up
   ■ Psychosocial: heavy workloads and insufficient staff

5. The major focus of an occupational hygienist is on the work environment. Their specialty is in conducting objective evaluations and measurements of the hazards in the work environment such as noise, temperature extremes, or chemicals. Their work provides the background data necessary to establish relationships between hazard exposure and health effects. The major focus of an OHN is on worker health. Along with the exposure information, the OHN considers signs, symptoms, and the effects of hazards on worker health and considers individual factors such as age and health history that can impact the health effects of work hazards on a particular worker. Both professionals are responsible for minimizing or eliminating hazards to protect worker health and prevent work-related illnesses and injuries.

6. Benefits to employees of having access to an OHN at their workplace are many. OHNs provide services that help workers prevent work-related injuries and illnesses resulting in a decreased risk of workplace illness and injury. OHNs also provide training and education in health and safety that protects health both on and off the job. Programs in occupational health help to place workers in jobs they can perform safety both on initial hire and after returning to work from injury or illness. All this can lead to more job satisfaction and higher morale.

Employers have both direct and indirect benefits as well. In addition to the direct human and economic cost savings of fewer injuries, illnesses, and sickness-related absences, employers with OHNs have increased compliance with health and safety legislation. Supervisors and managers still have the functions of maintaining health and safety, but they likely will spend less time and resources in dealing with health and safety issues with which they may be unfamiliar. Effective health and safety programs that are delivered by OHNs result in improved employee morale and productivity, improved labour relations, and an enhanced corporate image. There are also indirect savings related to decreased employee turnover, which reduces the costs of recruiting and training staff.

7. ■ Working alone: safety, possibly psychosocial
   ■ Hepatitis B: biological
   ■ Needlesticks: safety
   ■ Dog bites: safety

■ Cold sterilization solution: chemical

Chapter 13

1. The steps in the planning–evaluation cycle do not always occur in a linear fashion because previous steps may need to be repeated as one develops a better understanding of an issue and as one obtains additional input from collaborators and partners. The steps usually involve:
   a. Conducting a situational analysis or community assessment
   b. Identifying the problems or issues of concern
   c. Considering possible solutions or actions to address the problem
   d. Selecting the best alternative(s)
   e. Designing and implementing the program
   f. Monitoring and evaluating the program
   g. Analyzing and interpreting results of the monitoring and evaluation process
   h. Using results to make modifications to the program or to inform decisions about other programs

2. The four factors influencing selection of program planning and evaluation framework are:
   a. Use of a standard planning framework that is used across departments as this will allows for a coherent and consistent approach to planning within an organization.
   b. Use of a particular framework may be a requirement of those who fund programs as this allows them to compare results across funded programs.
   c. A framework may be chosen because it helps detail a particular aspect of the planning process that is vexing or challenging
   d. The selection of a framework may be influenced by a set of underlying values or principles such as an intention to use participatory approaches

3. The tools commonly used in planning program are:
   a. Environmental scans, using an assessment of strengths, weaknesses, opportunities, and threats; key informant interviews, focus groups, and round tables are examples of ways to engage partners efficiently and fully in a planning process.
   b. Examples of tools used to organize information include use of matrices, content analysis of qualitative data, graphs and tables to display quantitative data, and priority-setting.

4. Three uses of quantitative data in program planning and evaluation are:
   a. Documenting the magnitude of the problem and contributing factors.
   b. Helping to estimate program costs and the potential return on investments.
   c. Evaluating short-term and long-term results of the program.

5. The three principles of priority setting are:
   a. Buy-in
   b. Transparency
   c. Communication

6. The five main elements of MIP are:
   a. Identification of community health issue
   b. Description of socioecological determinants
   c. Intervention options
   d. Optimizing intervention strategies
   e. Monitoring and evaluating impacts, spin-offs, and sustainability

Chapter 14

1. For evidence-based decision making, consider research evidence, patient preferences, nurse skills, and resources available.

2. The most critical attitude for a nurse practising in an evidence-based way is a critical questioning approach to care planning and evaluation.

3. You might:
   - collect data for outcomes of care or for process indicators such as number of visits, hours of care, attendance at a session, or number of sessions delivered;
   - deliver experimental intervention, e.g., smoking cessation, sexual health intervention, comprehensive stroke care; or
   - work collaboratively to develop an important clinical question and to write a proposal to conduct the research.

4. Individual studies can produce different results, including no significant effect of treatment if the sample size was not large enough. By reading a systematic review, you get a more complete picture of the literature, both published and unpublished, compiled in a way that minimizes bias. This pre-appraised literature will save you time, money, and resources from doing the complete literature review yourself.

5. Factors to consider when planning to implement a clinical practice or policy change:
   - characteristics of the change (or innovation) itself, e.g., how different it is from current practice, will it save time or add to the time needed to give care
   - characteristics of the people involved in adopting the change, e.g., how open they are to change and their attitudes toward research and research utilization, age, time since graduation, and level of education
   - characteristics of the organization where the change will take place, e.g., how research-intensive the organization is, its culture of using research and "keeping up to date," and its culture of evaluating care given
   - characteristics of the organization's environment, e.g., rural or urban, in an academic setting

Chapter 15

1. The digital divide was first identified in the late '90s as the "haves" and "have nots," referring to populations with no access to digital information. Since its initial use, the term has been refined to describe people with *no access* at all, compared with those with *modest access* (slow dial-up connections) and the *broadband elite* (fast connections). Others have also revised the categories to provide more contextual information including the following: "net-evaders" live in connected homes but do not connect to the web themselves; "net-dropouts" used the internet in the past but have stopped due to technical problems or dislike of the web; "intermittent users" dropped out for a while and are back using the internet; "truly disconnected" have never used the internet and do not know any or many internet users.

2. Screen readers turn text into speech and are therefore very useful to support individuals with visual impairments.

   OCR (optical character recognition) software is useful for visually impaired individuals who want to read text not available in digital form. They can scan the document, and with the OCR software convert the scan to digital text; they can then use a screen reader to have it read aloud.

   Windows users can adjust the operating system in the Control Panel's accessibility tools to adjust various settings such as text magnification, screen resolution, and image contrast.

   There are many other tools to enhance accessibility. A reputable Canadian source of information to stay updated on software and products is the Canadian Adaptec Network Project website.

3. The HON code is a set of criteria developed by a group of internet experts to assess the credibility of health information websites. Eight criteria comprise the code: authority, complementarity, confidentiality, attribution, justifiability, transparency of authorship, transparency of sponsorship, and honesty in advertising and editorial policy. These criteria can be used to judge the usefulness of the information provided to health information consumers and health care professionals. These criteria reflect an emphasis on evidence-informed practice and the use of health information that is provided in an objective, unbiased format to support client decision making. This code has been widely accepted as a means of evaluating health information websites. It is made more useful to public consumers through the use of the "WRAPIN" website (www.wrapin.org), which applies these criteria to website URLs that users submit to the website for assessment.

4. There are many promising e-health promotion interventions that are gaining popularity and show promising results. They generally enable individuals, groups, and/or communities to take control over their own health. A few such interventions that will be interesting to continue to watch and study are online social support groups, online

screening tools, especially those that use tailored messaging, e-counselling, and interactive websites that involve local citizens in driving policy change. It is important to note that many of these interventions have not been rigorously evaluated, and further research is needed to draw firm conclusions about their effectiveness.

5. This is bit of a moving target as repositories of research findings, communities of practice, and portals continue to develop and evolve over time. There are some key web services and sites to visit, including the Canadian Best Practices Portal for Health Promotion and Chronic Disease Prevention, the Canadian Nurses Association's NurseONE portal, the Effective Public Health Practice Program Health-Evidence.ca: Promoting Evidence-Based Decision-Making, and the CHNET Works! Community of Practice.

6. Review Table 15.1, which describes a number of actions for CHNs to take into account. Some of the key actions include developing your own skills in online health information retrieval and evaluation, fostering discussions with clients regarding health information they found online, and teaching clients how to evaluate quality and appropriateness of health information on the internet.

Index

Note: *f* denotes a figure, *t* denotes a table, *i* denotes an image